# Davis's Patient–Practitioner Interaction

This best-selling textbook, now in its seventh edition, is the essential resource to foster the self-awareness and communication skills needed by health professionals in providing ethical, compassionate, and professional care for their patients.

The book begins by encouraging readers to understand, change, and evaluate their patterns of response so that they can adapt to patients in a range of stressful or contentious situations. Through holistic self-awareness, taking into account one's family history and personal values, the book then discusses methods of stress management before moving through the most effective ways to support and communicate with patients. There are chapters on establishing rapport, assertiveness, and conflict resolution, cultural sensitivity, leadership, spirituality, and patient education. Specific issues around communicating with terminally ill patients or those with disabilities are also covered.

Fully updated throughout, the seventh edition now features a new chapter devoted specifically to Justice, Equity, Diversity, and Inclusion, plus a new chapter covering professional formation in transitions from classroom to clinical education, including telehealth patient–practitioner interaction (PPI), interprofessional education, and early career pathways. The new edition is informed by the national Healthy People 2030 objectives, while also offering further coverage of the social determinants of health, biopsychosocial aspects of health and healing, and sexuality and sexual health.

Featuring interactive and online learning activities based on real-life clinical situations, as well as vignettes designed to make learning active and engaging, this invaluable text is ideal for any developing professional in the health professions.

**Gina Maria Musolino**, PT, DPT, EdD, MSEd, is an experienced educator, consultant, scholar, author/editor, and advocate clinician. Currently, Dr. Musolino is serving as Clinical Professor and Director of Curriculum of Physical Therapy with the Department of Physical Therapy, University of Florida, College of Public Health and Health Professions. She has served as tenured Professor, Program Director/Chair, and Director of Clinical Education. Dr. Musolino's scholarly works include impacting, peer-reviewed articles, and textbook chapters examining critical components of the scholarship of learning and teaching with focus areas of professional formation and holistic admissions. Dr. Musolino is co-editor/author of *Clinical Reasoning and Decision-Making in PT: Facilitation, Assessment, and Implementation* (2020) and *Patient Practitioner Interaction: An Experiential Manual for Developing the Art of Health Care*, 6th ed. (2016). In collaboration with colleagues, Dr. Musolino has earned over 130K in funded research and teaching grants. Dr. Musolino has served as Review Panel Chair and Reviewer for the US Department of Health and Human Services (US HHS), Office of the Assistant Secretary for Health (OAHS), Office of Minority Health (OMH) and Office of Population Affairs (OPA), and the US Congressionally Directed Medical Research Program and US Army Combat Readiness-Medical Research Program (CRRP).

**Carol M. Davis**, DPT, EdD, MS, FAPTA, is Professor Emerita of the Department of Physical Therapy in the Miller School of Medicine at the University of Miami and past Vice Chair for Curriculum. She retired from her academic responsibilities in 2015. Dr. Davis is an internationally known speaker and consultant in teaching and developing curriculum in professional behaviors, attitudes, and values, and holistic integrative therapies in rehabilitation for physicians and all health professionals. In addition to being the co-author of *Patient Practitioner Interaction: An Experiential Manual for Developing the Art of Health Care*, 6th ed. (2016), she is the editor of *Integrative Therapies in Rehabilitation: Evidence for Efficacy in Therapy, Prevention, and Wellness*, 4th ed. (2017), and co-editor of *Therapeutic Interaction in Nursing* (2004).

**Seventh Edition**

# Davis's Patient–Practitioner Interaction

## An Experiential Manual for Developing the Art of Health Care

Gina Maria Musolino and Carol M. Davis

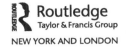

Routledge
Taylor & Francis Group

NEW YORK AND LONDON

Designed cover image: Getty Images

Seventh edition published 2025
by Routledge
605 Third Avenue, New York, NY 10158

and by Routledge
4 Park Square, Milton Park, Abingdon, Oxon, OX14 4RN

*Routledge is an imprint of the Taylor & Francis Group, an informa business*

First edition published by Slack 1989
Sixth edition published by Slack 2016

ISBN: 9781638220039 (hbk)
ISBN: 9781032942735 (pbk)
ISBN: 9781003525554 (ebk)

DOI: 10.4324/9781003525554

Typeset in Minion Pro
by codeMantra

Access the Support Material: www.routledge.com/9781638220039

To Susan Emily Davis Doughty—my twin sister, Master Women's Health Nurse Practitioner, a person beloved by all who interact with her.

In memory of Geneva R. Johnson, PhD, DPT (hon), FAPTA—revered mentor and friend, the person who insisted and inspired me to write the first edition of this book in 1985.

In gratitude to my graduates over 34 years who contributed to the many improvements of this material each time I taught them.

In gratitude to Gina Maria Musolino who accepted the task of adopting this work and carrying it on because she believed in the value of this work.

And again, to my friend Jamie, for the seventh time, with gratitude seven times as great as with the first edition in 1989.

Thank you.

*Carol M. Davis*


With much gratitude to Carol M. Davis, DPT, EdD, MS, FAPTA for sharing her treasured gift with me—I am and remain forever humbled.

With deep gratitude to all colleagues in health care, near and far, who dedicate themselves to teaching both the intangible and tangible, in support of the patients and clients we serve in health care.

With sincere gratitude to my dear and daring clinical and academic educators in health care who never stop learning, never stop asking questions, never stop truly listening, and lead by example; for those who embrace an open mind and positive attitude, even when facing the impossible, and for remembering that the art of healing and the affective learning domain are as important as the cognitive science and psychomotor aspects of practice.

For all in advocacy, may we never lose perspective and continue to tirelessly work to keep the care in health.

For my student learners and graduates, from whom I continue to learn—may you each endeavor to learn what matters most to your patients and clients, take the time to know them as a person first, find out what they understand and what their goals are and why, and continue to do your best as partners in the care of their health. May you have empathic ears in the face of discomfort and not be discouraged by the negativity. Health care is gratifying, and you have made the right choices. Learn from all your patients—keep asking why? And why not? Dare to dream of possibilities, stay curious. Keep an attitude of gratitude in all you do.

For my patients—thank you for all you have taught me and changed in me for the better, and for entrusting me with your care. May your stories serve to help others seeking care.

And deepest of gratitude to my dearly departed parents and my beloved family members—you have made all the difference in my life, and I thank you immensely for my delightful formative years that allowed me to be self-aware and taught me faith, hope, and values in life, love, and profession. Thank you for the many blessings we have shared and wishing you all tenfold in return.

*Gina Maria Musolino*

# Contents

# ABOUT THE AUTHORS

**Gina Maria Musolino**, PT, DPT, EdD, MSEd, is an experienced educator, consultant, scholar, author/editor, and advocate clinician. Currently, Dr. Musolino is serving as Clinical Professor and Director of Curriculum of Physical Therapy with the Department of Physical Therapy, University of Florida, College of Public Health and Health Professions. She has served as tenured Professor, Program Director/Chair, and Director of Clinical Education. Dr. Musolino's scholarly works include impacting, peer-reviewed articles, and textbook chapters examining critical components of the scholarship of learning and teaching with focus areas of professional formation and holistic admissions. Dr. Musolino is co-editor/author of *Clinical Reasoning and Decision-Making in PT: Facilitation, Assessment, and Implementation* (2020) and *Patient Practitioner Interaction: An Experiential Manual for Developing the Art of Health Care*, 6th ed. (2016). In collaboration with colleagues, Dr. Musolino has earned over 130K in funded research and teaching grants. Dr. Musolino has served as Review Panel Chair and Reviewer for the US Department of Health and Human Services (US HHS), Office of the Assistant Secretary for Health (OAHS), Office of Minority Health (OMH), and Office of Population Affairs (OPA) and the US Congressionally Directed Medical Research Program and US Army Combat Readiness-Medical Research Program (CRRP).

Dr. Musolino was recognized as Distinguished Manuscript Reviewer (2023) for the renowned *Physical Therapy & Rehabilitation Journal* (*PTJ*) of the American Physical Therapy Association (APTA). She is in her second term, as appointed by the APTA Board of Directors in service with the APTA Credentialed Clinical Instructor Program Advisory Work Group (2020–26) and currently serves as Florida Delegate to the APTA House of Delegates. For over 20 years, Gina has served and continues with colleagues as an APTA Level 1 & 2 Credentialed Clinical Trainer fostering best practice for clinical instructors' service in clinical education. Dr. Musolino is a frequent national speaker and has presented collaborative scholarly works at the international level with the World Confederation of Physical Therapy. She has previously served as two-term President of the APTA Academy of Education; two-term Chief Delegate-FL (2012–16) and Director, Board of Directors (BOD), Florida Physical Therapy Association; Scholarship Director for two-terms with the APTA Academy of Leadership & Innovation, BOD; Federal Affairs Liaison for the Academy of Neurologic PT; and Congressional Key Contact. Gina received the APTA Lucy Blair Service Award (2012) for service of exceptional value to the profession, was honored with the APTA Academy of Education, Feitelberg Journal Founders Award (2005) and recognition as a distinguished, senior manuscript reviewer with *PTJ*. Dr. Musolino serves as a contributing editorial board member with the Association of Schools Advancing Health Professions, *Journal of Allied Health*. Dr. Musolino has previously served two editorial board member terms with the APTA Academy of Education, *Journal of Physical Therapy Education*. In 2007, Dr. Musolino was recognized by her alma mater, Washington University, School of Medicine, Program in Physical Therapy with the Alumni Award and previously recognized upon her graduation with the Beatrice F. Schulz Award for Outstanding Clinical Achievement. She received her AS from John Wood Community College (Quincy, IL), her BS in Physical Therapy from Washington University School of Medicine, Program in Physical Therapy (WUMS PT; St. Louis, Missouri), her MSEd from Southwest Baptist University (Bolivar, Missouri), her EdD with specialization in Curriculum Design, Development, and Evaluation from Nova Southeastern University (NSU), Fischler College of Education (Ft. Lauderdale, Florida), and her post-professional DPT from Utica University (Utica, NY).

**Carol M. Davis**, DPT, EdD, MS, FAPTA, is Professor Emerita of the Department of Physical Therapy in the Miller School of Medicine at the University of Miami and past Vice Chair for Curriculum. She retired from her academic responsibilities in 2015. Dr. Davis is an internationally known speaker and consultant in teaching and developing curriculum in professional behaviors, attitudes, and values and holistic integrative therapies in rehabilitation for physicians and all health professionals. In addition to being the co-author of *Patient Practitioner Interaction: An Experiential Manual for Developing the Art of Health Care*, 6th ed., she is the editor of *Integrative Therapies in Rehabilitation: Evidence for Efficacy in Therapy, Prevention, and Wellness*, 4th ed, and co-editor of *Therapeutic Interaction in Nursing*.

Dr. Davis continues to teach internationally online, primarily focusing on the new science of fascia, biotensegrity, and therapeutic presence. She has published several research articles in peer-reviewed journals and is the author of 18 book chapters. She served six years as a commissioner on the Commission on Accreditation for Physical Therapy Education and was a team leader and site visitor. She also served on the Ethics and Judicial Committee for the American Physical Therapy Association (APTA) and was Chair (2004–05). She was awarded the Outstanding Teacher award by the Section on Geriatrics of the APTA (2003), was named Linda Crane Lecturer, Cardiovascular and Pulmonary Physical Therapy (2005), and was awarded the Lucy Blair Service Award (1991) and designated APTA Catherine Worthingham Fellow (2003). In addition to teaching and consulting, Dr. Davis maintains a part-time clinical practice in Portland, Maine, primarily treating patients with pain using J. F. Barnes sustained myofascial release and exercise.

# CONTRIBUTORS

**Kathleen A. Curtis**, PT, PhD, is Dean and Professor Emerita of the College of Health Sciences, and former Charles H. and Shirley T. Leavell Chair in Health Sciences at the University of Texas at El Paso. Dr. Curtis brings more than 35 years of leadership experience in clinical, education, research, and higher education administration roles in the health and rehabilitation sciences. Her background includes clinical appointments at Tufts–New England Medical Center, Santa Clara Valley Medical Center, and Cedars-Sinai Medical Center. She has held faculty appointments at Mount Saint Mary's College, the University of Southern California, the University of Miami School of Medicine, and California State University–Fresno, where she was honored with the university President's Award of Excellence. She is the author of many research publications and three physical therapy textbooks. Her research in the area of prevention of secondary disability in persons with spinal cord injury has been internationally recognized. Dr. Curtis received the Public Citizen of the Year award for her work in the El Paso community in support of the development of a Master of Social Work program. Dr. Curtis received her BS in Physical Therapy from Northeastern University (Boston, Massachusetts), her MHS from San Jose State University, and her PhD in education from the University of California (Los Angeles, California). Dr. Curtis currently serves on the Board of Directors, Friends of the Elephant Seal, which has been featured in the Smithsonian Magazine for their volunteer efforts to educate visitors to prevent conflicts, inspire awe, and prevent disturbances to elephant seals and other marine life.

**Solange Dagress**, PT, DPT, is a graduate of the University of Miami, Class of 2022. She received her Bachelor of Science in Exercise Science from Adelphi University prior to her move to Miami. She is a registered yoga teacher and has taught both in the United States and abroad. She has practice interest in both cardiovascular pulmonary and geriatric physical therapy and practices in West Palm Beach, FL. As a member of the LGBTQIA+ community, she is a passionate advocate for sexual and gender minorities. She hopes to raise awareness of the unique health care challenges that affect this population and improve clinicians' understanding and compassion for LGBTQIA+ patients.

**Sherrill H. Hayes**, PT, PhD, is Professor and Chair Emerita of the Department of Physical Therapy at the University of Miami, Miller School of Medicine. She was Assistant Dean for Women's Health in the Miller School of Medicine and has had a long career of involvement in women's issues, physical therapy, and obstetrics. She has a bachelor's degree in physical therapy, an advanced master's degree in allied health/neuroscience education from the University of Connecticut, and a PhD in higher education/administration from the University of Miami. She is a former president of the APTA Education Section (Academy of Education) and an international consultant in physical therapy education. Her clinical specialties are in neuroanatomy and neuropathology, acute care practice, neurological dysfunction, and women's health. She has been teaching about sexuality, rehabilitation, and pelvic floor physical therapy for over 40 years. She continues to teach in the entry-level doctorate (DPT) program at the University of Miami.

**Helen L. Masin**, PT, PhD, is Associate Clinical Professor Emerita of Physical Therapy in the Department of Physical Therapy and the Department of Pediatrics at the University of Miami Miller School of Medicine. She currently teaches in the DPT and PhD programs. In her teaching role, she has taught Communications in Physical Therapy, Pediatric Physical Therapy, Professional Socialization and Leadership, and Self Defense for Women. In her research role, she has investigated cultural aspects of patient care and taught a wide variety of health professionals how to enhance their cross-cultural communication skills. In her service role, she has provided consultation to the Deaf and Hard of Hearing program at the Mailman Center for Child Development in the Department of Pediatrics at the University of Miami. She also served as an Academic Coordinator of Clinical Education and supervised DPT students during their clinical internships. To assist in resolving challenges in the clinic, she became a certified practitioner in Neurolinguistic Psychology (NLP). Using her NLP background, she developed and published several articles on participant-centered problem solving (PCPS) as a method for resolving challenges in the clinic. In addition, she consults in continuing education and teaches PCPS to professionals interested in enhancing their problem-solving skills with patients, families, and colleagues.

**Mica (Mee-kuh) Mitchell**, PT, DPT, is an Assistant Professor of Physical Therapy at the College of Saint Mary's Doctor of Physical Therapy (DPT) Program in Omaha, NE. Since 2003, she has dedicated her career to working as a pediatric physical therapist in a variety of pediatric settings and has been involved in academia since 2017. Her passion for pediatrics led her to earn her DPT degree with a specialization in pediatric science from Rocky Mountain University of Health Professions. She earned her master's degree in physical therapy from East Carolina University. Dr. Mitchell's expertise is recognized by the American Board of Physical Therapy Specialties (ABPTS), where she is recognized as a Board-Certified Pediatric Clinical Specialist. Beyond her clinical expertise, Dr. Mitchell is deeply committed to community service, as exemplified by her volunteer work as a FUNfitness Clinical Director with Special Olympics. Driven by a profound desire to foster a sense of belonging for minoritized individuals and underrepresented groups, Dr. Mitchell champions representation and justice in all her endeavors, which include her advocacy efforts with the Ujima Center. She guides individuals and groups in mindfulness practices, supporting their wellness journeys, and has launched related podcasts. Dr. Mitchell's dedication to her work would be impossible without the unwavering support and exceptional examples of excellence she receives from her family.

**Darina Sargeant**, PT, PhD, is Professor Emerita in the Department of Physical Therapy and Athletic Training in the Doisy College of Health Sciences at Saint Louis University. Her areas of research included spirituality in physical therapy practice, interprofessional, and clinical education. Dr. Sargeant published articles and contributed to textbook chapters on spirituality in patient care; publications on interprofessional, and clinical education development in physical therapy and in family practice medicine. Dr. Sargeant received her Bachelor of Science in physical therapy at Saint Louis University (1975) and has practiced in the acute inpatient, orthopedic outpatient, and home care settings. Dr. Sargeant earned a Master of Education degree in curriculum (1983) and her PhD in educational studies (2003) with an emphasis on spirituality from Saint Louis University. Dr. Sargeant is retired.

**Alecia Helbing Thiele**, PT, DPT, ATC, MEd, is an Associate Professor and the Director of Clinical Education (DCE) in the Physical Therapy Department at Clarke University in Dubuque, IA. She has been in this position since 1999 and served as Assistant ACCE at the university in 1997. She received her BSPT degree in Physical Therapy (1991) from the University of Wisconsin La-Crosse, her MS in Education from the University of Wisconsin Platteville (2001), and her Clinical Doctorate from Clarke (2006). She is a certified athletic trainer and generational trainer. Dr. Thiele has published and presented on professional behaviors, generational influences, clinical education, integrated clinical education, interdisciplinary medicine, technology, and her experiences with Post Intensive Care Syndrome. She obtained her APTA Certification as a trainer for the APTA Credentialed Clinical Instructor Program (CCIP) Level 1 (2000) and the Advanced Level 2 APTA CCIP (2007). She is former two-term Treasurer for the Academy of Physical Therapy Education Section (APTE) and has also served as the two-term Secretary, National Clinical Education DCE Co-Chair, Clinical Education Special Interest Group (CESIG) Secretary and CESIG Programming Chair for the APTE. She is a member of the Iowa Clinical Education Collaborative and has also served as the Site Coordinator for Clinical Education in her sports medicine practice area for the past 30 years. Her specialty area of clinical practice is sports medicine and athletic training. Alecia has been practicing physical therapy for the past 33 years and athletic training for the past 29 years.

# FOREWORD

Clearly, medical care has expanded from an almost exclusive focus on the biological and physiological aspects of illness to a biospsychosocial approach. The biopsychosocial model is getting increased attention in health care by all providers. In fact, just referring to health care rather than medical care is reflective of the important expansion to consideration of the psychosocial aspects of the individual receiving care. Davis and Musolino recognized the importance of considering the whole human being in 1989, and through the years have expanded the pertinent information. This book is very comprehensive, dealing with aspects of understanding patients from a wide variety of psychosocial perspectives. In addition, they also provide expansive and important ways for practitioners to understand themselves and the many factors influencing the development of attitudes and behaviors. Dealing with how communication skills are so important and yet require insight, and usually modification, is another critical component of this book.

The authors even mention sitting on a stool when communicating with a patient to be at eye level and not always looking down on the patient. This comment reinforced my practice of squatting down to put on the shoes of my patients. I would purposely look up at them, so they could look down at me. I wanted to convey that I was going to help them with both large and small tasks. I just wish I had benefitted from the perspective of the information from this book to be more effective in my interactions. Having a systematic exam allows the provider to focus their attention on patient behavior and reactions and further implement the information in this book. The physical therapy provider has the challenging task of motivating patients to do exercises, change the way they do their basic activities, or recover from a variety of physical dysfunctions. This book covers all aspects of human qualities including self-awareness, behavior, interactions, and communication in a comprehensive way. Of value are the case reports within every chapter and the exercises. There are suggestions for journaling and assessing the success of gaining insight about the patients and the practitioner. Everyone reading this book will find it invaluable for optimizing the knowledge of the psychosocial aspects of both the provider and the patient. With the knowledge obtained from this book, the interaction between the patient and practitioner will be more effective, as will be the effectiveness of treatment. This updated version addresses the current issues of a pandemic, telehealth, and AI. This book is invaluable.

*Shirley Sahrmann, PT, PhD, FAPTA*
*Professor Emerita Physical Therapy*
*Washington University School of Medicine—St. Louis*

# PREFACE

How does one improve on a bestseller? Since the first edition, *Patient Practitioner Interaction: An Experiential Manual for Developing the Art of Health Care* has remained of high value for health care professionals and educators. With each new edition, the text has been improved with updates and progressions, and the seventh edition is no exception. All chapters have been significantly refined and updated with contemporary evidence, legislative updates, and experiential insights. There are also additional chapter exercises for both basic and more progressive applications of the skills needed for patient–practitioner interaction (PPI). *Patient Practitioner Interaction: An Experiential Manual for Developing the Art of Health Care*, 6th ed. (*PPI6*) added two new chapters, one devoted to peer and self-assessment and the other to leadership and advocacy for health care. The seventh edition (*PPI7*) has also added two new chapters: one devoted specifically to Justice, Equity, Diversity, and Inclusion (JEDI), and one dedicated to professional formation transitions from classroom to clinical education, including telehealth PPI, interprofessional education, and early career pathways. The new additions address important aspects of acculturation with transitioning from didactic to clinical environments with perspectives encouraging growth mindsets and intergenerational engagement, the unique aspects of telehealth and PPI, along with ethical and legal considerations with respect to artificial intelligence (AI). An emphasis on peer and self-assessment leading to reflective practice continues to be blended throughout the text, specifically addressing these aspects of professional formation and professional development of leadership and advocacy for health care. *PPI7* specifically incorporates Healthy People 2030, Social Determinants of Health, with expanded approaches for adversity adaptations, moral courage, and considerations for cultural humility. The biopsychosocial aspects of health and healing are addressed through an expanded lens, along with Sexuality and Sexual Health.

A companion electronic format for exercises is included. While keeping with the low-tech need for developing PPI skills, multimedia and website resource links for applications to provide broader perspectives for a digital generation are provided as key resources to enhance the content.

As in the last six editions, early chapters are devoted to students' self-awareness and understanding of their own history in developing their values and communication skills, along with exercises to analyze the effectiveness of those skills. The chapter on differentiating personal values and professional values remains and has been updated with contemporary evidence and exercises (Chapter 3). The chapter exploring peer and self-assessment has been retained to continue to plant the seeds for developing reflective practice capabilities for the health care professional, for it is in education that the process of education is so closely tied to the process of healing (Chapter 10). The word *education* derives from the Latin *educare*, meaning to mold, rear, or bring up; and/or *educere*, meaning to lead out, pull out, or lead forth. Genuine education for our students, patients, clients, families, and caregivers fosters self-awareness, self-knowledge, creativity, and self-trust, along with a realization of one's own abilities and identity. The barriers and challenges to peer and self-assessment are discussed, and current evidence and practical applications are incorporated to begin to develop the capabilities in thoughtful and meaningful ways. Learners are guided not only in habitual effectiveness, but also in how to write goals for their own personal and professional development, to facilitate the development of mindfulness, which is important as a foundation for expertise and decision making.

The chapter on identifying and resolving ethical dilemmas with problem-solving processes is enhanced and includes conceptual frameworks and suggested new models to consider for more in-depth ethical applications (Chapter 4). This chapter emphasizes the awareness that traditional biomedical (principled) ethical reasoning is not a sufficient process for those of us caring for patients day to day as we become embroiled in their histories and stories. Empathy, sympathy, and an ethic of care and discernment are described as virtue tools to assist in making sound ethical decisions within the framework of traditional ethical discourse that supports this process. Data are included elucidating the relationship of health care errors and everyday ethics in real-world health care examples. The vital chapter examining stress management (Chapter 5) has been expanded due to the exponential rise in the mental health and stress adaptation needs of today's generations; with ties to the final chapter (Chapter 20) content examining the multi-generations in the learners' transition to clinical environments. In addition, the plethora of increasing demands in health care has led to the need to further examine cases of risk management, fraud, and abuse, and to ensure that developing health care providers are aware of the relationship of stress and integrity in practice. Many additive considerations have also evolved because of the Covid-19 pandemic and the lasting impacts on health and health care.

The much-needed intentional chapter was added to address matters of Justice, Equity, Diversity, and Inclusion (JEDI), providing the opportunity for learners and future health care professionals to explore their abilities to actualize JEDI efforts (Chapter 7). JEDI descriptions, definitions, awareness, and educational exercises are provided to increase knowledge and capacities with pathways and plans for self-action. The chapter creates a dedicated space for this work serving society, rather than just being embedded into the text. Educators and learners will appreciate the opportunity to shine a lens on these matters in a more intentional way to dismantle barriers, consider allocation of resources, understand "isms" that exist, appreciate differences, and further examine bias and prejudice, along with precise efforts for how health care providers may foster a sense of belonging for all persons who may experience barriers to access based on their identity. The chapter also includes an examination, and indicators of the violation of basic human rights with respect to human trafficking, smuggling, physical, mental, and sexual abuse, and neglect. Challenging, eye-opening resources and activities are provided to assist learners in examining their own biases, applying JEDI principles, and examining scenarios based upon real-world experiences.

We have built upon the most recent edition's updates and address the frustrations of the generations by continuing our conversation and discussion of the much-needed development of face-to-face skills while encountering multiple generations in and outside of the health care workplace. We more deeply examine each of the generations and share perspectives for healthier work environments with an effort toward mutual understanding.

The remaining chapters teach actual skill development in communicating with people who trust the professional to offer therapeutic presence as well as skills in clinical reasoning, diagnosis, prognosis, and treatment progressions. The ever-popular exercises in assertive communication and challenging scenarios remain, with contemporary additions and with clear frameworks to assist the novice's development. The focus on bullying is expanded with deeper linkages codifying the challenges of moral integrity, moral distress, moral injury, and moral courage. Methods to confront and identify the targeted problems are included, with an exploration into how these behaviors undermine the culture of safety and meaningful progress in health care environments, including burnout of health care professionals (HCPs). A renewed focus on stress management, and moral injury with an emphasis on mental health, has been reflected in the related chapters to assist in fostering healthier health care professionals.

In addition, the chapter on communicating about spiritual needs with an exploration of the relationship with the Human Movement System (Chapter 15) has been refreshed with the expansion of evidence in this realm. This is not a chapter on religion but a chapter focusing on helping health care professionals to better assess the needs of patients and families in dealing with hope, faith, and despair. New research related to faith and mental health is included along with suggested frameworks as guides for the novice HCP, as well as additional case examples incorporated throughout the text's chapters.

The chapters on patient education (Chapter 16) and communicating with cultural sensitivity (Chapter 13) have been enhanced with updates on the application of the transtheoretical model of change and expanded patient/client education activities. The chapters further consider the appropriate use of interactive technology for patient/client education, along with tips and resources for health literacy considerations and fostering health promotion. Content has also been updated to address contemporary inclusive and identity terminology. The chapter on promoting effective health education (Chapter 16) has been updated to include higher level objectives, new evaluation tools, and comprehensive, enriching exercises.

The well-received chapter on leadership and advocacy for health care, added to the sixth edition, continues, asking the developing professionals to understand the importance of incorporating leadership skills with patient health care, with links to the societal generations (Chapter 11). Through guided reading and writing pre- and post-chapter exercises, learners are asked to proactively consider one's future as a leader while also appreciating the benefits of knowing when to lead and when to follow. Contemporary and classic leadership guidance is provided with application exercises. Both interprofessional and intraprofessional aspects of teamwork and advocacy are highlighted, with key exercises to facilitate professional formation with applications for taking advocacy action.

Additional chapters explore mindful practice and well-being activities while examining the influence of neurolinguistics, culture differences, cultural awareness, and special populations, contexts, and environments. New exercises exploring a patient's progression within the health care system are included, as well as an extensive list of media resources to supplement learning and reflection.

There is a changing face to health care. Increasing numbers of our developing professionals come from other cultures. Our patients and clients represent a variety of cultures and backgrounds. This text helps HCPs to develop assertiveness skills for those who are shy or from another culture that may emphasize less actively direct ways of communicating. Instructors can use this text (and its accompanying Instructor's Manual) to teach skills such as how to communicate therapeutically with patients from a different culture, identity, background, biological sex, sexual orientation, and expression spectrums; those who are depressed, those trying to cope with increasing disability, those who are facing death, those who have learned that they will not be able to be the same sexually as before injury, those with changed lives due to changed family dynamics from caretaker to caregiver or care receiver, those who are raging with anger and hostility, and those who are inappropriate sexually with the professional. A new final chapter has been added to address the transition that occurs with professional learners moving from didactic to full-time clinic settings (Chapter 20). The chapter offers prudent advice, pearls of wisdom, and tips from real-world experiences for setting the stage for success for further transitions in professional formation. This final chapter is designed to help students bridge from classroom to clinical learning and teaching environments. Their changed role is examined with an emphasis on the utility for maintaining a growth mindset. The roles of clinical instructors are examined as well as career pathways from novice-to-early career professional, including the pathways to clinical instruction and the benefits of specialization. Opportunities to explore residency and fellowship education are provided. Considerations of the unique aspects of telehealth and artificial intelligence are discussed in terms of augmenting clinical practice for the patients/clients we serve. The generations and biopsychosocial matters of holistic, patient-centered care are once again emphasized for clinical reasoning and interactive, therapeutic alliances.

And, as always, exercises at the end of each chapter encourage an essential element in the inculcation of these fundamental skills—reflection and personalization of the material to one's own story. These exercises are also available online at www.routledge.com/9781638220039.

Those who have used this text sometimes email, call, or send letters expressing gratitude for *Patient Practitioner Interaction* (*PPI*). Some of the unique benefits and features of this text are that it helps to develop self-awareness and communication skills for those situations with patients and colleagues where the health care professional might think to themselves, "What in the world do I say now? They never taught me in school how to deal with *this* situation." *PPI* remains the answer to every curricular need to develop interpersonal professional behaviors in health care providers' professional development, and we are grateful to say it has been so effective at this task that it has been a bestseller for nearly four decades.

This is material that is not easily or happily taught but is required by accreditation standards in all programs because effective professional health care requires these skills in professional formation. An Instructor's Manual accompanies the text to guide faculty how to best use this text to facilitate learning the material in a learner-friendly and patient-centered manner. Hints are provided on how to facilitate group interaction, helping developing health care professionals to grapple with the information personally and make the necessary changes in PPI to serve them well with patients and clients.

We all want to enjoy ourselves, and we should be able to as we learn and grow as professionals. One of the forces that interferes with that enjoyment is not knowing what to say in an uncomfortable or highly emotional situation with patients, colleagues, or professional learners. Once you start practicing the self-awareness and skills that this text is designed to teach, life will be much more enjoyable, and that's as it should be; we are all adaptive learners in this process, and it remains our wish for all who read this text to put these words into practice.

# ACKNOWLEDGMENTS

My immeasurable gratitude goes to Dr. Gina Maria Musolino, who skillfully took the helm for this latest edition of *Patient Practitioner Interaction*, and to Tony Schiavo from SLACK Incorporated, editor of our dreams. The two of you together, once again, have produced a wonderful addition to this lineage, which began with the first edition in 1989. Thank you both for your outstanding work, and for the richness of our interactions and our friendship.

*Carol M. Davis*

The completion of *Davis's Patient–Practitioner Interaction: An Experiential Manual for Developing the Art of Health Care*, 7th ed. (*PPI7*) was far from an individual undertaking. There are many students, faculty, colleagues, family members, and friends with whom we share credit.

The SLACK Incorporated staff have done it once again and remain a dedicated and classy team.

Special recognition to Kayla Whittle, former Acquisitions Editor, Slack Books, who assured timely peer reviews, and outstanding organization of files for the unexpected hand-off procedures. I am deeply thankful once again for the opportunity and pleasure to work so closely with Anthony (Tony) P. Schiavo Jr, former Senior VP Slack Books, now Senior VP. Tony was always responsive in his guidance, shared his astute wisdom and experiences, exercised formidable patience through the pandemic journey, and assured success. Thank you, dear Tony, for always being willing to have deep discussions, giving truthful guidance, and always being willing to lend a listening ear. Thank you for being there beyond the hand-off—a true friend and professional! Thank you also for sharing your family with me; your six children and wife are truly blessed to have such a dedicated father and husband. Being one of six myself, your sharing your family with me continues to take me back in time to the wonderful and carefree days of childhood and now collegiate and professional school years!

To Madaline (Madii) Cherry-Moreton, Editorial Assistant, Health & Social Care, Routledge, Taylor & Francis, and Russell George, Senior Editor, Public Health and Allied Health, Routledge, I am forever grateful for your unwavering assistance through the transition, adept and efficient responsiveness to manuscript checks and reviews, prompt follow-up queries and consultations, along with reassurances through the hand-off to production processes! Thank you as well to Jeremy North, Managing Director, Taylor & Francis Advanced Learning, for the warm welcome and swiftly providing the needed networks for transitioning. A multitude of gratitude to Sarah Webb, copyeditor, for her quality work, detailed acumen with a keen sense of connections. Sarah, your deep-seated passion for the work and finesse for *PPI* did not go unnoticed! Thank you to Cathy Hurren for bringing PPI home as Senior Production Editor, Taylor & Francis Group; assuring ease for the reader, attention to the details, and quality in production. Your guidance and patience with the process remain admirable!

I would like to specially acknowledge my co-author, Carol M. Davis, DPT, EdD, MS, FAPTA, for sharing her treasured gift of *PPI* with me, and handing-off to me for continued care. Dr. Davis is a celebrated leader, remains a tireless advocate for the profession, and fearlessly addresses the affective domain of learning for developing health care professionals for the patients and clients we serve. Although Carol's *PPI* text has been around since 1989, I did not discover it until later editions. I have used the *PPI* textbook since the mid-1990s with new and developing programs, where having no near peers makes the professional acculturation even more challenging and with long-standing and established programs that have benefited greatly from the deep dive into the affective domain as the solid foundation and springboard for reflective expertise in practice. Early in my career as a faculty member, I never would have survived teaching the content without the book's guidance to facilitate the eye-opening exercises and often amazing teachable moments in the classroom and clinics and to prepare future health care providers to connect with themselves and their patients. I never dreamed I would have the honor to carry the torch, and I hope that I have continued to do your early works justice while updating for contemporary practice in this thirty-sixth year of *PPI* with this seventh edition. Thank you for your trust in me and for allowing me the freedom to expand the text beyond the formative years. *PPI* has made a difference in so many lives, and I trust the novel contributions in this edition shall carry on your celebrated works to continue to produce changes in professional behaviors and to develop sensitive, caring, inclusive, and empathic health care professionals who serve as strong advocates to meet their patients' diverse needs, promote equity and accessibility, and serve as dedicated leaders in health care teams. Thank you, Carol, for seeing in me what I did not even see in myself! Your generative spirit is without question continuing to influence those that follow. Thank you for catalyzing me to soar to new heights I had never dreamt of reaching. Thank you, once again, for entrusting this work to me to carry on your legacy. I hope I continue to make you proud.

To our long-standing contributing authors Dr. Helen L. Masin, Dr. Darina Sargeant, Dr. Kathleen Curtis, and Dr. Sherrill H. Hayes—you too have each provided the foundational works from which *PPI* has continued to evolve. Your exceptional works have been revitalized, and you each remain deeply dedicated to PPI; for this we are all thankful. You are not only superb teachers and inspiring leaders and scholars, but you are also all willing to consider new perspectives and help others to not only learn best practices but also to enjoy them and have a thirst for more learning! Even though now retired, we are deeply grateful for your lasting and continued influence in challenging content areas for professional development of health care professionals.

Much gratitude is extended to our experienced, new, and continuing contributing authors for *PPI7*, Dr. Sherrill H. Hayes, Dr. Solange Dagress, Dr. Mica Mitchell, and Dr. Alecia Thiele. What a pleasure it has been to work with each of you. Your exceptional revitalization and novel contributions assure contemporary perspectives for *PPI7*. You each remain deeply dedicated to PPI; for this we are all thankful. Your fresh perspectives as creative educators, motivating leaders, specialized clinicians, and scholars made all the difference for *PPI7*. Being able to teach by example, share your experiences through story, and facilitate through guided exercises is a true gift, and each of you has this gift and can capably catalyze others in the desire to learn and apply. We are deeply grateful that you have chosen to continue to answer the call for *PPI7*. Without your continued dedication to the work of PPI, it would not be possible, and your responsiveness, even amid the pandemic, and publishing transitions, has made my work as co-author and editor a sheer delight! I commend each of you for your dedicated time, diligent efforts, and professionalism along the way, even when facing your own real-life challenges and transitions. Thank you for sharing your compassion and caring insights so graciously. Your unique expertise has helped to produce high-value learning and significant application exercises for professional formation within *PPI7*.

We cherish the Foreword previously provided by our dear departed Dr. Helen Hislop, PT, PhD, ScD, FAPTA, and although not included in this edition, it is preserved for historical purposes within *PPI5–6*. She now belongs to the ages and shall always be missed and remembered.

My sincere thanks to our esteemed colleague, Dr. Shirley Sahrmann, PT, PhD, FAPTA, for her continued contribution of the Foreword to *PPI7*. We all know Shirley is the remarkable one in moving forward the profession, especially in matters of Movement Science, and she has done it once again. We appreciate her taking time out from retirement and travels, and from her own high-impact, internationally renowned scholarly works to provide her insights again for *PPI7*. One glorious fall semester, when I was but a neophyte student physical therapist, I had the incredible honor of spending Wednesday afternoons with Dr. Sahrmann with one of my peers at Washington University School of Medicine, Program in Physical Therapy (WUMS PT) in the then Irene Walter Johnson Institute of Rehabilitation. Dr. Sahrmann was patient with us as novice learners (we were shaking in our lab tunics yet wore the name badges that said we had the right to be there), at least as much as any seasoned professional ought to be with true rookies. Dr. Sahrmann provided needed encouragement and spirited critique and was certain to cajole when we thought we had it all figured out already. She enlightened us on her patients' movement imbalances and Movement Impairment Syndromes and taught us to truly think on our feet. Thank you, Dr. Sahrmann, for sharing your discerning eye and words of wisdom on the important aspects of movement in every facet of health care and your personal patient–practitioner interaction insights! Your recognition of the significance of the role of the biopsychosocial influence for movement is genuinely appreciated. Your wisdom is highly valued, and we thank you for taking the time and effort to assure that we, as lifespan practitioners, keep the Human Movement System at the forefront for the benefit of our patients and clients. Thank you also for always bringing joy, incorporating laughter with your lecture and being able to laugh at oneself.

Special thanks to the many dedicated educators and leaders in my life who provided important professional foundations, especially those at Utica University, Utica, NY (post professional DPT); Washington University, School of Medicine, Program in Physical Therapy, St. Louis, Missouri; Nova Southeastern University, Abraham S. Fischler College of Education, Ft. Lauderdale, Florida; John Wood Community College; Quincy High School, and St. Peter School and Church of St. Peter, Quincy, Illinois. Thank you to the genuine people and multitude of inspiring places of Adams, Charlotte, Coconino, Levy, Moore, Nassau, Pasco, Salt Lake, Sarasota-Manatee and Yavapai Counties.

Thank you to the countless dedicated colleagues who have given me the incredible opportunities to serve with the American Physical Therapy Association (APTA), *Physical Therapy Journal*; Academy of Education, *Journal of Physical Therapy Education*; Association of Schools Advancing Health Professions, *Journal of Allied Health*; APTA Florida Physical Therapy Association, APTA House of Delegates; California Physical Therapy Association, Florida Consortium of Clinical Education, Northwest Intermountain Consortium of Clinical Education, The University of Utah, The University of South Florida, Morsani College of Medicine, School of Physical Therapy & Rehabilitation Sciences, and the University of Florida, Department of Physical Therapy, College of Public Health & Health Professions—the *Gator Nation*! Much gratitude as well to the many administrative staff members with these fine organizations who do so much to support our endeavors. To my many dear colleagues in academics and in the trenches of clinical education—thank you for sharing your stories and allowing us to influence your works. I am indebted to the tremendous support and dedication of nationwide clinical instructors and site coordinators of clinical education who hold their protégés accountable for compassionate care and empathic patient–practitioner interactions—keep making a difference! You are the ones who continue to ensure that we translate PPI for patient care, advocacy, and leadership. Thank you!

We are in a blessed profession when we can call our colleagues our friends, and so it is in physical therapy. With enormous heartfelt gratitude to my cherished colleagues who continue to believe in me and connect with me at important touchpoints in my life and career: Rita Pierson, Executive Associate, California Physical Therapy Association; Dr. Shontol Torres Burkhalter, PT, DPT; Dr. Alecia Thiele, PT, DPT, MSEd, ATC/L, DCE; Dr. Catherine Page, PT, MPh, PhD; Dr. William "Sandy" Quillen, PT, PhD, Professor Emeritus; Dr. Sarah Maher, PT, DPT, DScPT, OMT; Dr. Michael Simpson, PT, DPT, Board-Certified Cardiovascular and Pulmonary Clinical Specialist; Anna V. Howard, PT, Board-Certified Pediatric Clinical Specialist; Dr. Mark Bishop, PT, PhD, FAPTA; Dr. Marilyn Moffat, PT, DPT, PhD, DSc, FAPTA; Dr. Krista Vandenborne, PT, PhD; Dr. Dennis W. Fell, MD, PT; Dr. Michael Mueller, PT, PhD, FAPTA; Ronna Delitto, PT and Dr. Anthony Delitto, PT, PhD, FAPTA; Dr. Gail M. Jensen, PT, PhD, FAPTA; Dr. Elizabeth Mostrom, PT, PhD, FAPTA; Dr. Karen Hayes, PT, PhD, FAPTA; Dr. R. Scott Ward, PT, PhD, FAPTA; Dr. Edelle Field-Foote, PT, PhD, FAPTA; Dr. Mary Rogers, PT, PhD, FAPTA, FASB; Dr. Kathleen Rockefeller, PT, ScD, MPH; Dr. Katherine J. Sullivan, PT, PhD, FAHA; Dr. Susan S. Deusinger, PT, PhD, FAPTA; and Dr. Shirley Sahrmann, PT, PhD, FAPTA. You have each encouraged me in abundant ways! Your professional influence and friendship remain cherished.

Memorable thanks to those mentors gone too soon: the dearly departed Dr. Steven J. Rose, PT, PhD, FAPTA; Charles Magistro, PT, FAPTA; Dr. Linda M. Howard, RN, PhD; and Beatrice F. Schulz, PT. Dr. Rose taught me the value of discerning the useful, useless, and harmful aspects of health care and research and taught me that putting our pencils down is not a bad thing! Linda shared her undying enthusiasm, effervescent inspiration, and dedication to students, along with change-hardy leadership. Charles always had a twinkle in his eye, sharing his administrative words of wisdom and genuine leadership. Bea taught me that it was always okay to have joy in your work and to keep smiling.

I remain especially grateful to my graduates, student learners, and patients, who have taught me more than I ever imagined possible! Thank you for your enthusiasm, support, and willingness to share your journeys with me and for the privilege to assist you in yours. Thank you for giving back and continuing your dedication to professionalism.

I especially thank my first teachers—my parents. My father, the late Dr. Joseph L. Musolino, DVM, had the true gift of being able to listen to his patients. Thank you, Dad, for allowing me to go on "country calls" with you and being a true supporter of my every endeavor. For my dear departed and wonderful M.O.M. (Mother of Many), who dedicated herself daily to the challenges of movement—you never ceased to inspire and motivate. Thank you both for making sure I continued to reach my full potential. Thank you for your undying love, kindness, respect, tolerance, patience, playfulness, hope, faith, and understanding; you have never hesitated to share them all. I thank you both for your dedication to your children, to whom you gave eagles' wings. You navigated the challenges of life with true grace. Thank you to my family members and nieces and nephews who are always there, sparkling, constantly listening, supporting, sharing, and laughing, facing the unfortunate in life and love, doing the hard work of living and loss, and being passionate while dedicating yourselves to others, and pulling out all the stops in your learning and lifetime endeavors; you remain my deepest of inspirations. Especially for my cherished siblings, Adam, Renée, Christopher, Tony, and Lisa Jo, stay courageous! All my love for always sharing your unique talents and abilities—you have each taught me so much!

Once again, and especially to the many inspirational people and places of the great state of Florida, Sedona, AZ, Glacier National Park, King County, WA, Moore County, NC and Adams County, IL—stay beautiful!

And, finally, for each of you who cares to deeply dive in with PPI7 and dares to continue your professional transformation as an adaptive learner: may your health care experiences bring you joy, and, when they are challenging, may you rely on PPI7 to guide and enrich you once again, to cherish the human spirit and ensure care is at the forefront of your patient–practitioner interactions for health. We wish you courage and strength on your journey.

*Gina Maria Musolino*

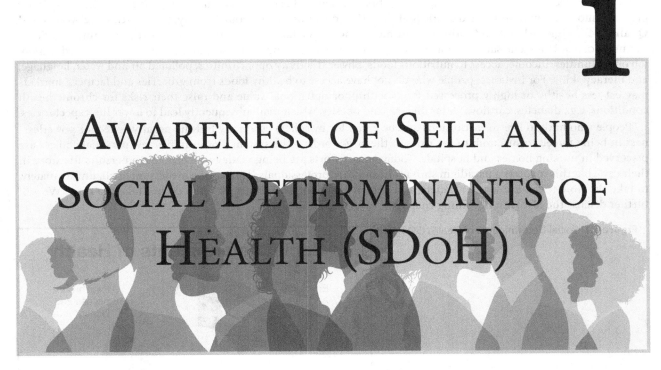

# AWARENESS OF SELF AND SOCIAL DETERMINANTS OF HEALTH (SDoH)

*Gina Maria Musolino and Carol M. Davis*

## OBJECTIVES

*The learner should be able to*:

- Conceptualize the multi-dimensional construct of the self.
- Assess the importance of self-knowledge in relation to one's quality of life and the choices one makes.
- Become cognizant of the Social Determinants of Health.
- Describe potential barriers to self-awareness.
- Apply helpful resources for self-awareness.
- Exemplify self-awareness through reading, exercises, and journaling about oneself.

## WHAT IS THE SELF?

Take a moment to reflect on this quote and consider how it relates to your sense of self:

*Nobody sees a flower, really—it's so small—we haven't time, and to see it takes time.* —Georgia O'Keefe

How well do you know yourself? Why would anyone ever ask that question? Some would say that the better you know yourself, the more aware you are of your thoughts and feelings, your strengths and weaknesses; the more you feel in control of your life, the less stressed and helpless you feel, and the less surprised you are by your responses to life. Yet, it takes time to know one's self through self-examination and reflection. Thus, the quality of one's life is, in part, measured by the amount of personal control one feels over day-to-day happenings and choices.

One's **Social Determinants of Health (SDoH)**, which are "the conditions in the environment where people are born, live, learn, work, play, worship and age, affect wide ranges of health functioning, quality-of-life outcomes, and risks."[1]

DOI: 10.4324/9781003525554-1

In fact, one's SDoH often have a very high impact on one's available choices and ultimate well-being. The SDoH[1] are grouped into five domains: **(1) Economic Stability, (2) Education Access and Quality, (3) Health Care Access and Quality, (4) Neighborhood and Built Environment, and (5) Social and Community Context** (see Figure 1.1). Some examples of SDoH include safe housing, transportation, neighborhoods, violence, discrimination, racism, education, job opportunities, income, access to nutritious foods, physical activity opportunities, polluted air and water, language, and literacy skills. For instance, people who do not have access to healthy foods from groceries and farmers' markets may eat less healthy or highly processed foods with poor nutritional value and raise their risks for chronic health conditions, e.g., diabetes, cardiovascular disease, and obesity, which may subsequently lead to lower life expectancies.

People who have to live in institutions and be cared for by others especially feel the negative effect of powerlessness in being forced to succumb to the rules of the larger order—the system. For example, few personal choices are preserved in nursing homes and hospitals. Today, more efforts are being made to incorporate a person's life story in their care, but this involves a paradigm shift for health care professionals (HCPs) who are less inclined, unfortunately, to take the time to get know their patient as a person first and, unfortunately, often do not take the time. We will further discuss the SDoH in upcoming chapters.

**Figure 1.1** Social Determinants of Health (SDoH).

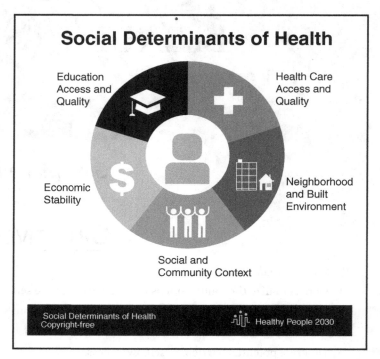

This chapter asks you to take the time to get to know yourself better as a person first so that you may better care for yourself and your well-being and, therefore, be more available and present to care for others as a health care professional. You are becoming a HCP, so it is important to know who you are and who you are becoming. *Who am I?*

What is the self? How is the self different from the body? What are people asking when they ask, "Who am I, really?" and "Why am I here?" These are timeless questions that become more the focus of concern during the second half of life than during the first. It has been said that, for many of us, the first half of life is the "doing" half and the second half is the "being" half. When we are busy achieving and working for security and happiness, questions such as "Who am I?" seem distracting. Beyond our mid-thirties, these questions take on greater importance as we reflect on the meaning of life as we begin to recognize and realize our own mortalities.

Young children are unable to be truly self-aware. But you may remember that delicious moment when you first discovered, all by yourself, that you were uniquely different from anyone else in the entire world. You were probably 6 or 7 years old. Zaner, in *The Context of Self*,[2] described a colleague's recounting of this moment:

> *As far as I can tell, I must have been younger than 8 years old when I began having what I now call I-am-me experiences. On such occasions I would tell myself insistently, "This is me, me …" The inner pronouncing of these words and especially the repetition of the personal pronoun were accompanied with the feeling of a cave-in, a dropping down from a surface level of self-awareness to a more and more personal me-myself. Along with it went a feeling of being sucked down as by a whirlpool into a bottomless depth. As I repeated the pronoun "me" I felt as if one mask after another fell off, until the actor behind these masks was stripped to the naked core.*

To be able to reflect upon the full nature of one's self, however, seems to require the cognitive skills and experiences of a person with a mature nervous system. To become aware of oneself, one must go outside of one's self and ponder the self and, for example, analyze one's motives for behavior. According to Piaget,[3] becoming self-aware occurs at the stage of formal operations.

# THE DESIRE FOR SELF-AWARENESS

The wish to become self-aware often has to do with the search for meaning in life and the desire to experience a choice in the process of whom one is becoming. In other words, the question "Who am I?" is necessary before one can truly be who one chooses. Parents tell children how to act most often with good intention. Most children are socialized into becoming what their parents or guardians believe are good human beings who will live happy and productive lives. The influence of the family, along with the generations, on one's self-esteem and self-concept is of utmost importance and covered in more depth in Chapter 2.

The goal of education for HCPs is to assist students in becoming a certain way: **professional**. What does it mean to be professional? Any description of a professional would contain the integration of a body of knowledge and skills and the proficient and effective delivery of the same. In the profession of health care, proficient and effective delivery requires a therapeutic use of one's self while interacting with patients and/or clients. Superior skill in the technology of the profession *must* be balanced with the *art* of relating to those who request our services in such a way that *healing is facilitated*, rather than interfered with, in the provision of care.

If health care consisted of working on bodies alone, perhaps a consideration of the self would not be necessary. But the fact remains that health care involves people and interacting with people in such a way that what is not right is correctly analyzed and appropriately influenced so that it is changed to approximate more closely what is right. This analysis and influence occurs between human beings who have not just brought their bodies to us but have also brought their feelings, fears, hopes, frustrations, and pain. Illness is meaningful only as it is lived, moment to moment. When we care professionally, we care for people living with their illnesses, not for broken bodies. There are numerous traits, entailing development of the prefrontal cortex (regulation of thoughts and emotions), both cognitive and meta-cognitive, that influence our abilities for positive performance as a professional, including ethical and legal practice, active learning and teaching, critical thinking and clinical decision making, inclusive and interpersonal communication skills, professionalism, and taking responsibility for one's own actions.[4]

Let us take a closer look at the nature of the self: what it is; what it is not; how it grows and is influenced; and how it performs as we mature into healthy, more self-actualized human beings.

# THE SELF

Human beings are tremendously complex organisms, capable of portraying various identities or roles, depending on the demands of a situation. Much study has been devoted to the way we can divide ourselves into various parts or take on different roles and remain essentially the same person, or whole. Transactional analysis literature teaches about the "parent, adult, and child" in each of us.[5] We each portray various roles throughout the day, such as employee, boss, sister, brother, and friend. Jung,[6] in attempting to explore the nature of the unconscious, described archetypal elements present in all personalities. Among them were the persona, the shadow, and the self. Freud is famous for his explications of the ego, the id, and the superego. All these now-common terms were created to help explain the complex behavior of humans.

The psychology literature informs us about the nature of the self and its role in human growth. Figure 1.2 represents the various layers of a person or the various aspects of a personality. The outermost layer is the *persona*, or the public face, each of us puts on in the world to appear in control, intelligent, witty, sensitive, and lovable. We act in the ways that we believe are going to bring us love and recognition. But, deep inside, we know that the persona is really a mask. Underneath that mask is another aspect of ourselves that is filled with doubts and insecurities. Almost all of us are dissatisfied with living our lives totally from behind the mask. Each of us desires to drop our false fronts and to become who we truly are, to express ourselves more honestly, to be more truly ourselves, and to be loved for who we truly are inside.

The second layer is composed of the *ego*, or the center of the conscious mind as described by Freud, and the *shadow*, the unconscious, natural side of our personalities. The ego is the part of us that gets the job of living done. It is the force that gets us through school and makes choices for us that are designed, as best we know, to bring us happiness.

**Figure 1.2** The nature of self.

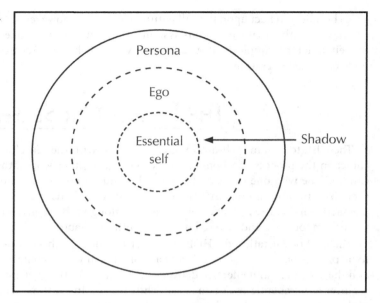

The ego problem solves for us and helps us have the courage to act and the patience to wait. But the ego is made up of all kinds of misinformation about ourselves and about the world. Egos tend to be very protective; they tend to move us toward safety, toward the status quo. The ego believes in its own omnipotence. But it must sustain that belief by using a lot of energy and by ignoring many messages that would refute that omnipotence. The feeling of a god-like ego is an illusion. In fact, the ego is filled with erroneous ideas and fears about the world and about ourselves. Our egos tell us we are highly intelligent one minute and totally naïve and stupid the next. First, they tell us the world is a wonderful, loving place, and then that it is a dangerous, destructive place.

Each of us tends to listen to the still, small voice of the ego when we must make important choices, but we become very confused about what is important and true. This is because we tend to allow the voice of the ego to reflect what we have heard from important people in our lives about ourselves. If we heard, "You are so stupid, you'll never amount to anything" when we were young, we believed that for a time until we had the power to prove that it was not true. As we achieved success, we told our egos, "See, I really am bright. I can succeed!" But instead of dropping the old data and incorporating the new, the ego holds on to the whole package and spits both messages at us at times when we feel most unable to modify that quiet voice.

Tolle[7] shares with us that, in awakening our life's purpose, we need others to give us a sense of ourselves. How we are seen by others evolves into how we come to see ourselves:

> *If you live in a culture that to a large extent equates self-worth with how much and what you have, if you cannot look through that collective delusion, you will be condemned to chasing after things for the rest of your life in the vain hope of finding your worth and completing of your sense of self there. … The ego isn't wrong, it's just unconscious.*

The *shadow* is Jung's[6] term for another aspect of the unconscious part of this second layer. It is our inferior side, the part of us that wants to do all the things our ego tells us we cannot do. When we say things like, "I wasn't myself" or "I don't know what came over me," we are acknowledging the presence of our unconscious shadow that tricks us into behaving in ways we say we abhor. Underneath these outer two layers, at the center of the person, lies the rest of us, the "more" that the outer two layers cannot fully incorporate: the *self*. The self is the essence of the person and incorporates conscious and unconscious elements of the person into itself. I have my persona, I have my ego, I have my personality, I have my body, I have my possessions in life … I am my self. The self is the irreducible energy of my uniqueness. It is the thing that makes me absolutely unique in the universe, even though one may be an identical twin, and thousands of people share your name. It is that marvelous essence of me that I approach as the masks are, one by one, stripped away in the search for what is undividable, what is at my core. It is the unfolding answer to the eternal question, "Who am I, really?"

The self is that energy that can linger for days before the moment of the "crossing over" into death of the physical body. Those who care for the terminally ill have often experienced the phenomenon that, for a time before the body stops functioning totally, it is more accurate to say that all that remains in the bed is a shell that looks like the person's body. The essence of the person seems to come and go, little by little, spending more time gone than present. Often in this stage, we acknowledge that it is "okay" for the person to go, and we express this, or we see the spark leave their eyes in an instant as they cross over. We will explore death and dying further in Chapter 19.

The self has to do with the energy inside each human that reincarnationists say is a piece of the deity that is never created nor destroyed.[8] It is my "higher self." Christians would call it the "Christ self" within each of us, and Buddhists would call it the "Buddha self." It exists for all time; it always has and always will, and the task of human beings on Earth is to house this energy as we grow and change, lifetime after lifetime, with the end goal of becoming more like God, like truth (of course those who are atheist or agnostic would likely not agree).

Jung said this about the nature of the self:[6]

> *The self ... can include both the conscious and the unconscious. It appears to act as something like a magnet to the disparate elements of the personality and the processes of the unconscious and is the centre of this totality as the ego is the centre of consciousness, for it is the function which unites all the opposing elements in man and woman, consciousness, and unconsciousness, good and bad, male, and female, etc., and in so doing transmutes them. To reach it necessitates acceptance of what is inferior in one's nature, as well as what is irrational and chaotic. This state cannot be reached by a mature person without considerable struggle; it implies suffering, for the Western mind, unlike the Eastern, does not easily tolerate paradoxes. [The self] consists ... in the awareness on the one hand of our unique natures, and on the other of our intimate relationship with all life, not only human, but animal and plant, and even that of inorganic matter and the cosmos itself. It brings a feeling of "oneness," and/or reconciliation with life, which now can be accepted as it is, not as it should be.*

Thus, the self, once uncovered, seems to hold the truth about us as human beings. It is our connection with the Truth, and it is out of this center of our existence that we come to feel at one with our fellow human beings. It is the self that can cross over in empathy and experience and feel what a moment in life must be like for another person. It is the self that we return to as we quieten our working minds in meditation. It is the self that allays our fears, that gives us true courage rather than braggadocio or false bravado; it is the self that feels the essential goodness of our humanness, in the face of our incompleteness; it is the self that grows in wisdom and becomes more as we mature, approaching the all-knowing goodness of Truth; it is the self that enables us to laugh at our egos and forgive the well-meaning unkindness visited upon us by parents and relatives as they tried desperately to get us to "act right" as children and thereby systematically helped to destroy our inborn connectedness with our true selves.

# SELF-AWARENESS

Rogers[9] has said, "It appears that the goal the individual most wishes to achieve, the end which one knowingly and unknowingly pursues, is to become oneself." How do we become ourselves? How do we discover our true nature? How do we access the self? How do we get close to it, get right up next to it? It begins when we recognize the burning desire to be known for who we are, not for who we believe others want us to be. It begins when we are willing to shed the roles we have assumed to win attention, affection, and acceptance and instead commit to being truthful and honest. Often the first steps we take in this direction come with our challenges to our parents and the "rules of the house."

Self-awareness requires reflection to ascertain who we truly are. The ego will work overtime to tell you about yourself, but it takes time and effort of a different sort to reflect deeper to the messages of the true self. We will further explore self-awareness in Chapter 10 for reflective practice as a developing professional, striving for expertise.

Often, we need help in this process of becoming more self-aware because our perceptions are unavoidably influenced by the messages we heard when we were incredibly young. To sift through unchallenged truths that were reinforced for years (e.g., all women are emotional, all men are insensitive) requires, for example, the perspectives of literature, art, and music and the professional preparation of counselors and psychologists to help us examine our habitual assumptions. The goal of growth of this sort is to expand the narrow, parochial views we held as children and to become more aware of a wider world view; a view that incorporates diversity and trades limited binary, dualistic thinking for the wonderful hues of ambiguity, free from the need to be right and the fear of being wrong, able to consider the multiplicity of perspectives. It is, in a sense, the search for truth that we are after as we mature in our world views. We want to enfold all possibilities, rather than leave out information that might be critical for comprehending the complexities of ourselves, our lives, and the world we live in. In the search for the self, the goal becomes to give up beliefs that entrap us in negativity, doubt, and self-centered behavior and replace them with beliefs that enlarge our consciousness and help us feel compassion for our oneness with all of life and sincere interest in the needs of those we serve.

# PATIENT-CENTERED SELF-AWARENESS

When we find ourselves distracted from the moment, or if we have never participated in self-awareness activities, patients can suffer from our insensitivity. Let us consider an example.

A recently graduated physical therapist was having a particularly difficult day and was not taking regular check on his emotions. He went into his patient's room and found the patient engrossed in a conversation with his nurse. The patient was trying to understand the various medications he was taking and their possible side effects. He was anxious and could not seem to understand what the nurse was repeating over and over to him. As the physical therapist waited for this discussion to be completed, he became increasingly impatient, recognizing that he was becoming more behind in his patient treatments for the day. He interrupted the conversation rudely and stated, "Look, I've been waiting patiently here for 5 minutes. I am on a tight schedule, and I have to see this patient next. Please wrap this chat up and let me get to work, will you?"

Had the physical therapist stopped for a second and taken a deep breath, he might have realized, first, that he was annoyed and, second, that this was an important conversation, and he had several choices available to solve his problem. Because he lacked self-awareness and tact, he saw the problem not as his, but as the nurse's.

This lack of self-awareness brought a negative energy into the entire situation, and this could have been completely avoided had the physical therapist, once he recognized his emotion of annoyance and impatience, reviewed his options, and invited the nurse and patient to help him decide when would be a suitable time to return. This was obviously an important conversation between the patient and nurse that needed to continue, and the needs of the patient are more important than the therapist's schedule. Very often, the major goal of those early or newly beginning health care professionals, as they become socialized into acting professionally, is to recognize that patient care is about patients, not about "me." *Patients and their needs come first.* Patient-centered care may be a new perspective for early career HCPs to accept; all part of growth and development for maturation in becoming a collaborative health care professional. This professional formation is highly important as, when patients entrust their care to HCPs, a holistic or "whole person" care approach is the expectation.[10] As advocates for all patients, HCPs are to ensure that patients' self-determination and autonomy are respected.[11] The concept of patient-centered care includes the following attributes:[10]

- Respect for patients' values, preferences, and beliefs
- Coordination and integration of care
- Information, communication, and education
- Physical comfort
- Emotional support and alleviation of fear and anxiety
- Involvement of family and friends
- Transition and continuity
- Access to care

# SEARCH FOR THE SELF

This text is designed to help you examine your values, beliefs, and communication patterns to assist you in the search for your self and to broaden your world view. It is from the *self* that we give health care of the highest quality. The *self* has the capacity to see clearly and to display compassion in the face of threat or fatigue, which crosses over into empathy. It is the *self* that sets appropriate boundaries and refuses to attempt to have personal needs met by patients. The *self* has unlimited patience and great understanding. The *self* comprehends the need to be ethical and to act with integrity. It is the *self* that has the desire and the capability to feel unconditional positive regard and oneness with all living beings, which cancels out judgment and prejudice.

However, it is the frightened ego that pities and pretends that it is displaying compassion; it is the frightened ego that becomes impatient and defends itself rather than offering a healing response to the angry patient; it is the ego that needs to be puffed up and made to feel important at the expense of others' feelings. It is the frightened ego that *requires* our patients to do as we say, to get better, and to thank us for helping them.

All of us want essentially the same thing: to be respected and to be treated with unconditional positive regard. But all of us want that positive acceptance of our whole being, not just of our persona (i.e., our ego). We want others to love and accept us as we are wholly, in all of our incompleteness. The more the ego tries to defend itself, the more difficult it is to catch a glimpse of ourselves and our essential natures. If you have been told that you tend to respond defensively to people, you developed this coping skill out of necessity. However, defensiveness is not particularly useful for patient care. This will be a good opportunity for you to examine the messages you are receiving that make you feel as if you must defend yourself. Defensiveness always obliterates the truth. It is noisy and useless and has no sense of humor at all. It is the mark of a person responding to life from an insecure ego, not the sign of a whole and integrated self who might respond to criticism with, for example, "I did not know I was coming across that way. I will take a closer look at my behavior now."

As HCPs gain expertise, they find that it becomes important to regularly take stock of one's feelings during the day. Emotions are key to what we experience, and sometimes we find ourselves disassociating from people in response to feeling overwhelmed with work or feeling insecure or angry with the system. Regularly experiencing our feelings as they arise during our day becomes a critical component of a HCP's well-being and keeps us connected with ourselves and able to focus on our patients and the task at hand. One must not lose track of normal emotional responses because this is what makes us sensitive and caring providers. Yet, as HCPs, we must learn to cope and manage appropriately by taking the time to recognize and respond to our own feelings, too. Sometimes we must take a personal time-out to make sure that this happens in a healthy manner. Again, caring for others means first caring for yourself.

Patients appreciate demonstrations of personal caring and responding with emotion to their stories and situations of the day. The expert clinician knows how to do this and how to set appropriate boundaries at the same time, which allows for therapeutic presence without burdening the patient with our feelings. The more connected we are with our own selves, the more connected we become with our patients and colleagues and the higher the quality of our caring and efforts.[12]

# Signs of Growth in Self-Awareness

As people struggle to become more themselves, usually out of the painful realization that the masks they have been using are no longer bringing them happiness and love, they change in noticeable ways. As described by Rogers,[9] they seem to do the following:

- Drop the defensive mask with which they have faced life and begin to discover and to experience the stranger who lives behind these masks—the hidden part of self.
- Emerge with a tendency to be more open to all elements of experience, growing to trust in one's organism as an instrument of sensitive living.
- Accept the responsibility of being a unique person.
- Develop the sense of living in life as a participant in a fluid, ongoing process, continually discovering new aspects of one's self in the flow of experience.

When we live daily with an awareness of our true selves, negative feelings are confronted, and the beliefs behind them are analyzed and replaced with beliefs that are more positive and cosmic. Thus, we take responsibility for creating our own reality, moment to moment. No longer do we allow ourselves to get away with such beliefs as, "You make me so angry." We acknowledge that we make ourselves angry in response to someone because of a belief we have about that person or that behavior, and then we search for a larger, more hopeful and understanding belief that will replace feelings of negativity.

Tolle[7] reminds us that "[t]he primary cause of unhappiness is never the situation but your thoughts about the situation. … Perceive the link between your thinking and your emotions. Rather than being your thoughts and emotions, be the awareness behind them."

Be conscious in today's society that the use of technologies may prohibit us from fully realizing who we are or can be as a person. Do not allow technology to keep you from knowing your self. Do not "fall prey to the illusion of companionship through the gathering of thousands of social media followers and friends, and confusing tweets, shares and posts with authentic communication."[13] As Turkle[13] described, this "relentless connection with technology leads to a new solitude." Technology may serve to connect people who might not otherwise connect, but it is not a replacement for knowing your true self. We may be more connected but more disconnected. Take time to get to know yourself and others in more connected ways. You will find greater happiness in life making true connections and using technology to enhance your relationships and expand your circle, but do not use it as a substitute for first-hand communication, whenever more appropriate. Do not allow technology to be another mask. As future HCPs, we must make every effort to be as connected as possible in the two-, three-, and four-dimensional world in which we live today.

As developing HCPs, selecting the most appropriate means of communication to ascertain the most meaningful ways to communicate is key. Do not allow objects to replace who you are as a person; experience your humanness.[14] Be fully present with those you are with, and engage in meaningful and deep conversations so as not to be depleted by the hype. Superficial communication shall leave you wanting. You will be more self-aware by not succumbing to a pure persona of social media, but by being yourself. Above all, as you develop as a HCP and engage in the often-hectic environments of health care delivery, take time in your life to do nothing, disconnect from technology, contemplate your navel, take a moment, take a minute, and pause for the cause of just being and for self-awareness. Take brief time-outs to aimlessly wander, by being in the here and now.[15] In this "stopping, we discover the vast spaciousness of life, of love, of connection."[16]

# CONCLUSION

Following most chapters in the text, including this one, you shall find additional helpful resources and references to further explore the topical content for each chapter. As a developing professional, you will want to revisit the textbook chapters and additional resources as you progress in your development and especially as you transition to more clinical works. It will be particularly relevant for you to follow up and revisit the workbook, learning in more depth as you begin and continue your patient–practitioner interactions (PPIs). Seeking out and exploring these resources, now or in the future, will continue to catalyze your personal development and professional formation, while reinforcing your continued self-awareness and learning. As a health care professional, it is important to maintain your sense of self and to stay centered, so you are able to help others reach their full potential. Even your posture, the way you carry yourself, and being able to truly pay attention to your own movement, emotions, and sensations are key to your own self-awareness.[17,18] Again, in this technologically driven society, people are losing touch with their bodies and may be compromising their own health status and self-awareness; as a health care professional, it is even more important for you to realize this in yourself, your patients, and your clients. Continuing to examine how your own mind–body–spirit connections work and how we use technology to enhance or detract from the human interface is something we need to be aware of and tuned into for our preferred PPI, as adaptive HCPs.[19-22] A cognitive neuroscience of self-awareness continues to emerge in the past few decades, with growing evidence shedding light on our capacities into the phenomenon of self-awareness processes of interoception (sense of the physiological conditions of the entire body), proprioception (mapping of the position of body parts and the feeling of knowing the body respectively within space and time), agency (sense of generating our own actions), metacognition (monitoring, knowledge and regulation of cognition), emotional regulation (monitoring and regulation of emotion), and our autobiographical memories (records of self-information, including specific episodes and general knowledge about oneself).[22] By continuing to explore these mechanisms of self-awareness, we will grow in a finer understanding of our brain function, expansion of our cognitive processes, and enhanced understandings within our health care practitioner–patient provider interactions.

Our journey together is just beginning; in Chapter 5, we will look to explore stress management; in Chapter 9, we shall discover mechanisms to resolve conflict in PPIs; and in Chapter 15, we shall specifically delve into aspects of spirituality in health care and the impact on PPIs.

The goal of this entire text is to assist you in learning more about yourself so that the way in which you relate to patients and clients who come to you for help might be sensitive, compassionate, and free from prejudice and negativity. Central to this goal is the assumption that our true or essential selves reflect the essential goodness in all of us and can be covered up by the persona, the many masks we wear, and the ego that sees the world through lenses that were originally set when we were incredibly young and helpless. The behaviors that facilitate healing, as we apply our technology, are those behaviors and underlying beliefs that bring about wholeness and oneness. Behaviors that interfere with healing result in fragmentation, discord, and negativity. It is possible to grow such that the nature of our essential selves is accessible to us and that, out of a connectedness with our essential selves, we are empowered to provide health care of the highest order. In that connectedness with our essential selves, we have the power to realize the fears and shortcomings of our egos, the falseness, and manipulation of our personas. Out of that connectedness with our essential selves, we can be the people we were created to be—capable of *unconditional positive regard* for all humans[9,23] and especially those we serve as our patients and clients. This is the greatest calling of HCPs. It is a tremendously challenging task to grow to this goal, but the rewards are indescribable. Be open to the possibilities on your journey to becoming a patient-centered, health care professional.

# REFERENCES

1. Healthy People. U.S. Department of Health and Human Services, Office of Disease Prevention and Health Promotion 2030. https://odphp.health.gov/healthypeople/priority-areas/social-determinants-health. Accessed October 23, 2024.
2. Zaner RM. *The Context of Self.* Athens, OH: Ohio University Press; 1981.
3. Piaget J. *The Construction of Reality in the Child.* New York, NY: Basic Books; 1954.
4. Cook C, McCallum C, Musolino GM, Reiman M, Covington JK. What traits are reflective of positive professional performance in physical therapy program graduates? A Delphi study. *J Allied Health.* 2018 Summer;47(2):96–102. PMID: 29868693.
5. Berne E. *Transactional Analysis in Psychotherapy.* New York, NY: Grove Press; 1961.
6. Fordham F. *An Introduction to Jung's Psychology.* Baltimore, MD: Penguin Books; 1953.
7. Tolle E. *A New Earth: Awakening to Your Life's Purpose.* New York, NY: Plume Books; 2008.
8. Challoner HK. *The Wheel of Rebirth.* Wheaton, IL: Theosophical Publishing House; 1969.
9. Rogers CR. *On Becoming a Person.* Boston, MA: Houghton Mifflin; 1961.
10. Frampton S, Guastello S, Brady C, Hale M, Horowicz S, Smith B, et al. *Patient Centered Care Improvement Guide.* Derby, CT: Planetree; 2008.
11. Gerber L. Understanding the nurse's role as patient advocation. *Nursing.* 2018 Apr;48(4):55–58.
12. Gordon GH. Giving Bad News. In: Feldman MD, Christensen JF, eds. *Behavioral Medicine in Primary Care: A Practical Guide.* 2nd ed. New York, NY: McGraw Hill Medical; 2003:17–22.
13. Turkle S. *Alone Together: Why We Expect More From Technology and Less From Each Other.* New York, NY: Basic Books; 2012.
14. Boyer J. *This "Me" of Mine: Self, Time & Context in the Digital Age.* Bloomington, IN: Xlibris Corporation; 2013.
15. Parent, J & Parent, N. *A Walk in the Wood: Meditations on Mindfulness with a Bear Named Pooh.* Los Angeles, CA: Disney Editions; 2018.
16. Kundtz D. *Quiet Mind: One-Minute Retreats From a Busy World.* York Beach, ME: Red Wheel/Weiser; 2002.
17. Rosen M. *Method Bodywork: Accessing the Unconscious Through Touch.* Berkeley, CA: North Atlantic Books; 2003.
18. Fogel A. *Body Sense: The Science and Practice of Embodied Self-Awareness (Norton Series on Interpersonal Neurobiology).* New York, NY: WW Norton & Company; 2009.
19. Popescu AM, Balica RŞ, Lazăr E, Buşu VO, Vaşcu JE. Smartphone addiction risk, technology-related behaviors and attitudes, and psychological well-being during the COVID-19 pandemic. *Front Psychol.* 2022 Aug 16;13:997253. doi: 10.3389/fpsyg.2022.997253. PMID: 36051208; PMCID: PMC9424853.
20. Thangavel G, Memedi M, Hedström K. Customized information and communication technology for reducing social isolation and loneliness among older adults: Scoping review. *JMIR Ment Health.* 2022 Mar 7;9(3):e34221. doi: 10.2196/34221. PMID: 35254273; PMCID: PMC8938833.
21. Lage CA, Wolmarans W, Mograbi DC. An evolutionary view of self-awareness. *Behav Processes.* 2022 Jan;194:104543.
22. Mograbi DC, Hall S, Arantes B, Huntley J. The cognitive neuroscience of self-awareness: current framework, clinical implications, and future research directions. *WIREs Cognitive Science.* 2024;15(2), e1670.
23. Gaines AN, Constantino MJ, Coyne AE, Farber BA, Hart NJ, Kmetz HM, Westra HA, Antony MM. Do patients internalize the positive regard they are offered? A dyadic test of a Rogerian condition. *Psychother Res.* 2024 May 8:1–11. Epub ahead of print. PMID: 38718140.

# SUGGESTED READINGS

Bobinet K. *Unstoppable Brain: The New Neuroscience That Frees Us From Failure, Eases Our Stress, and Creates Lasting Change.* Charleston, SC: Forbes Books; 2024.

Frankl VE. *Man's Search for Ultimate Meaning.* New York, NY: Basic Books; 2000.

Heatherton TF, Baumeister RF. Binge eating as an escape from self-awareness. *Psychol Bull.* 1991;110(1):86–108.

Kushner, HS. *When Bad Things Happen to Good People.* New York: NY: Knopf Doubleday Publishing Group; 2004.

Malik K. Collaboration between self and Self. *Bridges: International Society for the Study of Subtle Energy and Energy Medicine.* 2002;13.

Masterson JF. *The Search for the Real Self: Unmasking the Personality Disorders of Our Age.* New York, NY: The Free Press; 1988.

Peck, SM. *The Road Less Traveled.* New York, NY: Simon & Schuster; 2003.

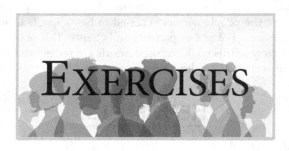

# EXERCISES

## REFLECTIVE RUMINATIONS: JOURNAL ACTIVITY

At the conclusion of the chapter exercises, begin a journal about yourself during this time. Journal entries are most useful in learning about yourself if they relate to what you learned from the experience. Most of us confuse the concept of a journal with a diary. A diary is designed to record noteworthy events in one's life. A journal is a letter to yourself that is designed to stimulate *reflection* about an experience, rather than just record the experience.

One way to keep from simply recording the event is to begin each entry with the following phrases:

- What I felt during the exercise.
- What I learned about myself.
- So what? Significance or meanings of my learning.

Your journal should be kept in a book or notebook with a cover and pages that do not easily become dislodged, or you may wish to keep a reflective, electronic journal utilizing document files for each chapter's exercises. Ideally, entries are to be written following each chapter. Many find it useful to journal as a way of privately discussing the chapter and its personal significance as well. Your journal is what *you* make it. Most university students are unaccustomed to this sort of activity, and some abhor writing. Make a commitment to this activity; it is the beginning of becoming a reflective health care professional, a strong characteristic of expertise, which we will discuss more in Chapter 10. Use the Feeling Wheel (Figure 1.3) to assist you in your reflective writings to get connected and be in touch with your affective domain, your true sense of self.

Remember, this reflective journal is by you for your personal use. Set aside the time on your calendar, and, once you get into it, the journal will become rewarding. This is the beginning of your professional formation journey to your preferred future professional self. Your course instructor may wish to glance at and see your entries now and again to be sure that you are keeping up. In that case, confidentiality may become more limited. You will not be graded on your journal. Because it is a collection of your feelings and reflections, a grade would be wholly inappropriate. However, the value of the activity is such that your instructor may wish to quickly view it to check your discipline with the activity. Actively reflect on your experiences attained through the chapter learning and exercises, rather than simply describing what happened.

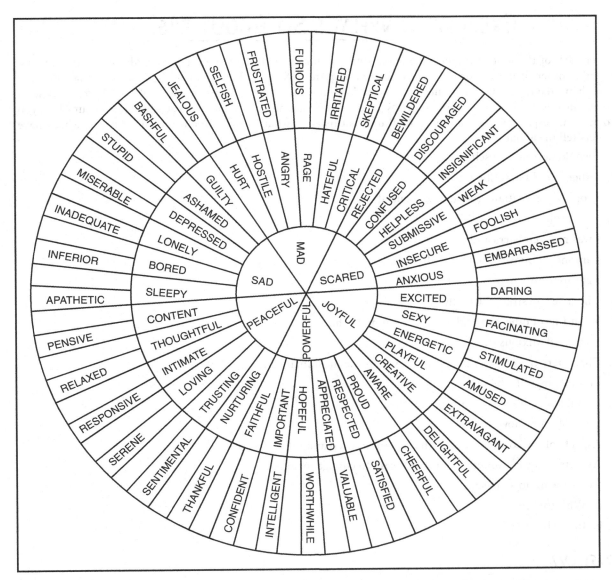

**Figure 1.3** The Feeling Wheel. (Reprinted with permission from Willcox G. The Feeling Wheel: a tool for expanding awareness of emotions and increasing spontaneity and intimacy. *Transactional Analysis Journal.* 1982;12[4]:274–276.)

# EXERCISE 1: WHAT'S SO ABOUT ME?

Answer each of the following queries as honestly as you can for this moment and record your responses in a confidential manner (just for your use). Each question requires reflection, but jot down the first thing that comes to mind and then take time with each question to clearly communicate your awareness (or lack of it!). You may wish to complete the question set over a period of a week or so, taking one or two questions at a time. Ask yourself as you reflect over your responses, "Is that my ego talking? Is this truly what I believe about myself, or is this what I have heard others tell me about me?"

1. I would describe myself as…

2. Others would describe me as…

3. People are essentially (good, bad, neutral) …

4. I am proudest of…

5. I was most embarrassed when I…

6. I am most annoyed about myself when I…

7. I get angriest when…

8. Under severe stress, I usually…

9. What I want others to understand about me is that…

10. I am most anxious that…

11. Characteristics of other people that impress me most include…

12. I protect myself when…

13. I would be willing to die in six months if…

14. I do not know how to say…

15. Aspects of my communication that I want to keep and refine are…

16. Aspects of my communication that I want to change include…

17. Goals I want to achieve…

    a. With this course…

    b. In my lifetime…

## Discussion

Once you have answered these questions, write a description about yourself from what you have discovered. Are you totally happy with yourself at this point? What would you change? What did you learn about yourself that will assist you in being a health care professional? What may detract from your effectiveness? How aware are you of the messages from your ego, of your shadow? How aware are you of your self? Identify responses that have a negative aspect to them. What is the belief that you hold that makes that answer true for you? What is an alternative belief that you also hold that would replace the negative one so that your response might be more positive and hopeful?

**Example:** I protect myself when I am criticized for being too unscientific, naïve, or idealistic. Negative belief: I lack the intellect to scientifically prove what I believe is true and important. Replacement belief: The scientific method holds one way of verifying what is true. The balance of logic and facts with intuitive knowing, together, frames a larger truth. I have proven skills as a scientist, and I have faith in my intuition. Both serve me well in my work.

# EXERCISE 2: CLINIC WAITING ROOM EXERCISE

This exercise is designed to help you recognize nonverbal indicators of emotion and, thus, keys to inner values that are often subtle and overlooked but, when recognized, can be of valuable importance in communication. It also reinforces what Tolle[7] said about recognizing that we are more than our emotions, and our emotions reflect our thoughts, which often are not accurate or appropriate to a situation but are false beliefs, things that we tell ourselves over time that we never question but should, because the source of much unhappiness is often erroneous beliefs and emotions that simply feel bad and are not even true.

The instructor writes one word describing an emotion on a 3×5 file card—words such as impatient, lonely, sad, eager, peaceful, relaxed, satisfied (see the Feeling Wheel [Figure 1.3] for suggestions). There is one card for each member of the class, and it is kept secret, known only to the holder of the card. A minimum of three chairs are placed side by side in the front of the classroom to represent the waiting room in a clinic. The exercise starts by having one person come forward spontaneously, and their task is to act out the word on their card. Then another person comes forward and joins the first person, acting out their word. You can use verbal expressions, but you cannot use the word on your card. The goal of the rest of the class is to guess what emotion or behavior each person is representing (refer to Figure 1.3). When you have correctly "guessed" a person's emotion being portrayed, replace that person in the waiting room. So that another person comes forward, spontaneously, and the other person gets up and leaves, so there are always two people interacting in the "clinic" (20 persons or fewer work best per waiting room).

Once everyone has had a chance to act out their word, the entire class forms a circle for discussion. Discussion should be focused on the nuances that each person used to convey an exact meaning (e.g., depressed in contrast to sad) of the emotion. Finally, discussion should center on how this would be helpful to students in interaction with their patients and, even more importantly perhaps, for self-awareness. How does each student convey feelings of joy? Anger? Impatience? Fear? What about being a health care professional is joyful, frustrating, and fearful, and how would that look in your behavior? How will you know this?

# EXERCISE 3: COLLAGE

With the use of any material, construct a collage that represents you as you know yourself at this moment. Your collage may comprise pictures and colors as in a traditional collage, or you may wish to use other materials such as digital images or 3D objects to construct a less traditional montage. Do not choose representations of your persona only. Search your heart for symbols of your true self, the part of you that you hold dear but that you do not readily reveal. Also, choose representatives of your ego and your shadow as well. You may want to use video or digital pictures to represent yourself. If you do decide to do that, be comprehensive. For example, the exercise would not be complete if you simply streamed one song and played it and declared, "This is who I am," without going into more detail.

Bring your creation to class wrapped or covered so that others cannot identify it. Gather in small groups or learning teams. Place one creation in the center of the group and observe it carefully without speaking for 2 or 3 minutes. Gather a private impression of what the creator was trying to convey. Then, in turn, offer observations that you perceive about the person for 5 minutes or so. After this anonymous discussion, identify the creator. Then the creator of that collage will respond to what was observed by classmates, what was on target, and where classmates missed the mark. Finally, group members should share what each learned about this classmate before bringing forth the next collage.

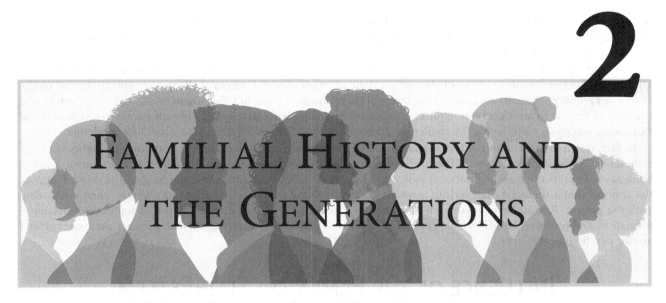

# 2

# FAMILIAL HISTORY AND THE GENERATIONS

*Gina Maria Musolino and Carol M. Davis*

## OBJECTIVES

*The learner should be able to:*

- Describe, in general, the role families play in the formation of identity and self-esteem.
- Examine the development of a mature personality as described by Erikson.
- Explain the concept of the false self in relation to the true self as it develops in dysfunctional families.
- Recognize the dangers inherent in being raised by overly attentive parents and those who, because of addictions to drugs, alcohol, or work, cannot truly parent.
- Differentiate the concept of the generations in relation to families and the work system.
- Value the importance of self-awareness for authenticity or the awareness of the true self as opposed to the false self.
- Seek authenticity for effective, mature helping.

It has been said that a clinician's most valuable tool is the effective use of self. Let's reflect on the effective use of self by taking a moment to consider these quotes:

> *You can often change your circumstances, by changing your attitude.* —Eleanor Roosevelt

> *Life is what you make it. Always has been, always will be.* —Grandma Moses

How do these quotes speak to you? Why do you think they are relevant for health care professionals (HCPs) in contemporary practice?

Our personalities and our styles of relating have everything to do with how effective we are in facilitating the healing process. No one wants to be treated unkindly, least of all when we are not feeling well. Yet, unkindness abounds in health care settings. If we were to ask HCPs to assess their abilities to relate effectively with people, few would admit to the inability to establish good rapport and eye contact with patients, lapses in temper, prejudicial behavior, irritability,

DOI: 10.4324/9781003525554-2

or cutting sarcasm. Yet, unfortunately, negative behaviors occur with great frequency. More difficult to observe are HCPs' negative behaviors of dishonesty, breaking confidences, lack of fidelity with colleagues, and causing patients to become overly dependent on oneself.

You might ask, "Why be a health care professional if you cannot act in ways that are positive and assist healing?" Often, clinicians are unaware of their behaviors or their effect on others. Patients challenge our sensitivity and maturity in unique ways. Patients react out of the stress of their illness or pain, but HCPs also must work under stress and the stresses unique to health care. It requires great maturity and patience to respond in healing ways in less-than-ideal situations, especially considering the challenges and burdens on HCPs due to the global Covid-19 pandemic.

In fact, researchers[1] discovered that worse outcomes in physical therapy were linked to therapists' higher neuroticism scores on the Big Five Index (BFI) score.[2] A lower neuroticism score (emotional stability, impulse control, and the tendency to express unpleasant emotions) indicates being more "calm, relaxed, secure, and hardy." The studies support the concept that a therapist's not feeling mentally stable may have consequences for their attitude when interacting with the patient. Researchers support self-awareness and reflection training during the initial stages of professional formation; and recommend additional exploration of the interplay of personality traits with patients' personality traits and/or psychological factors.[1,3]

# INFLUENCE OF THE FAMILY ON SELF-ESTEEM

Before reading any further, turn to Table 2.1, "Characteristics of Families," and skim through each column. Which column best describes your perception of the family dynamics you grew up with? Place a checkmark beside the phrase in column 1, 2, or 3 that best describes your family for each item listed.

Each of us views the world from a unique perspective. I like to use the analogy of a pair of lenses to illustrate one's world view. You and I can be looking at the exact same thing, but what I see, hear, feel, and experience will be different from what you experience because my lenses are set differently from yours. We receive our lenses as small children. One's world view evolves out of what one hears and experiences as a child growing up in a unique family unit. We develop in the ways that our parents would have us develop because we are, to them, an image on their lenses. Even twins, growing up under the same circumstances, will develop differences in their lenses based on what each chooses to attend to, ponder, and emphasize.

Children are not little adults, as Piaget first clearly described.[4] Children have underdeveloped nervous systems and lack the capacity to move, think, and act in the ways that adults can. Children live in a land of make-believe, enjoy fantasy, and are egocentric. They are unable to manage abstract logic and are present oriented and concrete. If you ask a child which of two parallel, identical pencils is longer, they will say, correctly, that both are the same length. But then, if you slide one pencil so that it is ahead of the other, although still parallel, and then ask, "Which pencil is longer?" they will say the pencil that is ahead of the other is longer. In other words, children cannot conserve information. Likewise, children are unable to come outside of themselves and view themselves, as we discussed in Chapter 1. Ask a child who has a brother if he has a brother, and he will say, "Yes." If you ask him if his brother has a brother, he will say, "No."[5] Finally, children idolize their parents. Feelings of helplessness and dependence are coped with by believing that Mommy and Daddy are perfect, and no harm can come to me as long as they are with me in life.

Erikson[6] developed a useful description of the development of personality that centers on the successful resolution of tension, in a series of dialectical steps, encountered by the growing person from birth onward. A certain degree of accomplishment is required with each stage as it is encountered, or the child will have to master the goal later. This is similar to the child who skips crawling, wherein critical movements necessary for an accomplished gait remain absent. There is a certain level of suffering or pathology that results even if one seems to function adequately. Table 2.2 summarizes Erikson's theory of development.[6] We will return to this theory when we discuss the development of effective helping behaviors.

Human beings are among the few living creatures born without the capacity to crawl, wiggle, or walk to a source of food. It might be said that for 9 months in the womb and 9 (or more) months out, we are totally helpless to move about to a source of food or nourishment. We lie there like blobs and must wail and cajole to get the attention of the big people around us to get our basic survival needs met. The fact that we are born totally dependent on others for our survival is a critical aspect of the development of our world view because who we are and how the world is for us depends totally on how we are responded to, in our profound neediness, and on what we hear others say to us and about us. As a child, I have no identity save what others say about me. It is obvious that the maturity of the parent and the extent to which the child is wanted and anticipated have a great deal to do with how the parent responds to the child and thus fosters or inhibits the development of a sense of self-identity and self-esteem.

| | TABLE 2.1 | |
|---|---|---|
| **CHARACTERISTICS OF FAMILIES** | | |
| **OPEN/HEALTHY** | **TROUBLED** | **CLOSED/UNHEALTHY** |
| ○ Open to change<br>○ Flexible responses to each situation | ○ Nothing can be done<br>○ What's the use? | ○ Rigid, fixed, harsh rules<br>○ Right vs. wrong, no exceptions |
| ○ High self-worth<br>○ People are valued as individuals | ○ Shaky self-worth<br>○ Covers feelings of low self-control | ○ Evasive responses<br>○ Low self-worth, lots of shaming behavior<br>○ Low ownership—blaming |
| ○ Functional defenses<br>○ Uses defenses as coping skill with insight | ○ Uses defenses to hide pain<br>○ Defenses more often deny real feelings<br>○ Choice is lost<br>○ Always smile or cry or complain | ○ No choice—reacts compulsively and rigidly out of fear<br>○ Short fuse<br>○ Lots of avoidance or rage |
| ○ Clear rules discussed<br>○ Hours, respect for property, telephone use, chores, etc., regularly negotiated | ○ Unclear—rules inconsistent<br>○ Depends on who is asked, what day, which child, etc. | ○ Edicts or no rules at all<br>○ Chaos—rules cannot be followed |
| ○ People take risks to express feelings, ideas, beliefs | ○ Not safe to express feelings or give opinions—"Don't rock the boat"<br>○ Can't disagree | ○ Denial of problems<br>○ Ignores bizarre behaviors<br>○ No-talk rule, even about serious problems, especially drinking, drugs |
| ○ Can deal with stress, notice others' pain<br>○ Nurturing and caring for each other<br>○ Seek out those in pain to support, encourage | ○ Avoid pain<br>○ Do not see it in others<br>○ Sweep problems under the rug<br>○ Pretend all is okay | ○ Denial of stress<br>○ Can't cope with anymore—glazed eyes don't see pain<br>○ Ignore basic need to be seen, acknowledged<br>○ Children become early helpers |
| ○ Accepts life stages, welcomes them<br>○ Celebrate growth—sexuality, new friends, accomplishments | ○ Parents may compete with kids<br>○ Growth is accepted painfully—don't talk about sex, try to keep children dependent | ○ Adults treated as children<br>○ Children may try to act like adults<br>○ Children ridiculed, teased but try to become helpful |
| ○ Either clear hierarchy or egalitarian<br>○ Strong parental coalition<br>○ Less need to control<br>○ Can negotiate | ○ Hidden coalitions across generations<br>○ Parental coalition weak<br>○ Rigid or shifting pattern of domination | ○ Either upside-down family—children may run it, or chaotic, no giving out of rules—or one parent in charge of all and can't cope |
| ○ Affect is open<br>○ Direct expression of feelings<br>○ All feelings are okay<br>○ Anger is in context of awareness of another person<br>○ Considerate of others | ○ Negativism, low feeling, bickering, argumentative controlled mood, some feelings okay, some not, inconsistent acceptance of feelings | ○ Cynicism, open hostility, violence, sadism—actually try to manipulate and hurt each other<br>○ Only happiness is allowed |

| TABLE 2.2 |
|---|
| ## PSYCHOSOCIAL THEORY OF DEVELOPMENT: A SUMMARY OF ERIKSON'S EPIGENETIC STAGES OF DEVELOPMENT |

**TRUST VERSUS MISTRUST (0 TO 12 MONTHS)**

From birth to approximately 1 year, this stage is the basis for all future development of personality. A feeling of physical comfort accompanied by minimal fear and uncertainty results in a sense of trust for the infant. The quality of the relationship with mother or maternal figure is more important than quantity of food or love demonstrations. Experiences with one's body are the first and primary means of social interactions for the baby; thus, they provide the foundations for psychological trust. The issues involved in trust and mistrust are not settled for all time during this phase of life; they may arise repeatedly during development and later life. Later confrontation with trust may shake one's basic trust or provide another opportunity for further development if these needs were not met adequately the first time.

**AUTONOMY VERSUS SHAME AND DOUBT (2 TO 4 YEARS)**

As the child of 2 to 4 experiences the world around him, he begins to discover that his behavior can bring about certain results. Out of these encounters with reality grows a sense of autonomy. At the same time, the child has some conflicts about asserting or remaining dependent and in which situations. Exploring is a primary goal of this growing and increasingly coordinated physical being. It becomes increasingly difficult to remain in a confined place. The child is occupied with activities involving retaining and releasing—manipulating objects, expressing himself, making new friends and letting them go, and bodily functions. The degree to which the child will allow others to regulate his behavior is regularly tested, leading to a greater sense of self-understanding and responsibility or, in the case of being overly controlled, leading to shame and doubt.

**INITIATIVE VERSUS GUILT (4 TO 5 YEARS)**

During the fourth and fifth years, language development and locomotion have reached a sufficiently high level to permit expansion of imagination. Play activities are more interesting and companionship with peers is sought. There is curiosity and comparison with others around size and skill issues, who is the better tree climber, who is biggest or best at—almost anything. The child in this stage is into everything and seeks attention verbally and physically. Sexual curiosity and genital stimulation are apparent. Adult treatment of the curiosity will reinforce the initiative or result in shame and guilt. Because of a highly active imagination, the child may feel guilty for the mere thoughts and for activities that no one has observed. The evolving conscience is becoming established and will ultimately control initiative. If the child's activities are perceived as a nuisance, whether motor or verbal, hemay develop feelings of guilt over self-initiated activities that may last a lifetime. Healthy identification with parents, teachers, and peers help resolve some of the guilt problems.

**INDUSTRY VERSUS INFERIORITY (6 TO 11 YEARS)**

Between the ages of 6 and 11, the child moves seriously into the world of competition and the separation of work and play. Individuals who impact on the developing sense of self now include many other adults and a wider sphere of peers. As the lessons of work are learned, the child often needs to slip into the familial play world to bolster what may feel like flagging initiative. The developing industry evolves from efforts and achievement rewarded by significant others and leads to a sense of social worth. When the child learns that social worth is linked to background of parents, color of skin, or the label on his clothes, identity with those conditions rather than self may result. These first four stages form the base upon which the adolescent builds a sense of identity.

**IDENTITY VERSUS IDENTITY DIFFUSION (12 TO 18 YEARS)**

During this stage of changes, the consistent task is striving to be oneself and to share oneself with something else. The beginning of separation from parents finally becomes a serious agenda. The adolescent experiences the need to be master of his own affairs and to be free of dependency. The emerging young adult is eager to know his abilities and to have the adult world recognize them as well. The adolescent also fears that the demands of adulthood will exceed the capacities to meet them. Time

*(continued)*

| TABLE 2.2 (CONTINUED) |
|---|
| ## PSYCHOSOCIAL THEORY OF DEVELOPMENT: A SUMMARY OF ERIKSON'S EPIGENETIC STAGES OF DEVELOPMENT |
| perspective versus time diffusion becomes the dilemma. When the adult world offers the adolescent responsibilities and privileges at an appropriate pace, commensurate with capacity and desires, there is resolution of some of the issues with a sense of time perspective, as opposed to urgency and hopelessness. The derivatives of the second stage of "autonomy versus shame and doubt" are reworked in the adolescent in the form of establishing a sense of self-certainty. When adult(s) can offer reinforcement appropriately to build the adolescent's self-esteem, feelings of inferiority diminish. The remains of "initiative versus guilt" reappear with the need to discover individualized and unique talents and interests. There seems to be a need to experiment with different roles and express initiative in different ways. If stymied in this dimension, it may seem easier to resolve the conflict by seeking behavior or roles in conflict with parents or the community, thus achieving a negative identity, which is preferable to an "identity diffusion," which is experienced as being nobody at all. Most authorities agree that the period of adolescence brings with it an increase in psychic energy. The young person who uses these energies effectively can experiment in many ways and have experiences of achievement. If much of the energy is used to resolve feelings resulting from earlier unresolved crises, which often reappear at this time, the rather fragile sense of self may be seriously threatened, with introspection interfering with concentration. The successful resolution of adolescent tasks and the development of a strong sense of identity may require many years beyond age 18. During this time, the young adult experiments with new behavior and may ignore some societal mores in the process. It is important for this process to work itself through, especially with talented and creative persons. Negative labeling may reinforce a temporary identity, which, given time, will work itself into something else. |
| **INTIMACY VERSUS ISOLATION** |
| The first phase of adulthood comes into being after the adolescent has worked out a sense of identity. Dealing with sexual and psychological intimacies between two people while retaining one's own identity is the primary task of this stage. This goal is sought through forms of friendship, leadership, and athletics—even combat. Unwillingness or inability to achieve intimacy will result in distancing oneself from others who pose a threat to identity. Achievement is characterized by the ability and willingness to share with another in mutual trust, to regulate cycles of work, and to participate in society in self-satisfying ways. This stage continues through early middle age. |
| **GENERATIVITY VERSUS STAGNATION** |
| The basic agenda of the middle years is aimed at guiding the next generation, whether in parenting or through employment and enjoyment situations. The critical question of this time occurs when the individual looks back to examine what has happened up to that time in life and whether it was good. If the individual turns inward and becomes self-absorbed, stagnation results. |
| **INTEGRITY VERSUS DESPAIR** |
| The primary task of the later years is the acceptance of one's self and one's life. When the individual has experienced the feelings that accompany a share of the good things of life without being overwhelmed by its tragedies, disappointments, and frustrations, ego integrity is the result. There is acceptance of one's existence with full responsibility and commitment to a certain way of life and its values. Having experienced what is felt to be a full life, the individual can accept giving it up with "integrity." If, on the other hand, the person feels that there has been little good from life and there are few prospects of any coming, there is a sense of despair often accompanied by fear of death. |
| Reprinted with permission from Ramsden E. Affective dimensions in patient case. In: Payton O, ed. *Psychosocial Aspects of Clinical Practice*. New York, NY: Churchill Livingstone; 1986. |

Few of us grew up in ideal homes or environments. Perhaps you think you are the exception. The fact is that we experience denial, and many of us have difficulty remembering the negative things about our childhoods. Remember that little children all think that their parents are perfect. Adolescents give up those notions but replace them with strongly held mores to honor parents and respect them. If parents were emotionally or physically abusive to a child, the child will automatically believe that it was their fault because they must have been bad. Part of maturation is to give up our idealized views of our parents. No parents are perfect. Ironically, however, the more abandoned the child was, the more they cling to the fantasy of how perfect their parents were. To idealize your parents is to idealize the way they raised you.[2] It is important to look back at what was happening in your family when you were growing up as one mechanism to increase your awareness of your self and your world view. What do you remember about the circumstances of your birth? Were you a wanted child? How did your birth order influence things? Did you have others who served in the roles of parents?

Each child is born into a unique and complex family situation and encounters various challenges, as described by Erikson,[6] as they develop day by day. If I, as a newborn, experience feelings of physical comfort, emotional calm, and joy at my presence and if my needs are addressed with love and compassion, I will develop a sense of trust and the view that the world is essentially a warm and loving place. If, for example, something happens to my mother and I become a burden to others left to care for me, and people are mourning the loss of my mother and harbor resentment toward me for causing her loss, I will experience a distinct set of feelings and may believe that the world is uncertain and chaotic in nature. If I am born to a 15-year-old girl who still needs love and attention from her parents and who has little love to give and should be giving it to herself, the situation becomes cruelly different. Highly likely, she cannot stand to hear me cry and may physically harm me when I do. If that is the case, I will experience the world as a hostile place, and I will mistrust from the very first days of my life. This scenario is the genesis of violent adolescents who are out of control, which is so prevalent in our contemporary society.

And so, we develop inwardly; we set our emotional lenses in response to the way our maturing nervous systems take in the information around us. At about age 2, we are confronted with the need to be toilet trained. This is reflected in Erikson's[6] second stage, Autonomy Versus Shame and Doubt (see Table 2.2). Some children are placed on the potty at 6 months, before total head control occurs, let alone complete myelination of the nerves. As the description in Table 2.2 suggests, critical learning at this stage is the child's appropriate and balanced willingness to allow others to regulate and control their behavior. Autonomy results in the feeling of success, free from shame and guilt. Shame and guilt result when the child is unable to succeed and consequently allow the adult to be overly controlling of their behavior. Only shame, or the feeling that "I am bad," can result when a child is placed on a potty and told to urinate when they do not even know what that means or how it feels to control that function because they cannot yet feel sensation in those nerves. However, when the child is fully ready for this learning, a marvelous feeling of success and pride results with being able to "make bubbles" in the water on command.

It is unrealistic to believe that each stage of development might be totally, successfully conquered. Children will have successful resolution at times and will suffer unsuccessful resolution at times. The point to stress here is that the balance toward more successful resolution, rather than unsuccessful resolution, has a great deal to do with parents and other adults who do not set children up to fail. Parents who do not parent well were, themselves, not parented well. Dysfunctional parents learned to be dysfunctional from the families in which they were raised.

Current self-awareness is assisted by an attempt to remember (and to ask for the help of others who watched one grow through) critical stages in development over the years. How we respond to the world today is greatly influenced by our sense of ourselves and the adequacy of our self-esteem. The development of a healthy self-esteem requires more successful than unsuccessful resolution of the tensions described by Erikson,[6] either as we mature or later. As adults, we can examine our growing up experiences, gain insight into our dysfunctional views, and consciously change our distorted world views or correct our lenses to give us a more true and accurate focus of the world and of ourselves. However, we usually enter into this examination only because we are experiencing emotional pain or are bored with our lives.

# HEALTHY OR OPEN FAMILIES

Healthy families interact in ways that have been described as open in contrast to the rigid or closed functioning of troubled or dysfunctional families (see Table 2.1). A family functions to provide a safe and supportive environment for all of its members, to help them learn basic values, grow, and become more fully human. In healthy families, members feel empowered to adapt to change and feel supported in coping with the stresses of the world, outside the home and within. The stress inside the home is usually perceived to be less than the stress faced outside in the world, except in transient phases of family crisis. Individuals are recognized as being unique and having worth. There is value to the family unit, and there is open communication in which members feel free to speak their opinions but do so with concern and caring for others. In sum, family members feel safe, supported, encouraged, and appreciated. Roles and responsibilities of members are flexible but clear. People function well day to day and in crisis. Finally, quality time is shared by parents and children and is enjoyed.[7]

# DYSFUNCTIONAL OR CLOSED FAMILIES

Whitfield[8] believed that many people grow up in families that stifle the development of the true self and, instead, cultivate in the child a false or codependent self. Children need to feel as if they are safe and always protected. They need to feel free to ask questions, to run and play, and to know that the boundaries that parents set for them are fair and consistent. Children need to feel as if they can be children, learning and growing without fear of being ridiculed or punished cruelly for making mistakes. Children need to be invited to feel their feelings and put words on them so they can learn gently how not to be impulsive and controlled by their feelings.

However, dysfunctional families respond to the neediness and dependence of children in ways that interfere with the development of authenticity. In the dysfunctional family of the twentieth century, and perhaps some even now, children were to be seen and not heard. They did not feel free to make mistakes but felt that if they were not right, they would be called stupid. "Children are virtuous when they are meek, agreeable, considerate, and unselfish."[8] Adults assumed the role of authoritarian masters intent on breaking the child's will at any cost, or they tended to be absent totally from parenting, escaping in alcohol, work, mental illness, or travel. Children, who want to think of their parents as perfect, soon began to realize that they were not free to act naturally or to be children and so adopted another way of being, usually that of comforting and nurturing the parent. The child thus became a parent to the parent. As a result, a false self emerged in the child. According to Miller,[9] the persistent denial of the true self and true feelings takes its toll in the development of the coping mechanisms of depression or feelings of grandeur, neither of which is facilitative to a realistic view of the world or to healing. Such was the more common parenting pattern for current, mid-career, and later career or what is considered by many as their "prime-time" professionals' parents and grandparents: the Traditionalists (born 1925 to 1945), the Baby Boomers (born 1946 to 1964), and the Generation Xers (born 1965 to 1981).[10] Many early career professionals (Millennials) have grown up with what is referred to as helicopter parenting.

# MILLENNIAL GENERATION

With the advent of the technology age and the ubiquitous presence of cell phones and instant communication, even at a distance, Millennial children (born between 1982 and 2000) were parented in ways that are 180 degrees opposite from the authoritarian ways of previous generations. Their parents are often referred to as *helicopter parents*, due to their hovering. Millennial children were encouraged to be unique and were often rewarded and celebrated for any and all accomplishments, no matter the level of achievement. As often happens, parents are loathe to inflict what they perceived as poor parenting on their children and, as often happens, difficulties in establishing healthy parent–child relationships continue to occur but with a different twist.

According to Mueller:[11]

> *The renewed enthusiasm and concern for the welfare of the nation's children that began in the late 1980s was a dramatic contrast to the prevalent "antichild" attitudes of the previous 2 decades. Millennial children were treated as precious commodities, protected at every turn. Beginning with their births, ubiquitous "Baby on Board" stickers adorned their parents' cars, loudly and proudly exhorting other drivers to be mindful of the priceless human cargo within. … the millennials' parents became known as the "helicopters," hovering, continually at the ready to answer every question at the speed dial ring of a cell phone.*

As a result, instant access to parental advice and guidance helps to enable children's dependency and unwillingness to stand on their own under difficult circumstances, which can, in turn, delay a young person's readiness to assume responsibility as an adult health care professional responsible for the well-being of patients entrusted to their care.[12] Described herein are the extremes of older and newer patterns of parenting, but both can be envisioned to present difficulty in assisting with the maturation of children and adolescents to the point where they feel confident and self-reliant when it comes to assuming responsibility for those trusting in them for their care.

# HEALTH CARE PROFESSIONALS' SELF-ESTEEM

It has been said that many people enter the health professions for a variety of poor, although unconscious, reasons. On the surface, most applicants to health care professions admit that they have a great desire to help people. Among more subconscious or unconscious reasons might be a need to be depended upon, a need to control people, and a need to get one's natural attention and affection needs met. Some may be looking for emotional healing themselves by way of making life easier for others. Few people are conscious of these motives, however. Nonetheless, they act in ways that are responsive to their unconscious needs and do things that are harmful overall to patients and are contrary to the healing process, as is characteristic of early helpers. In addition, young Millennial adults admit to a dearth of practice in establishing one-on-one communications with strangers, let alone family members, and feel somewhat inept at personal interactions.

The bottom line is this: dysfunctional families breed early helpers and dysfunctional interactions. One example of a dysfunctional family is a family in which one or both parents are addicted to alcohol. It is estimated that "76 million Americans, about 43% of the US population, have been exposed to alcoholism in the family. Almost 1 in 5 adult Americans (18%) lived with an alcoholic while growing up."[13] The literature that has developed from the Adult Children of Alcoholics movement in the United States has shed needed light on the distorted world view of the adult who grew up in a home where one or both parents were not able or willing to parent. This circumstance encourages the development of the false self, stifles the successful resolution of the tensions described by Erikson,[6] and contributes to chronic low self-esteem and feelings of being, if not unbelievably bad, then never good enough. All children experience shame, but children in dysfunctional families take on shame as part of their identity. Children in dysfunctional families are never free to be children; they have to be grown up and helpful. It seems as if, because this is a perplexing task indeed, they are always doing something wrong. Shame is different from guilt. Whitfield[8] described shame as "the uncomfortable or painful feeling that we experience when we realize that part of us is defective, bad, incomplete, rotten, phony, inadequate, or a failure." Thus, guilt says, "I made a mistake" and shame says, "I am a mistake."

Self-esteem can be viewed as the extent to which we are able and willing to own our essential goodness (our true self) in the face of our own incompleteness or lack of perfection. More than simply self-acceptance, self-esteem includes pride in the promise of ongoing growth and change with maturity and the hope of a richer and more peaceful and congruent life as a result of honest, day-to-day struggle. Children reared in dysfunctional families feel the shame of never being quite good enough rather than confidence and pride in doing the best they can. Because they were ridiculed and punished just for being, they grow up repressing hurtful feelings, thus believing that they had a marvelous family life as a child. But underneath the repressed feelings lie severe self-esteem problems that must be admitted and talked about for one to identify the lenses. Feelings of shame must be identified, confronted, and replaced with a more humane, realistic acceptance of one's own imperfections and essential goodness.

Parental dysfunction may or may not be due to alcohol or drug dependence. The critical factor seems to be how well the parent was genuinely present for the growing child in such a way as to encourage the natural curiosity of the child and the natural desire to learn and grow and explore the world; how well the parent nurtured and protected the child; and how safe and free from potential harm the child felt.[8] When the parent absents themselves from those responsibilities, for whatever reason (drug dependence, workaholism, depression or mental illness, absence of a good model for parenting, too much concern with activities outside the home), the child starts parenting the parent, and an early helper emerges. A common description given by children from dysfunctional families is that they feel that they were a burden and that they were being bad when they simply showed natural curiosity or asked questions. In fact, it was their very existence that seemed to bring unending pain and suffering to their family.

Children are not meant to be parents. When they take on this role, they take on a false self, and authentic feelings of curiosity, fear, and need become repressed, covered by feigned feelings of bravery and affection in an attempt to please the needy parent. Common characteristics that materialize from the distorted world view and false view of the self that then emerge include the following:[14]

- Fear of losing control
- Fear of feelings that seem overwhelming
- Fear of conflict
- Fear of abandonment
- Fear of becoming alcohol or drug dependent
- Fear of becoming dependent on another person for survival
- Overdeveloped sense of responsibility
- Feelings of guilt and grief
- Inability to relax and have fun spontaneously
- Harsh self-criticism

- A tendency to lie, even when it is not necessary
- A tendency to let one's mind wander, lose track of a conversation, and figuratively leave the room
- Denial and/or the tendency to create reality the way you want it to be, rather than the way it is
- Difficulties with intimacy and getting close to people
- Feelings of vulnerability, of being a victim in a harsh world
- Compulsive behavior, tendency to become addicted to things that alter mood
- Comfort with taking charge in a crisis; panic if you cannot do something in a crisis
- Confusion between love and pity
- All good or all bad perspectives (nothing in-between)
- Internalizing (taking responsibility for others' problems)
- Tendency to react rather than act
- Experiencing stress-related illnesses
- Overachievement

Despite this, "we have a marvelous ability to survive and cope."[14] Children from dysfunctional families are often the heroes in health care, the ones who, at great personal sacrifice, go beyond the call to fix things for everyone else and are praised and admired for their Herculean efforts. They thrive on rescuing others and creating order out of chaos. Often, these are the people whom others admonish to lighten up because they take every aspect of their lives seriously.

As Miller pointed out, having a world view that necessitates the coping behaviors (noted previously)—the behaviors of a false self, not the true self—inevitably leads to depression and often to the desired comfort of addiction as well.[9] Addictive behavior is repeated, and habitual behavior that is designed to bring comfort and take attention away from experiencing what appears to be the negative, intense feelings of the true self attempt to break through in a given situation. For all the comfort that the addiction brings, the dependence it brings on chemicals (often depressants), on experienced highs, or on a kind of numbness simply reinforces a denial and continues to reinforce the false self, making the authentic or true self even more difficult to locate. Whenever the true self is blocked, our life energy, authenticity, and capacity to truly respond to the question "Who am I?" are blocked. We cannot grow and become who we were created to be. We are stuck like a mouse on an exercise wheel.

# CODEPENDENCE AND THE GENERATIONS

For many young people, addictive impulses are focused not only on substance abuse, drugs, and alcohol but on another person and/or virtual connections, a potential source of affection to help ease the pain of never feeling as if one received enough authentic recognition, affection, and unconditional love as a child. Discomfort emerges when one nervously admits that one cannot live without the other person because the dependency has become so great. Millennials often admit, with mixed feelings, that their parents were their best friends growing up and they did not want to have to live without them. Because the true self of the person has been underdeveloped or lost long ago, it is a false self that has "fallen in love" and proceeds to do its best to please the other, indeed, to live for the other, much as it did for the parents. This phenomenon of living for (being addicted to) the happiness and well-being of another person is termed *codependence*. In fact, codependency is experienced with more than just a person. It has been described as "an exaggerated dependent pattern of learned behaviors, beliefs, and feelings that make life painful. It is a dependence on people and things outside the self, along with neglect of the self to the point of having little self-identity."[8] The person demonstrating codependent behavior looks outside themselves to discover what they want, need, and believe in for identity, security, power, and belonging. They look *outside* themself to feel whole and get what is missing inside. The codependent person often says yes when they mean no.

The greeting card industry has done us a great disservice through expressions of this pathological view with sentimentalities, e.g., "Even before I knew what my needs were, you were there to help me. You alone taught me the meaning of true love." These are leftover fragments, memories of immature needs from our totally dependent infant. Adults must mature and take responsibility for knowing what their needs are and setting an appropriate course to get them met beyond destructive dependence on others. The goal of maturation is to develop autonomy, self-control, self-reliance, and interdependence on others.[15] For life to be lived in an authentic way, one's identity, power, self-worth, and individuality must be experienced as coming from *within*.

TABLE 2.3

## GENERATIONS DEFINED

| GENERATION NAME AND YEARS OF BIRTH | BUILDERS 1925–1945 | BABY BOOMERS 1946–1964 | GENERATION X 1965–1979 | GENERATION Y 1980–1994 | GENERATION Z 1995–2010 | GENERATION ALPHA 2010–2024 |
|---|---|---|---|---|---|---|
| Iconic Technology | Radio (Wireless), Motor Vehicle, Aircraft | TV (1956), Audio Cassette (1962), Transistor Radio (1955) | VCR (1976), Walkman (1979), IBM PC (1981) | Internet, Email, SMS DVD (1995), Playstation, XBox, iPod | MacBook, iPad, Google, Facebook, Twitter, Wii, PS3, Android | PS4, FaceTime, Zoom, Air Pods, Nintendo Switch, Oculus Quest, Artificial Intelligence Networks & Learning, Metaverse, Predictive Analytics, Convolutional Neural Networks, Haptic Technolologies, Telehealth, Non-Fungible Tokens (NFTs), Driverless Transportation, Aerial Ridesharing, Smart Devices, Translation Earbuds |
| Music | Jazz, Swing, Glen Miller, Frank Sinatra | Elvis, Beatles, Rolling Stones, Johnny O'Keefe | INXS, Nirvana, Madonna, Midnight Oil | Eminem, Britney Spears, Garth Brooks, Puff Daddy, Jennifer Lopez | Kanye West, Rhianna, Justin Bieber, Taylor Swift | Ariana Grande, Beyoncé, Drake, Lady Gaga, The Kid Laroi, The Weeknd, Billy Eilish, Lizzo |
| Media | *Gone With the Wind*, Clark Gable, Advent of TV | *Easy Rider, The Graduate*, Color TV | *ET, MTV, Star Trek, Brady Bunch, Sesame Street* | *Titanic, Back to the Future, Star Wars*, Oprah, Reality TV, Pay TV, Hooked on Phonics | *Avatar*, 3D Movies, Smart TV, *American Idol* | Streaming Services, YouTube, *Inception, Ted Lasso, Game of Thrones, Spiderman Series, Ryan's World, ABCMouse* |
| Popular Culture | Flair Jeans, Roller Skates, Mickey Mouse (1928) | Roller Blades, Mini Skirts, Peanuts Cartoon, Barbie®, Frisbees (1959) | Body Piercing, Hyper Color, Torn Jeans, Rubik's Cube (1974) | Baseball Caps, Men's Cosmetics, Havaianas, SimCity, All Terrain Bikes, Skateboarding | Skinny Jeans, V-necks, RipSticks, Call of Duty, Harry Potter, Drones, Folding Scooters | Athleisure, Sustainable, Baggy Clothing, Cold-shoulder tops, Baby Shark, Snapchat, Fortnite, Minecraft, Fidget Spinners |

|  | | | | | | |
|---|---|---|---|---|---|---|
| **Social Markers/ Landmark Events** | Great Depression (1930s), Communism, World War II (1939–45), Pearl Harbor (1941), Darwin Bombing (1942) | Decimal Currency (1966), Neil Armstrong (1969), Vietnam War (1965–73), Cyclone Tracy (1974) | Challenger Explodes (1986), Halley's Comet (1986), Stock Market Crash (1987), Berlin Wall (1989), Newcastle Earthquake (1989) | Thredbo Disaster (1997), Columbine Shooting (1999), New Millennium, September 11 (2001), Bali Bombing (2002) | Euro (1999) Iraq War (2003–11), Afghanistan Longest War (2001–22), Asian Tsunami (2004), Global Financial Crisis (2008), WikiLeaks, Arab Spring (2011) | Mass Shootings, Covid-19 Pandemic, Social Justice Movements, Russian Invasion—Ukraine War, 70 yr. Monarch Queen Elizabeth II Passes, Crises: Climate, Homelessness, Hunger, Culture, Immigration, Refugee, Political, Economic |
| **Influencers** | Authority Officials | Evidential Experts | Pragmatic Practitioners | Experiential Peers | User-generated Forums | Chatbots, Globally Hyperconnected, Social Issues/Activists, Kid-Powered/ Social Media Influencers, Crowd-Sourced |
| **Training Focus** | Traditional On-the-job, Top-down | Technical, Data, Evidence | Practical, Case Studies, Applications | Emotional, Stories, Participative | Multi-modal, eLearning, Interactive, Adaptive, Competency-based | Multi-modal, Multiple Perspectives, Virtual Problem-solving, Logical Abilities, Physical Interactions, Self-regulation, Goal Setting |
| **Learning Format** | Formal, Instructive | Relaxed, Structured | Spontaneous, Interactive | Multi-sensory, Visual | Student-centric, Kinesthetic, Service-oriented | Holistic, Personalized, Haptic Virtual Realities, Meta-Learning, Digitally Intertwined |
| **Learning Environment** | Military Style, Didactic & Disciplined | Classroom Style, Video-based, Quiet Atmosphere | Round-table Style, Relaxed Ambience | Cafe-Style, Music & Multi-modal | Lounge Room Style, Multi-stimulus | Flexible Smart Spaces, Mobile, Artificial Intelligence |
| **Marketing** | Print & Radio, Persuasive | Broadcast (mass) | Direct/Targeted media | Online (Linked) | Digital (Social) | In Situ (Real-time) Interactive, Voice Assist, Visual & Experiential, Individualistic & Ever-changing, Click-bait |
| **Purchase Influences** | Brand Emergence, Telling | Brand-loyal, Authorities | Brand Switches, Experts | No Brand Loyalty, Friends | Brand Evangelism, Trends | Brand Influencers, Parent & Kidfluence |
| **Financial Values** | Long-term Saving, Cash, No Credit | Long-term Needs, Cash, Credit | Medium-term Goals, Credit Savvy, Life-stage Debt | Short-term Wants, Credit Dependent, Life-style Debt | Impulse Purchases, E-Stores, Life-long Debt | Kidpreneurs, Chores for Higher Allowance, Financial Literacy Efforts, Fractional Shares, Smart Contracts, NFTs |
| **Ideal Leaders** | Authoritarian, Controlling Commanders | Directors, Thinkers | Co-ordinating, Doers | Guiding, Supportive, Interactive | Empowering Collaborators | Inspiring, Co-creators |

Adapted from McCrindle Research. ©2012, 2021 McCrindle Research, et al.16–21

Just as families are dysfunctional, the influence of the generations has an impact on the workplace and families. Today's contemporary workplace also asks us to be able to function as mature individuals with different generations of influence. In today's workforce system, up to six different generations[16–21] are in play, sometimes working side-by-side, sometimes collaborating virtually. Sociologically, the generational demographics have been trended and categorized by timelines, and some slight variations[10,16–21] exist in the timelines depending on whose classifications you are viewing, nationally and internationally.

A taxonomy of the generations defined[19,21] has been published (Table 2.3) with slightly different year spans from the categories introduced earlier in the chapter, based upon contemporary trending and historical data. The generations are defined as the following: the Traditionalists or Builders (born prior to 1946), the Baby Boomers (born 1946 to 1964), Generation X (born 1965 to 1979), Generation Y or the *Millennials* (born 1980 to 1994), Generation Z (born 1995 to 2009), and Generation Alpha (born 2010 to 2024).[19,21] Social markers and landmark events vary greatly and traverse the generations.

Regardless, from a psychosociological perspective, the vast differences between iconic technologies alone are reason to recognize the need to bridge the divide, ranging from the Traditionalists using rotary telephones and radio to the Boomers using television and audio cassettes and to the Millennials and Gen Alpha growing up with Snapchat, FaceTime, Twitter, and iPads. Most grandparents have initially learned everyday technology-use from their grandchildren, so they can communicate and stay in touch. While most generations continue to adapt to modern and innovative technologies, the Covid-19 pandemic forced technologies upon those who may not have been adopters, stretching and stressing these capacities, yet also providing a means to connect when in person, face-to-face (F2F) communication was not viable. Understanding the differences in generations assists in key communication perspectives. Some may have a challenging time imagining why others would want to communicate primarily virtually, whereas others can hardly imagine what a rotary telephone is or what to do when presented with one. For some generations, texting may be preferred over talking and virtual game friends may be relied upon to make decisions; whereas other generations would prefer to "stand on their own feet" to make decisions.[16–26]

# GENERATION Z

Generation Z, also known as Gen Z or Zoomers, succeeds the Millennials with most being children of Gen X or older Millennials. Gen Z is the first generation to have grown up with Internet access and digital technologies and therefore Gen Zers are often referred to as "digital natives," while the Millennial generation had largely finished puberty when this re-wiring with phone-based (rather than play-based) childhoods emerged. Gen Z overall has lower rates of teen pregnancies and many Gen Zers have experienced "sexting," with less consumption of alcohol and delayed gratification than former generations. Gen Z has many nostalgic-based youth subcultures and many in this generation enjoy volunteering at greater rates than those from prior generations.[21–23,26] Yet, unfortunately, Gen Z, shaped in a pandemic-era, is more vulnerable to mental health issues, including depression and anxiety (anticipation of future threats) due to the brain influences from phone-based rather than play-based childhoods. Many companies have utilized psychological trickery to engage youngsters in "click bait" to maximize their engagement ratings. These digital hooks roped youngsters into inappropriate and addictive content with visual and auditory stimulations, replacing normal development in physical play and in-person socializations. This rewiring from childhood, along with the impacts of the Covid-19 pandemic and remote learning, have resulted in a host of challenges including sleep deprivation, attention fragmentation, addictions, loneliness, social contagion, social comparison, and social perfectionism. These impacts are more pronounced, especially from the influences of social media, in girls than in boys, resulting in a public health emergency due to sharp rises in depression, anxiety, self-harm, and suicide.[26] Anxiety manifests in both the mind and body, with muscular and organ tensions, and often exhaustion.[26]

Some of this anxiousness is likely spilling over into Generation Alpha, especially with the advent of immersive artificial intelligence (AI), as society has not yet fully addressed these harmful impacts, with efforts underway to monitor, restrict, and de-escalate the culprits and educate parents regarding the impacts of hyper viral social media, excessive digital-use, and endless scrolling.[26] To counteract these harmful impacts, efforts to limit access to social media and smartphones in adolescence and early teens, along with phone-free schools and increased play opportunities are much needed reforms being implemented and advocated for across the nation. Haidt specifically noted two trends, impacting Gen Z: *overprotection in the real world and under protection in the virtual world*.[26] Hence, children born after 1995 became the Anxious Generation.[26]

While Gen Z has been digitally compromised, those belonging to it are resilient and facing these challenges without denial. Gen Z is striving to grow stronger and healthier and is open to new ways of interacting, which is typical of former generations. When given the opportunity, through real-world interactions and psychological support (including

Cognitive Behavioral therapies) the gloominess, depression, and withdrawal from society can be changed, and anxiety lessened, with less need for unproductive ruminations and catastrophizing.[26] Parents, family members, educators, and HCPs should be aware of the challenges of Gen Z and assist in supporting and advocating for the proposed reforms and have patience with the process. Gen Z is resilient!

# GENERATION ALPHA

Generation Alpha (or Gen Alpha) are the Children of Millennials who will be parents to Generation Gamma (spanning those born from 2040–2054). According to McCrindle,[21] Generation Alpha represents an entire new, global generation born in a new century, hence, following scientific nomenclature, naming moved to the Greek alphabet. Generation Alpha is represented by 2.2 billion people globally, as the *largest generation* in history. In 2025, the top Gen Alpha countries of birth are predicted to be India, China, and Indonesia.[21] Generation Alpha is keen on high-quality, sustainable products. Gen Alpha is health conscious, and has communicated via social media, gaming platforms, and Snapchat from an incredibly young age. Gen Alpha prefers interactive gaming with friends and making purchases via experiential retail. Other labels being attributed to Gen Alpha include: Multimodals, Generation Glass, Screenagers, The Alphas, and Global Gen.[21] Generation Beta will be born 2025–2039.[21] Generation Alpha is predicted to surpass Gen Z in high school completion (90%) rates, with 1 in 2 obtaining a university degree.[21] Gen Alpha is predicted to have 18 different jobs over six careers, many that do not yet exist, or in emerging industries, e.g., nanotechnology, block-chain, cyber security, autonomous transport, or virtual reality.[21] Shifts in demand will continue in caring roles for the aging, changing family structures, childcare services, and shifts in cultural diversity. We will talk more about the impact of technology for health care providers and influences of the generations in health care settings in Chapter 20.

Gen Alpha is curious and adaptable yet, as with the Millennials, requires improvement in leadership skills.[21,23–26] Screen saturation will be evident, and Gen Alpha will require greater focus on well-being for their health and quality of life function, simplification (apps), and customization for their penchants and unique priorities, as they will live and work later in life.[21]

# BRIDGING GENERATIONS

With respect to the generational classifications, timelines, and categorizations, the social markers and landmark events vary greatly and traverse the generations.[16–22] Some purport that it is not these landmark, historical events that define generations, yet the ever more rapid evolution of technological advances that is differentiating generations.[16–22]

Learning and on-the-job formats for the generations range from the traditional top-down focus, with formal classroom-based instructions to contemporary lounge room, café-style learning, and work environments, mixed in with gaming, with a multimodal media and e-learning emphasis. Historical timeline events for the generations range from the Great Depression of the 1930s to World War II, the Vietnam War of the mid-1960s to early 1970s, the September 11 attacks in 2001, school and mass-gathering shootings, and Operation Desert Storm and Shield, the Gulf Wars (Iraq and Afghanistan Wars), and the Russian invasion of Ukraine. Suffice it to say that the need to bridge these generational divides in the workplace system[19] is similar to perspectives and variations within families. From traditional nuclear families to blended families, generational differences are evident in many aspects of life and personal and lifestyle characteristics: core values, reward systems, and expectations; family; education and media; methods of communication; and how we manage financial matters. Generational differences also take their toll on workplace systems and continue to be a major source of financial and management strain. Understanding the generational perspectives will help us become better health care professionals and improved collaborators in health care work environments, through more effective interactions with all generations. Our patients, too, shall be representative of all generations.

We will talk more about the generations in relation to health care leadership and advocacy in Chapter 11 and in terms of communication in Chapter 12. However, knowing your own *self first* remains key to being able to relate more effectively with others, no matter the generation; this must come from *within*.

# THE NEED TO KNOW OURSELVES

The mature health care professional must know themself well, as emphasized in Chapter 1. HCPs must be aware of behaviors that result in harmful dependence on patients, in having personal needs for intimacy met, or in behaviors that fail to facilitate therapeutic presence and listening due to undeveloped rapport-building skills that have taken a backseat to the impersonal nature of technology. When one spends a great amount of time communicating with the thumbs or emojis (i.e., texting or emailing), face-to-face, deep listening skills are not learned and practiced. Multitasking is not an effective method to facilitate therapeutic communication with your patients. The end goal of all healing is the restoration of independent function for the highest and deepest quality of life possible for the patient. Patients who never feel adequately listened to and patients who depend on us, rather than on themselves, for this independence, struggle to make it on their own. We foster this destructive dependence when we ourselves depend on our patients to meet our needs for attention, affection, and/or power and authority. We do patients a huge disservice when we fail to **establish good rapport** and **truly listen** to their unique stories. Our patients entrust the care of their health to us, and to understand their needs we must listen carefully and closely during each encounter and assist by interacting with them through their preferred communication methods.

**Self-awareness** helps us to identify whether our lenses need resetting, cleaning, or replacing. It is difficult to help others effectively if we need help ourselves. Help is available through the insights gained in this course; through feedback from your classmates and faculty; in the excellent literature now available for those who grew up in dysfunctional families; and through counseling and participation in stress and support groups and 12-step groups that meet throughout the United States, such as Al-Anon, Addiction Recovery, Overeaters Anonymous, Narcotics Anonymous, Alcoholics Anonymous, and Adult Children of Alcoholics; or through other support measures. Seeking help is a sign of strength and self-recognition. Cognitive Behavioral Therapies have been successful in assisting those experiencing anxiety and depression. The goal of seeking help is always to become acquainted with the true self that was repressed many years ago. In this process, one gains insight into the distortion of one's lenses and then, often for the first time as an adult, clearly discerns that there are choices in behavior and that many of the choices one has habitually made in the past have contributed to a chronic feeling of chaos and victimization. Another goal would be to identify negative shame-based beliefs and replace them with more accepting, cosmic beliefs as described in Chapter 1. Recognize when your negative, undesired behaviors emerge, work on strategies to address and replace them with more positive thoughts and behaviors. It takes practice, and collaborating with professionals and trusted peers is a start.

The specific support groups listed previously were formed by people who realized that compulsive behavior and addictions serve to blunt one's awareness of the true self. In order to rid oneself of addictions, support is necessary. These groups are devoted to helping people heal from their addictive behavior and live authentic and genuine lives in the search for the true self, lost long ago in an effort to cope with the unfair stress of childhood. It takes courage to seek support, yet the return on that investment leads to self-awareness and finding the true self.

# SELF-AWARENESS THROUGH ACTION

The exercises for this chapter are designed to help you review your family history, your growth and development, the messages you received, and the values you adopted from growing up in your particular setting and circumstances. Try to withhold judgment on what you remember and experience. Remember, feelings *are*—they exist. Feelings are neither bad nor good, appropriate nor inappropriate; they just are. However, what we do with our feelings and how we respond to them are open to our evaluation and choice. Allow yourself to feel. One's emotions determine where we are directing our attention, what we learn and remember.[25] Persistent emotions may lead to potentially damaging or harmful circumstances (e.g., anxiety, anger, hopelessness) and limit our brain's capacity to a narrow, perilous focus.[25] The ability to identify, express, and harness all feelings can be the path to allow our emotions to help each one of us to create positive, more productive, and more satisfying lives.[25] Through regulating our own emotions, we are then available to more effectively interact and understand our patients. Being aware of our feelings is the first step. No family is perfect, and parents often parent the way they were parented and are often influenced by societal influences and events. Use these Chapter 2 exercises to gain insight into your experience and to set goals for your personal growth and professional formation that will help you become a mature health care professional.

# CONCLUSION

The next chapter discusses values in more depth. We develop our values initially by learning what to value from significant people in our lives, but a value cannot be said to be our own until we accept it for ourselves and act on it. In your journal, reflect on your values that you caught from significant people in your life. How many of them can you say you have truly reflected upon or assessed and have adopted as your own? Do you hold any values that would be perceived as negative? By whom? How does that make you feel?

# REFERENCES

1. Buining EM, Kooijman MK, Swinkels IC, Pisters MF, Veenhof C. Exploring physiotherapists' personality traits that may influence treatment outcome in patients with chronic diseases: a cohort study. *BMC Health Serv Res.* 2015;15:558.
2. John OP. History, measurement, and conceptual elaboration: the big five-trait taxonomy. In: John OP, Robbins RW, eds. *Handbook of Personality: Theory and Research.* 4th ed. New York, NY: Guilford; 2021:35–82.
3. Kooijman MK, Buining EM, Swinkels ICS, Koes BW, Vennhoff C. Do therapists' effects determine outcome in patients with shoulder pain in a primary care physiotherapy setting? *Physiotherapy.* 2020;Jun;107:111–117.
4. Piaget J. *The Construction of Reality in the Child.* New York, NY: Basic Books; 1954.
5. Bradshaw J. *Bradshaw On: The Family: A New Way of Creating Solid Self-Esteem.* Deerfield Beach, FL: Health Communications; 1996.
6. Erikson EH. *Identity, Youth and Crisis.* New York, NY: WW Norton; 1968.
7. Krysan M, Moore KA, Zill N. *Identifying Successful Families: An Overview of Constructs and Selected Resources.* Washington, DC: Department of Health and Human Services; 1990.
8. Whitfield CL. *Healing the Child Within: Recovery Classic Series.* Baltimore, MD: Health Communications; 1987.
9. Miller A. *The Drama of the Gifted Child: The Search for the True Self.* 3rd ed. New York, NY: Basic Books; 2008.
10. Raines C. Managing millennials. In: Raines C, ed. *Connecting Generations: The Sourcebook for a New Workplace.* Menlo Park, CA: Crisp Publications; 2003:171–185.
11. Mueller K. *Communication From the Inside Out: Strategies for the Engaged Professional.* Philadelphia, PA: FA Davis; 2010.
12. Tyler K. The Tethered Generation shrm.org. Accessed July 13, 2024.
13. National Association for Children of Alcoholics www.nacoa.org. Accessed September 13, 2023.
14. Malone M. Dependent on disorder. *MS Mag.* 1987;15:50.
15. Greenberg LS, Johnson SM. *Emotionally Focused Therapy for Couples.* New York, NY: Guilford Publications; 2012.
16. Lancaster LC, Stillman D. *When Generations Collide: Who They Are, Why They Clash, How to Solve the Generational Puzzle at Work.* New York, NY: Harper Collins; 2003.
17. Twenge, JM. *Generations: The Real Differences between Gen Z, Millennials, Gen X, Boomers and Silents—and What They Mean for American's Future.* New York, NY: Atria Books; 2023.
18. Lancaster LC, Stillman D. *The M-Factor: How the Millennial Generation Is Rocking the Workplace.* New York, NY: Harper Collins; 2003.
19. McCrindle Research. Generations defined. The Generations Defined Report—McCrindle https://mccrindle.com.au/resource/report/the-generations-defined-report/ Accessed July 13, 2024.
20. Zemke R, Raines C, Filipczak B. *Generations at Work: Managing the Clash of Boomers, Gen Xers, and Gen Yers in the Workplace.* 2nd ed. New York, NY: Amacom; 2013.
21. McCrindle M, Fell A. *Generation Alpha: Understanding Our Children and Helping Them Thrive.* Sydney, NSW, Australia: Hachette Book Group; 2021.
22. Howe N, Strauss W. *Millennials Rising.* New York, NY: Vintage; 2000.
23. Bittner A. Mentoring millennials for nursing leadership. *Nursing.* 2019 Oct;49(10):53–56. doi:10.1097/01.*NURSE.* 0000580656.81188.ee. PMID: 31568084.
24. Desy JR, Reed DA, Wolanskyj AP. Milestones and Millennials: a perfect pairing—competency-based medical education and the learning preferences of generation Y. *Mayo Clin Proc.* 2017 Feb;92(2):243–250. doi: 10.1016/j.mayocp.2016.10.026. PMID: 28160874.
25. Brackett M. *Permission to Feel: The Power of Emotional Intelligence to Achieve Well-being and Success.* New York, NY: Celadon Books; 2020.
26. Haidt J. *The Anxious Generation: How the Great Rewiring of Childhood Is Causing an Epidemic of Mental Illness.* New York, NY: Penguin; 2024.

# SUGGESTED READINGS

Anderson FG. *Transcending Trauma: Healing Complex PTSD with Internal Family Systems.* Eue Claire, WI: PESI Publishing & Media; 2021.

Brackett M. *Permission to Feel: The Power of Emotional Intelligence to Achieve Well-being and Success.* New York, NY: Celadon Books; 2020.

Kaslow FW. *Handbook of Relational Diagnosis and Dysfunctional Family Patterns.* Hoboken, NJ: John Wiley & Sons; 1996.

Kushner HS. *When Bad Things Happen to Good People.* New York, NY: Anchor Books; 1978.

Peck MS. *The Road Less Traveled: A New Psychology of Love, Traditional Values and Spiritual Growth.* New York, NY: Simon & Schuster; 1978.

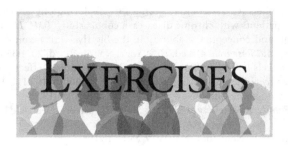

# EXERCISE 1: MAGIC CARPET RIDE

This exercise is best conducted with the instructor reading the instructions to a group. It is intended to help participants remember what it was like as they were growing up in their families. The magic carpet is a symbol for a ride back into time and memory. Thus, this is a type of guided imagery exercise followed by personal reflection on the content that concludes with a group discussion where participants can share with one another, at their own level of comfort, what insights they gained.

## *Instructor*

"So, sit back in your chairs, feet flat on the floor, and breathe deeply three times, each time feeling more and more relaxed. Concentrate on your breathing, have your mind go blank as you focus on the air going in through your nostrils and back out through your mouth. With each breath you feel increasingly relaxed." (Pause.)

"I want you to go back in time to when you were a little child in elementary school." (Pause.)

"You are inside your house with your family all gathered together; your parents are there, or those who reared you, and any brothers and sisters are also there." (Pause.)

"People are having a conversation." (Pause.)

"What are they talking about?" (Pause.)

"Now, ask them to stop talking for a second because you want to ask each of them an important question. Starting with the adults, ask each one, in turn, to tell you something about you. You're so—what? Listen carefully to the descriptions each gives you and pay attention to the feelings each person seems to display as each answers your questions." (Pause for 2 or 3 minutes.)

"As you get ready to leave the group, say goodbye to each person and come gently forward in time to the present, opening your eyes slowly as you return." (Pause.)

"Before talking, write down the names of each person with whom you spoke, then jot down what each told you about yourself, the feeling or attitude conveyed in that message, and how that made you feel." (Pause for 2 or 3 minutes.)

"Now, choose one person with whom to share your experience. Remember, your fantasy was a very private adventure. Some of what you remembered you may decide to keep private. You choose, carefully, the extent to which you want to reveal things about yourself and your family." (Pause for 5 minutes for discussion in groups of two or three.)

"Now, return to your written comments. Search each message for the values that underlie each. For example, if you heard from your mother, 'You're so messy! I wish you'd clean up your room,' you might discern that she values neatness or obedience to her values. 'You're so helpful' naturally leads one to the value of helping, or perhaps altruism, unless said with sarcasm. Then search for the message behind the message. Perhaps what was meant was, 'I wish you'd stop interfering in my life by always trying to do things for me.'"

## Large-Group Discussion

1. Discuss various messages and feelings. How many heard essentially negative messages about themselves? How many essentially positive? How many half and half?

2. How many people live up to the description heard from one or both parents? Negative or positive? Give examples.

3. Discuss values inferred from messages.

## Exercise Conclusion

Record what you learned and felt about the exercise in your journal. Explore the impact that the messages you heard have on your current self-esteem. How do you feel about yourself today in general? How does that relate to the messages heard? Was this exercise a positive or a negative one for you? What made it so?

# EXERCISE 2: FAMILY GENOGRAM

1. Draw your genogram for at least three generations (Figure 2.1). Label anything that seems important to you. See if you can locate pictures of family members to go with the circles and squares on your page.

2. Try to identify any addictions, family tension, conflicts, or incidents of children parenting their parents. What patterns emerge? What do you now know about yourself that you failed to see before? What stories are important enough to be handed down? Who/what is the family proud of? What secrets does the family hide from others?

3. Discuss your genogram with two other people in your class that you choose. Each of you should take 5 minutes to describe the people represented and 25 minutes to discuss the family dynamics as you understand them.

4. Perhaps questions came up for you about various family members' lives and habits. Write to relatives asking them to fill in the missing pieces to help you better understand your heritage.

**Figure 2.1** A family genogram is a map of a family for several generations. It is a very useful picture that reveals multigenerational patterns.

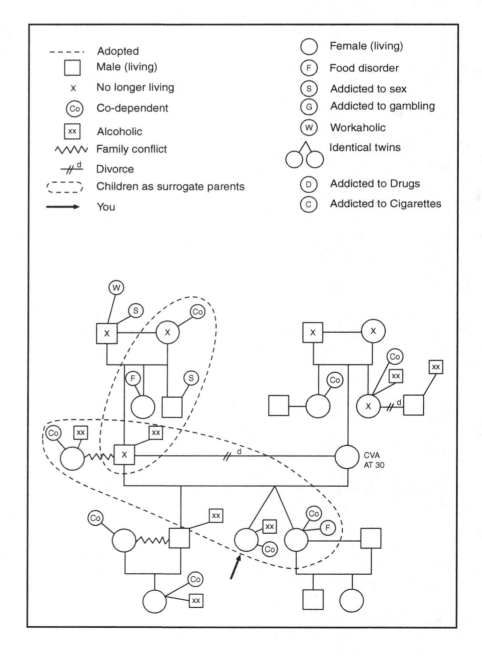

5. Remember, with this exercise in particular, the importance of confidentiality. Nothing revealed should ever leave the classroom. Be worthy of the trust placed in you as others take the risk of discussing private and sensitive material with you.

6. Journal about your feelings and your awareness from this exercise. Can you identify behaviors that you have developed from your family that may interfere with mature healing? Comment on any, and problem solve ways in which you might be able to work through those behaviors.

# Exercise 3: Value Boxes

1. Figure 2.2 is a diagram of eight boxes surrounding a circle that represents you. Each box represents a significant person in your life. Envision a person who corresponds to the descriptor at the top of each box and place that person's initials in the upper right corner. If there is no one who meets that description right now in your life, cross out the descriptor and simply put another important person's initials there. One person should not appear in two boxes.

**Figure 2.2** Value boxes.

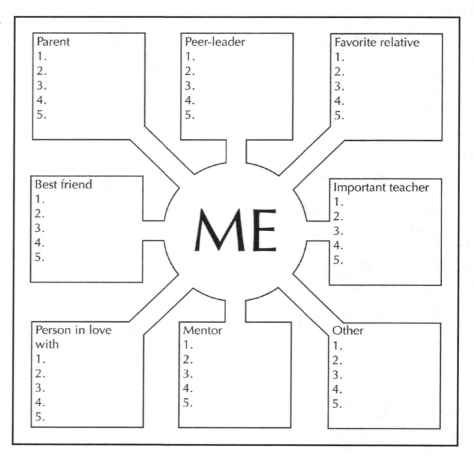

2. Now list four or five things you perceive each person would want you to value. What do they count on you for? What demands do they place on you? What do they want you to do, think, and be? What do they want you to value?

3. Now, look for similarities from various people. Are there values that are repeated often? List them in the lower right of the diagram as recurring values.

4. Underline each value that you want for yourself and place those values in the center circle.

5. Now, list the conflict areas to the lower left of the diagram. What do others want for you that you do not desire? What values seem most important to you?

These exercises are also available online at www.routledge.com/9781638220039.

# 3

# VALUES AS DETERMINANTS OF BEHAVIOR

*Gina Maria Musolino and Carol M. Davis*

## OBJECTIVES

*The learner should be able to*:

- Examine personal and professional values.
- Explore personal and professional values in determining one's behavior.
- Value integrating critical thinking and self-reflection for professional formation.
- Analyze values underlying behaviors that prohibit or enhance healing.
- Differentiate between being morally aware and morally conscious.
- Contrast nonmoral and moral values.
- Correlate evidence supporting the importance of values for health care professionals (HCPs) in service to society.

The process of professional socialization is a process of growth, of becoming a professional person. Ideally, that growth is holistic and permeates ourselves at deep levels. We realize that we have grown and that we have learned when we can observe changes in our thoughts and in our behaviors. Most obviously, we know more as we become a professional. We incorporate an entire new body of knowledge (cognitive learning domain) and skill (psychomotor learning domain) and deploy most of it daily in our professional care; while simultaneously continuing lifelong learning, driven by patient/client needs. But we also develop different attitudes and values (affective domain of learning) as we grow professionally; while simultaneously seeking to expand our professional acumen, striving for expertise in collaborative clinical decision making that is patient informed. We transform as health care professionals (HCPs) with an innate desire to continue our professional development. The learning domain frameworks for the Affective, Cognitive and Psychomotor Learning Domains are included at the end of this chapter (Appendix—Bloom's Taxonomy) so you may start to realize and become familiar with the classifications of each of these components of professional growth and development. Each learning domain is defined and then detailed in 5–6 major process categories (skills and abilities) in a hierarchical fashion with action verbs that may be utilized to produce learning and teaching goals for assessment in a scaffolding manner. We will refer to them in subsequent chapters and application exercises, along with learning about the Spiritual Domain in Chapter 15. Take a moment to review the learning domains in the Appendix at the end of this chapter.

DOI: 10.4324/9781003525554-3

Professional growth involves changes in our knowledge, skills, attitudes, thoughts, values, and beliefs. You may not realize it, but you are becoming someone different as a result of your professional development as a HCP. You should be changed through the process, and you are encouraged to consider who you are becoming in the development and formation of your professional identity. Let's reflect upon this now in your journal by responding to the query "Who are you becoming?" As you continue your professional formation journey, refer to this entry every six months or so. Consider how you are changing, and journal your feelings.

We will get to the definition of what a value is in a moment, but first, here are some general observations. All people, after a certain age, can be said to have values. Some of those values we examined in Chapter 2. Consequently, you are now more aware of some of the values you have learned and adopted or introjected from your family and/or guardians. It is appropriate for family members to help us grow as children by teaching us what to believe and value when we are too young to choose critically for ourselves. Babies are not born with the values needed to live peacefully in the community. We appreciate this when we eat at a restaurant with a 4-year-old child who has not yet been socialized adequately and runs around the room playfully throwing food at people.

Now let's pause for a moment and consider our own values. Do you believe this quote holds true:

*It's not hard to make decisions once you know what your values are.* —Roy E. Disney

Why or why not? Consider an encounter where your values were not the same as another's or an organization's. What transpired? How do values influence decisions?

Sometimes we introject the values of those who raised us so completely that we do not even know what we truly value or, more importantly, why. The story is told of a young couple starting life together cooking a special dinner for guests. As one partner prepared the roast, he cut the two ends of the ham off before putting it in the oven. His wife chided him for wasting so much meat, and he defended himself by saying that his mother taught him always to cut the ends off. "Why?" she asked. He responded that he did not know, but he thought it was important and probably had something to do with the proper cooking and circulation of juices. The next time they visited his parents' home, the new wife asked her husband's mother about cutting the ends off the ham. "Oh, yes," she replied, "My mother always taught me to do that. It's critical to the cooking of the meat." Still not satisfied, the grandmother was called on the phone. "Grandma, tell our new daughter-in-law why it is so important to cut the ends of the meat off the ham before cooking it!" Grandma replied, "Oh, that old trick. It's just a habit I got into. When I first married, we did not have a big enough pot to fit all the meat in, so I just trimmed the ends. After a while, it just became a habit, I guess."

And so it is with some of the values and/or beliefs we "catch" from our parents, without thinking about them. Cutting off the ends of ham is not a good example of value-based behavior, but the analogy is important. A clear definition of value-based behavior follows.

Rogers and Stevens[1] indicated that immature people, in an attempt to gain or hold love, approval, and esteem, place the locus of evaluation of values on others. They learn to have a basic distrust for direct experiencing as a valid guide to appropriate behavior. They learn from others what values are important and adopt them as their own, although they may be widely discrepant from personal experience. Because these introjected values are not based on genuinely experienced personal feelings, they tend to be fixed and rigid, rather than fluid and changing.

Culturally accepted values change over time as society changes. The dawning of the age of information technology has brought with it a whole new set of values and a vocabulary to match. Rogers and Stevens[1] disclosed a list of what they termed the commonly adopted or *introjected* values, and their associated beliefs found often in the subjects from the United States (U.S.) they studied in the 1950s and 1960s. Consider how times have changed over the years:

- Sexual desires are mostly bad. Source: Parents, teachers, the church.

- Disobedience is bad. To obey is good; to obey without question is better. Source: Parents, teachers, the church, the military.

- Making money is the highest good. Source: Too numerous to mention.

- Aimless, exploratory reading for fun is undesirable and lazy. Source: Teachers, the educational system.

- Abstract art is good. Source: "The sophisticated people."

- To love your neighbor is the highest good. Source: Parents, the church.

- Cooperation and teamwork are preferable to acting alone. Source: Companions.

- Cheating is clever and desirable. Source: The peer group.

- Coca-Cola, chewing gum, electric refrigerators, and automobiles are utterly desirable. Source: Advertisements (still reinforced by people in many parts of the world).

This list reveals that commonly held values reflect the cultural mores of the time a half-century ago. Now, in the twenty-first century, it is much more difficult to find broadly held cultural values than it was when the U.S. was emerging from the great Depression and World War II. Individualism has become even more valued, sometimes to the detriment of the society as a whole. Next generations are more group focused, likely as a result. What values can you identify that are broadly held in this era? Surely the commonly held sanctions against killing and abuse hold true. The entrepreneurial spirit and creativity are robustly honored. Unfortunately, the value of making a lot of money as an end, no matter what means are used, seems to prevail. However, ongoing national and global crises, tragedies, and subsequent increasing global terrorism with cybersecurity issues (refer to Table 2.3) have caught the attention of our entire world and have demanded that we as citizens reevaluate prevailing value-based beliefs and behaviors that endanger the whole of society in ways not even imagined by most people years ago.

"Having a lot" in these times is mistaken for self-worth and intrinsic value. The health care system saw a decline from a service profession to a business as an economic-driven health care system took shape in the mid-1990s. Universal access to health care in the U.S. has now become law. Nonetheless, health care is still a privilege for many and still not a "right" in America, nor providing for equal access to care[2]; often as a direct result of the Social Determinants of Health (SDoH) as discussed in Chapter 1 (SDoH Figure 1.1). Not all agree on the values that were codified in the health care reform law that passed in Congress; discussion continues, and is debated, with efforts to repeal or implement health care and access to care differently at state and national levels. The Covid-19 global pandemic further brought to light health care inequities, the impact of politicization of public health matters, and the challenges of personal beliefs and values clashing with what may be in the best interests of all.

Perhaps we are getting ahead of ourselves. Let us take a closer look at what constitutes values.

## DEFINING VALUES

What is a value? Values have been defined in many ways. The term value refers to an operational belief that one accepts as one's own and that determines behavior. Morrill[3] was far more specific, however, and defined values as follows:

- Standards and patterns of choice that guide persons and groups toward satisfaction, fulfillment, and meaning.
- Constructs that orient choice and shape action.
- Concepts that call forth thought and conduct that have worth, that lead (under the right conditions) to the fulfillment of human potential or to the discovery of a variety of types and levels of meaning.
- Concepts that are not themselves beliefs or judgments but come to expression in and through thought.
- Concepts that are not themselves feelings or emotions but inevitably involve desires and fears and that cannot be defined as deeds but are always mediated through specific acts.

Thus, values orient our choices and inspire our actions. Because this is a text devoted to developing appropriate professional ways of being, it becomes critical to examine and clarify the values you now hold in relation to the values that form ethical and sensitive professional caregiving as you progress in your professional formation.

## VALUES VERSUS NEEDS

Values can be distinguished from needs, which also influence our behavior. If you are thirsty, without thinking much about it, you get something to drink. Needs push us into behaving in certain predictable ways. A theory of human behavior based upon a hierarchy of needs has been outlined in detail by the psychologist Maslow.[4] However, for behavior to be value based, I must reflect upon the choices I have and act according to my reflection. Thus, need behavior is more automatic and driven, whereas value-based behavior takes place upon reflection.[5] Implied in this distinction is the idea that value-based behavior is more mature and less impulsive, especially when compared with behaviors that are based on the more basic or lower-level needs. People with chronic conditions that impact their endurance and ability to walk may want to get a drink when they are thirsty and value the need for hydration. However, they may be considering instead how much effort it will take them to get the water and how it will make them later need to urinate and, therefore, need to walk again, which is a challenge. They may also be dreading the impact of potential incontinence in their efforts to make it timely to the bathroom. Their values are affected and now changed dramatically by the influences of their chronic condition on their quality of life, and they may require assistance to meet their daily needs and reinforce their true values. Scheduled bathroom breaks with planned assistance may be in order and less catastrophizing, replaced by positive thoughts of the benefits of hydration and movement.

The example from earlier—cutting off the ends of the ham—does not represent value-based or reflective behavior but an introjected behavior based on the tendency to distrust one's own experience as a guide. Perhaps the value underlying this behavior was to follow the example of elders despite logic. Indeed, two generations of the family distrusted their own experience! It may be motivated out of respect or tradition, and possibly even love, but the *why* was not really known or questioned. And so it goes in our families.

# MORAL VERSUS NONMORAL VALUES

The professional socialization process requires the clarification and prioritization of currently held values and the adoption of new values that are consistent with the values of the profession. Deciding how to prepare ham or what clothes to wear to a party is a decision-making process of a different sort from deciding whether a patient is a viable candidate to successfully utilize an above-knee prosthesis. The differences are important. The first category is an example of personal choice or preference; the second is a professional decision. Personal and professional choices can be based on reflection of values, but professional choices are different from value preferences. The first is a choice that bears little consequence for the chooser if the less-than-best decision is made. However, the decision about the prosthesis has profound consequences for another person if the less-than-best decision is made.[6]  Mueller and Rose expound on the need for self-regulation and self-discipline for professional growth for best practice and emphasize the value of compassion in professional decision making: "a compassionate approach … is critical to quality patient care. Science does not preclude compassion, and each patient must be treated as an individual in a sensitive, caring manner."[7]

Values that lead to personal preference are termed *nonmoral values*, whereas values that have to do with the way we relate to and interact with fellow human beings are termed *moral values*.[8] Moral values, such as compassion, trust, justice, honesty, love, and faithfulness to one's professional colleagues, form the heart of a profession's value structure. Moral values take on more importance than value preferences and must be regarded with greater seriousness because the needs of human beings are more important than what food, music, and hairstyle we prefer.

# PROFESSIONAL FORMATION AND PROFESSIONAL VALUES

Professionalism is grounded in core values. In days past, professions assumed that new members would automatically pick up professional values and behaviors, but this is no longer the case.[9] We now know we must encourage ourselves and each other to consistently demonstrate the behaviors characteristic of a professional as lifelong learning professionals. Professionalism is the social contract with society, founded upon altruism, morality, and virtue.[10]

Professional formation is an ongoing, dynamic, and iterative process of internalizing a profession's core values and beliefs, developing professional behaviors and actions essential for HCPs to accept responsibility for the profession's social contract.[10,11] Professional formation occurs through reflection and analytical thinking, through personal involvement with value integration through a consciousness of one's own and the profession's values.[12,13]

Professional formation often requires one to act courageously,[12] and the leaders of the community of practice are responsible for negotiating the social contract on behalf of the profession, ensuring devotion for the public good,[12,14] which we will further discuss in subsequent chapters. Attributes of being a healer and professional explicitly overlap, and the intersection reveals not only competence but the core values and ethics of the profession.[15]

According to Kolb,[16] "The values of a society, a group such as the American Physical Therapy Association (APTA), and each individual are the culmination of all that has gone before."[(870–71)] Kolb[16] cautions, however, that "the group must be in step with the society, or its influence diminishes and may become nonexistent."[(872–73)] Hence, at the time of the association centennial, the APTA House of Delegates revised the core values for the Physical Therapist (PT) and Physical Therapist Assistant (PTA) to encompass the professional behavior incumbent to provide the best quality of physical therapy services: accountability, altruism, collaboration, compassion and caring, duty, excellence, inclusion, integrity, and social responsibility.[17] Even a cursory look at these values reveals that they might be universally held values rather than unique to physical therapy alone. The APTA's Core Values for the PT and PTA and each descriptor follow:[17]

- **Accountability:** Accountability is active acceptance of the responsibility for the diverse roles, obligations, and actions of the physical therapist and physical therapist assistant including self-regulation and other behaviors that positively influence patient and client outcomes, the profession, and the health needs of society.

- **Altruism:** Altruism is the primary regard for or devotion to the interest of patients and clients, thus assuming the responsibility of placing the needs of patients and clients ahead of the physical therapist's or physical therapist assistant's self-interest.

- **Collaboration:** Collaboration is working together with patients and clients, families, communities, and professionals in health and other fields to achieve shared goals. Collaboration within the physical therapist–physical therapist assistant team is working together, within each partner's respective role, to achieve optimal physical therapist services and outcomes for patients and clients.

- **Compassion and Caring:** Compassion is the desire to identify with or sense something of another's experience, a precursor of caring. Caring is the concern, empathy, and consideration for the needs and values of others.

- **Duty:** Duty is the commitment to meeting one's obligations to provide effective physical therapist services to patients and clients, to serve the profession, and to positively influence the health of society.

- **Excellence:** Excellence in the provision of physical therapist services occurs when the physical therapist and physical therapist assistant consistently use current knowledge and skills while understanding personal limits, integrate the patient or client perspective, embrace advancement, and challenge mediocrity.

- **Inclusion:** Inclusion occurs when the physical therapist and physical therapist assistant create a welcoming and equitable environment for all. Physical therapists and physical therapist assistants are inclusive when they commit to providing a safe space, elevating diverse and minority voices, acknowledging personal biases that may impact patient care, and taking a position of anti-discrimination.

- **Integrity:** Integrity is steadfast adherence to high ethical principles or standards, being truthful, ensuring fairness, following through on commitments, and verbalizing to others the rationale for actions

- **Social Responsibility:** Social responsibility is the promotion of a mutual trust between the profession and the larger public that necessitates responding to societal needs for health and wellness.

As you review these core values, do you believe that you have the ability to exhibit these as a developing professional? Can you imagine the challenges if you are not able to acculturate to these values that the profession has accepted and deemed omnipotent? Developing HCPs are often challenged by the core values because they mismatch with their personal beliefs and values for their generation or personal upbringing. You can see how a clash of values might transpire, especially if you were not aware in comparison with the expected core values for the profession. Now that you are cognizant of the values of the profession, where do you see that you might have areas that you may need to evolve and be more mindful, or are the values congruent with your personal values and beliefs? Take a moment to journal your reflections on the core values.

Peterson and Seligman[18] published a list of six overarching virtues that many people world-wide aspire to achieve. These enduring virtues and their accompanying character strengths can be viewed as values that are advantageous for clinical therapeutic presence, promoting virtuous practice:[18]

1. **Wisdom and knowledge:** Creativity, curiosity, love of learning, perspective.

2. **Courage:** Authenticity, bravery, persistence, zest.

3. **Humanity:** Kindness, love, social intelligence.

4. **Justice:** Fairness, leadership, teamwork.

5. **Temperance:** Forgiveness, modesty, prudence, self-regulation.

6. **Transcendence:** Appreciation of beauty, gratitude, hope, humor, religiousness.

# VALUES CONFLICTS

There are times when the behavior of HCPs comes into direct conflict with patients' behaviors. The moral or interpersonal values that the profession espouses, for example, in its code of ethics or its core values statements, and the behavior observed in many hospitals and patient/client care settings, often seem far removed from each other. Often, the behavior exhibited in conflict situations is not value based or based on reflection at all, but is highly impulsive and defensive.

Values conflicts are always rich in their lessons for learning, although many of us shy away from them because we are afraid of doing the wrong thing. In tense times, most of us want someone to tell us what to do. Debriefing when conflicts occur is also another rich learning opportunity for our own professional development and reflection.

A moral dilemma exists when we do not know what choice to make from two or more conflicting choices; thus, we have difficulty choosing which value should have priority. Chapter 4 focuses on the examination of ethical dilemmas and their resolution, but a brief example here will illustrate this point. Respect for life is the central value for advocates of a woman's right to choose abortion, as well as for those opposed to abortion. The difference in opinion and belief of these two groups is not the value of life, but the importance of the mother's life over the fetus's life. The antiabortionists claim the primacy of the fetus's life above all considerations, whereas the reproductive freedom advocates claim the primacy of the mother's choice for the quality of her life and resist outside interference with her right to choose.[6] Likewise, those who favor capital punishment value the lives of those who might become victimized over the life of the person convicted of murder.

The set of moral norms or societal responsibility statements adopted by a professional group to direct value-laden choices, in a way consistent with professional responsibility, is termed a *code of ethics*. One might follow the code without internalizing it or introjecting it, just as one did in younger years with parents' values. For a code of ethics to function as a set of professional moral values, one must reflect on it and decide that it forms a values complex around which one is willing to organize professional choices. Thus, as stated previously, reflection is necessary to the internalization of values to make them truly one's own, whether personal or professional. Those who make the smoothest transitions into professional practice are likely to be those whose personal values and priorities greatly overlap with the values inherent in their chosen professional practice. Given that one's basic human survival needs are met, the more one reflects on one's choices and on which choices result in a good and meaningful life, the more one is apt to experience consistent reward from choices made; while learning from the opposite.[8]

# VALUES DETRACTING FROM THERAPEUTIC PRESENCE

Often, patients and clients end up needing the help of rehabilitation professionals because of impulsive, poor choices reflecting an immature and inconsistent set of values that have been introjected, but not clarified or claimed as one's own. An example might be a young person who comes to physical therapy needing relief from low back pain incurred from lifting a heavy railroad tie while showing off in front of peers in an attempt to impress. Many patient and client problems in movement and function are not the result of fate but the result of a lifetime of choices that reveal little attention or value to behaviors that preserve physical and emotional health. Thus, it sometimes becomes difficult to avoid becoming judgmental, and, as professionals, we sometimes feel resistance to treating people who may not practice wellness behaviors and have become, for example, obese, drug addicted, or chronic vapers/smokers.[6]

Professional ethics demand that, when a feeling of criticism and negative judgment of a patient occurs, we must be aware of it and consciously work to not let it interfere with our commitment to compassionate, quality care. Common behaviors that reveal difficulty in this task include the following:[6]

- Acting cool or aloof, obviously paying more attention to other patients. **Underlying value:** Prejudice or indifference.
- Overly criticizing the patient so they feel as if nothing is right. **Underlying value:** Prejudice, perfectionism, rigidity.
- Treating the patient as an object rather than a person with feelings of pain, worry, and insecurity. **Underlying value:** Depersonalization.
- Treating the patient like a child, incapable of understanding or making wise choices. **Underlying value:** Patronizing, adopting an air of condescension.
- Being unable or unwilling to help the patient in treatment, leaving the patient alone most of the time. **Underlying value:** Indifference or prejudice.
- Gaslighting or making fun of the patient in their presence and/or behind their back. **Underlying value:** Depersonalization, Cruelty.
- Telling others things that the patient shared in confidence. **Underlying value:** Breaking confidentiality.
- Refusing to let the patient work on their own, constantly supervising and instructing. **Underlying value:** Fostering dependence, having own need to be needed and met by patients.
- Guessing what is best to do, refusing to find correct and best treatment alternatives, and acting on habit. **Underlying value:** Refusing to recognize and act based on one's own limits of knowledge, Incompetence.
- Always fitting the patient in as if everything else is more important. **Underlying value:** Selfish interest over needs of patients.

- Refusing to listen to a patient's story of pain and difficulties dealing with pain and dysfunction. **Underlying value:** Importance of defending oneself against personal feelings of fear and insecurity around pain and possible addiction.

Most of us would read this list of behaviors and say to ourselves, "I'd never act like that!" But as much as we would never want to act in ways that interfere with healing, when we are unclear of our values—or, more important, when we are not in touch with our feelings and when we do not know ourselves—we often end up doing and saying things, especially under stress, that we regret later. These regretful behaviors stem, in part, from impulsive and immature needs to be spontaneous and egocentric and arise from feelings of criticism and the judgment that our patients do not deserve our help. Or perhaps they grow out of unrecognized fears, such as not knowing the right thing to do. Perhaps they stem from not having clarified the values underlying a therapeutic presence.

# VALUES THAT REINFORCE HEALING

Essential to a therapeutic use of self is the capacity to feel compassion for those who need our help. Compassion is quite different from pity, wherein I feel sorry for this poor person (and secretly feel smug and am thankful that this is not my problem). Compassion in a mature HCP is a value that is fueled with imagination and the ability to envision what is possible from the other person's perspective. When we truly value our patients as human beings, we express behavior based on moral values that enhance healing, such as sincere, active listening and a desire to treat patients as adults, in charge of their own lives and capable of making wise and appropriate decisions for themselves. We treat what they say with confidence and respect, attend to them with interest, and obtain their informed consent for therapeutic procedures. We convey to them that their choice to come to us was well founded and that we will help within clearly set boundaries and expectations. In other words, we work to be able to feel sincere, genuine positive regard for all our patients and relate to each with sensitivity to their uniqueness.

When we become professionals, we gain many things, but we also give up some things. One of the things we give up is the right to walk away from people we would rather not treat. What patient would be your most dreaded? Would it be the rapist? The child abuser? The alcoholic? The obese? The person who is HIV positive or who has AIDS? The person who has Covid? When we judge our patients, we cannot help but treat them as less than human. What is required is a sense of oneness with all human beings, regardless of the mistakes they may have made. Deciding that the mistakes *you* have made are far less evil only distances you from your patient. We all make mistakes; how we respond and recover from them is what remains relevant. We should be prepared to assist our colleagues in these efforts too, not bringing further shame or judgment and defamation of character. How will you collaborate to assist those in need?

As professionals, we also give up the right to say whatever we feel at any moment. We give up the right to speak and act impulsively and take on the responsibility to act in accordance with core values and the code of ethics or, in similar terms, to act according to the moral values that facilitate healing. No longer may we claim the luxury of spontaneous outbursts or selfish indifference. No longer may we put our own needs before the needs of our patients. No longer may we be run by unclear values or fears that have not yet been examined and resolved. Is it challenging? Yes. Will we likely falter? Yes. Again, we learn from our errors and experiences and become better as a result, when taking the time to reflect on and regain our professional values.

Professional rehabilitative care requires problem solving that is initiative-taking; based on scientific data; and demonstrates a consistent, conscious value of choosing behavior that is conducive to healing. As a HCP, you must become an informed reasoner. You must continually be open to collaboration and communication with your patients and their families/caregivers. We always have more to learn that may be vital to their progress. You must learn to value the systematic gathering of facts and compassionately relate to people who come to you for help. You must value taking the time to reflect on your behavior and choose to act in ways that reinforce healing. Central to this process is the courage to carefully examine your values and the values of healing, and to make a commitment to change behaviors that interfere with effective and compassionate care. Feedback from others is important, but at this point in the *Patient Practitioner Interaction* (*PPI*) text, you are asked to focus on self-examination.

# DEVELOPMENT OF AN ETHICAL CONSCIOUSNESS

We are not born knowing the right thing to do; we develop the ability to solve moral problems in conjunction with cognition. There are three common approaches to teaching children the right thing to do:[3] *objectivism*, or *legalism*; *ethical subjectivism*, or *values clarification*; and *ethical relativism*. The most common is *objectivism*, or *legalism*, which asserts that to do the right thing is to obey the rules. The rightness of the value is within the value itself; therefore, it is always right, for example, to love people and to act justly, honestly, and with compassion. Organized religion teaches this approach to values education. To do the right thing, one should obey the higher authority, do as the Bible says, follow the Torah, the Qur'an, The Ten Commandments, etc. But objectivism offers little help in reconciling the contradictions that can be found in the Bible or in resolving the dilemma, for example, between honoring your parents and following your own conscience in developing your career when your choice and the choice your parents would have you make are at odds. Likewise, objectivism fosters the development of a moral belief system based on outside authority. For these reasons, it does not adequately serve the purpose of dilemma resolution in health care.

The second approach, *ethical subjectivism*, or *values clarification*, offers an alternative that approaches ethical relativism.[19] The third approach, *ethical relativism*, is the view that each person's values should be considered equally valid. Subjectivism suggests that one examine the conflicting values to make sure that each is, indeed, a value. If a belief or idea does not meet true value status, it is relegated to a position of less importance than a true value. To satisfy the definition of value, Raths et al.[19] suggested a value must satisfy the seven criteria listed in Table 3.1. The content of a value, so important in objectivism, becomes secondary to the process of determining whether something is, indeed, a value.[19]

How well does subjectivism assist us in making value-based decisions? It probably does not make that much difference if one begins treating patients at 8:00 a.m. or 7:30 a.m. People will (and often do) argue the importance of their priorities, but nonmoral values, or value preferences, are just that—relative preferences. Moral values present a different story. Moral relativism renders an ethical code meaningless.[8]

Thus, in a moral or ethical dilemma, in which one must choose between doing the loving thing and following the rules, it does little good to use a subjectivist approach, clarifying whether both compassion and justice fit the criteria of a value. What is needed is a way of weighing the relative goodness of each value *in the situation*. Thus, subjectivism and objectivism both fall short of informing us clearly how to decide between two conflicting values.

Gilligan[20] and Kohlberg[21] developed theories that assist us in our task. Their theories each fall under the category of *contextualism*, in which they assert that as people develop their ability to think, they also develop their ability to reason about the right or best thing to do *in each situation*. This approach to dilemma resolution has been termed contextualism because the *context of the situation* provides the key information in deciding the right thing to do *in that situation*. Certain values are, as the objectivists suggest, always going to assume great importance, but the key to resolving the dilemma is to collect all the pertinent data about this particular situation and then weigh alternatives for the best thing to do according to the best and most mature debate. How do we discover the most adequate reasoning, the most mature debate? Developmental psychology and philosophy inform us here.

## MORAL DECISION MAKING: DEVELOPMENTAL ASPECTS

In general, developmentalists assert that as people grow and change, they pass through predictable stages in which new behaviors are formed and stabilized. The maturation process consists of a progression through a series of

| TABLE 3.1 |
|---|
| **RATHS' 7 REQUIREMENTS FOR A VALUE** |
| **CHOOSING ONE'S BELIEFS AND BEHAVIORS** |
| 1. Choosing freely |
| 2. Choosing from among alternatives |
| 3. Choosing after considering consequences of choice |
| **PRIZING ONE'S BELIEFS AND BEHAVIORS** |
| 4. Prizing and cherishing |
| 5. Publicly affirming when appropriate |
| **ACTING ON ONE'S BELIEFS AND BEHAVIORS** |
| 6. Acting |
| 7. Acting repeatedly, showing consistency |
| Adapted from Raths LE, Harmin M, Simon S. *Values and Teaching*. Columbus, OH: Charles E. Merrill; 1966. |

passages or stages, which reflects the increasingly sophisticated changes occurring in a person's nervous system. Thus, children are not little adults and should not be treated as such, nor should they be asked to act like adults before they know what that means.

Perhaps the most famous developmentalist, Piaget,[22] suggested that as cognitive abilities develop, the ability to know the right thing to do also develops. Piaget[22] suggested four stages of development of a moral conscience (Table 3.2): amoral (ages 0 to 2 years), egocentric (ages 2 to 7 years), heteronomous (ages 7 to 12 years), and autonomous (ages 12 years and older). Kohlberg[21] based his work on that of Piaget[22] and further refined the stages, based on research conducted around the world. Kohlberg[21] suggested six stages that most people go through in developing a mature moral consciousness (Table 3.3). Earliest and most immature is the punishment and obedience stage, in which that which is wrong is that for which I get punished. Tables 3.2 and 3.3 illustrate the progression stages through to stage 6, an autonomous stage of knowing the right thing based on a decision of conscience in accord with self-chosen, well thought out ethical principles appealing to logical comprehensiveness, universality, and consistence and that flow from the basic principle of justice.[21] When faced with dilemmas, Kohlberg[21] observed that males did not just work out the right answer for themselves by guessing or by trial and error. Rather, depending on their age and maturity, they appealed to a category of reasons outlined in the stages in Table 3.3. Kohlberg[21] and Piaget[22] believed that children progress from a total abdication to an outside authority to an autonomous stage, wherein they make their own choices.

Gilligan,[20] also a contextualist and student of Kohlberg,[21] reacted to the fact that Kohlberg only studied men and boys and then generalized his theory to girls and women. Kohlberg[21] stated that some get stuck in the stage 3,

| TABLE 3.2 | | | | |
|---|---|---|---|---|
| **DEVELOPMENTAL MODEL COMPARISON** | | | | |
| **PIAGET'S MORAL DEVELOPMENT MODEL** | **KOHLBERG'S MORAL DEVELOPMENTAL COMPARISON** | | | |
| | **Level** | **Orientation Stage** | **Characterized by** | **Personally Stated as** |
| **Amoral stage** (ages 0 to 2) | | | | |
| **Egocentric stage** (ages 2 to 7): Lacks morality, bends rules, and reacts instinctively to environment | **Pre-conventional** | 1. Punishment and obedience orientation 2. Instrumental relativist orientation | Satisfying one's own needs | I must obey the authority figure or else... |
| **Heteronomous stage** (ages 7 to 12): Based on total acceptance of a morality imposed by others | **Conventional** | 3. Good boy–nice girl orientation 4. Law and order orientation | ○ Conformity to social conventions and expectations ○ Respect for authority and society's laws | ○ I probably should because everyone expects me to ○ I ought to because of duty to obey the rules |
| **Autonomous stage** (ages 12 and older): Based on an internalized morality of cooperation | **Post-conventional or autonomous** | 5. Social contract orientation 6. Universal-ethical principle orientation | ○ Conformity to the ever-changing values and demands of society ○ My conscience holds me responsible for doing what is right | ○ I may because of my role in society, but I often question the relative values of society ○ I will because I know it is the right thing to do |

Reprinted with permission from Piaget J, Kohlberg L. Comparison of the stages in two models of moral development. In: Francoeur RT. *Becoming a Sexual Person*. New York, NY: John Wiley and Sons; 1982:673.

| TABLE 3.3 |
| --- |
| **KOHLBERG'S STAGES OF MORAL DEVELOPMENT** |
| **1. PRECONVENTIONAL LEVEL (3–7 YEARS OF AGE)** |
| Child is responsive to cultural rules and labels of good and bad or right and wrong as they relate to physical consequence of action (reward of punishment). |
|     **Stage 1: Punishment and obedience orientation.** Avoidance of punishment and unquestioning deference to power valued in their own right, not in terms of respect for underlying moral order supported by punishment and authority (stage 4). |
|     **Stage 2: Instrumental relativist orientation.** Right actions are those that satisfy one's own needs. Reciprocity is not a matter of loyalty or justice but of "You scratch my back and I'll scratch yours." |
| **2. CONVENTIONAL LEVEL (8–13 YEARS OF AGE)** |
| Maintaining the expectations of the individual's family, group, or nation is valuable in its own right, regardless of consequences. |
|     **Stage 3: Interpersonal concordance or good boy–nice girl orientation.** Good behavior is that which pleases others and is approved by them. Behavior is often judged by intention. One earns approval by being nice. |
|     **Stage 4: Law and order orientation.** Right behavior consists of showing respect for authority, following the rules, doing one's duty, and maintaining the given social order for its own sake. |
| **3. POSTCONVENTIONAL, AUTONOMOUS, PRINCIPLED LEVEL (ADULTHOOD)** |
| Clear effort to define moral values and principles that have validity and application apart from authority of groups or other persons holding these principles. |
|     **Stage 5: Social contract, legalistic orientation.** Right actions are defined as those that have been critically examined and agreed upon by the whole society. Emphasis placed on procedural rules for reaching consensus in the face of relativism. Aside from what is constitutionally and democratically agreed upon, what is right is a matter of personal values and opinion. It is possible to change the law when it is to the benefit of society. Outside the law, free agreement and contract are the binding elements of obligation (the "official" morality of the U.S. government and Constitution). |
|     **Stage 6: Universal–ethical principle orientation.** Right is defined by the decision of conscience in accord with self-chosen ethical principles appealing to logical comprehensiveness, universality, and consistency. The basic universal principles are those of justice, the reciprocity and equality of human rights, and respect for the dignity of human beings as individual persons, no matter which nationality, race, color, or creed. |
| Adapted from Kohlberg L. The cognitive development approach to moral education. *Phi Delta Kappa.* 1975; June: 670–677. |

"good–nice" orientation, which reveals conformity to social expectations because some are socialized to stay at home and tend the house, yielding to the decisions of others predominating outside the house. Right is that which pleases others. This is changing in today's contemporary society, but many still hold these values; yet gender-associated roles and norms continue to evolve. Gilligan's[20] work challenged the rigid assumptions. She revealed that some "appear to frame moral problems in terms of conflicting personal responsibilities, rather than conflicting rights and the concept of justice." Thus, as a function of social conditioning, adolescent males may well focus first on achievement and self-identity and much later focus on developing a value of intimacy and friendship, whereas females do just the opposite. All people have the same ability to mature to higher stages of moral conscience; however, some seem to mature not linearly as Kohlberg's[21] scale illustrates, but horizontally, in a net-like fashion, favoring the higher importance of relationships over abstract goals such as social justice and achievement. As we mature and enter relationships, we may also tend to demonstrate these value scales, whereas "men are motivated when they feel needed, while women are motivated when they feel cherished."[23] These classic studies are limited in that they did not account for any other distinctions in gender identity types.

# MORAL AWARENESS VERSUS MORAL CONSCIOUSNESS

To be morally aware is to know what the dictionary says about, for example, compassion, and to be somewhat aware of whether your behavior fits that description at any given time. To be morally conscious, however, is to examine how compassion weaves its way through your behavior, how it influences you in your various decisions, and how you feel about compassion with regard to justice, for example, in a moral dilemma. Thus, moral consciousness represents a deeper way of knowing and thus a firmer commitment to consistency in moral behavior or the way we interact with other human beings. The goal of this text is, at the least, to confirm your moral awareness and, ideally, to help stimulate a moral consciousness that is consistent with quality and compassionate health care. Knowing the right thing to do does not guarantee doing the right thing, but it is a major first step. Pellegrino[24] suggested that quick self-examination on the effectiveness of one's therapeutic presence might be accomplished by answering these three questions **truthfully**:

1. **Do I listen and not only respond to but satisfy the fundamental questions each person who is ill and anxious brings to me?**

2. **Can I accept the patient for who they are, not for who I think they should be?**

3. **Can I manage my authority humanely to respect the patients' life and values?**

To be able to answer yes to any of these questions requires that we continue to grow as persons as we become HCPs. It behooves us to revisit Pellegrino's[24] self-examination questions as a reminder of the values of therapeutic presence, not only as we develop, but also as we mature as empathic, entrusted HCPs and self-monitor our values over the course of our careers and assure we do not need to change direction. Hopefully, you can find a mentor and/or trusted colleagues with whom you can debrief when needed. The value of a lifelong commitment to growth and increasing moral consciousness ensures a meaningful and peaceful professional as well as personal life.[24]

# AWARENESS THROUGH ACTIVITY

Most health care professions are adversely affected by lack of acculturation to the values of the health care disciplines.[25–27] In a retrospective study, Papadakis et al.[25] reported that 95% of the disciplinary actions taken by the state medical boards were linked with unprofessionalism exhibited in medical school. Hence, problem behaviors in medical school were directly associated with subsequent future disciplinary action by the state. In a subsequent study of three medical schools from 1990 to 2003, Papadakis et al.[28] found that 235 graduates were disciplined by medical state license boards. The disciplinary action was strongly associated with prior unprofessional behavior while in medical school. The most strongly linked unprofessional behaviors were severe irresponsibility, followed by diminished capacity for self-improvement; the practicing medical school graduates who were disciplined also demonstrated low scores on the admissions tests and poor grades in the first two years of medical school. Wynia et al.[26] stated that lists of desirable professional attributes and characteristics are incredibly important for education and to begin to understand the implications of values within the health professions that are needed for real-world practice, yet they are not by themselves sufficient. Even in the early phase of health professions education, the respect that is provided with the gift of a human cadaver is the opportunity to begin to demonstrate appropriate values and professionalism.[29]

In her Linda Crane Memorial Lecture entitled "Integrity: At the Heart of Our Profession," Frese,[30] focused on integrity related to professionalism, ethics, and core values, and associated professional responsibilities; she described the calling for developing HCPs:

> *Students are growing up in a society with declining ethical values, and we cannot expect students to have strongly developed moral behaviors. Unfortunately, students may see dishonest, unethical behavior in the world, as a normal part of life. Evidence supports a high correlation between academic cheating and deviant behavior in the workplace … our professional responsibility has increased even more with the growth of autonomous practice and the increased complexity of ethical situations … physical therapists must adhere to the rules and regulations of state and federal institutions, insurance companies, and employers, but they also are expected to deliver high-quality, patient-centered care. The emphasis on productivity, can conflict with quality, but it can also challenge the moral behavior of a therapist. With integrity being "at the heart of our profession" we must emphasize integrity in our professional education, and professional socialization. We cannot separate who we are from what we do.*

As future HCPs, we must first examine our own personal values before we can begin to ascribe to the values of our profession. It remains relevant that we are able to adjust to the values of our health care discipline so as to avoid the potentials for disciplinary actions that might range from loss of your professional license to fines and reprimands that may require restitution and, once again, supervised practice. We must also recognize the problematic behaviors in others and assist in their professional socialization.[31] We may need to reconcile our own personal values, such as embracing computerized technologies[32] and social media platforms[33] and/or the use of assistive technology,[34] with those that vary from the culture of the clinical practice arena. We may also need to be open to the values of our patients/clients, who may or may not be accepting of new technologies or cutting-edge research or accessibility to assistive technologies.[34] Reconciling our personal values, professional values, and the patients'/clients' values and beliefs, along with considerations of aspects of social justice, are paramount to the patients' experiences.[34] Many decisions we must make as HCPs are not value neutral,[34] and first knowing your own values is key. This is so you can best determine how to interface with the profession, the cultural values of the systems we work within, colleagues, and the people who are to be your patients and clients. Each of these people comes with their own values and belief systems and looks to you to provide appropriate clinical reasoning to effect a positive change in their preferred life.[30,33–39] Traits such as critical thinking, promoting and engaging in an active learning process, ethical practice, good communication skills, conveying professionalism, and responsibility for one's own actions are the skills that are predictive criteria for positive professional performance;[40] you cannot attain these without first knowing yourself and then being prepared to be flexible and adaptive in learning as you grow and change through your continued professional socialization and professional formation.

Hopefully, you are now motivated to examine your own values, self-assess, and realize the importance of professionalism and the implications of values for true reflective practice.[35] We will further examine the concepts of self-assessment and reflective practice in Chapter 10. The exercises at the end of this chapter are designed to help you further analyze important personal values you currently hold and to help you learn which of your values you regard more highly or what your highest order value is today. A visit to a clinic or patient care area (or reflection upon these), where you will be asked to make careful observations of behavior and to comment on the values that seem to underlie the setting and PPI interactions, will help sensitize you to the stresses of patient care and will illustrate various kinds of interactions that take place with patients. Finally, a forced-choice exercise will pull out some introjected values that you may not even be aware that you hold.

# REFERENCES

1. Rogers CR, Stevens B. *Person to Person: The Problem of Being Human*. Lafayette, CA: Real People Press; 1993.
2. 2021 National Healthcare Quality and Disparities Report. Content last reviewed January 2022. *Agency for Healthcare Research and Quality*, Rockville, MD. https://www.ahrq.gov/research/findings/nhqrdr/nhqdr21/index.html. Accessed September 13, 2022.
3. Morrill RL. *Teaching Values in College*. San Francisco, CA: Jossey-Bass; 1980.
4. Maslow A. *Motivation and Personality*. New York, NY: Harper and Row; 1954.
5. Beck C. A philosophical view of values and value education. In: Hennessy T, ed. *Values and Moral Development*. New York, NY: Paulist Press; 1976:13–23.
6. Davis CM. Influence of values on patient care: foundation for decision making. In: O'Sullivan S, Schmitz T, eds. *Foundations of Rehabilitation*. 2nd ed. Philadelphia, PA: FA Davis; 1988:31–37.
7. Mueller MJ, Rose SJ. Physical therapy director as professional value setter: a special communication. *Phys Ther.* 1987;67(9):1389–1392. doi: 10.1093/ptj/67.9.1389. PMID: 3628493.
8. Wehlage G, Lockwood AL. Moral relativism and values education. In Purpel D, Ryan K, eds. *Moral Education … It Comes With the Territory*. Berkeley, CA: McCutchen; 1976:334–335.
9. Hensel WA, Dickey NW. Teaching professionalism: passing the torch. *Acad Med.* 1998;73(8):865–870.
10. Cruess RL, Cruess SR, Boudreau SR, Donald J, Snell L, Steinert Y. Reframing medical education to support professional identity formation. *Acad Med.* 2014;89(11):1446–1451. doi: 10.1097/ACM.0000000000000427.
11. Sullivan KJ, Wallace JG Jr, O'Neil ME, Musolino GM, Mandich M, Studer MT, Bottomley JM, Cormack JC, Nicholson SK, Jensen GM. A vision for society: physical therapy as partners in the national health agenda. *Phys Ther.* 2011;91(11):1664–1672. doi: 10.2522/ptj.20100347.
12. Haugland BØ, Lassen, RM, Giske, T. Professional formation through personal involvement and value integration. *Nurse Educ Practice.* 2018;29:64–69.
13. Clark D, Wainwright S, Tschoepe BA, Green-Wilson J, Sebelski C, Zeigler S, McGinnis P. The relationship between professionalism and leadership: parent–child or sibling? *Phys Ther.* 2022;102(9):1022022, doi: 10.1093/ptj/pzac089.
14. Cruess RL, Cruess SR. Professionalism, communities of practice and medicine's social contract. *J Am Board Fam Med.* 2020;33S(S50–56); doi:10.3122/jabfm.2020.S1.190417.

15. Cruess SR, Cruess RL. Teaching professionalism—Why, what and how. *Facts Views Vis Obgyn.* 2012;4(4):259–265. PMID: 24753918; PMCID: PMC3987476.

16. Kolb ME. A sense of values: The 1965 Presidential Address. *Phys Ther.* 1965;45(9):870–876, doi: 10.1093/ptj/45.9.870.

17. *Core Values for the Physical Therapist and Physical Therapist Assistant.* American Physical Therapy Association. https://www.apta.org/apta-and-you/leadership-and-governance/policies/core-values-for-the-physical-therapist-and-physical-therapist-assistant Accessed July 13, 2024.

18. Peterson C, Seligman MEP. *Character Strengths and Virtues: A Handbook a Classification.* Washington, DC: American Psychological Association; 2004.

19. Raths LE, Harmin M, Simon S. *Values and Teaching.* Columbus, OH: Charles E. Merrill; 1966.

20. Gilligan C. *In a Different Voice: Psychological Theory and Women's Development.* Cambridge, MA: Harvard University Press; 2016.

21. Kohlberg L. The cognitive development approach to moral education. *Phi Delta Kappa.* 1975; June:670–677.

22. Piaget J. *The Construction of Reality in a Child.* New York, NY: Basic Books; 1954.

23. Gray J. *Men Are From Mars, Women Are From Venus: The Classic Guide to Understanding the Opposite Sex.* New York, NY: Harper Collins Publishing; 2012.

24. Pellegrino ED. Educating the humanist physician—an ancient ideal reconsidered. *JAMA.* 1974;227(11):1288–1294.

25. Papadakis MA, Hodgson CS, Teherani A, Kohatsu ND. Unprofessional behavior in medical school is associated with subsequent disciplinary action by a state medical board. *Acad Med.* 2004;79(3)224–229.

26. Wynia MK, Papadakis MA, Sullivan WM, Hafferty FW. More than a list of values and desired behaviors: a foundational understanding of medical professionalism. *Acad Med.* 2014;89(5):712–714.

27. Papadakis MA, Osborn EH, Cooke M, Healy K. A strategy for the detection and evaluation of unprofessional behavior in medical students. University of California, San Francisco School of Medicine Clinical Clerkships Operation Committee. *Acad Med.* 1999;74(9):980–990.

28. Papadakis MA, Teherani A, Banach MA, et al. Disciplinary action by medical boards and prior behavior in medical school. *N Engl J Med.* 2005;353(25):2673–2682.

29. Talarico EF Jr. A change in paradigm: giving back identity to donors in the anatomy laboratory. *Clin Anat.* 2013;26(2):161–172.

30. Frese E. *Integrity: at the heart of our profession.* Linda Crane Memorial Lecture presented: APTA Combined Sections Meeting; February 5, 2015; Indianapolis, IN.

31. Lowe DL, Gabard DL. Physical therapist student experiences with ethical and legal violations during clinical rotations: reporting and barriers to reporting. *J Phys Ther Educ.* 2014;28(3):98–111.

32. Foreman KB, Morton DA, Musolino GM, Albertine KH. Design and utility of a web-based computer-assisted instructional tool for neuroanatomy self-study and review for physical and occupational therapy graduate students. *Anat Rec B New Anat.* 2005;285(1):26–31.

33. Gagnon K, Sabus C. Professionalism in a digital age: opportunities and considerations for using social media in health care. *Phys Ther.* 2015;95(3):406–414.

34. Greenfield B, Musolino GM. Technology in rehabilitation: ethical and curricular implications for physical therapist education. *J Phys Ther Educ.* 2012;26(2):81–90.

35. Musolino GM. Fostering reflective practice: self-assessment abilities of physical therapy students and entry-level graduates. *J Allied Health.* 2006;35(1):30–42.

36. Rindflesch A, Hoverstien K, Patterson B, Thomas L, Dunfee H. Students' description of factors contributing to a meaningful clinical experience in entry-level physical therapist professional education. *Work.* 2013;44(3):265–274.

37. Wong CK, Driscoll M. A modified jigsaw method: an active learning strategy to develop the cognitive and affective domains through curricular review. *J Phys Ther Educ.* 2008; 22(1):15–23.

38. Noteboom JT, Allison SC, Cleland JA, Whitman JM. A primer on selected aspects of evidence-based practice relating to questions of treatment. Part 2: interpreting results, application to clinical practice, and self-evaluation. *J Orthop Sports Phys Ther.* 2008; 38(8):485–501.

39. Simoneau GG, Allison SC. Physical therapists as evidence-based diagnosticians. *J Orthop Sports Phys Ther.* 2010;10(40):-603–605.

40. Cook C, McCallum C, Musolino GM, Reiman M, Covington JK. What traits are reflective of positive professional performance in physical therapy program graduates? A Delphi Study. *J Allied Health.* 2018 Summer;47(2):96–102. PMID: 29868693.

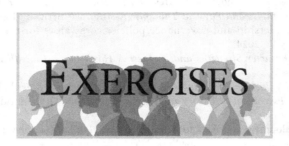

# EXERCISE 1: VALUES PRIORITY

This exercise takes place in four parts:

1. First, with each of the values listed in Step 1, indicate its degree of importance to you.
2. Then, list your five least and five most important values from this list.
3. Then, complete the Five-Sort Value Inventory.
4. Then, transfer the numbers from the Five-Sort Value Inventory to the Value Inventory Rating Summary.

## Step 1

Read through the complete list. This is not a semantics test, so feel free to cross out the definition and add your own if you wish. Then, circle each item's level of importance to you.

**Achievement (accomplishment; results brought by resolve, persistence, or endeavor)**
          Not very important         Important         Very important

**Aesthetics (appreciation and enjoyment of beauty for beauty's sake, in both arts and nature)**
          Not very important         Important         Very important

**Altruism (regard for or devotion to the interest of others; service to others)**
          Not very important         Important         Very important

**Autonomy (ability to be a self-determining individual; personal freedom; making own choices)**
          Not very important         Important         Very important

**Creativity (developing new ideas and designs; being innovative)**
          Not very important         Important         Very important

**Emotional well-being (peace of mind, inner security; ability to recognize and manage inner conflicts)**
          Not very important         Important         Very important

**Health (the condition of being sound in body)**
          Not very important         Important         Very important

**Honesty (being frank and genuinely yourself with everyone)**
          Not very important         Important         Very important

**Justice (treating others fairly or impartially; conforming to fact, truth, or reason)**
  Not very important  Important  Very important

**Knowledge (seeking truth, information, or principles for the satisfaction of curiosity)**
  Not very important  Important  Very important

**Love (want, caring; unselfish devotion that freely accepts another in loyalty and seeks the other's good)**
  Not very important  Important  Very important

**Loyalty (maintaining allegiance to a person, group, or institution)**
  Not very important  Important  Very important

**Morality (believing and keeping ethical standards; personal honor, integrity)**
  Not very important  Important  Very important

**Physical appearance (concern for one's attractiveness; being neat, clean, well-groomed)**
  Not very important  Important  Very important

**Pleasure (satisfaction, gratification, fun, joy)**
  Not very important  Important  Very important

**Power (possession of control, authority of influence over others)**
  Not very important  Important  Very important

**Recognition (being important, well-liked, accepted)**
  Not very important  Important  Very important

**Religious faith (having a religious belief; being in a relationship with God)**
  Not very important  Important  Very important

**Skill (being able to use one's knowledge effectively; being good at doing something important to me/others)**
  Not very important  Important  Very important

**Wealth (having many possessions and plenty of money to do anything desired)**
  Not very important  Important  Very important

**Wisdom (having mature understanding, insight, good sense, and judgment)**
  Not very important  Important  Very important

# Step 2

After completing Step 1, pick out and list in the spaces provided the five items that you feel are the most important to you and the five items that are the least important.

Five Most Important:
1.
2.
3.
4.
5.

Five Least Important:
1.
2.
3.
4.
5.

# Step 3—Five-Sort Value Inventory

The following are 21 sets of 5 values each. Within each set, rank the values from 1 (favorite value of the set) to 5 (least favorite value of the set).

1.  ( ) Achievement
    ( ) Altruism
    ( ) Justice
    ( ) Religious faith
    ( ) Wealth

2.  ( ) Altruism
    ( ) Autonomy
    ( ) Loyalty
    ( ) Power
    ( ) Recognition

3.  ( ) Creativity
    ( ) Love
    ( ) Pleasure
    ( ) Recognition
    ( ) Wealth

4.  ( ) Aesthetics
    ( ) Justice
    ( ) Pleasure
    ( ) Power
    ( ) Wisdom

5.  ( ) Altruism
    ( ) Honesty
    ( ) Love
    ( ) Physical appearance
    ( ) Wisdom

6.  ( ) Achievement
    ( ) Aesthetics
    ( ) Health
    ( ) Honesty
    ( ) Recognition

7.  ( ) Achievement
    ( ) Autonomy
    ( ) Physical appearance
    ( ) Pleasure
    ( ) Skill

8.  ( ) Autonomy
    ( ) Emotional well-being
    ( ) Health
    ( ) Wealth
    ( ) Wisdom

9.  ( ) Honesty
    ( ) Knowledge
    ( ) Power
    ( ) Skill
    ( ) Wealth

10. ( ) Achievement
    ( ) Emotional well-being
    ( ) Love
    ( ) Morality
    ( ) Power

11. ( ) Aesthetics
    ( ) Autonomy
    ( ) Knowledge
    ( ) Love
    ( ) Religious faith

12. ( ) Aesthetics
    ( ) Loyalty
    ( ) Morality
    ( ) Physical appearance
    ( ) Wealth

13. ( ) Creativity
    ( ) Health
    ( ) Physical appearance
    ( ) Power
    ( ) Religious faith

14. ( ) Health
    ( ) Justice
    ( ) Love
    ( ) Loyalty
    ( ) Skill

15. ( ) Aesthetics
    ( ) Altruism
    ( ) Creativity
    ( ) Emotional well-being
    ( ) Skill

16. ( ) Emotional well-being
    ( ) Justice
    ( ) Knowledge
    ( ) Physical appearance
    ( ) Recognition

17. ( ) Altruism
    ( ) Health
    ( ) Knowledge
    ( ) Morality
    ( ) Pleasure

18. ( ) Morality
    ( ) Recognition
    ( ) Religious faith
    ( ) Skill
    ( ) Wisdom

19. ( ) Emotional well-being
    ( ) Honesty
    ( ) Loyalty
    ( ) Pleasure
    ( ) Religious faith

20. ( ) Achievement
    ( ) Creativity
    ( ) Knowledge
    ( ) Loyalty
    ( ) Wisdom

21. ( ) Autonomy
    ( ) Creativity
    ( ) Honesty
    ( ) Justice
    ( ) Morality

# *Step 4—Value Inventory Rating Summary*

To summarize the results in Step 3, begin entering the numbers you recorded for the first set of five values in the first box of each of those values below. Each value occurs five times, so when you are through recording all 21 sets of five values, you will have five entries for each value. Add those five numbers across. The Totals column will then give you some ideas of the respective weights you give to the values involved. Remember, the lower the number in the Totals column, the higher that value ranks in your priorities.

| | | | | | | TOTALS |
|---|---|---|---|---|---|---|
| Achievement | | | | | | |
| Aesthetics | | | | | | |
| Altruism | | | | | | |
| Autonomy | | | | | | |
| Creativity | | | | | | |
| Emotional well-being | | | | | | |
| Health | | | | | | |
| Honesty | | | | | | |
| Justice | | | | | | |
| Knowledge | | | | | | |
| Love | | | | | | |
| Loyalty | | | | | | |
| Morality | | | | | | |
| Physical appearance | | | | | | |
| Pleasure | | | | | | |
| Power | | | | | | |
| Recognition | | | | | | |
| Religious faith | | | | | | |
| Skill | | | | | | |
| Wealth | | | | | | |
| Wisdom | | | | | | |

Top three values:

1.

2.

3.

Are you surprised? If yes, why? If no, why not?

# EXERCISE 2: ENVIRONMENTAL CRISIS

This is another exercise designed to help you learn more about the values you learned at home, some of which you may not have given much thought but accept as true and often believe that everyone accepts them as true.

## The Situation

You are a young HCP in a moderately sized metropolitan hospital that has an entire unit devoted to the care of patients with kidney disease. The kidney unit can accommodate five people at a time on dialysis and is the only unit within a 500-mile radius that has dialysis capability. At times, there are scheduling difficulties, at which time a committee is called together to help resolve decisions of priority. The committee is made up of health personnel from the hospital and community and of laypeople from the community. You are on that committee.

The community in which you live and work has had a crisis. A toxin has leaked into the water supply for the city and has made more than half of the citizens terribly ill. Those most vulnerable to the toxin are people with kidney disease. Ten people are near death (within 1 hour) unless their blood is dialyzed. There are only five machines.

The committee has been called together to decide who should receive priority. It is impossible to save the lives of all the victims, but you must make the decision of which five will be saved.

Your group has only minimal chart information about the ten people, and 30 minutes to make the decision. Your group realizes that there is no alternative to making this choice if five people are to be saved. With no decision, all ten people will die.

Here is what you know about the ten people:

1. Bookkeeper, 31-year-old man
2. Bookkeeper's wife, 30 years old, 6 months pregnant
3. Second-year medical student, man, African American
4. Famous historian and author, 41-year-old woman
5. Hollywood actress/actor, 50 years old
6. Biochemist, 35-year-old woman
7. Rabbi, 54-year-old man
8. Olympic athlete, shot put, 19-year-old man
9. College student majoring in health profession other than medicine, woman
10. Owner of a topless bar, 56-year-old man, prison record

## Instructions

1. Read the situation carefully.
2. Working alone, decide which five people are to go on dialysis. You have 10 minutes to make your personal decision.
3. At the instructor's signal, join with three others in the room and, working as a group of four, decide on the five people to receive dialysis. You have only 20 minutes to make your decision. Argue strongly for your ideas and opinions. The future of these people's lives depends on your group decision. Make sure that your group is satisfied with the final list. Agree with other group members only if they truly convince you that their idea is better than yours.
4. Decisions by majority vote are not permitted. Every member of your group must agree with, and be committed to, the decision.
5. Group discussion: At the end of 30 minutes, one member of each group comes forward and places a mark in the data summary box on the board in the front of the room. Discuss as a group.
   a. Why did you decide on each person? What were the assumptions you made that convinced you and others of the worth of each person's life?

b. What process did you go through to decide? Once you accepted the responsibility for the decision, was it difficult to decide on the final five? Who in the group was most convincing? How vocal were you in arguing for what you felt was right?

c. What values emerged as you decided on the worth of a person's life and the opportunity for that person to continue living? Where did those values come from? When your decision was challenged, were you surprised that someone placed a different value higher than yours? Or did you assume that most everyone would agree with you?

d. After reflecting for a few minutes, comment on this exercise and what it teaches us about the nature of stereotype, labeling, and prejudice. How might this affect our decisions as clinicians?

e. Did everyone agree that every life has equal value and therefore suggest a lottery? How do you feel about that idea?

| GROUP | 1 | 2 | 3 | 4 | 5 | 6 | 7 | TOTAL |
|---|---|---|---|---|---|---|---|---|
| Bookkeeper | | | | | | | | |
| Bookkeeper's wife | | | | | | | | |
| Medical student | | | | | | | | |
| Historian/author | | | | | | | | |
| Hollywood actress/actor | | | | | | | | |
| Biochemist | | | | | | | | |
| Rabbi | | | | | | | | |
| Olympic athlete | | | | | | | | |
| Health profession student | | | | | | | | |
| Topless bar owner | | | | | | | | |

Journal about what you felt as you completed the exercise and what you learned about yourself with regard to what you believe is true and worthwhile and what you learned about your style of arguing for what you believe in. What are you feeling? Compare and contrast how you approached this situation vs. how the Covid-19 pandemic was handled in the distribution of life-saving vaccinations.

# EXERCISE 3: CLINICAL FIELD TRIP

This is an exercise designed to deepen your understanding of the nature of health care behavior and, specifically, of patient–practitioner interaction. Read over the questions below carefully and then visit a facility where patients are being treated by HCPs from the profession you have chosen. Visit as an observer only, and carefully make observations, from which you will respond to the questions asked. Once the questions are answered, journal about what you learned and felt with this experience.

1. What pleased you about what you saw?

2. What bothered you?

3. How did this experience impact your choice to be a HCP?

## Clinical Interaction Observation

1. Observe the environment. Describe how things are ordered and how things appear, and comment on possible underlying values.

2. Is efficiency a value? How do the HCPs perform or function in relation to a wise use of time?

The patient–practitioner relationship is one of the major factors that affects the success of treatment. This relationship is based on the establishment of sound, professional judgment. No two practitioners approach a patient in exactly the same manner. With experience, you will develop your own personal style of rapport. By observing interactions between experienced HCPs and their patients, you will be better prepared to form your own approach to patient–practitioner interaction.

Use the following questions as a guide to direct your attention to specific aspects of patient treatment. You will be concerned primarily with the verbal and nonverbal communication that exists between the HCP and patient.

## Attending Skills

1. What did the HCP do to attend to the patient's personal needs and/or comfort before, during, and after treatment?

2. How did the HCP maintain the patient's dignity during treatment?

3. Did the HCP seem to really listen to the patient's description of their illness/disability as it is lived by that person?

# *Communication Skills*

## NONVERBAL BEHAVIOR

1. Did the HCP exhibit any personal mannerisms/behavior that might have added to or detracted from gaining the patient's confidence?

2. Could you explain why any additional behaviors might have been effective?

3. Was the HCP a good listener? What behaviors make you say that?

4. Did the HCP maintain eye contact while talking with the patient? If not, did it seem to detract?

5. Were the HCP and patient at the same eye level for most of the time? Comment.

## VERBAL BEHAVIOR

1. Describe and comment on the HCP's voice quality as they communicated with the patient (soft-spoken, brusque, rapid, etc.).

2. How did the HCP seem to motivate the patient? Was the method effective?

# *Summary*

1. What impressed you most about your visit?

2. What impressed you least?

3. What did you learn that you did not know before?

(Adapted from material developed by Marilyn DeMont Philips, MS, PT, at that time Assistant Professor, Sargent College, Boston University and retired, following 20 years as Director of Professional Development, American Physical Therapy Association. She served on the Parkinson's Disease Foundation Advisory Council as a research advocate and volunteer ensuring PDF grants meet patient needs.)

# APPENDIX

## BLOOM'S TAXONOMIES: AFFECTIVE, COGNITIVE, AND PSYCHOMOTOR LEARNING DOMAINS

## Bloom's Taxonomy: Affective Domain

**Affective domain:** emotional response concerning one's attitudes, values and appreciation for motivation in learning

**Characterization**
Value that will control the outcome and behaviour

**Organization**
Intergrating and comparing values, ordering them according to priorities

**Valuing**
Finds value and worth in one's learing and is motivated to continue

**Responding**
Actively participating and engaging to transfer knowledge

**Receiving**
Being willing to listen and be aware to receive knowledge

| Receiving | Responding | Valuing | Organization | Characterization |
|---|---|---|---|---|
| acknowledge | agree to | accept | adapt | act |
| ask | answer | approve | arrange | arrange |
| attend | ask | complete | categorize | behave |
| choose | assist | choose | classify | characterize |
| describe | clarify | commit | compare | defend |
| follow | communicate | describe | complete | display |
| give | contribute | debate | defend | exemplify |
| identify | cooperate | demonstrate | explain | function |
| listen | discuss | differentiate | establish | incorporate |
| name | help | explain | formulate | influence |
| reply | indicate | establish | generate | justify |
| select | inquire | identify | identify | listen |
| | participate | initiate | integrate | maintain |
| | question | justify | modify | modify |
| | | prepare | order | practice |
| | | refute | prepare | perform |
| | | | rank | preserve |
| | | | relate | propose |
| | | | | question |
| | | | | revise |

Developed by the Centre of Teaching Excellence, University of Waterloo
**References:** Krathwohl, D.R., Bloom, B.S., and Masia, B.B. (1964). *Taxonomy of Educational Objectives: The Classification of Educational Goals. Handbook II: Affective Domain.* New York: David McKay Company University of Mississippi School of Education. (2007). Bloom's Taxonomy: Affective Domain. Retrieved from: http://www.olemiss.edu/depts/educ school2/docs/stai manual/manual9.htm

| | Receiving | Responding | Valuing | Organization | Characterization |
|---|---|---|---|---|---|
| **Learning Activities** | • Attend focus groups<br>• Listen as audience to a presentation<br>• Read articles/papers/ textbooks<br>• Watch a video | • Active participating in classroom activities<br>• Brainstorm ideas<br>• Group discussions<br>• Present in front of audience<br>• Problem solving activities<br>• Role-play<br>• Written assignments (essays, reports etc.) | • Debates<br>• Opinionated writing piece<br>• Reflection exercises (reflection paper)<br>• Self-report | • Analyze and contrast (with charts, tables, Venn diagrams)<br>• Concept map (report formal and informal experiences and identify skills) | • Critical reflection<br>• Group projects<br>• Self-report goals (personally and academically) |
| **Assessments** | • Feedback forms<br>• Fill-in-the-blanks<br>• Knowledge survey<br>• List<br>• Match<br>• Memory tests<br>• One-minute paper<br>• Qualitative interviews<br>• Test activities (recall and verbalize reactions)<br>• Write summary on key points of presentation | • Answer questions<br>• Ability to follow procedures<br>• Critical questioning<br>• Feedback and peer evaluation<br>• One-minute paper<br>• Questionnaires<br>• Willingness to participate | • Attendance<br>• Neatness and carefulness (with minimal errors) of submitted work<br>• Meet deadlines<br>• Proposals of new plans<br>• Questionnaire<br>• Rating scale<br>• Reflection piece<br>• Report on extra-curricular activities<br>• Ungraded paper | • Develop realistic aspirations<br>• Prioritize time to meet goals<br>• Focus groups<br>• Questionnaires<br>• Ability to solve new problems | • Criteria for group projects<br>• Self-evaluation<br>• SMART goals |

Developed by the Centre of Teaching Excellence, University of Waterloo
**References:** Krathwohl, D.R., Bloom, B.S., and Masia, B.B. (1964). *Taxonomy of Educational Objectives: The Classification of Educational Goals. Handbook II: Affective Domain.* New York: David McKay Company University of Mississippi School of Education. (2007). Bloom's Taxonomy: Affective Domain. Retrieved from: http://www.olemiss.edu/depts/educ school2/docs/stai manual/manual9.htm

## Bloom's Taxonomy: Cognitive Domain

**Cognitive domain:** intellecutal skills and abilites required for learning, thinking critically and problem solving

**Create**
Compile information to generate new solutions

arrange
calculate
compose
construct
design
develop
devise
formulate
generate
hypothesize
plan
prepare
produce
propose
revise
summarize
synthesize

**Evaluate**
Make judgements based on evidence found

attribute
argue
assess
check
compare
conclude
contrast
criticize
critique
defend
examine
justify
measure
recommend
support
reflect

**Analyze**
Break down information to look at relationships

categorize
contrast
compare
criticize
debate
differentiate
experiment
inspect
infer
investigate
organize
outline
question
separate
test

**Apply**
Apply knowledge to different situations

calculate
complete
demonstrate
execute
illustrate
implement
modify
organize
practice
prepare
solve
show
use
write

**Understand**
Translate and interpret knowledge

compare
classify
describe
discuss
explain
give examples
interpret
paraphrase
predict
present
report
rewrite
summarize

**Remember**
Retain, recall and recognize knowledge

arrange
define
identify
indicate
label
list
match
memorize
recall
recite
recognize

Developed by the Centre for Teaching Excellence, University of Waterloo
References: Anderson, L., & Krathwohl, D. A. (2001). *Taxonomy for learning, teaching and assessing: A revision of Bloom's Taxonomy of Educational Objectives.* New York: Longman.
IUPUI Center of Teaching and Learning. (2006). Bloom's Taxonomy "Revised" Key Words, Model Questions, & Instructional Strategies. Retrieved from: www.center.iupui.edu/ctl/idd/docs/Bloom_revised021.doc

| | Remember | Undestand | Apply | Analyze | Evaluate | Create |
|---|---|---|---|---|---|---|
| **Learning Activities** | • Flashcards<br>• Highlight key words<br>• List<br>• Memory activities<br>• Reading materials<br>• Watching presentations and videos | • Case studies<br>• Concept map<br>• Demonstrations<br>• Diagrams<br>• Flowcharts<br>• Group discussions<br>• Mind map<br>• Matrix activity<br>• Play/sketches<br>• Summarize<br>• Think-pair-share | • Calculate<br>• Case studies<br>• Concept map<br>• Creating examples<br>• Demonstrations<br>• Flipped classroom<br>• Gallery walk<br>• Gamification<br>• Group work<br>• Lab experiments<br>• Map<br>• Problem-solving tasks<br>• Short answers<br>• Role play | • Case studies<br>• Compare and contrast (with charts, tables, Venn diagrams)<br>• Concept map<br>• Debates<br>• Discussions<br>• Flowchart<br>• Graph<br>• Group<br>• Investigation<br>• Mind map<br>• Questionnaires<br>• Report/survey<br>• Think-pair-share | • Debates<br>• Compare and contrast (with charts, tables, Venn diagrams)<br>• Concept map<br>• Journal<br>• Pros and cons list<br>• Mind map<br>• Review paper | • Brainstorm<br>• Decision-making tasks<br>• Develop and describe new solutions or plans<br>• Design project<br>• Performances<br>• Presentations<br>• Research projects<br>• Written assignment |
| | • Clicker questions<br>• Fill in the blanks<br>• Label<br>• Match<br>• Multiple choice<br>• Quizzes<br>• True and false questions | • Concept map<br>• Create a summary<br>• Essay<br>• Diagrams<br>• Infographics<br>• Matrix activity<br>• One-minute paper<br>• Presentation<br>• Provide examples<br>• Quizzes<br>• Short answers | • Discussion board post<br>• E-portfolio<br>• Lab reports<br>• One-minute paper<br>• Presentation<br>• Problem-solving tasks<br>• Short answers | • Analysis paper<br>• Case study<br>• Evaluation criteria<br>• Critique hypothesis, procedures etc.<br>• Muddiest point<br>• One-minute paper<br>• Research paper<br>• Review paper | • Argumentative or persuasive essay<br>• Debates<br>• Discussions<br>• Presentation<br>• Provide alternative solutions<br>• Report | • Develop criteria to evaluate product or solution<br>• Grant proposal<br>• Outline alternative solutions<br>• Research proposal |

Developed by the Centre for Teaching Excellence, University of Waterloo
References: Anderson, L., & Krathwohl, D. A. (2001). *Taxonomy for learning, teaching and assessing: A revision of Bloom's Taxonomy of Educational Objectives.* New York: Longman.
IUPUI Center of Teaching and Learning. (2006). Bloom's Taxonomy "Revised" Key Words, Model Questions, & Instructional Strategies. Retrieved from: www.center.iupui.edu/ctl/idd/docs/Bloom_revised021.doc

**Bloom's Taxonomy: Psychomotor Domain**

**Psychomotor Domain:** ability to use motor skills that includes physical movement, reflex and coordination to develop techinques in execution, in accuracy and time

**Set**
How ready one is to act (physically, mentally and spiritually)

arranges
begins
demonstrates
displays
explains
moves
prepares
proceeds
reacts
responds
shows
states

**Guided Response**
Beginner level, learns through trial and error by practicing

assembles
attempts
builds
copies
follows
imitates
reacts
reproduces
responds
traces
tries

**Mechanism**
Intermediate level, develops proficiency and action becomes habitual

assembles
constructs
dismantles
displays
fastens
fixes
grinds
measures
mends
mixes
organizes
sketches

**Complex Over Response**
Expert level, high proficiency and performs with accuracy

assembles
builds
calibrates
constructs
dismantles
displays
fastens
fixes
grinds
heats
measures
mends
mixes
organizes
operates
performs
sketches

**Adaptation**
Skills strongly developed and can be modified in different situations

adapts
alters
changes
modifes
rearranges
reorganizes
revise
varies

**Origination**
Create new procedures and solutions to approach various situations

arranges
builds
combines
composes
constructs
creates
designs
formulates
initiates
makes
modifies
originates
re-designs

**References:** Clark. D.R. (1999) Bloom's Taxonomy: The Psychomotor Domain. Retrieved from http://www.nwlink.com/~donclark/hrd/Bloom/psychomotor domain.html
Simpson, E.J. (1966). *The Classifications of Educational Objectives, Psychomotor Domain.* University of Illinois. Urbana, Illinois.

| | Set | Guided Response | Mechanism | Complex Over Response | Adaptation | Origination |
|---|---|---|---|---|---|---|
| **Learning Activities** | • Attend project exhibition<br>• Cognitive rehearsal of a physical task<br>• Observe demonstrations through audio, videos, visuals<br>• Listen to music<br>• Prepare blueprints and designs for construction<br>• Set-up and warm-up before exercise<br>• Set-up machine<br>• Set-up lab equipment for experiments | • Complete training<br>• Experiment using new tools/instruments through trial and error<br>• Follow manual to run and program machine<br>• Games and hands-on activities<br>• Use new tools by following demonstrations or being guided by mentor | • Perform gross motor movements (ex. dead lift, squats etc.)<br>• Practice instruments and use controlled movements<br>• Program and practice running machines<br>• Practice using equipment | • Control and use correct movements when playing instruments<br>• Final projects<br>• Operate and run machines efficiently (ex. drill press, band saw, pump etc.)<br>• Perform fine movements (ex. Adjust stopcock of a burette)<br>• Use equipment with confidence | • Control fine movement changes required for music dynamics and style<br>• Field-trips<br>• Strategic games<br>• Revise and improve procedures of movements<br>• Use tools for situations outside typical discipline | • Creates own choreography<br>• Create own process in executing physical tasks<br>• Strategically creates own workout plans |
| **Assessments** | • Pre-lab assessment<br>• Self-criteria<br>• Summary of demonstration and set-up process | • Evaluate accuracy with criteria on standard performance<br>• Give feedback | • Performance test (performance indicators)<br>• Self-evaluation on performance (based on progress and confidence) | • Clinical exams<br>• Final project (ex. Create project exhibition)<br>• Performance | • Assess and evaluate outcomes<br>• Self-criteria | • Assess and evaluate outcomes<br>• Rubric<br>• Self-criteria |

**References:** Clark. D.R. (1999) Bloom's Taxonomy: The Psychomotor Domain. Retrieved from http://www.nwlink.com/~donclark/hrd/Bloom/psychomotor domain.html
Simpson, E.J. (1966). *The Classifications of Educational Objectives, Psychomotor Domain.* University of Illinois. Urbana, Illinois.

These exercises are also available online at www.routledge.com/9781638220039.

# 4

# IDENTIFYING AND RESOLVING MORAL DILEMMAS

*Gina Maria Musolino and Carol M. Davis*

## OBJECTIVES

*The learner should be able to*:

- Analyze professional ethics that guide the health professions.

- Differentiate ethical situations, ethical problems, moral temptation, and true ethical dilemmas.

- Compare manners and etiquette with ethics and distinguish the continuum between moral obligations and nonmoral obligations as health care professionals (HCPs).

- Examine research that explores ethical and moral decision making in developing and licensed HCPs in everyday practice.

- Differentiate the numerous factors to consider in making sound ethical decisions.

- Compare discursive or principled ethical reasoning processes with nondiscursive aspects of ethical reasoning.

- Contrast the difficulties inherent in using the principles and rules of traditional biomedical, ethical reasoning alone in resolving dilemmas.

- Deconstruct the Realm–Individual Process–Situation (RIPS) model and Applied Ethics Model with individual, organizational, and societal dilemmas.

- Develop *active engagement* for ethical problem solving to incorporate traditional discursive ethical reasoning with nondiscursive elements, such as story, virtue, discernment, and meta-beliefs.

*Ethics* is the study of morality or moral behavior and moral principles. *Moral decisions* are decisions about what is right and wrong or better and best to do in a situation. *Descriptive ethics* discusses the moral systems of a group or culture; *normative ethics* deals with establishing a moral system that people can use to make moral decisions, and *meta-ethics* is the study of moral thoughts and moral language, the meanings of ethical terms and ethics itself.[1]

*Bioethics*, or *biomedical ethics*, is the application of ethics to health care. To reiterate, according to the American Nurses Association, *ethics* are "a theoretical and reflective domain of human knowledge that addresses issues and questions about morality in human choices, actions, character and ends,"[2(xii)] while the *applied* ethics of HCPs are about considering what is wrong versus what is right while using clinical judgment for clinical decision making.[2-4]

DOI: 10.4324/9781003525554-4

Ethics are not only described by their type, but also by the setting in which decisions are made, for example, organizational or systems.

Why should HCPs have to consider the ethical? HCPs are faced with many decisions each day. Professionals must interrelate professional ethics with clinical judgments to make clinical decisions frequently and daily. Most HCPs place immense importance on making sound clinical or therapeutic decisions in practice. At times, the legal ramifications of a clinical decision become apparent, but less seldom do HCPs consider the ethical or moral implications of decisions unless they come face to face with a difficult moral dilemma that is not easy to resolve with confidence. Perhaps Mark Twain's thoughts best summarize the inherent challenges: "It is curious that physical courage should be so common in the world, and moral courage so rare." Do you believe this holds true today? Why or why not?

## ETHICAL DECISIONS APPERTAIN TO CLINICAL DECISION-MAKING

Whereas clinical decisions are based on weighing and considering facts (e.g., given these laboratory values and these symptoms, the diagnosis is likely to be X), moral decisions are based on weighing and considering values, so there is no such thing as a true or false moral decision. However, just as it is incredibly important for HCPs to make the right clinical decision, it is assumed that practitioners would rather act ethically than not, choosing the highest or best moral alternative in a value-laden dilemma.

Clinical decisions, no matter how purely factual they seem, still deal with people making decisions about what is best and true for other people. Few clinical decisions, especially those that deal with integrative or alternative treatment choices, are void of a moral component because most clinical decisions necessitate weighing the value of various outcomes. Different people may place varying importance on the values aspects of any decision.[5] Value-laden ethical decisions, like factual clinical decisions, are better made if they are made thoughtfully and rationally, not based solely on intuition or the emotion of the moment.

## MANNERS ARE MINOR MORAL BEHAVIORS

The value-laden decisions we make at any one moment in the clinical setting can be analyzed as stemming from two main circumstances. Genuinely moral situations, which we discussed in Chapter 3, are those situations pertaining to how we interact with our fellow humans vs. nonmoral choices or value preferences, which relate more to social convention and personal predilection.

But the social and cultural rules that can be observed in patient care settings often have grown up around moral choices while working with patients and colleagues. A common example would be the rules around dress and appearance, which can be directly associated on a continuum of individual preference to responses to one's appearance and attire that lead to trust, comfort, and confidence (or its opposite). For example, students who push professional dress code and appearance regulations by wearing attire more suited to leisure may risk losing patients' respect and trust.

Mueller[6] made the excellent point that often "the lines between etiquette, laws, and ethics are difficult to distinguish, leaving the individual to decide the best course of action." Proper behavior in the professional cultural setting often must be learned in much the same way that we learned manners and rules in our families (Chapter 2). Many of the habitual behaviors will be in direct conflict in the patient health care delivery settings, and some could be determined to be unethical or immoral (e.g., accepting a large gift from a grateful patient without realizing the ethical ramifications of this, texting one's friends or family while supervising a patient carrying out an exercise program, or leaving a patient abruptly because you put in your time for the day).

The professions mandate moral behaviors in a way that occupations do not. A clinical decision that results in *not* putting the patient first—or, in moral language, not showing *beneficence*—doing good or the best for the patient— must be able to be justified only on the grounds that there is a higher competing value. Let's examine the various ethical situations that call for decisions by HCPs.

## ETHICAL SITUATIONS, PROBLEMS, AND DILEMMAS

There are three major kinds of ethical decision-making opportunities in clinical practice: *ethical situations*, *ethical problems*, and *ethical dilemmas*. Ethical situations contain important values or duties but require no problem solving or difficult decision making, but ethical action may be part of the situation. Many ethical decisions are simple to solve. In the same or comparable situation, most people would do the same thing, say, in deciding between good and evil (e.g., refusing to assist—or trying to prevent—a depressed person from taking their own life).

Then there are ethical problems. *Ethical temptations* fall into this category, where we know what we should do but do not want to do it, often because we stand to profit, or self-interest takes precedence over doing good for others (or beneficence). Another kind of ethical problem is *ethical distress*, where we know what we would like to do but are prohibited or constrained from doing it by organizational policies and procedures (e.g., you want to have your patient seen on a Sunday before discharge, but institutional policy does not allow patient care on Sundays) or societal laws or rules (e.g., you would like to be able to treat your Medicare patients, but you are prohibited from seeing them and charge for providing services because you do not have a Centers for Medicare and Medicaid Services, National Provider Identifier number).

Ethical dilemmas, more difficult ethical decisions, deal with which is better, and which is worse—do I continue to treat (and bill) a terminally ill patient even when my treatment is of little benefit for their impairments, and functional limitations, but my visit seems to make a substantial difference in the quality of the patient's existence? This example might be seen to be a struggle between the ethical principles of beneficence (contribute to the good of each patient) and *distributive justice* (just distribution of limited resources to those who would benefit most). Ethical thinking is initiating when one asks *why* something is considered bad or good.

The choice of the right thing to do is not only very unclear, but acting on one moral conviction can mean breaking another.[1] For example, as a physical therapist, if I act on behalf of my patient recovering from a traumatic brain injury, who is emerging from a coma state, yet in a plateau phase, and document in the medical record that the patient is still progressing with physical therapy, I am not telling the truth because the patient is not in a stage of progression. However, if I tell the truth, the best interests of my patient are compromised because the third-party insurance reimbursement may be justified to be withdrawn, and the patient may not be able to pay for therapy and then, in my professional opinion, the patient will regress. This illustrates a dilemma where beneficence—acting in the best interest of my patient—means breaking a moral conviction to tell the truth. Which is the higher moral alternative? How do I decide?

Some would say that the most difficult of all moral decisions in health care have to do with allocation of scarce resources. Examples to consider are the scarcity of patient ventilators early on during the Covid-19 pandemic and the lack and provision of proper personal protective equipment (PPE) for health care providers. Who deserves to receive help, and on what do we base our decision?[5]

# WHAT DO WE DO WHEN FACED WITH NOT KNOWING WHAT TO DO?

When faced with an ethical decision, what choices do we have? We could ignore it, follow our ideas or perceptions of current custom (what everyone else would do in this situation), ask our superior what to do, search for a policy that speaks to our problem or a rule to follow, do what feels emotionally best or right, follow our perception of the dictates of our religion, follow our perception of the dictates of our family rules, or apply traditional methods of ethical dilemma resolution in the search for the best moral alternative.[5] Bioethicists advocate for the best moral alternatives; unfortunately, many HCPs elect the former alternatives and hope for the best.[7]

Ethical dilemma resolution has not received the same attention in professional curricula that clinical decision making has received. Teaching developing HCPs how to decide the best moral alternative remains challenging, as there is no one principle that binds us, and there is no absolute dictum against which we can measure the adequacy of our moral choice as being best.

# BIOMEDICAL ETHICS VERSUS EVERYDAY ETHICS

What issues come to mind when we speak of biomedical ethics or health care ethical decisions? The media favors reporting life-and-death moral dilemmas that deal with issues that reflect the increasing impact of high technology on health care (e.g., organ transplants, fetal tissue research, euthanasia, genetic engineering, and abortion). Granted, these ethical dilemmas are important, and we all benefit from studying the ethical treatment given these issues from ethicists who help direct us in our own decision making. Our task is to read the various arguments and decide which argument and conclusion seem to match our own evaluation of the best alternative in terms of logical soundness and consistency and what we feel in our hearts is the highest moral alternative.

Many bioethicists would tell us that our hearts should have nothing to do with this problem solving because our hearts contaminate our reasoning with subjectivity that cannot be substantiated with logic.[8] This would seem more acceptable if we were robots dealing with robots. Because we are people—HCPs dealing with everyday issues of deciding the best thing to do for people, our patients, as well as their families—it is impossible for many of us to find comfort solely in the rationalistic, discursive resolving of dilemmas according to principles alone. The compelling facts of each situation, our own personal priorities, our personal knowledge of the individuals and situation involved, and our own personal integrity developed over time by making decisions and weighing the consequences will all come into play to help us decide which is the best decision in this situation with the limited information we have in that moment.

The ethical dilemmas we face day to day have to do with trying to do the best thing for our patients within the organization or institution of health care delivery, created mainly to meet the needs of vast numbers of people, not necessarily individuals. These dilemmas often have to do with maintaining or improving the quality of a single patient's life. In discussing quality of life in the nursing home, Kane and Caplan[9] said it this way:

> *In one sense the disproportion of time and energy spent discussing transplants, artificial hearts, and other issues of high technology, acute care medicine, is appropriate. Matters of when and whether life should be maintained are of fundamental ethical importance, but the seemingly small stakes involved in the nursing home context—setting mealtimes and bedtimes, use of the phone, the right to keep personal property in one's nightstand—should not lull anyone into thinking that daily life in a nursing home lacks either ethical content or importance.*

The content of ethical concerns in health care parallels shifting cultural mores and values. A survey of the most common ethical issues faced by physical therapists in New England listed issues such as which patients should be treated, the obligations entailed by that decision, who should pay for treatment, and what duties are incumbent on physical therapists as they relate to physicians and other professionals.[10]

Triezenberg[11] published data which indicated that there was a shift in the most common ethical issues toward concerns about overutilization, supervision of support personnel, informed consent, protection of patients' rights to confidentiality, justification of appropriate fees, truth in advertising, preventing sexual misconduct and abuse, maintaining clinical competence and ethical guidelines for the use of human subjects in research, and inappropriate endorsement of equipment and products by physical therapists. A panel of experts listed what they felt would be future ethical issues and included responses of physical therapists to environmental issues of pollutants and health hazards associated with specific treatment modalities (e.g., the effects of fluoromethane sprays on the ozone layer), employment discrimination, duty of physical therapists to report misconduct in colleagues, defining the limits of personal relationships in physical therapy, encroachment on practice, use of treatments not validated by research, use of advertising, and sexual and physical abuse of patients by physical therapists and those whom they supervise.[11]

The actual retrospective data analysis of physical therapist professional liability claims was elucidated by a claims study[12] examining the decade of the mid-1990s to the mid-2000s. Claims were made in all practice settings, most frequently in hospitals and patient homes, followed by nursing homes, schools, and outpatient service areas. The most frequently cited injury claims were: trauma, including fractures; burns; delayed recovery; not providing additional needed procedures; injury; loss of limb use; abrasions/lacerations; emotional distress; bruises and contusions; and sprains and strains. The most frequently claimed (7% to 15%) primary allegations were: failure to supervise treatments and procedures; injury during manipulation; improper techniques; injury due to heat therapies; and injury during stretching or exercise. Less frequently (4% to 5%) cited primary allegations were: failure to monitor the patient; improper management of the course of treatment; injury during electrotherapy; and inappropriate behavior by the clinician, including physical, sexual, or emotional abuse/misconduct. These were followed by even less frequent (< 2% to 3%) primary allegations claimed of: improper use of equipment; equipment malfunction or failure; improper performance of a test; injury during passive range of motion; and improper positioning. Even less frequently cited (< 1% to 2%) were primary allegations of: failure to refer/seek consultation; injury from cold therapies, manipulation, or massage; failure to report patients' changed condition(s); and injury during traction. Even less frequently cited (< 1%), yet no less relevant to point out, were allegations of: failure to maintain proper infection control; failure to follow established policy; failure to diagnose; breach of confidentiality/privacy; inadequate record keeping/documentation; failure to treat; lack of informed consent; and failure to respond to the patient.[12] HCPs are encouraged to be mindful of the primary claim concerns as a matter of ethical obligation and safety and obligation to **first do no harm.**

Because the provision of health care remains a hands-on profession, the need to continue to seek informed consent, not just initially, and educate your patients/clients, as therapeutic touch evolves during care, is continually reemphasized based on the prior claims alleged and in the suggested self-assessment for risk management. However, HCPs must not forgo high touch with the high tech merely due to fear of litigation. Establishing an appropriate therapeutic presence in our patient–practitioner interaction (PPI) remains paramount, and effective communication is important for diminishing risk. We shall cover these topics related to communication and therapeutic presence more in-depth in subsequent chapters.

Physical therapy was further examined retrospectively, from 2001–10, with the liability underwriter[13] examining closed liability claims. As a result of the study, physical therapists were "encouraged to examine their own practice and policies to discern areas of possible improvement and dedicate themselves to maximizing patient safety and minimizing risk."[13] Similar outcomes studies[9,13] have been completed for nurses, nurse practitioners, pharmacists, counselors, and other HCPs. Interestingly, the highest average paid claims were in a hospital setting, yet the highest total paid claims were in offices or clinics.[13] The most common allegations were improper performance using therapeutic exercise, improper performance using a physical agent, and failure to supervise or monitor.

Many of the recommendations to decrease risk are related to components of PPIs. To minimize risk, the Healthcare Providers Service Organization (HPSO) recommended a Risk Control Self-Assessment Checklist risk management overview:[13]

- ☐ Communicate effectively with patients, families, and colleagues.
- ☐ Delegate patient therapy services only to the appropriate level of staff.
- ☐ Provide appropriate supervision for all delegated patient services.
- ☐ Adopt an informed consent process that includes discussion and demonstrates that the patient understands all the risks associated with treatment.
- ☐ Ensure that clinical documentation practices comply with the standards promulgated by professional associations, state practice acts, and facility protocols.
- ☐ Avoid documentation errors that may weaken legal defense efforts in the event of litigation.
- ☐ Maintain clinical competencies specific to the relevant patient population.
- ☐ Be vigilant about protecting patients from the most common types of injuries.
- ☐ Recognize patients' medical conditions and comorbidities that may affect therapy.
- ☐ Know and comply with state laws regarding scope of practice.

Licensing board outcomes, as a result of the claims, ranged anywhere from license probation, stipulations, reprimands, suspension, and fines, to prescribed continuing education. Everyday ethics can have far-reaching impacts, and it remains in the HCP's best interest to complete self-assessment activities to ensure currency and management of risk related to PPIs while considering ethical and legal implications of decision making related to patient care.

Health professions students in educational settings in classroom and clinical education environments are not without ethical challenges in terms of environmental influences and practice exposures. Remarkably, in terms of environmental toxins exposures in HCPs education, Cope[14,15] discovered and confirmed the hazards of air quality in educational anatomy laboratories for formaldehyde exposure and pleaded for the removal of the health hazard. The ethical decision making relates to the cost benefits of an exposure to a known carcinogen compared with alternative forms of instruction, combined with availability of anatomical structures with fewer exposures and/or decreasing the exposure risk with improved air quality management. Efforts to monitor the risk of exposures are significant in anatomical laboratories. As haptic technologies continue to improve, the need for excessive exposures is lessened, with alternative instructional formats.

Lowe and Gabard[16] gained insight into students' experiences with ethical and legal violations during clinical education with reporting and barriers to reporting. The survey included many of the commonly claimed areas, such as inappropriate use of resources, improper supervision, lack of truth telling, sexual harassment, blatant wrong doing, and medical billing fraud. They surveyed 70 clinical students who noted violations but who oftentimes failed to report due to "low hierarchical position, fear of not being a team player, and personal consequences."[16] The researchers recommended that all students complete a mandatory competency test on the state practice act prior to clinical affiliations and that coursework include instruction in moral reasoning, options, and outcomes for reporting, with process steps, to diminish barriers.[16]

In 2016, HPSO's *Physical Therapy Professional Liability Exposure* summary report (retrospectively covering 2011–15) provided an updated *Risk Control Self-Assessment* in the commonly claimed areas of *Scope of Practice*, *Supervision of Personnel*, *Documentation*, and *Communication*. Malpractice claims rose to $42 million in the 5-year period.

Claims allegations included improper management with treatment, therapeutic exercise, biophysical agents, manual therapy, and failure to supervise or monitor; including *failures to* follow practitioner orders, diagnose, cease treatment following excessive/unexpected pain, obtain informed consent, and report the patient's condition or change in condition to the referring practitioner.

Released in 2020, the most recent HPSO *Physical Therapy Professional Liability Exposure Claim Report: 4th Ed.* (2015–19) detailed ten key findings:[17]

1. The average total incurred of closed claims increased more than 12% in the 2020 claim dataset ($134,761) from the 2016 claim dataset ($119,893).

2. The proportion of closed claims that resolved between $100,000 and $749,999 has increased 8.1% since the 2016 claim dataset.

3. Physical therapy private offices/clinics (nonhospital) continue to experience the highest percentage of closed claims.

4. Fractures, increase or exacerbation of injury/symptoms and burns continue to be the three most common patient injuries in the 2011, 2016, and 2020 claim datasets, representing more than 60% of all closed claims.

5. Patient burns represented 16.4% of all closed claims. While the proportion of claims has decreased since prior reports, burns continue to be one of the most frequent injuries.

6. Patient falls comprised 30.6% with re-injury representing 33.8% of all closed claims.

7. Claims associated with re-injury represented 33.8% of all PT professional liability closed claims, per the 2020 claim dataset.

8. The average cost ($6,420) of defending allegations asserted against a physical therapist's or physical therapist assistant's license increased 33.0%.

9. Three out of every five (59.4%) of license protection matters involved an allegation related to the physical therapist's or physical therapist assistant's professional conduct.

10. Approximately 52% of licensing board matters led to some type of board action.

It is recommended that you visit the HPSO claims report firsthand and review the outcomes (www.hpso.com/getmedia/843bca04-caa8-47aa-be5d-52d307495944/physical-therapy-claim-report-fourth-edition.pdf) and recommendations to gain additional insights now, for your continued professional formation, and again, as a reminder as you enter clinical experiences. Risk control resource highlights for key areas include the following: burns, license protection, documentation, home care, telehealth, falls and supervisors, along with self-assessment resources. Keeping current in this area is essential for all HCPs. Now that we have piqued your ethical interest from a personal, professional, and everyday standpoint, let's look more closely at the need for approaches aimed at ethical action and moral decision making.

# FOUR COMPONENTS OF ETHICAL ACTION

The ability to make a mature moral or ethical decision requires four behaviors that are often viewed as progressing developmentally: *moral sensitivity, moral judgment, moral motivation,* and *moral character/courage.*[18]

Table 4.1 illustrates why simply knowing the best or right thing to do does not ensure that a person will do it. Most difficult of all the components is *moral character/courage.* Moral sensitivity, judgment, and motivation can be encouraged and taught, but standing up for what you believe in in the face of adversity requires self-discipline, impulse control, and resistance to the fear of rejection and losing one's position.

| TABLE 4.1 |
|---|
| **FOUR COMPONENTS OF MORAL ACTION** |
| **MORAL SENSITIVITY** |
| ○ Ability to interpret a situation correctly and appropriately |
| ○ Awareness of how our actions will affect others |
| ○ Awareness of all possible lines of action and their effects on others and self |

○ Ability to imagine various scenarios with limited facts
○ Ability to role play and take the other's part

**MORAL JUDGMENT**

○ Judging which action is right or best, wrong or worst
○ Judging which line of action is more morally justified given the facts
○ Grasping the importance of the context of the situation that will point to the higher, more caring, more morally justified value

**MORAL MOTIVATION**

○ Prioritizing moral values over personal values
○ Wanting to do the caring or beneficent thing over self-interest

**MORAL CHARACTER OR MORAL COURAGE**

○ Having the strength of your convictions, courage, and persistence in overcoming distractions, pressures, and obstacles, no matter how large
○ Having implementation skills, focus, and ego strength: "Here I stand. I can do no other." (Martin Luther, 1483–1546)
○ Resisting fatigue, the morality of the day, the morality of expedience
○ Having self-discipline, impulse control, and skill to act according to one's highest goals
○ Resisting the need to be approved of and liked

Adapted from Rest JR. Background: theory and research. In: Rest JR, Narvaez D, eds. *Moral Development in Professions*. Hillsdale, NJ: Lawrence Erlbaum Associates; 1994:1–26.

# INGREDIENTS OF A MORAL DECISION

A moral statement says that, in situation X, person Y should do Z. Thus, a moral statement includes what should be done (Z), who is to do it (Y), and the conditions under which the statement is applicable (X).[5] Most decisions made each day in health care are working decisions based on the facts of the situation. The decision is subject to modification or reversal when more facts become known. Decisions must be provisional when each day brings new facts to bear. This is the reality of day-to-day health care. "Our task then," according to Francoeur,[19] "is to collect as much information as possible and then refer to the principles involved and choose the highest or best moral alternative in light of the situation at hand."

Let's look at discursive or principled ethical reasoning and see how it can guide us in deciding the highest or best alternative and then look at nondiscursive methods that will help us discover our own meta-beliefs that underlie and influence our final decisions about what is absolutely right and best in each situation. Basically, ethical reasoning is recognizing, analyzing, and clarifying ethical problems.[1] It assists HCPs in making decisions about the right thing to do for each particular case and considers the *why* in the process.[20] Ethical reasoning is the moral basis for professional actions and behaviors; the focus being on what should be (not what could be) done for the patient.[20]

# TRADITIONAL BIOMEDICAL ETHICS

Traditional discursive or principled ethical reasoning requires adherence to four levels of thinking: (1) the particular ethical decision will be made by (2) favoring an ethical rule that (3) sits within an ethical principle that (4) evolves out of an ethical system. Ethical systems grow out of how we tend to view the world or how we "set our lenses." We try on and adopt points of view about right and wrong as we are growing up and following the dictates of higher authorities, such as our parents, church, and other authorities.

Two ethical systems predominate: (1) ends- or results-oriented systems, which say that the best way to decide the right thing to do is to act to bring about the best result or the maximum good (teleological systems) and (2) duty- or principle-oriented systems or deontological systems, which say that the proper decision should not simply be decided by the results. The highest moral alternative should be situated in principles or rules known to be right whether or not they serve good ends.[5] In sum, in deciding the best thing to do, does the end (commonly the greatest good) most of the time justify the means, or do the means need to be carefully weighed without primary concern for the outcome?

An example of a principle that stems from a teleological or consequential way of looking at an ethical problem (ends are the most important) would be to act so that the greatest good can be brought about for the greatest number. That which is best is that which benefits everyone. Individuals come second to the good of the group. Hospital and nursing home administrators often make decisions based on this principle (e.g., when all patients are required to go to bed at a certain time for the convenience of the staff). Another question that could be asked to weigh the good of an action from this perspective is, "Would I be satisfied with the consequence of this action if it were done to me?" Many principles exist, and in each situation we appeal to the most relevant and appropriate principle to generate the highest moral action.[21]

# MORAL PRINCIPLES AND RULES OF PROFESSIONAL CODES OF ETHICS

Four moral principles and three rules that stem from those principles make up the foundational ethical framework for the professions (law, theology, and medicine), each one of which provides service to the community.[19,22] A scan of most code of ethics documents will reveal ethical standards based on the following principles and rules:

1. **Autonomy**: Do that which enables the patient's or client's right to choose for one's life and to voice that choice for as long as possible. Informed consent, or the freedom to act on one's own behalf and to implement one's free decision, is a right situated in the principle of autonomy.

2. **Beneficence**: Do that which is best for your patient or client. Professionals are obliged to act in the best interests of the patient when the benefit to the patient outweighs harm it may cause the professional. At first glance, it may seem as if beneficence and nonmaleficence are the same, but they are not.

3. **Nonmaleficence**: Above all, do no harm. Do not do anything that may cause injury to, disable, or kill a person or undermine the person's reputation, property, privacy, or liability. In all cases, prevent any harm from happening. This principle is often the one that is cited as the higher alternative to not allowing a patient to die because removing life support is seen as causing harm rather than allowing a natural event to occur (allowing death to take place rather than stopping it). The key question to be answered is, "By your action, are you preventing harm (an untimely death) or preventing death from taking place when it is inevitable, and no semblance of meaningful life is probable?"

4. **Social justice**: Act with equality and fairness to all, regardless of age, gender, identity, social orientation, religion, race, ethnicity, socioeconomic status, or education, and so on.

    a. *Distributive* justice: Equal distribution of goods (attention, service) to all members of a group. (All qualified disabled drivers receive the same vehicle placard for parking privileges.)

    b. *Compensatory* justice: Act to make up for past injustice (affirmative action).

    c. *Procedural* justice: First come–first served or alphabetical order are the most common procedures used to be fair to several.

The three ethical rules that follow from these four principles include the following:

1. **Veracity** (from autonomy and beneficence): Tell the truth; do not lie. Most often, this rule is challenged with the question of just how much of the truth the patient should hear and when.

2. **Confidentiality, privacy** (from beneficence): Moral obligation to keep confidential all information concerning patients/clients *even if not specifically requested by the patient or client*, except when doing so would bring harm to innocent people or to the patient or client personally. In addition, patients or clients have the right to keep privileged information not relevant to care.

3. **Fidelity** (from beneficence): Actions should, at all times, be faithful not only to one's patient or client but to one's fellow colleagues. Criticizing the opinion of a colleague to a patient or family members undermines the whole of health care. If you disagree with a colleague, you can simply say that you have formed a different opinion.[19,23]

In sum, these principles and rules serve as a beacon to all HCPs when confronted with a moral dilemma. Owing to the nature of the professions (bound in service), these values turn out to be the higher ones in principled decision making. At times, we are confronted with a patient who requests one thing (autonomy), and we feel that it is not in the patient's best interest to comply (beneficence). Then we must guard against paternalism, or choosing for the patient what is best because we think we know better. Instead, we must strive to inform the patient to ensure their best choice. Then, we must do what we can to ensure the patient's right to choose, even if we disagree.

Unfortunately, most often the common dilemma is between autonomy or beneficence and self-interest (i.e., moral temptation that becomes disguised or rationalized).[21] For example, the physical therapist indicates that all ten or more episodes of care are necessary to meet the patient goals to ensure the income from those visits, whereas if the patient had been placed on an adequate home program, some of those visits may have been unnecessary. The extra income is a self-interest decision that would be rationalized as necessary treatment for quality care. Today, it is more the exception than the rule to be fully reimbursed by third-party payors. Currently there are more serious concerns with professional integrity related to fraud, abuse, and waste in health care, which we will address further in subsequent chapters.

# PRINCIPLE UTILIZATION: ADVANTAGES AND CHALLENGES

When one must decide what the highest moral action to take is in any given situation, it helps to be freed up from the intensity and confusion of spontaneous feelings. This is true whether we are deciding a true biomedical dilemma, such as distributive justice (i.e., who should be treated and who should not) or a day-to-day dilemma, such as the head nurse who has to decide whether the dying patient on the unit can have a visit from his grandchildren from out of town who arrived after visiting hours were over.

Using a reflective, problem-solving process that considers all the given facts and uncovers all of the principles and rules that might apply is a way to rise above the subjective moment in an attempt to articulate an objective and defensible rationale for your decision. Trying to discern the *best* rule or principle or the *highest* moral action is often the most difficult decision, especially when you have limited information and must act right away.

We have stated that a teleologist will adopt the point of view that the facts should be weighed and the action that is best would be the action that benefits the greatest number. (The head nurse decides that the visit of young grandchildren might be disruptive to other patients—the greatest number—and decides not to allow it.) Meanwhile, the duty-oriented person will refer to a list of principles and pull out all of those that seem to bear on the case and, weighing the facts, decide which principle is the highest in this situation. (The head nurse decides that beneficence, contributing to the good of the patient, is more important than worrying about future decisions; if all patients ask for this privilege, chaos might result [justice].)

# THE INHERENT CHALLENGES OF PRINCIPLED DECISION-MAKING

Well-known medical ethicists Pellegrino and Thomasma[23] asked, "Is there a set of obligations which bind all who practice medicine? Is there one rule, or set of rules, that HCPs will find almost always is the highest moral alternative in health care?" Adherence to principles does not always work because people disagree about which principles are most acceptable. Gilligan[24] posits, "The way people define moral problems, the situations they construe as moral conflicts in their lives, and the values they use in resolving them are all a function of their social conditioning." Thus, even recognizing a problem as having an ethical aspect has a lot to do with how we were raised and view the world, and how our lenses are set.

# NONDISCURSIVE APPROACH TO ETHICAL DILEMMA RESOLUTION

"While acknowledging the power of such rational systems, nondiscursive ethicists … challenge the narrowness of a strictly applied, formal system of ethical reasoning."[22] Nondiscursive ethicists do not claim that discursive ethics is too theoretical or difficult to perform. Rather, their complaint is that theories, principles, and rules alone promote a formalized, purely objective, cognitive way of thinking that is excessively rational and unbalanced. Nondiscursive ethicists attempt to balance the process of dilemma resolution by incorporating such aspects of thought as imagination, virtue, character, role, power, discernment, and liberation in their search for an adequate method to decide the highest moral alternative.[22]

## The Importance of a Person's Story

The final ethical choice, which theory seems more compelling, ends vs. means, derives from within a personal moral narrative developed over time that we all inherit. Nash[22] believed that to restrict ethical decisions to rules and principles alone "sends out the false message that a person's story is irrelevant to (or worse, destructive of) the 'proper' formation of a moral self." A person's story is a "moral necessity because it provides one with the ethical skills to form one's life truthfully, committedly, and courageously. ... Objective discursive systems allow for rational, step-by-step deliberation and decision making. But the individual's moral intentions and motives originate in, and are formed by, significant people and events in the individual's life."[22]

The key perspective in discussing the nondiscursive aspect of dilemma resolution is to make clear that a choice of the highest moral alternative can be seen to be seated in a rather consistent system of values that can be uncovered by proving one's moral convictions in a deliberate fashion or by writing a personal, ethical autobiography. Once this story is better understood, important questions of character and virtue (What kind of a person am I? What kind of a person should I be as a HCP?) can be asked. HCPs must be helped to recognize the way their lenses are set so that they can adjust to a more professional perspective. For example, if what emerges on self-examination is a preoccupation with self-interest or a fear-laden perspective that takes precedence over autonomy, nonmaleficence, or beneficence, which are critical to professional health care value decisions, the HCP must realize that decisions made very often will not be with the highest concern for the welfare of the patient.

One must also be cautious about over-analyses leading to paralyses of action, too. There is merit in being exhaustive of possibilities, however over-laboring the options may prevent appropriate and timely action and inefficiency.

Deontology and teleology *presume* personal integrity. Principled ethicists believe that one develops moral character and integrity by making rule-based decisions, justified by ethical principles. Nondiscursive ethicists insist that moral character and integrity consist of more. To be moral requires constant training as a child and young person, and that training is more than applied ethics. "Integrity is the lifelong outcome of actions that shape particular kinds of character. ... And the character that develops is like the narrative of a good novel: it gives coherence to ethical decisions, and forces individuals to claim their actions as their own."[22]

As we learned in the previous chapter, cognitive developmental psychologists, such as Kohlberg,[25] favor a type of training to be moral, maintaining that children are only able to learn how to make higher or more adequate ethical decisions as they develop their cognitive reasoning skills. Moral developmentalists advocate teaching children how to reason morally by teaching them how to solve moral problems. The best moral decisions, according to Kohlberg,[25] are those that are logically consistent and admit to fewer exceptions, respect the dignity of all persons, and aim toward just treatment of all people, regardless of the law or of the person's race, creed, color, gender, or sexual orientation. Finally, cognitive developmentalists[18,25] offer methods of assessing the developmental level of moral consciousness of a person by asking the person to comment on the moral aspects of a dilemma that they identify as being most relevant. In this way, subjects reveal whether they have progressed in their reasoning to an understanding of moral principles or remain stuck in simply obeying the law or doing that which is socially appropriate.[26]

# VIRTUE ETHICS: THE DEVELOPMENT OF INTEGRITY OR CONSISTENT MORAL BEHAVIOR

What kind of a person should I be? Integrity is built from a continuum of choices, some important enough to be remembered, some almost habitual and unreflective. Each time a student cheats in class, or a citizen cheats on reporting income for tax purposes, that choice to behave unethically, no matter what the rationale, wears away at the development of integrity. Choice is not only about what to do in each situation; choice in making moral decisions is about **who I want to become and be**. The key question in self-examination is, "How does a truthful examination of my moral actions fit my moral image of myself?" Do I claim to be a person of virtue and integrity but choose to participate in gossip, judge others with prejudice, lose my temper, break my promises if I believe they are stupid promises, hurt people under the guise of trying to help by being honest, or lie when it is expedient to my goals? Answering truthfully requires our lenses to be set to listen carefully to the essential self; the ego must be still. The ego, the pragmatic goal seeker, will act to get ahead and rationalize that action so that it sounds acceptable and even clever.

How does this detrimental pattern of choice make sense? It makes sense if in my autobiography I remember the moral axioms of a parent who repeated such phrases to me as, "Get them before they get you," "If you don't look out for yourself, no one else will," "People get what they deserve," "The only thing that matters is who wins," "The winner is the one with the largest or most possessions or salary." Fear-based axioms are often behind this behavior, and, over time and with repeated exposure, this negativity will seat itself in one's conscience. Feelings of guilt and shame will then surface when you feel that someone is out ahead of you or is better than you are in class, or when you feel as if you have acted naïvely or allowed yourself to be taken advantage of in life.

In a conflict over altruism or beneficence vs. self-interest or personal gain, it will be difficult to act for the good of your patient when doing so makes you feel as if you have been taken advantage of in the situation. Often, daily ethical decisions are made by deferring to policies and procedures to assuage guilt. For example, a decision of what to do about a walker, paid for by the patient but left behind after her discharge, may not be seen as an ethical decision, if one refuses to deal with this mistake because one is "too busy with more important things." "It is just too bad that the walker was left behind. Thanks for the donation to the department. I do not have time to chase down discharged patients. They are not our concern once they have left this facility." This treatment of a decision ignores the ethical aspect entirely. Selfish concern over the value of one's time vs. concern over returning property to its rightful owner and then "passing the buck" by claiming that it is not your fault or problem are attempts to brush away the inadequacy of this mistaken choice. Or, following repeated patient falls, a HCP who defends themself based on the "system" that patients are expected to fall because it is a dementia unit, rather than proactively working to prevent falls, is blaming the system rather than taking accountability and responsibility to provide best practice for promoting and being accountable for a culture of safety and falls prevention. Thus, one's character, built up over the years by listening to important moral statements and making little decisions day after day, will dictate whether a clinical decision has a moral component. If a value-laden decision is not recognized, the process of solving the dilemma for the highest good will never begin.

In other words, being moral means (1) being able to identify the moral aspect of a problem as well as (2) being a certain kind of person who wants to be able to reason adequately, and, finally, (3) doing the right thing. Virtue ethicists claim that virtues such as compassion, generosity, fidelity, graciousness, justice, and prudence should be cultivated in people so that doing the right thing becomes consistent with one's character.[27] A person will choose their ethical behaviors more wisely if they choose in accordance with commonly held virtues.[28] Virtue ethicists argue about which are the most important virtues. Lebaqcz[29] argued that the virtues of fidelity and prudence should be central to the professions. Fidelity to clients includes trustworthiness, promise keeping, honesty, and confidentiality; prudence has to do with "an accurate and deliberate perception that enables professionals to perceive realistically what is required in any situation."[29]

## DISCERNMENT AS A VIRTUE

The common criticism of virtue theory is that cultivating virtue in one's being does not dictate that one will act virtuously in all instances. One might argue that a virtuous person, by definition, would tend to act in a virtuous way, but character traits alone are not enough to ensure the highest moral action.[28] But, if one has reflected on one's values, paid attention to moral choices, and developed integrity and compassion over time, it becomes easier to act with moral consistency, and inconsistencies serve to stir one's conscience in a way not as available to the morally unaware.[30] As detailed in Table 4.1, moral character or courage is more assured following components of moral actions, through moral sensitivity, judgment, and motivation.

The concept of *discernment* is integral to the development of character because discernment is the ability to assert that there is more than objective rationality to moral decision making. The best truth is found within the human decision maker, within the essential self, and that every moral decision should combine the best of logic and justification methods with attention to the various impulses and movements that occur within a deliberative consciousness. Again, ethical decisions are not an easy accomplishment and require courage. Just consider the dilemmas faced by HCPs because of natural disasters and pandemics.

Following Hurricane Katrina, many residents of New Orleans, and HCPs, either did not or could not comply with the order that had been issued to evacuate. The events surrounding Katrina raised critical legal and ethical questions about the use of mandatory evacuation orders, especially in consideration of the social determinants of health (SDoH).[31] Following Katrina, the surrounding levees broke, leading to devastating flooding and loss of power for many days in New Orleans and the surrounding parishes. Memorial Hospital was severely impacted, having a lack of adequate disaster planning, being surrounded by chaos, and being deficient in needed support and supplies, which led to the HCPs making life-changing decisions for debilitating, critically ill patients.[31] HCPs had to make critical decisions related to rationing food, water, and medical care throughout the post-Katrina emergency, determining the prioritization of treatment, while enduring not knowing when or even what kind of help would be on the way.[31] Many overstressed, overheated, and sleep-deprived HCPs became health care delivery heroes and stepped up to the unbelievable challenges and rescue demands; comforting and caring for patients, evacuating multiple disabled and obese patients who were severely dependent on oxygen, manually lifting and transferring them through parking garages, and up hundreds of stairs to the heliport,[31] while other HCPs' actions were called into question. The treatment of patients, or lack thereof, by some HCPs at Memorial Hospital during the incredibly horrific conditions and resulting complex crisis, was brought before a grand jury to consider, due to the taking of human lives by lethal injections.[31] The resultant outcomes were settled out of court on appeal, for some, and led many to question the value of a human life.[31] Furthermore, what conditions could possibly justify the taking of human lives? These were the questions raised due to the failures of local, state, and the federal government to lend timely and adequate support, and the resulting horrific circumstances endured that were not their fault.[31] Fortunately, according to the Florida Governor's office, HCPs and administrators learned from the Katrina experiences, and prior to the 2022 landfall of Hurricane Ian in Florida, made a truly Herculean effort in the 48 hours prior to successfully evacuate 61 babies in the neonatal intensive care unit and 8,500 patients in over 200 health care facilities, keeping them from harm's way.

In 2019, especially early on during the Covid-19 pandemic, HCPs were asked to compromise their own health and safety without proper PPE, for the good of their patients. Today, many HCPs and patients are still coping with Long Covid, a potentially long-term, and life-changing, multisystem (sensory, neurological, cardiorespiratory) illness due to prolonged recovery from the Covid-19 respiratory infection.[32–36] Large numbers of people, including HCPs, are carrying the illness burden. While even one vaccine may reduce the number of new cases of Long Covid, yet as of this writing, it will not fully eliminate it.[33] The public did not always comply with the recommended scientific guidelines for prevention, as in pandemics past. Health care advisement became politicized and even when a vaccine became available many were and still are reluctant to comply due to fear, beliefs, personal freedoms claimed, and/or overwhelming misinformation presented over social media outlets. Lockdowns and isolation became the norm for some time, in an effort to arrest the spread of the virus, leading to additional challenges of declines in mental health, education and routine health care, as well as loss of income for many nonessential workers. Despite the indifference of many, who later succumbed to Covid sequelae, HCPs pressed on, providing needed care. Many health care heroes emerged, suiting up daily in PPE, even those personally considered at high-risk, health-wise, putting their own lives and health on the line, in care of others; while others opted out. Some were shamed for their decisions, while others were heralded. Many HCPs became disenchanted with being called "heroes" but not being supported by the public in everyday actions to assist in reducing the spread of the virus (e.g., masking, vaccinations, handwashing). Many ethical circumstances led to changes, requiring tremendous moral courage.

What is required in day-to-day ethics is a balance of heart and head, founded in a virtuous moral character that places the good of our patients foremost. Ethical decision making should never be reduced to subjectivity and feelings or intuition alone. The nondiscursive aspects of moral decision making are not meant to replace the discursive, but to add to it, to approach a balance with head and heart. Attention to the nondiscursive elements in a moral decision helps one to gain a personal understanding of the moral life. It is in paying attention to this aspect of moral reasoning that one can decide, for example, "when one is willing to make or break a promise, when to tell only the truth, to decide what one is willing to die for."[22] To learn to live the consistent and good moral life is one reason we believe we are all here on this Earth.

# THE ETHIC OF CARE

The ethic of care suggests that we do what is most important to preserve the integrity of the therapist–patient relationship.[21] To care for the patient is to have regard for their views, interests, and cultural mores and to hold warm acceptance and trust for the other, rather than doing good simply because beneficence dictates it. Sensitivity to the deepest values and concerns of the patient in the context of the patients' life situation is what drives the decision making. To follow an ethic of care requires moral sensitivity and judgment, discernment, and excellent interpersonal skills. HCPs must listen carefully to the initial history and the patient's description of the problem and the meaning that this has in the person's life. The current economic pressures of the health care system commonly place restrictions on the ability of the HCP to engage with patients in such a way as the ethic of care requires. The institutional constraints on caring must be confronted as an ethical situation for HCPs to be able to practice without feelings of conflict or doubt. Once this is done, the quality of one's practice can be anticipated to improve. Take a moment to consider how this proclamation pertains to HCPs' moral *abilities and actions:* "You are what you repeatedly do. Excellence is not an event—it is a habit"—Aristotle.

# ETHICS AND THE LAW

Generally, ethics provide higher standards of the best to do than do state laws. Laws are created to protect the citizens of the state from unsafe practice; ethics bind HCPs to the highest care.

Each jurisdiction in the U.S. has laws and statutes called *practice acts* that guide the limits of professional obligation and responsibility for HCPs in that jurisdiction alone. The statute itself is accompanied by a document, usually referred to as the rules, that further clarifies the statute. The rules can be clarified and changed more easily than the statute itself, which was created by the lawmakers of that jurisdiction for its citizens. Refer to your specific profession and jurisdictional practice acts for more information regarding laws, rules, and regulations. Changes in health care are occurring so rapidly that HCPs constantly must refer to their practice acts to ascertain the specific scope of HCP practice and current presiding jurisprudence.

In the past, when no specific law existed to cover an action that ended up in the courts, the court (the judge) ruled according to interpretation of the facts of the case and their interpretation of the practice act. In fact, courts may hold HCPs to a higher standard than the state practice act dictates.[37] For example, even though not all physical therapists are members of the American Physical Therapy Association, which binds its members to a code of ethics for proper practice, the court is starting to accumulate case law decisions that all physical therapists are professionals who should be held to this code of ethics standard. Many practice acts today incorporate the codes of ethics and standards of practice espoused by the professional associations and, therefore, hold nonmembers to the same standards and ethical obligations from a legal standpoint. Students and licensed HCPs must comply with jurisdictional laws and rules; hence, it would behoove you to begin to become familiar with your practice act and/or the jurisdiction in which you are going to train or practice. The Federation of State Boards of your profession of practice provides extensive information and links to guide licensees, those applying for license, jurisprudence, and information for the public (e.g., the Federation of State Boards of Physical Therapy [www.fsbpt.org], with a mission to promote safety and competence).

The Federation works closely with the professional association and collaborates on efforts for Licensure Compacts for interstate license portability, to ensure greater access to care; yet state legislators must also be willing to adopt these changes. So, you can see the ethical need for health care advocacy with the legislative body, which we will address in Chapter 11.

# ETHICAL REALITIES

It is important that HCPs are able to carefully analyze their patients' needs and use sound moral reasoning and ethical dilemma resolution skills to decide on the appropriate actions for the good of the patient and for justice or appropriate fairness when there is a shortage of professional care available. The primary duty of the HCP is always to the patient and secondarily to the business contract. This can result in ethical distress when you know the best thing to do but are prohibited from doing it by the organization within which you practice. For example, if, under a capitation agreement, coverage is for only six visits and the goals set for the patient at the initial evaluation cannot be met in such a brief time, the HCP can be held liable for abandonment if their response is to discharge the patient short of the agreed-upon goals. Business cannot dictate to HCPs when to discontinue treatment.[37] HCPs are obligated to provide needed care. Likewise, HCPs have the right to maintain an adequate financial base of practice and thus should seek private or other reimbursement from the patient; some utilize the opportunity to fulfill pro bono services obligations, where appropriate. In fact, case law now indicates that the court's expectations are for the HCP to carry out the duty to continue to serve the patient pro bono or without compensation. Thus, each practice needs to develop a policy or guide outlining how it will determine the incidence and limits of pro bono care and, beyond that, the care of the patient who cannot pay but requires treatment should be transferred to colleagues who have pro bono capacity at that time.[37]

When health care as a service is managed only as if it were a business, where profit is the primary reason for its existence, a conflict is bound to emerge. We have seen the concept of facilitating the healing of the whole patient or client all but disappear from health care. Business executives, with their eyes on the bottom line and dictating to HCPs who they can treat, for how long, and what is reasonable to charge strip HCPs of their ethical foundations. The definition of a profession's autonomy requires that HCPs are the only ones who can make those judgments, and they are morally obliged to make them not with profit in mind but with service for those in need.[21]

It is important that you, as an early career HCP, stay current with local, state, and federal guidelines on health care practice and reimbursement and learn how to resolve the ethical dilemmas that result in these unstable times. Your professional association assists HCPs in timely updates regarding these matters, yet individual HCPs are responsible, as professionals, to stay current. Only time will tell just how the Affordable Care Act (ACA), which refers to two separate pieces of legislation—the Patient Protection and Affordable Care Act (P.L.111–148) and the Health Care and Education Reconciliation Act of 2010 (P.L. 111–152)—will affect all these issues. Even before the Covid-19 pandemic, 45% of working-age Americans either had no insurance or had insurance that carried deductibles and copays so high that they could not afford medical care anyway. Some predict that the negative impact of business on health care will become more restrictive to providing quality care before improvements begin. The ACA continues to be challenged with political challenges and the past decade has resulted in many efforts to repeal and replace ACA, along with ACA Medicaid expansion, leading to over a dozen state contentions. Continued health care reforms are needed. ACA has led to many state and federal battles and political divides, along with recent actions related to sexual and reproductive rights, with the U.S. Supreme Court overturning *Roe v. Wade* (2022), relegating to the states. Some providers have also further boycotted the ACA and set up boutique-type health care where providers are placed on robust annual retainers and you may use the service at any time, whereas others have implemented cash-only services, leading to additional ethical and access conundrums. In terms of the ACA, although the patient/client savings in health care costs are far less than were predicted, the current trend has resulted in isolated areas of cost containment, as well as a greater shift of the burden of care to patients and their families, some of whom are experiencing greater expenses. This results in more responsibility on the part of patients for their health and for prevention and maintenance of their own care. We will discuss the challenges of patients' health behavior change for HCPs in Chapter 16. Once again, the value of health care as a right vs. a privilege in the U.S. is changing and evolving, and it remains important that we monitor and advocate for our patients. We will discuss this more in Chapter 11.

Above and beyond all trends and reimbursement mechanisms, when the interests of the patient and the HCP collide, always remember that beneficence and autonomy ethically must outweigh self-interest.[21] If HCPs were engaged only in business, there would be no dilemma. But HCPs are bound by codes of ethics of service, not profit, that mandate advocacy for our patients who come to us because we have the education and the commitment to help them.

# REALM—INDIVIDUAL PROCESS—SITUATION (RIPS) CONCEPTUAL ANALYSIS MODEL

Professional behavior requires fulfilling a role in society in relationship to individual patients or clients, the institutions, and organizations in which we practice, and society as a whole. In the past, resolving ethical dilemmas concentrated on one aspect of this complicated relationship alone—the relationship with individual patients or colleagues. Although all ethics are interpersonal, the most compelling dilemmas we deal with today often concern our relationship with our organizations and institutions and with society. To be ethically competent, we must be able to resolve all kinds of ethical situations, taking into consideration the context of the situation (the realm), the individual process involved (moral sensitivity, judgment, motivation, and courage), and the kind of ethical situation that is before us (issue, problem, dilemma).

An amalgamated, theoretical model of ethical analysis[32] was developed that combines the prior work of Glaser[39] in the *realm* arena, Rest[18] in the *individual process* arena, and Purtilo[40] in the *ethical situation* arena. Glaser[39] first developed a model for exploring beneficence in three realms: individual, institutional, and societal. Glaser[39] posited that within the individual realm, a question might be, "May I deliberately and actively end my own life?" At the societal level, the appropriate question might be, "Does patient autonomy include the right to medically assisted death?" Once we determine the realms involved, we have a starting point for ethically based reasoning. The three realms are interdependent and help guide ethical decision making by providing guidelines or a partial map of ethics. The collective works of ethicists Glaser,[39,41] Rest,[18,42] Purtilo,[40] and Kidder[43] are combined in the conceptual model, termed the *RIPS conceptual model of analysis* (see Table 4.2).[38] The ethical rules of veracity or informed consent or confidentiality are well worked out at the individual level, but when it comes to the systems, policies, and procedures of organizations and institutions or the cultural dictates of society, it becomes less clear how to act. Each of the realms, at best, tries to promote the good and encourages moral behavior, but each realm will differ on definitions, priorities, authority, and what data are meaningful in coming to the decision of what is best and right in a given situation.[32] In other words, ethics becomes more complicated as you move beyond the concerns of individuals, and it is believed that you cannot resolve organizational and societal ethical distress and dilemmas with purely individual modes of action. For example, the inability of a person in a wheelchair to access an entrance to a public building is, in part, an issue of justice (individual), but it requires policy changes beyond simply changing the rules (organizational and societal). Likewise, the unwillingness of payors to reimburse for treatment based on faulty research or inaccurate reimbursement formulas goes beyond veracity. Policies and procedures, authority, laws, and bureaucratic customs all converge on decisions of federal reimbursement, and "organizational and social problems demand strategies and solutions appropriate to that realm."[38] For example, there are times when the best thing we can do to feel as if we have acted in good conscience is to email, phone, and/or meet with members of Congress and

| TABLE 4.2 | | |
| --- | --- | --- |
| **RIPS CONCEPTUAL MODEL: FRAMEWORK** | | |
| **REALMS** | **INDIVIDUAL PROCESS** | **SITUATION** |
| Individual | Moral sensitivity | Issue |
| Organizational | Moral judgment | Problem |
| Societal | Moral motivation | Dilemma |
| | Moral courage | Distress |
| | | Temptation |
| Adapted from Realm–Individual Process–Situation (RIPS) ethical analysis model.[38–40] | | |

their staffers to advocate on behalf of our patients, sharing their stories, or making phone calls to request payments for our patients from third-party payors and follow-up with appropriate appeals and evidence-based justification letters for care.

# SOLVING ETHICAL PROBLEMS: SUGGESTED PROCESS

Ethical issues, problems, and dilemmas occur frequently and require different problem analyses and solutions. The most difficult problem to resolve is a dilemma—when two or more ethical principles conflict with each other in a given situation and it is unclear what the best or highest moral action would be in this case or instance. The following problem-solving process method is suggested for application to solving ethical situations, including ethical dilemmas. It incorporates a rule-based method (deontology) with consideration of the consequences (teleology) and attends to nondiscursive elements (virtue theory and the ethic of care). The suggested method is a combined adaptation of the work of Seedhouse and Lovett[44] and the RIPS conceptual model of analysis.[38–40]

1. Gather all the facts that can be known about this situation.

2. Decide which realm is primary: individual, organizational, or societal (Table 4.2).

3. Then, decide the process that seems to be called for: sensitivity, judgment, motivation, or character (see Tables 4.1 and 4.2).

4. Decide what level of ethical situation is involved: issue, problem, temptation, distress, or dilemma (see Table 4.2).

5. If the situation is within the realm of individual, organizational, or societal, efforts for resolution should focus on identifying needed policy and systems changes. Suggest the values that are involved and the policies and procedures that contribute to the ethical problem. Tackle the problem at the individual process level required—sensitivity, judgment, motivation, or courage (see example that follows).

6. If the situation is a true ethical dilemma at the individual level, proceed to decide which ethical principles are involved (e.g., beneficence, nonmaleficence, justice, autonomy, confidentiality, veracity, and/or fidelity).

7. Clarify your professional duties in this situation (e.g., do no harm, tell the truth, keep promises, be faithful to colleagues, etc. Duties such as these are often outlined in one's code of ethics).

8. Describe the general nature of the outcome desired or the consequences. Which seems most important in this case—an outcome that is most beneficial for the patient, the family, or your colleagues?

9. Describe pertinent practical features of this situation—one or more of the following: disputed facts, the law, the wishes of the others, resources available, effectiveness and efficiency of action, the risk, your code of ethics and standards of practice, the degree of certainty of the facts on which you base your decision, and the predominant values of the others involved (which may or may not coincide with predominant values in U.S. health care).

When all the pertinent aspects that go into this particular decision are laid out before you, use your discernment to decide which action is the highest moral alternative. Justify your decision by explaining your ethical reasoning process and your conscious weighing of one value over another in this situation based on what you know about your moral character; the virtues, traditions, and beliefs that frame your choices in life; and your professional ethical mandates.

# APPLICATION OF THE SUGGESTED PROBLEM-SOLVING PROCESS

Let's take an example of an ethical situation that involves the expectation of a kickback or gift in exchange for referring patients.

> An occupational therapist certified in hand therapy visits a local orthopedic hand surgery practice with information about her skills and her practice in hopes of educating the physicians and office staff about the benefits of referring their patients to her for rehabilitation. She is told by the receptionist that unless she was prepared to offer regular golf outings at the local country club, she could not compete with the local physical therapist who got there before she did, although he was not board certified.

This surely is an ethical problem. Let's apply the problem-solving process to the case. The facts are that a highly qualified hand therapist would like to receive referrals from an orthopedic surgery practice, but she is told she must give a kickback, or pay for the referrals, in competition with another therapist who at face value seems less qualified to help the patients than she is based on advanced certification. Another fact is that kickbacks are against the law. But, unlike pharmaceutical manufacturers and medicine, exactly what constitutes a kickback and what constitutes an expense associated with promoting one's business have not been clearly delineated by physical or occupational therapy organizations.

Going to Table 4.2, we decide that the principal realm involved here is organizational. The ethical situation is between the occupational therapist and the orthopedic practice or the organization. The individual process required is one of moral courage or implementation. The occupational therapist is motivated to want to work for change but will need the courage to report this infraction and remain in her mind a viable therapist in the community. The situation would be one of distress. She may be tempted to just look away and not make waves and thus protect her business, but she knows that what is going on currently is unethical, illegal, and not good for patients. She knows what she must do, but she must work up the courage to take the appropriate course of action, reporting unethical behavior to the state boards of practice. So, this is not an ethical dilemma at all, but an uncomfortable ethical distress.

Now, let's illustrate how this process is used to solve a dilemma. One common ethical problem that occurs in spinal cord rehabilitation facilities is the ethical dilemma of what to do when a mentally competent patient refuses beneficial treatment. (We already know that this is at the realm of the individual.) But first, the facts:

> Alex is a 23-year-old patient with a cervical fracture and spinal cord lesion at the level of C6-C7. He has had a surgical fusion, is medically stable, and is ready to begin rehabilitation, but he refuses to allow others to transfer him from bed to begin the process of tolerating sitting. Testing has revealed normal intelligence and a suspected level of grief and depression following this accident. No active motion has yet been seen below the level of the lesion. The nurses have had problems with his refusal to eat, the physical and occupational therapists have been unable to get him out of bed, and the social worker has been unable to engage him in discussion about his depression. He lies in bed with the covers over his head and says, "Leave me alone. I want to die." The physician on the case refuses to take Alex's desires seriously but also shows little compassion or sensitivity and commands the orderly to bodily remove Alex from the bed and wheel him to physical therapy. The other members of the team, although not wanting simply to yield indefinitely to Alex's depression, believe that the physician's order is inappropriate and are struggling with what to do next. They feel a strong pull of loyalty to other members of the team, including the physician, but resist the command to force Alex to comply. They feel a loyalty to their patient but believe that his depression blocks him from making the best decisions for himself at this time.

# APPLICATION OF THE PROBLEM-SOLVING METHOD

1. Gather all the key facts.

    a. Cervical lesion, complete, at C6-C7.

    b. Young male, 23 years old. No committed relationship to a partner. Family (i.e., father, mother, sister) supporting and visit regularly.

    c. Completed two years of college, proven intelligence, taking a year off to "find himself," risk taker, athlete.

    d. Accident occurred showing off by diving into shallow water of friend's pool at a party late at night.

    e. From family history, suspected addiction to alcohol, history of risk-taking behaviors.

    f. Family has excellent health insurance.

    g. Friendly, bright personality, strong previous desire to contribute to society, active in Big Brothers and Boy Scouts.

    h. Without conferring with the team, the physician has ordered that they act in a way that seems to many to be abusive and insensitive to the patient's (hopefully) temporary feelings of depression and hopelessness.

2. Decide which realm—individual—between the team, the patient, and the physician.

3. Decide which process is required. It is not moral sensitivity. The team understands and recognizes the problem. But they do not know the best thing to do, so this requires a process of moral judgment.

4. Decide which situation is present. There is no moral temptation, really. The team genuinely does not know what is best to do. This is a problem that seems to come to the level of a dilemma. To act in fidelity to the physician who believes that he is doing the best for the patient will be going against what the team believes is beneficent for the patient.

5. Organizational or societal issues at work here are not primary, so we go to the following.

6. Ethical principles involved: Decision to allow the patient to have his freedom to act in his own interest (autonomy) vs. acting in a way to convince the patient to get motivated to begin rehabilitation (beneficence) contributing to the overall benefit of the patient. But the other factor is, what is the action that is most beneficial? The doctor's demand to bodily force the patient to comply with a rehab plan may be the end desired, but the means do not seem to be justified. Above all, do no harm (nonbeneficence) is an issue, and a logical question would be what harm might result from physically forcing the patient to comply. Fidelity to one's professional colleague seems to be less important than do no harm.

7. Clarify your duties in the situation: If I am the physical therapist, I have a different specific duty from if I were the social worker, occupational therapist, recreation therapist, or nurse. But each of us has the duty to act in such a way that the patient is supported in overcoming his natural depression and becoming invested in hope for a new life. Once Alex gets beyond his depression and understands, at the deepest levels, what his choices will be living with quadriplegia, then his decision to live or die will be his to make, free of interference. Right now, he does not have all the facts, and his depression keeps him from even considering what those facts might be and how important they are to his decision. In other words, his depression renders him mentally incapable of deciding adequately in his own best interest. My duty as a HCP is to contribute to the team's individual and collective effort to support Alex through his depression and to help him learn what he can expect from life living with quadriplegia. I am also obliged to be faithful to my colleagues so that we are united in our approach and work together for a good outcome, but I cannot be faithful to a plan that might cause the patient harm. The physician's order is not one that I can readily follow, so the desire to do no harm and the patient's beneficence seem more important than fidelity to my colleague, the physician.

8. Describe the general nature of the outcome desired: I want Alex to become involved in rehabilitation and to learn what it is like to be as independent as possible with his quadriplegia without having to go through the humiliation of being bodily forced to participate in rehabilitation.

9. Describe pertinent practical features of the situation.

   a. Disputed facts: (1) It is permissible to insist that patients not yield to depression by bodily forcing them to go to rehab. The end justifies the means. This fact can be disputed. (2) Alex is taking up someone else's bed who wants to be involved in rehab, and someone else deserves the bed more.

   b. Wishes of others: (1) Family wants everything done for Alex as soon as possible. (2) Mother has little tolerance for her son's depression. Concurs with physician's order. Father asks for patience and perseverance, plus treatment of depression.

   c. Resources available: Rehab beds are in demand, but money is not an issue for the family.

   d. Risk: Forcing Alex to be involved in rehab could cause injury to body or emotions. Also, it may backfire, causing more resistance.

   e. Degree of certainty of facts: The most uncertain of the facts concerns the nature of the cervical lesion. What will Alex's physical and emotional deficit look like in 6 months? In 1 year? How debilitated will Alex be, and how independent can we hope he can become? How successful will he be in reforming his core self-worth and values so that he might live a fulfilled life as a patient with a disability? Likewise, we are uncertain just how long Alex's depression will last. Even with the uncertainty of the future, the fact now is that he is physically ready to participate in rehab. Also certain is the fact that rehab cannot take place successfully without Alex's cooperation.

## Decision

1. Meet with the team physician to discuss unwillingness to carry out the order to force Alex to go to rehab.

2. Confer with the psychologist, physician, nurse, and/or social worker and agree on a plan to systematically confront Alex's depression in a supportive way, with the goal of helping him through it in as timely a way as possible. Commit as a team to giving him the time he needs.

3. Once rehab has begun, practice beneficence and guarded paternalism while Alex is gaining a sense of himself with his new identity, and then be careful to relinquish any paternalism as Alex becomes able to make decisions cognitively and emotionally for himself, even if the health care team and/or family disagree with those decisions.

Two things seem obvious at this point. Moral decision making takes time and practice, and we may not have considered aspects of this situation that seem quite apparent to you. What if the physician becomes enraged that the team has not followed his instructions and threatens to have each one fired? Sometimes moral stances come to this level of confrontation, but not often. When one's integrity is challenged, moral temptation becomes more compelling. It helps to have systematically thought through your decision to avoid this lapse in moral judgment.

Hopefully, the case application of the problem-solving approach has assisted you in further understanding the value of ethics in clinical decision making. The relevance of the impact of not considering ethical aspects of clinical decision making could lead to not only the incorrect decisions, but also sometimes more harmful or hurtful ones. Research studies of physical therapy students in ethics content demonstrate that students who consider case-based, ethical applications with ethical problem-solving processes in the classroom find that the material is easier to integrate with real-world practical applications and have improved critical thinking with respect to clinical practice scenarios encountered.[45,46]

Delany et al.[46] shared that "as moral agents, physical therapists are required to make autonomous clinical and ethical decisions based on connections and relationships with their patients, other health care team members, and health institutions and policies." Their study proposed an applied ethics model termed the *active engagement model* (Table 4.3) to further integrate clinical and ethical dimensions of practice. The active engagement model includes "3 practical steps: (1) to listen actively, (2) to think reflexively, and (3) to reason critically."[46] Step 3, critical reasoning, incorporates the components of realms in PPIs, organizations, and society. The model suggests within each of the three steps specific facilitating questions (or sideways questions[47]) to support the process. The questions facilitate HCPs to actively go deeper to consider the broader aspects of care. You may wish to revisit the prior case and/or consider a case of your own once you are in fieldwork or clinical experiences to apply these deeper and expanded steps of the active engagement model for ethics in professional practice.

| | TABLE 4.3 |
|---|---|
| **ACTIVE ENGAGEMENT MODEL: STEPS AND QUESTIONS** | |
| **STEPS** | **FACILITATING QUESTIONS** |
| **Step 1: Active listening** | ○ How has the patient and health care team member cast their story?<br>○ Within the story, how do they portray themselves?<br>○ Why are they telling the story in this way?<br>○ Whose voice in the story is dominant?<br>○ Whose voice in the story is not being heard?<br>○ How else might this story have been told?<br>○ What is ethically at stake in this story?<br>○ What are the ethically important moments in the story? |
| **Step 2: Reflexive thinking** | ○ What goals and values do I, as the physical therapist, personally bring to a given treatment?<br>○ What goals and values are inherent within the physical therapy treatment that I offer?<br>○ What influence do my language and my treatment methods have on the patient and others?<br>○ How do others (patients, colleagues, managers) know what they know?<br>○ What shapes and has shaped their world view?<br>○ How do they perceive me and why?<br>○ How do I perceive them?<br>○ How do they make sense of what I give them?<br>○ What perspectives do they bring to the findings I offer? |
| **Step 3: Critical reasoning** | **Realm of Patient and Therapist Relationship**<br>○ What values and goals do I bring to the therapeutic relationship?<br>○ How do my professional and personal values and goals differ from the patient's?<br>**Organizational Realm**<br>○ What is my relationship with the health care organization?<br>○ How does this relationship influence the clinical encounter?<br>○ How do institutional systems and structures affect the patient's ability to receive treatment?<br>**Societal Realm**<br>○ What are the health care structures, resources, and economic policies that influence the goals and provision of physical therapy? |
| Reprinted from *Phys Ther.* 2010;90:1068–1078, with permission of the American Physical Therapy Association. © 2010 American Physical Therapy Association. | |

# CONCLUSION

We hope you see that the systematic processes to examine ethical encounters work to raise the decision-making process up out of the murky waters of intuition and subjectivity alone, and that one could defend the decision as the best or highest decision one could make at the time with the facts provided. To go back on ethical decisions because of a threat would weaken one's integrity. We hope that the situations would not come to that end, but if they did, we would be confident in one's discernment and, one would hope, remain committed to one's decision.

Globally, HCPs are encountering messy, ambiguous,[31,48] "diverse and complex ethical landscapes where therapists grapple with ethical questions emerging from the impact of funding models, policies affecting clinical work, expanding boundaries, scope of practice, changing professional roles and relationships."[49] Codes of conduct remain foundational ethical knowledge but may not always be helpful for real-time ethical decision making, with support and preparation needed for ethical encounters.[31,48,49]

Never forget that this process of deciding the highest moral choice must always be reflective of the needs of the patient and the patient's family. The real-life person before you with whom you are interacting is who you are accountable to and responsible for in health care. As Greenfield and Jensen[50] so eloquently put it, "We are not well served by a rational principlist approach to ethical issues that excludes the possibility of contextual understanding from the perspectives of our patients." The starting point for all the processes of ethical clinical decision making must be the patient's own story if we are truly in service to meet the needs of society as partners in health care.[50–53]

The exercises that follow will give you a chance to discover more clearly the qualities of your discernment by asking you to write your moral autobiography, and will give you the opportunity to practice ethical dilemma resolution using the suggested processes. Remember, you have been making personal moral decisions all your life. Now, what is asked of you is to search for the values, beliefs, stories, myths, and parables that have informed those choices in a consistent way. How well will that way serve you now as a HCP? What changes must you make, if any, to remain true to a commitment to therapeutic presence and healing, to minimize preventable harm?[52] Do not forget to journal about your discoveries.

# REFERENCES

1. Doherty RF. *Ethical Dimensions in the Health Professions*, 7th ed. Philadelphia, PA: Elsevier; 2020.
2. American Nurses Association (ANA). *Code of Ethics for Nurses with Interpretive Statements*. Silver Springs, MD: ANA; 2015.
3. Musolino, GM, Jensen, GM. *Clinical Reasoning and Clinical Decision Making in Physical Therapy: Facilitation, Assessment, and Implementation*. Thorofare, NJ: Slack; 2019.
4. Purtilo, RB. Early markers of a 100-year journey toward the American Physical Therapy Association becoming an ethically grounded societal presence: An ethicist's reflection, *Phys Ther.* 2021;101(11)1–3.
5. Brody H. *Ethical Decisions in Medicine*, 2nd ed. Boston, MA: Little Brown and Co., 1981.
6. Mueller K. *Communication From the Inside Out*. Philadelphia, PA: FA Davis; 2010.
7. Nalette E. Constrained physical therapist practice: an ethical case analysis of recommending discharge placement from the acute care setting. *Phys Ther.* 2010;90(6):939–952.
8. Greenfield, B. The role of emotions in ethical decision making: implications for physical therapist education. *Phys Ther Educ.* 2007;21(1):14–21.
9. Kane RA, Caplan AL. *Everyday Ethics: Resolving Dilemmas in Nursing Home Life*. New York, NY: Springer;1990.
10. Guccione AA. Ethical issues in physical therapy practice. A survey of physical therapists in New England. *Phys Ther.* 1980;60(10):1264–1272.
11. Triezenberg HL. The identification of ethical issues in physical therapy practice. *Phys Ther.* 1996;76(10):1097–1107.
12. CNA/Health Providers Service Organization. Physical Therapy Claims Study, 1993–2006. CNA HealthPro. www.cna.com. Accessed June 1, 2015.
13. CNA/Health Providers Service Organization. Physical Therapy Liability 2001–2010. CNA. http://www.hpso.com. Accessed June 1, 2015.
14. Cope JM, Sanders E, Holt SM, Pappas K, Thomas KJ, Kernick E. Comparison of personal formaldehyde levels in the anatomy laboratories of 5 physical therapy education program. *J Phys Ther Educ.* 2011;25(3):21–29.
15. Cope JM. Comparison of two formaldehyde exposure assessment devices in a physical therapy education program anatomy laboratory. *J Phys Ther Educ.* 2014;28(3):15–20.
16. Lowe DL, Gabard DL. Physical therapist student experiences with ethical and legal violations during clinical rotations: reporting and barriers to reporting. *J Phys Ther Educ.* 2014;28(3):98–111.
17. CNA and HPSO. *Physical Therapy Professional Liability Exposure Claim Report: 4th Ed.*, 2020. https://www.hpso.com/Resources/Legal-and-Ethical-Issues/Physical-Therapy-Claim-Report-Fourth-Edition Accessed October 27, 2024.
18. Rest JR. Background: theory and research. In: Rest JR, Narvaez D, eds. *Moral Development in Professions*. Hillsdale, NJ: Lawrence Erlbaum Associates; 1994:1–26.
19. Francoeur RT. *Biomedical Ethics: A Guide to Decision Making*. New York, NY: John Wiley & Sons; 1983.
20. Devettere R. *Practical Decision Making in Health Care Ethics: Cases, Concepts, and the Virtue of Prudence*. Washington, DC: Georgetown University Press; 2016.
21. Pellegrino ED. Altruism, self-interest, and medical ethics. *JAMA.* 1987;258(14):1939–1940.
22. Nash RJ. Applied ethics and moral imagination: issues for educators. *J Thought.* 1987;22(3):68–77.
23. Pellegrino ED, Thomasma DC. *A Philosophical Basis of Medical Practice: Toward a Philosophy and Ethic of the Healing Professions*. New York, NY: Oxford University Press; 1981.

24. Gilligan C. *In a Different Voice: Psychological Theory and Women's Development*. Cambridge, MA: Harvard University Press; 2016.

25. Kohlberg L. The cognitive development approach to moral education. *Phi Delta Kappa*. 1975;56(10):670–677.

26. Munsey B. *Moral Development, Moral Education and Kohlberg*. Birmingham, AL: Religious Education Press; 1980.

27. Noddings N. *Caring: A Feminine Approach to Ethics and Moral Education*. 2nd ed. Berkeley, CA: University of California Press; 2003.

28. Pence GE. *Ethical Options in Medicine*. Oradell, NJ: Medical Economics Co; 1980.

29. Lebaqcz K. *Professional Ethics: Power and Paradox*. Nashville, TN: Abingdon Press; 1985.

30. Haddad A, Doherty RB, Purtilo RF. *Health Professional/Patient Interaction*. 10th ed. Philadelphia, PA: Saunders; 2023.

31. Fink, S. *Five Days at Memorial: Life and Death in a Storm-Ravaged Hospital*. New York, NY: Crown Publishing; 2016.

32. United Kingdom Government. Coronavirus (Covid-19) in the UK. *coronavirus.data.gov.uk*, 2022; April. Accessed May 10, 2022.

33. United Kingdom Health Security Agency. *The Effectiveness of Vaccination Against Long Covid: A Rapid Evidence Briefing*. United Kingdom Health Security Agency; gov.uk. 2022.

34. University of Oxford. Oxford to test potential treatment for fatigue in long Covid patients. *ox.ac.uk*. (2021); 29 October. Accessed May 10, 2022.

35. Heightman M, Prashar J, Hillman, TE, et al. Post-COVID-19 assessment in a specialist clinical service: a 12-month, single-centre, prospective study in 1325 individuals. *BMJ Open Respiratory Research*. 2021;(8): e001041.

36. Maxwell E. Unpacking post-covid symptoms. *BMJ*. 2021;(373): n1173.

37. Scott R. *Legal, Ethical, and Practical Aspects of Patient Care Documentation: A Guide for Rehabilitation Professionals*, 4th ed. Burlington, MA: Jones & Bartlett Learning; 2013.

38. Swisher LL, Arslanian LE, Davis CM. Realm-individual process-situation (RIPS) model of ethical analysis decision-making. *HPA Resource*. 2005;(3):1, 3–8.

39. Glaser J. *Three Realms of Ethics: Individual, Institutional, Societal: Theoretical Model and Case Studies*. New York, NY: Rowman & Littlefield Publishers; 1994.

40. Purtilo RB. A time to harvest, a time to sow: ethics for a shifting landscape. *Phys Ther*. 2000;80(11):1112–1119.

41. Glaser JW. Three realms of ethics: an integrative map of ethics for the future. In: Purtilo RB, Jensen GM, Brasic-Royeen C, eds. *Educating for Moral Action: A Sourcebook in Health and Rehabilitation Ethics*. Philadelphia, PA: FA Davis; 2005: 169–184.

42. Rest JR, Narvaez D, Bebeau MJ, Thoma SJ. *Postconventional Moral Thinking: A Neo-Kohlbergian Approach*. Mahwah, NJ: Lawrence Erlbaum Associates; 1999.

43. Kidder RM. *How Good People Make Tough Choices: Resolving the Dilemmas of Ethical Living*. New York, NY: Harper Collins Publisher; 2009.

44. Seedhouse D, Lovett L. *Practical Medical Ethics*. New York, NY: John Wiley & Sons; 1992.

45. Venglar M, Theall M. Case-based ethics education in physical therapy. *J School Teach Learn*. 2007;7(1):64–76.

46. Delany CM, Edwards I, Jensen GM, Skinner E. Closing the gap between ethics knowledge and practice through active engagement: an applied model of physical therapy ethics. *Phys Ther*. 2010;90(7):1068–1078.

47. Guillemin M, Gilliam L. *Telling Moments: Everyday Ethics in Health Care*. Melbourne, Australia: IP Communications; 2006.

48. Strum A, Edwards I, Fryer CE, Roswith R. (Almost) 50 shades of an ethical situation—international physiotherapists' experiences of everyday ethics: a qualitative analysis. *Physio Theory Practice*. 2022;1–18e doi: 10.1080/09593985.2021.2015812

49. Delany C, Edwards I, Fryer E. How physiotherapists perceive, interpret, and respond to the ethical dimensions of practice: A qualitative study. *Physio Theory Practice*. 2019(35):663–676.

50. Greenfield BH, Jensen GM. Understanding the lived experiences of patients: application of a phenomenological approach to ethics. *Phys Ther*. 2010;90(8):1185–1197.

51. Sullivan KJ, Wallace JG Jr, O'Neil ME, et al. A vision for society: physical therapy as partners in the national health agenda. *Phys Ther*. 2011;91(11):1664–1672.

52. Ofri D. *When We Do Harm: A Doctor Confronts Medical Error*. Boston, MA: Beacon Press; 2021.

53. Christ C. *Diving Deep and Surfacing*. Boston, MA: Beacon Press; 1995.

# SUGGESTED READINGS

Annas GJ, Grodin MA. *The Nazi Doctors and the Nuremberg Code: Human Rights in Human Experimentation / Edition 1*. New York, NY: Oxford University Press; 1995.

Banja JD. Ethics, outcomes, and reimbursement. *Rehab Manag*. 1994;7(1):61–65.

Clancy CM, Brody H. Managed care. Jekyll or Hyde? *JAMA*. 1995;273(4):338–339.

Curtin LL. Why good people do bad things. *Nursing Manage*. 1996;27(7):63–65.

Devettere R. *Practical Decision Making in Health Care Ethics: Cases, Concepts, and the Virtue of Prudence*. Washington, DC: Georgetown University Press; 2016.

DeGrazia D, Mappes TA, Ballard J, eds. *Biomedical Ethics*. 7th ed. New York, NY: McGraw Hill Higher Education; 2010.

Emmanuel EJ, Gluck AR., eds. *The Affordable Care Act: How The Affordable Care Act Transformed Politics, Law and Healthcare in America.* New York, NY: Public Affairs; 2020.

Finis J. *Rights Come to Mind: Brain Injury, Ethics, and the Struggle for Consciousness.* Cambridge: Cambridge University Press; 2010.

Gawande A. Why doctors hate their computers. *The New Yorker.* November 5, 2018.

Gawande A. *Being Mortal: Medicine and What Matters in the End.* New York, NY: Picador; 2017.

Gawande A. Overkill: an avalanche of unnecessary medical care is harming patients physically and financially. What can we do about it? *The New Yorker.* May 11, 2015.

Gawande A. The cost conundrum redux. *The New Yorker.* June 25, 2009.

Gray, FD. *The Tuskegee Syphilis Experiment: The Real Story and Beyond.* Montgomery, AL: NewSouth Books; 2002.

Grimaldi PL. Protection for patients or providers? *Nursing Manage.* 1996;27(7):12–17.

Jones JH. *Bad Blood: The Tuskegee Experiment.* New York, NY: Free Press; 1993.

Krimsky SK. *Stem Cell Dialogues. A Philosophical and Scientific Inquiry into Medical Frontiers.* New York, NY: Columbia University Press; 2017.

Ofri D. *When We Do Harm: A Doctor Confronts Medical Error.* Boston, MA: Beacon Press; 2021.

Pence G. *Medical Ethics: Accounts of Ground-Breaking Cases.* New York, NY: McGraw-Hill; 2024.

Rawal PH. *The Affordable Care Act: Examining the Facts.* Santa Barbara, CA: ABC-CLIO; 2015.

Rodwin MA. *Medicine, Money and Morals.* New York, NY: Oxford University Press; 1993.

Ruggiero VR. *Thinking Critically About Ethical Issues.* 11th ed. New York, NY: McGraw Hill; 2024.

Salladay SA. Rehabilitation, ethics and managed care. *Rehab Manag.* 1996;9(6):38–42.

Stahl DA. Risk shifting in subacute care. *Nurs Manage.* 1996;27(7):20, 22.

# SUGGESTED RESOURCES

American Physical Therapy Association. *Ethics in practice resources and modules*: https://learningcenter.apta.org/ (please see related professionalism modules within the APTA Learning Center)

Federation of State Boards of Physical Therapy Practice. www.fsbpt.org

Fink, S. *Five Days at Memorial: Life and Death in a Storm-Ravaged Hospital.* New York, NY: Crown Publishing; 2016 (also available on Apple TV+)

The *Deadly Deception. Nova* video written, produced, and directed by Denisce Di Anni, WGBH Boston, 1993 production. [Films for the Humanities and Sciences, P.O. Box 205, Princeton, NJ 08543-2053.]

The National Commission for the Protection of Human Subjects of Biomedical and Behavioral Research. *The Belmont Report.* OPPR Reports, NIH, PHS, HHS, last reviewed March 15, 2016. Available: https://www.hhs.gov/ohrp/regulations-and-policy/belmont-report/index.html Accessed September 11, 2022.

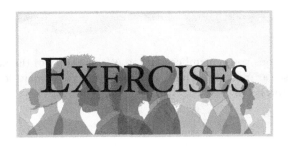

# EXERCISE 1: WRITE YOUR MORAL AUTOBIOGRAPHY

People reveal themselves in telling stories. We all have stories to tell about ourselves, our lives growing up, the choices we had to make, close calls we have had, funny incidents where we were caught off guard, a great (or terrible) date, a wonderful concert or movie, and an exciting time with an old friend.

Christ wrote, *in Diving Deep and Surfacing:*[53]

> *When meeting new friends or lovers, people reenact the ritual of telling stories. Why? Because they sense the meaning of their lives is revealed in the stories they tell, in their perception of the forces they contended with, in the choices they made, in their feelings about what they did or did not do. In telling their stories, people speak of parents, lovers, ecstasy, and death—of moments when life's meaning seemed clear or unfathomable.*

One of the most important aspects of your story is your perception of how, growing up, the values of your family provided a sense of orientation for you that perhaps became a taken-for-granted set of boundaries against which you played out your life, against which you had to contend, the currents in which you learned to swim, and the forces that helped you to define yourself. In this way, those values provided a sense of meaning. They grounded you in powers of being that enabled you to challenge the obstacles of the world to become who you are now.

Think back to when you were a child. You may want to interview parents and grandparents for more information.

1.  What were the rules of the family? Where did those rules seem to come from? The Bible? The church? From ancient wisdom passed down?

2.  For what do you remember being punished? For what were your siblings punished? Were you punished, or would you say you were "disciplined"? What is the difference to you?

3.  For what were you praised? What were you encouraged to do? How did that make you feel?

4.  Were there certain favorite virtues that were emphasized? For example, always refer to people with their preferred nouns, pronouns, always do your best, always tell the truth, get good grades, and go out for sports?

5.  What were the family rules for making decisions, or did that remain a mystery?

6.   What do you remember being most emotional about? Did you have a favorite cause? Have you ever participated in a march for a cause or in any actions of civil disobedience? Would you if you were challenged to? Why or why not?


Recount any major moral decisions you remember making. Write a story of the development of your moral consciousness. What values do you see as most important, and how, from your story, do you know this? Does this have implications for your choice of profession?

# EXERCISE 2: EXAMINE YOUR CODE OF ETHICS AND PRACTICE ACT

Locate a copy of your profession's code of ethics. Analyze the code statements to determine the values and ethical principles that are most esteemed by your profession. Next, examine the code and its accompanying rules for what seems to be missing. What would you wish the code and rules would speak to that is not present? Are the directions for moral action specific enough for your guidance? Why not?

Locate a copy of your licensing authority's practice act for your profession and its accompanying rules. Outline the scope of practice allowed by the Act. What are you able to do, and what are you prohibited from doing? What guidelines are given about delegation of care to aides and assistants? What might you be asked to do by an uninformed superior that would not be legal? What might you be asked to do that is legal but would not be ethical? How would you respond?

# Exercise 3: Ethical Dilemma Resolution

Below are several day-to-day ethical situations faced by HCPs. Choose one. Go through the process to solve it as illustrated in this chapter.

1.  A physical therapist colleague in private practice admits that he charges less money for patients who pay with cash because he never records his income for tax purposes. You have been working for this therapist for 6 months, and to keep your job, he is asking you to adopt the same system and offers you a cash bonus of $5,000 at Christmas because you deserve the money more than the Internal Revenue Service. Personal circumstances make this the only place where you can practice and still fulfill your family responsibilities. You are the only person in your family employed at this time, and you are supporting two children and an elderly mother.

    a.  Look at Table 4.2. Is this an individual, organizational, or societal problem?

    b.  What kind of ethical situation is described here—an issue, problem, dilemma, distress, or temptation?

    c.  Finally, what kind of process is required on the part of the physical therapist—moral sensitivity, judgment, motivation, or courage?

    d.  What should this physical therapist do? Why?

    e.  Consider the queries for active listening, reflective thinking, and critical reasoning in Table 4.3 applying the Active Engagement Model.

2.  You have agreed to fill in for a home care therapist for two weeks. At four of the five patients' homes in one day, as you evaluated and treated according to your standards, the patients have made comments that the other therapist never did any of this kind of therapy. It becomes apparent to you that the therapist you are filling in for is giving no professional care. You are scheduled to move out of this town to another state as soon as this two-week period ends. If you report this person, you would likely need to return to the state to testify, but the state would likely pay your expenses to do so.

    a.  Look at Table 4.2. Is this an individual, organizational, or societal problem?

    b.  What kind of ethical situation is described here—an issue, problem, dilemma, distress, or temptation?

    c.  What kind of process is required on the part of the physical therapist—moral sensitivity, judgment, motivation, or courage?

    d.  What should this physical therapist do? Why?

e. Consider the queries for active listening, reflective thinking, and critical reasoning in Table 4.3 applying the Active Engagement Model.

3. At 4:45 p.m., a woman in severe pain walks into the physical therapy department with a referral from her physician to be evaluated and treated for severe low back pain. The physical therapist in charge (and the only one present) had stayed late to see patients well after the usual closing time of five o'clock for the past week. Furthermore, the day care center had called just before the woman walked in, stating that the therapist's 6-month-old daughter was extremely sick with severe vomiting and diarrhea, and they were very worried about her. The therapist's wife is out of town. The therapist tells the patient, "I'm sorry, we're closed for the day, and I must leave. You'll have to come back in the morning." The woman bursts into tears and says she does not even know if she can make it home, she is in such pain.

   a. Look at Table 4.2. Is this an individual, organizational, or societal problem?

   b. What kind of ethical situation is described here—an issue, problem, dilemma, distress, or temptation?

   c. Finally, what kind of process is required on the part of the physical therapist—moral sensitivity, judgment, motivation, or courage?

   d. What should this physical therapist do? Why?

   e. Consider the queries for active listening, reflective thinking, and critical reasoning in Table 4.3 applying the Active Engagement Model.

4. You are treating a woman who recently had a stroke. Her insurance allows for payment for only ten treatments. What ethical implications are there when you cannot achieve agreed-upon functional goals in ten treatments?

   a. What is your professional responsibility? What is your legal responsibility? What would you do to resolve this problem short of refusing care?

   b. How might you go about working to change this organizational limitation from the insurance company? Would you do it? Why or why not?

   c. Consider the queries for critical reasoning in Table 4.3 applying the Active Engagement Model.

**These exercises are also available online at www.routledge.com/9781638220039.**

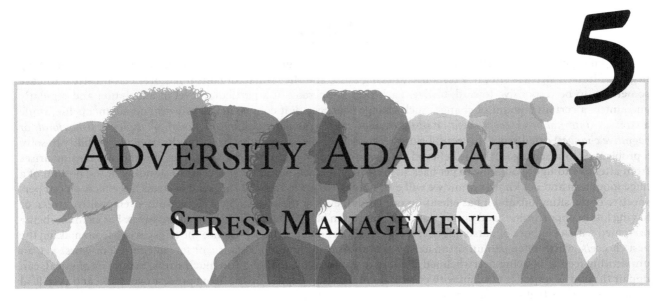

# ADVERSITY ADAPTATION
## STRESS MANAGEMENT

*Gina Maria Musolino and Carol M. Davis*

## OBJECTIVES

*The learner should be able to:*

- Discover personal sources of stress.
- Examine effects of stress on the body.
- Reflectively express one's perceptions of stress and stressful situations.
- Describe signs, causes, and examples of burnout.
- Apply the stress development model and related screening tools.
- Contrast external and internal factors that contribute to stress build-up for health professionals.
- Assess how stress impacts health care, quality of care, safety, and health care providers.
- Review contemporary mental health status data.
- Adopt an initiative-taking mindset of prevention for stress management.
- Explore mechanisms that interfere with stress accumulation to help control harmful impacts.

One of the most powerful rewards of the helping and healing professions is the tremendous professional satisfaction. Most people enter these professions to work with people who need help in overcoming illness or disability or to support well people to stay healthy. The expectation is a professional career in which one believes that each day will be interesting and rewarding, with the assumption of professional satisfaction and meaning in helping others through healing and preventative assistance. Few people ever anticipate or prepare for the tremendous amount of mental and physical stress that is inherent in the helping professions. Many patients experiencing physical conditions have co-existing mental health concerns.[1] Despite the deepest feelings of caring and altruism, caring for people who need help can bring with it substantial emotional and physical exhaustion to those who do not prepare for these challenges. While a bit of stress can be good, too much can be destructive.

DOI: 10.4324/9781003525554-5

# STRESS

Let's take a closer look at stress in general. Stress is a value-neutral word; that is, it need not indicate something negative. In fact, stress is simply a response to being alive, and the human organism requires certain stress to have something to be responsive toward, to live. Each person operates at a particular level of adaptation and regularly encounters a certain amount of change. Such change is expected; it contributes to growth and augments life, while a stressor (*internal or external event or situation that creates the potential for emotional, physiologic, behavioral, or cognitive changes*) can disrupt this equilibrium. What we perceive as negative stress results from our inability to solve a problem or to reach a goal that is believed (or feared) to be unattainable. We feel out of control, and tension arises from attempts to figure out how to get back in control and reach our goals,[2] similar to standing at the bottom of a huge mountain and not knowing how we will ever manage to get to the top. This kind of stress has effects on our perspective of the situation, and it has effects on our bodies, even at the cellular level. Sometimes even positive stress, or having lots of opportunities and options, at times, may even be more stressful than negative stress. For example, being presented with a plethora of outstanding career pathways and opportunities; hence the stress arises from making the best choice/s, which often can unfortunately, be paralyzing, leading to no choice, or forced choices; or worse yet, an unrelenting feeling of being overwhelmed, leading to paralysis by analysis. Too much stress, mental or physical, can impair the body's response to adapt with environmental changes, speed up the aging process over time, and even lead to certain diseases that increase degeneration.[3]

The desired response to stress is when a person appraises and copes with changing situations through adjustments and adaptations to the change/s. Coping is the behavioral and cognitive compensatory process. Stress can also deplete the reserve capacities, especially in older adults, and lessens one's ability to respond, and adapt to environmental changes. While no stage of life is stress-free, as we age, we are at higher risk of impacts from rapid environmental and/or lifestyle changes, illness, loss of significant others, financial hardships, and relocation/s.[3] Resilience is one's ability to recover and adapt appropriately following any stress, trauma, tragedy, or adversity in life—leading to a resilient disposition for both psychological and physical wellness.

When we feel the anxiety of negative stress, we tend to misread the situation at hand, blow things out of proportion, take on unrealistic guilt, or internalize and personalize thoughts that have little to do with us. For example, let's say you feel under the stress of seeing five more patients in the next 12 minutes (*an unattainable goal*), and a colleague comes into your office and is noticeably upset about something. There is a high likelihood that one of your immediate responses to your colleague would be, "Oh great! What did I do now?"

The fact is that often you are not the cause of another person's anger or frustration, and you increase your stress by making that erroneous assumption. Under stress, you have simply distorted a situation and, depending on the energy of your paranoia, blown it all out of proportion. Stress distorts our ability to see the world as it truly is, and this distortion then increases our stress, causing a positive progression or escalation of our anxiety. The greater the existing stress, the more likely the addition of more stress. In other words, a positive feedback loop is established.

Many aspects of day-to-day life, both positive and negative, cause some minor stress; e.g., change in sleeping habits, church, social activities, new school, vacation, personal achievement, etc. Many life events are sources of major stress; e.g., death, divorce, separation, injury, illness, change in health (self or family member), sexual difficulties, changing jobs, relocation, etc. Stressors on a day-to-day basis, e.g., getting stuck in traffic, familial arguments, technology challenges, in a cumulative fashion can also be as impactful as life events.[4] Major stressors also include historical events, e.g., hurricanes, wars, terroristic activities, population shifts, etc. Duration or time may also be of consideration with respect to stressors, e.g., chronic, daily hassles; chronic illness; food insecurity; disabilities; acute, time-limited practical examinations. Those under constant stress, especially those negatively impacted by the social determinants of health (SDoH; see Figure 1.1 in Chapter 1), e.g., lack of access to health care; have a higher incidence of disease.[5] Distress is associated with alterations in a person's physical and emotional health status, decreased or altered social support, changes in daily functioning abilities, and loss of significant others.[6]

It will come as no surprise that the Covid-19 pandemic challenged everyone in a variety of ways, with many unexpected stressors. These included: changes in roles, at work and at home; changes in the purpose of home environments constantly altered for competing school and work needs; more or less time with family members and/or significant others, caregivers, and friends; screen fatigue; sleep pattern alterations; fear of missing out; inability to attain needed goods and services; missed expectations; ever-changing requirements; employment losses, or excessive employment demands, especially for those deemed as essential workers; conflicting messages from authorities. Many of the stressors led to catastrophizing, and mental health needs quickly escalated, coming to the forefront, prevailing for all age groups, as a primary concern.[7]   A new emphasis has been placed upon the need to screen and manage mental health needs for all patients and to be aware of our own needs, as health care professionals (HCPs).[7,8] HCPs can offer suggestions for stress management and coping. As HCPs we need to be keenly aware of our own stress reactions for both personal and professional needs, and seek mental health care intervention, early and as often as needed. Seeking this care is a sign of strength. Our responsibility for our own actions as HCPs is a key ability for professional formation and preeminent practice.[7–9]

## Stressors Commonly Experienced by Health Care Professionals

The health care profession has undergone massive change in the last three decades and currently continues to reflect those changes. The impact of reimbursement and technological advances on the quality of care of patients has had a mixed review, but for the most part, patients now report more depersonalized care; are disappointed with the quality of the care they are receiving, particularly the lack of individual time spent with their providers; and resent the increasing cost of health insurance.[10–11] Today, more access to care is available, yet with varying quality and proximity. Less comprehensive coverage is available, but more preventative coverage is generally attainable. Catastrophic care is still problematic for those without private insurance and the federal and state governments continue to offer a range of plans. The burden is now on the public, more than in the past, to select a plan. Limited consultation is available to assist the public in selecting insurance coverage. Just making a choice about health care has now become a point of stress for the untrained public and many do not have any idea how to examine a policy to learn how various aspects of care, such as rehabilitation therapies, will or will not be covered. Often, the coding and billing staff in your practice setting may help to offer advice, and HCPs are often called upon for guidance. As policies change, HCPs are expected to keep up to date with changing payment models and a plethora of insurance types, while maintaining contemporary, evidence-based practice and striving for excellence in patient–practitioner interactions (PPIs). Health care is not for the faint of heart. HCPs are being challenged to do more for less. Evolving payment models and systems continue to be studied and considered, and more reform is needed, causing even greater stress on the HCP to provide accurate documentation to support the payment systems.[12] HCPs must select appropriate codes and provide standardized measures to support progressions of care. Ensuring compliance with federal regulations (e.g., Medicare [www.medicare.gov], third-party payers, Federal civil rights laws, and the Health Insurance Portability and Accountability Act Privacy Rule [HIPAA, www.hhs.gov/ocr/office]) may be a source of stress in everyday practice. Note, we will discuss some key legislation affecting patients and HCPs in Chapter 17.

Assessing risk for fraud and abuse and doing the right thing are part of practice management for all HCPs. If one does not manage these practice demands daily, they can become an escalated, negative, and unnecessary stress and potentially lead to devastating fines and even criminal charges or behaviors. The American Physical Therapy Association (APTA), The American Occupational Therapy Association (AOTA), and the American Speech-Language-Hearing Association (ASHA), together, have issued a consensus statement related to clinical judgment in health care settings regarding ethical service delivery, the need-to-know rules and regulations, evaluation, treatment, and documentation as well as upholding clinical integrity. The statement also provides information on the Office of Inspector General hotline for reporting fraud anonymously. You may access the joint statement via www.aota.org/-/media/corporate/files/practice/ethics/apta-aota-asha-concensus-statement.pdf as well as many other compliance tips and educational opportunities to assist in your efforts for integrity in practice (e.g., fraud, abuse and waste, via the APTA Learning Center [www.apta.org/your-practice/ethics-and-professionalism/preventing-fraud-abuse-and-waste]; understanding compliance [www.apta.org/your-practice/compliance]).

Knowledge is certainly a way to combat stress, and reassures that you are doing the right or best things in practice and conscientiously choosing to make the wisest possible decision. Staying active in your professional associations helps to keep you abreast of changing practice needs on both national and state levels. While the rewards of the profession, in assisting another human being accomplish therapeutic goals, is paramount, the stress of care management in an ever-changing health care world demands that HCPs manage their stressors daily. One cannot be like an ostrich, sticking one's head in the sand when it comes to regulating stress management in health care. Patients should also be informed and aware of their own rights in receiving health care (www.fsbpt.org/Secondary-Pages/The-Public/Understand-Your-Rights).

Now, let's consider select research studies, regarding the issue of stress in HCP practice. A study examining the impact of the changing health care environment on fieldwork education in occupational therapy revealed that levels of stress were raised by increased productivity expectations, number of hours worked, and time spent in documentation, with a decrease in job security, time for continuing education, and quality of patient care.[13] In a study of primary care physician practices, patients reported a lower rating on the quality of care from physicians in managed care practices.[14] Some of the most common sources of workplace stress for nurses included more intense workload, conflicts with leadership/management style, professional conflicts in general, and the emotional cost of caring.[14]

In sum, it remains a sign of the times that the environment of health care has changed significantly to become more stressful for health care professionals and their patients, and it will take a quantum shift for health care to once again be characterized by healing and less by business practices. When patients become a means to an end for profit, the stress on health care professionals who want to serve those in need becomes enormous when they are forced by organizations to pay more attention to the "bottom line."[15] Upcoming, in Chapter 11, we will discuss the role of the professions and HCPs in advocacy for our patients with regards to health policy and payment legislation.

# Stressors Commonly Experienced by Students

Ongoing anxieties are commonly experienced by students[1,2] due to similar stressors. Remember that negative stress is experienced in the presence of a fear that a goal that we have set is unattainable. Students respond most dramatically to three anxiety-provoking questions throughout their education[2]:

1. *Am I good enough?* Not only troublesome just before exams but also an ongoing fear related to questions of moral and intellectual competence—in other words, this is an issue of self-esteem and can be fueled by constant comparison of oneself with "more talented" classmates and professionals.

2. *Do I have what it takes?* Considers perceptions of and fears about one's physical and emotional limits. An anxiety that often appears the first time a student feels faint while in a hospital or experiences the exhaustion of long hours of upstanding physical work without breaks.

3. *Can I pay?* The cost of tuition is steadily rising, although some efforts to forgive some student loan debts are in motion. The anxiety of having to take out additional and override loans, pay for temporary housing, take on another job, or quit, weighs on students, and often affects their performance in classes and clinics. Research supports that certain professions must be cautious about raising tuition and fees due to the overburden of debt that may be recoverable over a course of a career.[16] Take a look at your professional association websites for additional information and resources for financial literacy and management (e.g., www.apta.org/your-career/financial-solutions-center). Most health careers are in high demand, hence taking out a reasonable amount of loans can reduce other burdens, enabling more focus on studies.

A review of the literature examining students' difficulties with stressors in medical school described sources of stress for medical students, varying by year in training:[17]

*First-year stressors:*

- Challenges of being uprooted from family and friends.
- Adapting to a demanding new learning environment.
- Human cadaver dissection.
- Substantially increased scholastic workload.
- Concern for academic performance.

*Preclinical years:*

- Attempting to master a large volume of information.
- Joining a peer group of equal motivation and intelligence, particularly for those who struggle academically.
- High-stakes examinations, e.g., National Board of Medical Examiners, Step 1, Step 2.
- Tests that must be passed before academic advancement.

*Clinical years:*

- Separation from peer support group/s.
- Frequent rotations to new work environments at different hospitals requiring a unique medical knowledge base and skill set, which tends to highlight students' deficiencies rather than their progress.
- Less or unstructured learning environments.
- Lack of time for recreation.
- Concerns about financial issues.
- Long on-duty assignments.
- Student abuse.
- Exposure to human suffering.

Life issues go on while students are in school, and as the age of students entering the professions increases, these issues can become more complex, with those related to families, partners, or caring for aging parents, for example, to be concerned about during professional school training. For example, illnesses, pregnancies, having to move, marriage, divorce, disconnecting from social networks, and marital and/or parent problems do not automatically disappear while the student finishes their education. The anxieties feed into the base level of life stress and can markedly affect students' abilities to learn and focus. Professional students are encouraged to utilize their student support services to assist in their educational endeavors when encountering stress management concerns. Counseling, both individual and group, and related support services are available to assist learners in the notable stresses of life and in being a professional student in training. Part of becoming a professional means the ability to effectively cope and manage your stress. Availing yourself of available resources is not a sign of weakness, it is a sign of courage and strength, and critical to you becoming the best HCP. Not only will you learn coping skills for yourself, but you can also gain insights into patient stress management, as you travel your personal and professional development journeys. Do not be afraid to seek support, rather embrace the learning and growth opportunity. Mental health support is often needed for your ability to be fully devoted to the necessary intensive learning and performance capabilities as a HCP advancing in professional formation. A little help goes a long way with those willing and interested to effect change in themselves for the good of their future patients and colleagues.

## Physical Effects of Stress

Stress takes its toll physically as well. Now that medicine has made great strides in eradicating many infectious diseases, most illnesses are of a chronic nature, and most chronic diseases have been found to be influenced by stress. When we perceive stress, the endocrine system goes into action.

This was quite useful when we depended upon the sympathetic nervous system for our survival in primitive times. "Fight or flight" was, at one time, our only alternative in stressful situations, most of which were, indeed, life threatening. However, it seems as if our nervous system has not kept up with our progress as a civilized society. Few wild animals threaten daily survival, but in some situations we respond as if that were exactly the case.[18] This outpouring of adrenaline and other neuropeptides acts as a stressor on our bodies.[19] People's physical responses differ. Some suffer from headaches, others from diarrhea, nausea, cardiac palpitations, panic, etc. Over time, organ systems break down under this constant stress, and the result might be a lowered immune system, diabetes, high blood pressure, ulcers, colitis, or arthritis, and/or chronic fatigue.

As a developing HCP, transitioning from classroom-based activities to more clinically based patient interactions, you will also find yourself both physically and mentally challenged. You are on your feet more throughout the day and thinking on your feet often, addressing competing clinical and patient management needs. You no longer can pull "all-nighters" and must practice good nutrition and sleep hygiene, and maintain your own physical health to assure that your patient encounters are as safe and effective as possible. Overuse of technology, especially with increased screen time, has wreaked havoc on many HCPs' ability to sleep properly. You will need to manage your devices in order to practice good sleep hygiene.[20] You will need to find ways to manage your daily stress with simple techniques. These can include practicing the art of deep breathing, continuing to maintain good physical health, even as simply as walking to decompress, and stay fit, while practicing to deeply focus without interruptions. Techniques such as meditation, yoga, relaxation training, massage, mindfulness, practicing gratitude, recreation, and hobbies, for example, have all been found to aid stress reduction.

Again, maintaining both your mental and physical health, as a HCP, is critical to your success. Do not skip your annual physical exams, well vaccines, and preventative screens, and seek medical care when needed. The Centers for Disease Control (CDC) maintains updated recommendations for all persons and ones specific to health care providers (www.cdc.gov/vaccines/index.html). Be sure to keep current for both your, and your patients', safety. Do not be your own worst patient, causing yourself unnecessary stress. Seek the expertise of those who can provide any required care needed. In this way you shall also serve as a role model for your patients and clients by maintaining your optimal physical and mental health status.

## Stress Development Model

The key to understanding stress, and preventing negative effects, lies in understanding a continuum model:

*Life Situation* ⇨ *Perception* ⇨ *Emotion* ⇨ *Physiological Response* ⇨ *Disease*

The life situation is *not* the key component in this model; it is the *perception* that I have that this life situation is a tiger that is going to eat me, unless I get out of here fast or fight like crazy for my survival. Some people live all day, every day, as if there were a tiger just around the corner. They have learned a world view that life is a hostile place, and one must always be on guard.[18] (Remember that Chapter 2 gives us insights into how people learn this world view.) Others simply periodically find themselves in situations where they realize that their stress is too high, that the world view has been distorted, and that it is time to get a grip on things and time to do what they must to get back in control of their lives.

## How Misperceptions Develop

When there is, indeed, a misperception of the current situation, it is most often a result of the influence of past experience. We become programmed, in a sense, based on unfortunate things that have happened to us in the past, and thus we misperceive what is happening right now and we fear the unknown of the future. As a result, we allow history or old data to distort the present and our anxiety mounts. Thought is at the heart of all stress. Our thoughts create our reality in the largest sense. When you think of it, there are four kinds of thoughts. Only one kind of thought is hugely beneficial to maintaining the quality of our lives—*positive* thoughts. Thoughts that are focused on optimism, possibility, connection with others and the world, gratitude, appreciation, and love are thoughts that will develop a feeling of oneness, confidence, and hopefulness. However, too often we are consumed by negative thoughts, wasted thoughts (if only I had …), and neutral thoughts (thoughts needed to get through the day). Thoughts lead to feelings, which lead to attitudes, which lead to actions and behavior, which lead to habits, which lead to destiny.

The key, then, to changing the negative effects of stress is to carefully examine the nature of our thoughts and our misperceptions. Negative thoughts and beliefs (thoughts we just keep telling ourselves over and over) leave us feeling exhausted, worried, frustrated, drained, combative, and angry. Positive thoughts leave us feeling hopeful, appreciative, optimistic, and caring. We have an internal mechanism that can help us recognize, immediately, whether our thoughts are helpful or stressful. If we can *interrupt* the stress build-up by changing what we think and what we believe about what is happening, then the emotion will be more realistic, and the sympathetic nervous system need not be overstimulated.[21] By reaching for the positive thought, or even just a more neutral thought, we can interrupt the sympathetic response and choose a more life-nurturing activity. We then can make the best of a situation; we can literally transform our day from stressful to uplifting, but this takes concerted practice.

Learning to stay in the present is a place to start. As soon as we begin to feel anxious, we should take a deep breath and simply say to ourselves, "Stay in the now. Do not be influenced by the past that is gone forever, or the future that has yet to happen. Listen carefully to what is going on now. Do not personalize or react. Listen."[22] This is not an easy thing to do, because our reactions are firmly set in place by years of habitual ways of thinking. To interrupt these entrenched habits takes conscious practice and commitment to change. According to Tolle[22] and Kabat-Zinn,[23] the skill of staying in the "now" is best learned by purposely quieting your mind. This can be done by learning meditation techniques such as Transcendental Meditation[19] or by practicing tracking your breath for 10 to 30 minutes every day.

Sit quietly and practice focusing 100% of your concentration on the breath, as it flows in and out of your nostrils. Quieten the "monkey chatter" and naysayers in your brain, let all thoughts float away in imaginary bubbles, and simply breathe. Soon your body will relax, and your parasympathetic nervous system will help you to slow down and feel more centered and peaceful. Be patient with yourself. When you find yourself thinking thoughts, just say to yourself "thinking," and then gently return your awareness to your breathing.[23]

# BURNOUT

*Burnout* is a term that has been popularized to indicate a state of emotional and physical exhaustion that results from intense and long-standing professional stress. Maslach[24] first described burnout. The subjects in her investigation were human service personnel, or people helpers. The fact is that, when we agree to help people, there are always professional demands that seem impossible to meet, and this creates stress and tension that builds over time. The professional stress and tension are termed burnout. Burnout is a dynamic process that is fed by a negative self-concept and negative job attitudes, which result in a loss of concern for people, a withdrawal from interaction, and alienation from the work environment.[25] The World Health Organization (WHO) recently redefined burnout as a "syndrome conceptualized as resulting from chronic workplace stress that has not been successfully managed."[26] The Maslach Burnout Inventory[24] (with career-specific assessments for health care providers, educators, and students) is one measure that aligns with the WHO's definition for burnout[26] and considers three dimensions:

1. Feelings of energy depletion or exhaustion.

2. Increased mental distance from one's job, or feelings of negativism or cynicism related to one's job.

3. Reduced professional efficacy.

# Signs and Symptoms of Burnout

Health professionals enter the professions with enthusiasm and optimism and often soon realize that the demands of the work far exceed their expectations. The common response is to double the effort, with little change in productivity.[14] Soon, fatigue and discouragement set in. The stress of the intense emotional demands of health care interaction builds, and a common coping mechanism is to distance oneself or become emotionally detached from work.[25] Detachment is often unconscious and can take the form of actual physical withdrawal, spending shorter amounts of time with people, or emotional withdrawal, objectifying people (e.g., by labeling them). A patient with back pain becomes "the low back in 343."

Other signs of burnout are the drawing of crisp boundaries between work and home; compartmentalizing one's life sharply; and demonstrating less creativity in treatment, offering more rigid, "by the book" responses to problems, lowering the risk of making a mistake. Feelings of personal inadequacy from not achieving (often unrealistic) goals can lead to self-dissatisfaction, which results in projected anger and frustration. People tend to stay away from you because of your "short fuse."

At-home burnout can contribute to marital tension, as well as tension with family members and/or close friends. There is a tendency to engage in compulsive behavior (addictions) to numb oneself from stress, so use of food, drugs, sex, gaming, alcohol, etc. may increase. Physical signs such as headaches, stomach ailments, or problems with elimination begin to appear. Sleep may be disturbed. By this time, one is well on the way to increased absenteeism and begins to job hunt or seriously consider applying to graduate school, often believing that finding the right place to work, or be, will solve all these problems.

Table 5.1 illustrates that the manifestations of burnout permeate several areas of our lives and build over time. As they escalate, they can be seen to fall into four stages.[27] Stage 1, enthusiasm, characterizes the symptoms of early burnout. Without appropriate intervention, a person inevitably progresses to stage 4, which carries many of the symptoms of a full-scale depression.[21] Stage 4 burnout is a serious condition, and very often professional help is needed to free oneself from this situation.

| TABLE 5.1 | | | | |
|---|---|---|---|---|
| **MANIFESTATIONS OF BURNOUT IN OCCUPATIONAL THERAPISTS**[27] | | | | |
| **COMPONENTS** | **STAGE 1: ENTHUSIASM** | **STAGE 2: STAGNATION** | **STAGE 3: FRUSTRATION** | **STAGE 4: APATHY** |
| **Personal characteristics** | Do I invest my whole self in my work? <br><br>Do I set extremely lofty goals for myself? | Am I beginning to question whether I like my job and whether it meets my personal needs? <br><br>Am I beginning to see that there are limitations in my work environment? | Am I not only questioning the value of my job but also the value of the entire profession? <br><br>Do I blame myself when a patient does not improve or return to treatment? | Am I feeling totally disinterested in my job? <br><br>Do I avoid work by using all my sick time? <br><br>Am I disinterested in patient progress? |
| **Modality use** | Do I work to increase my repertoire of activities and/or attempt to create new program ideas? <br><br>Do I verbally discuss with my patients the purpose of an activity and observed progress? | Do I find myself using the same activities repeatedly? <br><br>Do I focus with the patient on only 1 or 2 aspects of their performance? | Is my stress so great that I no longer feel creative? <br><br>Do I look at product versus process? | Do I always let the patients choose their activity, even when another modality may be more therapeutic? <br><br>Am I disinterested in my patient's response to the modality selected? |

*(continued)*

| | | TABLE 5.1 (CONTINUED) | | |
|---|---|---|---|---|
| | **MANIFESTATIONS OF BURNOUT IN OCCUPATIONAL THERAPISTS**[27] | | | |
| **COMPONENTS** | **STAGE 1: ENTHUSIASM** | **STAGE 2: STAGNATION** | **STAGE 3: FRUSTRATION** | **STAGE 4: APATHY** |
| **Use of theoretical** | Am I interested in learning about new theories and applying them to my practice? | Do I prefer to use the theory base with which I am most comfortable? Do I attempt to use new concepts after discussion with peers and supervisors? | Do I find new theories to be a waste of time and more professional jargon? | Do I find myself using no theoretical base at all? |
| **Inter-professional relationships** | Do I attempt to engage other disciplines in the activity process? Do I work to increase communication among team members and to effectively resolve conflicts? | Do I get annoyed when people from other professions ask to observe my groups? Do I feel that my domain is being stepped on by other team members? | Do I feel competitive with team members and avoid talking to them outside required meetings? Do I find myself expressing my anger about the team to the other therapists in my department? | Do I feel there is no need to deal with my team about unresolved issues because nothing helps? |
| **Education** | Do I enjoy the opportunity to educate others about what I do as an occupational therapist? | Do I get tired of always having to explain my practice? | Am I beginning to resent the need to always educate others, especially team members? | Do I avoid having to explain what to do? |
| **Budget** | Do I find it easy to adapt to a low budget by finding creative ways to use limited supplies? | Am I becoming tired of the constant need to adapt my programs to supply and budget constraints? | Do I find myself frequently complaining to my coworkers and supervisor about our limited budget and supplies? | Have I given in to our low budget by limiting my program to only those supplies that are readily available? |
| **Response to supervision and increased responsibilities** | Do I look forward to supervision and the opportunity to improve my job performance? | Do I become anxious when my supervisor suggests a change or that I take on additional responsibilities? | Do I resent changes implemented within the department and frequently discuss my resentment with peers? | Do I avoid work because of what will happen next? |
| **Professional development** | Do I actively pursue workshops, seminars, and courses to improve my skills? Do I put a lot of energy into my professional organizations? | Do I find that outside of work I always choose to pursue activities other than continuing education? Am I questioning the value of the profession and its organization? | Do I find suggestions to pursue continuing education to be an imposition? Will I pursue these activities only on work time? | Am I disinterested in professional activities and continuing education? |
| Reprinted with permission from Apter LC, Kolodner EL. Professional burnout—are you a candidate? *Phys Ther Forum.* 1987; 6:10. | | | | |

## Physical Stress Symptom Scale

In most families, people react to stress in similar ways. The data are inconclusive as to whether this is primarily due to genetic weakness or learned behavior, but it is common to see several people in a family respond to stress with similar symptoms. Refer to the Physical Stress Symptom Scale (Table 5.2).[28] Which of your organs or systems are most vulnerable to stress? You may want to compare results with other members of your family.

## Causes of Burnout

Factors that lead to burnout can be grouped into internal and external causes. External causes include conditions in the workplace that make it virtually impossible to experience consistent success, such as the following:[25]

- Work overload
    - Understaffed conditions
    - Lack of adequate, basic resources for safety
    - Overload of too many of one type of patient or one type of activity; not enough variety
    - Inability to use professional skills and creativity due to lack of time
- Role ambiguity
    - Less-than-clear guidelines of boundaries of responsibility
    - Nebulous expectations not communicated clearly
    - Scope of practice encroachment
- Role conflict
    - Conflicting advisement from authorities
    - Unwilling clinician collaboration for patient care
    - Several professionals perceive they are responsible for achieving the same goal; especially apparent in multidisciplinary team situations in which there is inadequate communication
    - Physicians make all decisions with no regard for input from other professionals

Internal causes of burnout are more difficult to identify and often are more challenging to influence. They include the following:[25]

- Professional's self-esteem. How individuals view themselves personally and professionally has an impact on their work. Low self-esteem facilitates imagined feelings of failure.

- Inability to set clear boundaries between personal and professional needs. Unclear ideas about the motives for wanting to help people (i.e., the desire to "fix it" for people rather than encouraging autonomy) result in inadvertently contributing to patients' neediness and dependence on health care workers, which results in a feeling of becoming too close or trapped in a relationship with a patient.

- The establishment of unrealistically optimistic goals for patients and the failure to meet them, which lowers self-image, a common event for overachieving new graduates. Intervention and guidance are required from more experienced mentors or supervisors.[25]

## Burnout Experienced by Health Care Professionals

In a pre-pandemic study[29] of burnout in practicing physical therapists in rehabilitation hospitals, the Maslach Burnout Inventory (MBI) scores indicated that 46% of the respondents scored high on the emotional exhaustion subscale, 20% scored high on the depersonalization subscale, and 60% scored low on the personal accomplishments subscale. Of the 250 therapists, 52% responded to the questionnaire, and the respondent sample presented with moderate burnout. Several factors were considered as contributing most: communication and connectedness, achievement, time constrains, variability in depersonalization, and personal accomplishment. Most of the physical therapists in this study[29] were in practice for fewer than four years.

Continuing to work toward recognition of burnout by HCPs, and addressing burnout syndrome, remain crucial. HCPs should be watchful for signs and symptoms of burnout, not only in themselves, but also in helping co-workers and patients, and suggesting appropriate referrals.

TABLE 5.2

# PHYSICAL STRESS SYMPTOM SCALE[28]

In the space provided, indicate how often each of the following effects happens to you either when you are experiencing stress or following exposures to a significant stressor. Respond to each item with a number between 0 and 5, using the following scale: 0 = never, 1 = once or twice a year, 2 = every few months, 3 = every few weeks, 4 = once or more each week, 5 = daily

## Cardiovascular Symptoms

_____ Heart pounding

_____ Heart racing or beating erratically

_____ Cold, sweaty hands

_____ Headache (throbbing pain)

_____ **Subtotal**

## Respiratory Symptoms

_____ Rapid, erratic, or shallow breathing

_____ Shortness of breath

_____ Asthma attack

_____ Difficulty in speaking because of poor breathing control

_____ **Subtotal**

## Gastrointestinal Symptoms

_____ Upset stomach, nausea, or vomiting

_____ Constipation

_____ Diarrhea

_____ Sharp abdominal pains

_____ **Subtotal**

## Muscular Symptoms

_____ Headaches (steady pain)

_____ Back or shoulder pain

_____ Muscle tremors or hand shaking

_____ Arthritis

_____ **Subtotal**

## Skin Symptoms

_____ Acne

_____ Dandruff

_____ Perspiration

_____ Excessive dryness of skin or hair

_____ **Subtotal**

## Immunity Symptoms

_____ Allergy flare-up

_____ Catching colds

_____ Catching the flu

_____ Skin rash

_____ **Subtotal**

## Metabolic Symptoms

_____ Increased appetite

_____ Increased craving for tobacco or sweets

_____ Thoughts racing or difficulty sleeping

_____ Feelings of crawling anxiety or nervousness

_____ **Subtotal**

_____ **Overall Symptoms Total (add all 7 subtotals)**

**Scale:**

0 to 5: *No predisposition in that symptom*

6 to 13: *Slightly higher risk of disease in that symptom*

14+: *Likely to experience psychosomatic disease in that symptom*

Adapted from Allen R. *Progressive Neuromuscular Relaxation*. College Park, MD: Autumn Wind Press; 1979.

Not unexpectedly, HCPs' burnout rates were exacerbated by the Covid-19 pandemic. In Missouri,[30] a study of primary care clinicians reporting higher rates of burnout. Unfortunately, only 17% sought help. Most did not take advantage of resiliency training (81%); of those that did, 16% stated sessions "made me feel less alone," while others found training less useful, due to lack of organizational support and available resources. Feedback focused on the need for dedicated support time that was included in working hours, ongoing assistance, and de-briefing, along with time for breaks and self-care. Also, according to a large Minnesota hospital association study[31] of clinicians' burnout, job demands were strongly related to burnout, whereas supporting resources were most related to work engagement. The greatest variables related to burnout were having sufficient time for work, values alignment with leaders, and teamwork efficiency; while the highest variables for engagement included values alignment, feeling appreciated, and autonomy.[31]

Likewise, physiotherapists in Poland,[32] during the pandemic, exhibited high occupational burnout rates on the MBI in all three domains: emotional exhaustion, depersonalization, and personal accomplishment. A comparative analysis of findings,[32] with related pre-pandemic published studies,[33,34] demonstrated that the burnout rates among physiotherapists significantly increased during the Covid-19 pandemic, with recommendations to employers to proactively address mental health needs for burnout prevention.

In fact, it's a health matter—burnout leads to safety issues and concerns. An attitude of humanism versus heroism has been encouraged by the National Academies of Practice,[35,36] as heroics did not best serve patients and providers, ultimately. Throughout the Covid-19 pandemic, HCPs were laser-focused on life-saving efforts for infectious patients in the face of equipment shortages and staffing inadequacies, facing challenges that led to the quality and safety of care being compromised.[36] For example, hospital-acquired infection rates rocketed; central line bloodstream infections in the final quarters of 2020 were 46–47% higher than in 2019.[35] The National Academies of Practice authors stated,

> *Rather than envisioning medicine as a province of brilliant individuals saving lives without a thought for their personal regard, the aim should be to achieve a culture of teamwork that acknowledges the human needs of clinicians and does not ask them to sacrifice their wellbeing on a routine basis.*[35]

Nash further implored:[36]

> *COVID-19 cast a spotlight on our woefully unprepared healthcare system and on the heroic responses of physicians and other healthcare professionals who put their own health at risk to care for overwhelming numbers of patients. I believe that the nation should be forever grateful to our courageous healthcare workforce. But I think we need to shift our perspective from heroic stories to acknowledging and addressing the systemic shortcomings that made heroics necessary. Going forward, what we need is support for a system in which skilled professionals have the resilience to respond heroically in an emergency because they would not have to do so every day.*

# ASSESSMENT, INTERVENTION, AND PREVENTION

Previously we have discussed the importance of perception in handling stress. Cultivating an ability to stay present or stay in the now, resisting the habit of interpreting present, ongoing events from history or fear of the future, will greatly assist one in remaining clear and realistic from moment to moment.[22,23] Asking clarifying questions and employing active listening skills will reduce the tendency to personalize and take undue responsibility for others' problems. Learning to inventory one's thoughts by checking on how you feel is critical to replacing negative thoughts with more energetic and hopeful thoughts that feel better.

However, the next step in reducing the problem of burnout is recognition that it is occurring, that it is happening right now to you, and choosing to believe that you have the power to stop its escalation. Because burnout has both internal and external antecedents, intervention must take place in both areas.[25]

Externally or organizationally, lowering staff–patient ratios remains critical, as does allowing for time away from contact with patients. Doing less stressful tasks such as record keeping, reading journal articles, planning patient research, clinical education, or quality assurance activities is an effective ways to lower the stress exacerbated by intense interaction with patients.[24] Required use of vacation/leave time also helps those who tend to overwork and deny the presence of burnout.[27] Mixing of patient loads and scheduling of regular staff rotations also helps to reduce the stress of seeing too many of any one type of patient.[27]

Organizationally sanctioned support groups are also an effective way to help reduce stress.[37] In these sessions, discussion of feelings is more important than discussion of patient problems. Many HCPs keep fears and feelings of personal failure to themselves, but most will welcome the opportunity to discuss frustrations concerning patients, especially if the organization encourages this opportunity for all its members.[37]

In rehabilitation we must maintain a constant awareness that strict adherence to the medical model of diagnose-treat-discharge "cured" very often does not apply to our patients. Most patients we see have multiple chronic illnesses, and we must learn how to expect an appropriate amount of effort from them, maintaining a more realistic goal than a hope for a cure. Patients' values, beliefs, and hopes must be clearly delineated and integrated into any collaborative plan of care.[38]

Studying burnout and its prevention while still in school gives you an added advantage before you get caught up in the confusing situations that your first position offers. You may also wish to become familiar with some of the scales and tools to screen for burnout, stress, depression, and work addiction for yourselves and your patients; e.g., Maslach Burnout Inventory,[24] Portuguese Dutch Work Addiction Scale,[39] Holmes-Rahe Life Stress Inventory,[40] Workplace Stress Survey,[41] Areas of Work-Life Survey,[42] Beck Depression Inventory,[43] and Pandemic Experiences Survey.[44] Self-monitoring and being able to screen for stress are important professionally, with our patients/clients, and for ourselves and often colleagues. Internally, or personally, health care professionals must develop a realistic view of helping and learn effective ways to manage repeated intense, emotional interactions with people.[25,26] Regular exercise is critical in reducing stress and addressing depression.[45] Increase in exercise is negatively correlated with the risk of depression. Randomized controlled trials provide clear evidence that exercise, resistance exercise, and mind–body exercise can improve depressive symptoms and levels.[45] Exercise has been proven to reshape the brain structure of patients with depression, activate the function of related brain areas, promote behavioral adaptation changes, and maintain the integrity of hippocampal and white matter volume, thus improving the brain neuroprocessing and delaying cognitive degradation in depression.[45] A lunch break, taken away from the patient care milieu, followed by a brisk walk, bike ride, or swim, has immediate and long-term positive benefits. Sufficient sleep and a nutritional diet also serve to keep one's internal stress low.

The logical, systematic left brain is the seat of the anxiety that leads to burnout. It is the left brain that cannot seem to figure out how to get the goal met. The right brain, however, is the source of relief from this pressure. The right brain functions by way of pictures, symbols, colors, and dreams. Meditation and activities that balance left–right brain activity and engage the right brain in activities such as daydreaming, painting, drawing, other hobbies, or imagery for relaxation during breaks in the workday also help. Tracking your breath, as described earlier, is one such activity.[23] Working at "play" increases creativity with resultant increases in solutions to life's problems and conditions.

Above and beyond all, however, is the importance of each health professional carefully examining their own needs in becoming a HCP to identify and curtail the tendency to overwork that is so common among us.[21] Work is just as addictive as alcohol, food, and drugs. We engage in compulsive behavior to keep us from dealing with our problems or from feeling the pain of normal growth and development. When work is used to keep us from growing, everyone suffers. Unfortunately, unlike drugs and alcohol, which do not carry public sanction, workaholics are often praised for their dedication and allow themselves to be taken advantage of by others. Instead, managers and employees should set boundaries and prevent colleagues and supervisors from infringing on personal time.[46] Advocating for boundaries (staying in one's lane) can prevent the extreme resultant reaction of "quiet quitting" with disengagement and decreased productivity.[47] This may occur to due to employee burnout, feeling undervalued, toxic work cultures, feelings of not being heard, being overwhelmed with responsibilities, or misalignment with doing what one was hired to do.[46,47] In a systematic and meta-analytical review of 170 studies of over 240,000 doctors experiencing burnout, researchers discovered that doctors were more than twice as likely to be involved in a patient safety incident (highest in those aged 20–30 years), four times less likely to have job satisfaction, and three times more likely to regret their career choice and consider leaving.[48] The review recommended that health care organizations should invest more time and effort in implementing evidence-based strategies to mitigate burnout, e.g., dedicated, restorative supervision time; flexible, compassionate scheduling; supportive, mentored career progressions; progressive pay, and benefits.[48]

Eventually, workaholics come to the realization that they are receiving from their efforts far less than they are contributing, and often this awareness leads to a temporary decrease in activity. But unless the original pain and the need for personal growth are examined and confronted at this time, a new addictive behavior will move in rapidly to fill the void. Chapter 2 focuses on the need to not only confront compulsive behavior, but to locate and communicate with the abandoned child within all of us, to begin the healing process before real change can be experienced.

Because stress occurs from the perception of the inability to successfully achieve goals, one way to prevent this from occurring is to set goals that are predictably attainable. Stewart[37] writes, "Unless the goals of therapy are agreed upon in the beginning, the therapist and the patient can be forced to work together over a long period of time attempting to achieve goals which are not shared by both." When collaborating with patients, Stewart[37] suggests the following steps to help lower stress:

- Establish a clear contract with the patient. This should contain an explicit description of the goals and responsibilities of both parties, ongoing, and should consider the patient's values and priorities.

- Do not promise more than you are prepared to deliver to the patient, the family, and/or significant others/ caregivers, or the referring practitioner.

- Be aware of the patient's feelings of dependency, loneliness, and fears of abandonment. Deal with feelings with active listening, encouraging open discussion. Give plenty of advance notice before taking time off or separating from patients in any way.

Another skill that is useful in helping to keep control over the work environment is assertiveness training, for those who lack the skills needed to communicate ideas for change. Learning how to speak up from a position of personal confidence can help revitalize an entire work setting.[49] Chapter 9 will assist you in developing these skills.

# MENTAL HEALTH IN THE UNITED STATES

The findings of an American Psychological Association (APA) 2015 national study[50] of over 2,000 individuals suggested that people in the United States were not receiving what they needed from HCPs to manage stress and address lifestyle changes to improve their health. The APA[50] study found that only 17% of Americans were having needed conversations with their HCPs about stress management. The study clearly demonstrated that Americans at that time were struggling with managing stress and that stress was on the rise. Millennials, in particular, were noted as having trouble managing stress, with their stress levels exceeding national averages, compared with those of other generations.[50] Regrettably, stress levels have not improved in the United States, with recent escalations due to the Covid-19 pandemic, war, inflation, money concerns, and stress challenging our abilities to cope.[51-54]

Let's examine the contemporary data with respect to mental health in the United States. American workers' rates of burnout intensified in 2021, according to the APA's Work and Well-being Survey[51] of 1,501 U.S. adult workers. Study outcomes indicated 79% of employees had experienced work-related stress; including lack of interest, motivation, or energy (26%) and lack of effort at work (19%). Additionally, 36% reported cognitive weariness, 32% reported emotional exhaustion, and an astonishing 44% reported physical fatigue—a 38% increase since 2019. The APA's pandemic survey found Covid-19-related stress was associated with unhealthy weight changes and increased drinking.[51,52]

The APA released survey outcomes again in March 2022,[53] confirming that these unhealthy behaviors have persisted, suggesting that coping mechanisms have become *entrenched*—and that mental and physical health may be on a continuing decline for many as a result. Close to half of adults (47%) said they had been less active than they wanted to be since the pandemic started, and close to three in five (60%) reported experiencing undesired weight changes (±15–26 pounds).[53] More than one in five Americans (23%) said they had been drinking more alcohol during the pandemic. Adults also reported separation and conflict as causes for straining and/or ending of relationships.[53] Half of adults (51%, particularly essential workers at 61%) said they had loved ones they had not been able to see in person in the past two years, due to the pandemic.[53] Strikingly, more than half of all U.S. adults (58%) reported experiencing a relationship strain or end because of conflicts related to the pandemic, including canceling events or gatherings due to Covid-19 concerns (29%); difference of opinion over some aspect of vaccines (25%); different views of the pandemic overall (25%); and difference of opinion over mask-wearing (24%).[53]

Strained social relationships and reduced social support during the pandemic made coping with stress more difficult. In fact, more than half of respondents (56%) said that they could have used more emotional support than they received since the pandemic started.[53] Most parents reported concerns regarding their child(ren)'s development, including social life or development (73%), academic development (71%), and emotional health or development (71%).[53] More than two-thirds of parents reported concern about the pandemic's impact on their child's cognitive development (68%) and their physical health/development (68%).[53] Healthy and supportive relationships are key to promoting resilience and building people's mental wellness; especially during periods of prolonged stress, it remains important that we connect socially, and that HCPs provide emotional support.

Owing to high stress levels, decision making has also been adversely affected.[52] About half of U.S. adults say that the uncertainty of the pandemic has made future planning feel impossible; while nearly a third say their stress levels are so high that they sometimes struggle with even basic decisions, such as what to wear or eat. Compared with other generations, Millennial and Generation Z adults reported the highest stress levels, the lowest ability to manage that stress, and the most difficulty with both day-to-day and major decisions,[52] while Hispanic, Black, and Asian American adults reported more Covid-related stress than did non-Hispanic White adults.[52]

In 2022, the APA[54] indicated that:

> *top sources of stress were the rise in prices of everyday items (e.g., gas prices, energy bills, grocery costs, etc.) due to inflation (87%), followed by supply chain issues (81%), global uncertainty (81%), Russia's invasion of Ukraine (80%) and potential retaliation (80%) from Russia (e.g., cyberattacks, nuclear threats).*

Enduring historic threats often results in lasting, traumatic impacts on generations. This means not only connecting those in distress with care, but also mitigating risk for those more likely to experience challenges and engaging in prevention for those who are relatively healthy.

# CONCLUSION

Health professionals are responsible for clearly understanding the patient's problem and, perhaps most important and most stressful, we are responsible for teaching the patient how to avoid future problems. We are responsible for helping people take responsibility for themselves and their health, physical and mental. This can be the most demanding of our obligations to those we serve. We must learn to manage situations that fail to respond to our interventions and understand the stress associated with compassion fatigue, when caring for others going through trauma and suffering. We must learn to do self-care and set realistic limits as to what we are willing and able to do to facilitate change and make appropriate referrals. We must learn to face the inevitability of terminal illness and death. Each of these realities in health care, if perceived as failure, will cause stress, because the ideal, hoped-for goal of cure and wellness is often unattainable. We set ourselves up to experience burnout if curing is our only goal in health care. Even as a HCP student, stress is inevitable. Notably, Smith et al.[55,56] validated the Oldenburg Burnout Inventory (OBI-S) for doctor of physical therapy (DPT) students and discovered in the midst of the Covid-19 pandemic that over 35% of a national representative sample of DPT students identified with being burned out (as measured by the OBI-S) while in the professional program and emphasized the importance of being self-aware, resilient, prioritizing time, having a supportive learning environment and faculty, along with utilizing counseling support to manage stress. In a 2024 world-wide systematic review of 31 studies and a meta-analysis of 32 studies reporting burnout prevalence in physiotherapists; a total of 5,984 physiotherapists from 17 countries were examined.[57] Pooled prevalence (95% confidence interval) of burnout was 8%. Prevalence figures for the MBI Inventory dimensions were: (i) emotional exhaustion, 27%, (ii) depersonalization, 23%, and (iii) low personal accomplishment, 25%.[57] Both overall and single component burnout prevalences were higher, although not significantly, in studies from developing, rather than developed countries.[57] The expansive worldwide study[57] reinforces that work-related burnout is a significant concern amongst HCPs, including physiotherapists. The occupational phenomenon of burnout does indeed have negative impacts for both staff well-being and the quality of care delivered to patients.[57]

When one enters the health professions, there must be an early commitment to taking care of oneself to prevent the negative effects of inevitable stress and working to prevent burnout. HCPs must work at being resilient, and compassionately assist their patients and clients in doing the same. Reflect for a moment now on Piemonte's[58] advisement: "Using only your head and hands in every encounter cannot sustain you. Connection to others can protect against burnout. Connection requires compassion, an ability to feel alongside another person."

We suggest that people can be seen to be composed of four quadrants: the physical, intellectual, emotional, and spiritual. To avoid stress, one must keep a *healthy balance* of activity and growth in all four quadrants (Table 5.3). This would include a commitment to eat well, get enough rest and sleep, take regular exercise, take time away from people, get emotional confirmation and support, and dedicate oneself to play and having fun. Some of us who become health professionals, who grew up in troubled homes, have had to be "serious" from the very start, and we lack the ability for spontaneous play. If that is true, we must find others to help us.

Our healthy survival depends on a true dedication to creative play and an assurance of having memorable fun. Do not hesitate to utilize mental-health professionals for help. The amount of compassion you receive will not only give you hope but allow you to be more compassionate with your colleagues and patients. Take care of yourself first, so that you can provide the best care for others. Do not be afraid to block out time for your fun activities![47]

Although stress has risen, and may seem insurmountable, Wellons,[59] pediatric neurosurgeon, reminds us, "It is not a surprise that we are all fragile. … The dark and unknown we all face make us more so. But life wants to live, and I have learned that we are also extraordinarily resilient."

Let's now pause to take a moment to reflect on this quote and consider how you will implement the adage as a developing HCP today and in your preferred future:

*We don't stop playing because we grow old; we grow old because we stop playing.* —George Bernard Shaw

The exercises that follow are designed to help you identify the amount of stress you are currently experiencing and how that stress affects you physically. Please also consider completing some of the life stress inventories as a baseline for yourself as a developing HCP. The final exercise addresses HCP Choosing Wisely[61] and Integrity in Practice[62] specifically, fraud, abuse, and waste, which may arise from HCP stress and burnout.

| TABLE 5.3 | |
|---|---|
| **BALANCING THE FOUR QUADRANTS OF NEED AND FUNCTION FOR STRESS RELIEF** | |
| **PHYSICAL QUADRANT CARE**<br>○ Eat breakfast; eat nutritious food<br>○ Drink plenty of water<br>○ Don't smoke; don't do drugs<br>○ Exercise regularly but moderately<br>○ Sleep at least 8 hours a night<br>○ If you drink alcohol, drink moderately<br>○ Alternate work with rest and play | **EMOTIONAL QUADRANT CARE**<br>○ Find and keep a confidant, and talk often<br>○ Join a group<br>○ Be a good listener who does not judge<br>○ Cherish a pet of your own<br>○ Make use of the counseling services<br>○ Journal |
| **INTELLECTUAL QUADRANT CARE**<br>○ Read material that adds energy to your life<br>○ Listen to good music<br>○ Crossword puzzles, chess, bridge<br>○ Design and build···write···create<br>○ Learn another language<br>○ Learn to play a musical instrument | **SPIRITUAL QUADRANT CARE**<br>○ Establish a regular meditation practice<br>○ Attend religious services<br>○ Read inspiring literature<br>○ Get out into nature regularly<br>○ Listen to inspiring music |

# REFERENCES

1. Heywood SE, Connaughton J, Kinsella R, Black S, Bicchi N, Setchell J. Physical therapy and mental health: scoping review, *Phys Ther.* 2022; pzac102, doi: 10.1093/ptj/pzac102.
2. Haddad A, Doherty RB, Purtilo RF. *Health Professional/Patient Interaction.* 10th ed. Philadelphia, PA: Saunders; 2023.
3. Smith CJ, Harris H. Caring for our nation's Veterans: a shared responsibility. *Nursing.* 2017;48(2);56–59.
4. Terrill AL, Molton IR. Frequency and impact of midlife stressors among men and women with physical disability. *Disability & Rehab.* 2019; 41(5);17660–17667.
5. Kalinowski J, Taylor JY, Spruill TM. Why are young Black women at high risk for cardiovascular disease? *Circulation.* 2019; 139(8):1003–1004.
6. Bhenhan G, Charak R. Stress and sleep remain significant predictors of health after controlling for negative affect. *Stress & Health.* 2019; 35(1):59–68.
7. Pfefferbaum B, North CS. Mental health and the Covid-19 pandemic. *New Engl J Med.* 2020;383(6):510–512.
8. Connaughton J. Working in general practice treating people with comorbid mental health problems. In: Probst M, Skjaerven LH. *Physiotherapy in Mental Health and Psychiatry E-book: A Scientific and Clinical Based Approach.* Philadelphia, PA: Elsevier Health Sciences; 2017.
9. Cook C, McCallum C, Musolino GM, Reiman M, Covington JK. What traits are reflective of positive professional performance in physical therapy program graduates? A Delphi study. *J Allied Health.* 2018 Summer;47(2):96–102. PMID: 29868693.
10. Barr DA. The effects of organizational structure on primary care outcomes under managed care. *Ann Intern Med.* 1995; 122:353–359.
11. Tu HT. More Americans willing to limit physician-hospital choice for lower medical costs. *Issue Brief Cent Stud Health Syst Change.* 2005; 94:1–5.
12. Emmanuel EJ, Gluck AR., eds. *The Affordable Care Act: How the Affordable Care Act Transformed Politics, Law and Healthcare in America.* New York, NY: Public Affairs; 2020.
13. Casares GS, Bradley KP, Jaffe LE, Lee GP. Impact of the changing environment on fieldwork education: perceptions of occupational therapy educators. *J Allied Health.* 2003; 32:246–251.
14. Grembowski DE, Patrick DL, Williams B, et al. Managed care and patient related quality of care from primary physicians. *Med Care Res Rev.* 2005; 62:31–55.
15. Nalette E. Constrained physical therapist practice: an ethical case analysis of recommending discharge placement from the acute care setting. *Phys Ther.* 2010; 90:939–952.
16. Cook C. 20th Pauline Cerasoli lecture: the sunk cost fallacy. *J Phys Ther Educ.* 31(3):10–14.
17. Dyrbye LN, Thomas MR, Shanafelt TD. Medical student distress: causes, consequences, and proposed solutions. *Mayo Clin Proc.* 2005; 80:1613–1622.
18. Keyes K. *Handbook to Higher Consciousness.* Coos Bay, OR: Living Love Publications; 1975.

19. Chopra D. *Ageless Body, Timeless Mind: The Quantum Alternative to Growing Old (Abridged)*. New York, NY: Penguin Random House; 2022.

20. Hereford JM. *Sleep and Rehabilitation: A Guide for Health Professionals*. Thorofare, NJ: Slack; 2013.

21. Lipton BH. *The Biology of Belief*. Carlsbad, CA: Hay House; 2016.

22. Tolle E. *The Power of Now: A Guide to Spiritual Enlightenment*. Novato, CA: New World Library; 2004.

23. Kabat-Zinn J. *Coming to Our Senses—Healing Ourselves and the World Through Mindfulness (Abridged)*. New York, NY: Hachette Audio; 2020.

24. Montgomery A, Panagopoulou E, Esmail A, Richards T, Maslach C. Burnout in healthcare: the case for organizational change. *BMJ*. 2019 Jul 30;366:l4774. doi: 10.1136/bmj.l4774. PMID: 31362957.

25. Wolfe GA. Burnout of therapists inevitable or preventable? *Phys Ther*. 1981; 61:1046–1050.

26. World Health Organization (WHO). *International Classification of Diseases, ICD-11 for Mortality and Morbidity Statistics*, Version 02/2022. QD 85 Burnout. Accessed May 1, 2023. Available: https://icd.who.int/browse11/l-m/en#/http://id.who.int/icd/entity/129180281

27. Apter LC, Kolodner EL. Professional burnout—are you a candidate? *Phys Ther Forum*. 1987; 6:6–10.

28. Allen R. *Progressive Neuromuscular Relaxation*. College Park, MD: Autumn Wind Press; 1979.

29. Donohoe, E, Nawawi, A, Wilker, L, et al. Factors associated with burnout of physical therapists in Massachusetts Rehabilitation Hospitals. *Phys Ther*. 1993; 73:750–756.

30. Sullivan EE, McKinstry D, Adamson J, Hunt L, Phillips RS, Linzer M. Burnout among Missouri primary care clinicians in 2021: roadmap for recovery? *MO Med*. 2022 Jul–Aug;119(4):397–400. PMID: 36118800.

31. Koranne R, Williams ES, Poplau S, Banks KM, Sonneborn M, Britt HR, Linzer M. Reducing burnout and enhancing work engagement among clinicians: The Minnesota experience. *Health Care Manage Rev*. 2022 Jan–Mar 01;47(1):49–57.

32. Pniak B, Leszczak J, Adamczyk M, Rusek W, Matłosz P, Guzik A. Occupational burnout among active physiotherapists working in clinical hospitals during the COVID-19 pandemic in south-eastern Poland. *Work*. 2021;68(2):285–295.

33. Bejer A, Domka-Jopek E, Probachta M, Lenart-Domka E, Wojnar J. Burnout syndrome in physiotherapists working in the Podkarpackie province in Poland. *Work*. 2019;64(4):809–815.

34. Pustułka-Piwnik U, Ryn ZJ, Krzywoszański Ł, Stożek J. Burnout syndrome in physical therapists—demographic and organizational factors. *Med Pr*. 2014;65(4):453–462.

35. National Academies of Practice National Academies of Sciences, Engineering, and Medicine; National Academy of Medicine; Committee on Systems Approaches to Improve Patient Care by Supporting Clinician Well-Being. *Taking Action Against Clinician Burnout: A Systems Approach to Professional Well-Being*. Washington (DC): National Academies Press (US); 2019 Oct. 23, 1, Introduction.

36. Nash, D. Frontline Health Workers: "Heroes" or casualties of a broken system? *MedPage Today*. December 27, 2021. Accessed January 15, 2023. Available: https://www.medpagetoday.com/opinion/focusonpolicy/96387

37. Stewart TD. Psychotherapy and physical therapy common grounds. *Phys Ther*. 1977; 57:279–283.

38. Pines A, Maslach C. Characteristics of staff burnout in mental health settings. *Hosp Com Psyc*.1978;29:233–237.

39. Borges E, Sequeira C, Martins T, Queirós C, Mosteiro-Díaz MP. Psychometric properties of the Portuguese Dutch Work Addiction Scale. *Rev Esc Enferm USP (University of São Paulo Nursing School Journal)*. 2021 Apr. 23;55:e03765. doi: 10.1590/S1980-220X2020029603765. PMID: 33909873.

40. Rahe, R. *Holmes-Rahe Life Stress Inventory: The Social Readjustment Scale-The American Institute of Stress*. Accessed March 9, 2023. Available: https://www.stress.org/wp-content/uploads/2024/02/Holmes-Rahe-Stress-inventory.pdf

41. The American Institute of Stress, 1998, *Workplace Stress Survey*. Accessed April 30, 2015. Available: http://www.stress.org/wp-content/uploads/2011/08/Workplace-Stress-Survey.pdf

42. Leiter MP, Maslach C. *Areas of Work Life Survey (AWS)*. Accessed May 1, 2022. Available: https://www.mindgarden.com/274-areas-of-worklife-survey

43. Beck Depression Inventory Beck AT, Ward CH, Mendelson M, Mock J, Erbaugh J. An inventory for measuring depression. *Arch Gen Psychiatry*. 1961;4:561–571. doi: 10.1001/archpsyc.1961.01710120031004

44. Leiter MP. *Pandemic Experiences & Perceptions Survey (PEPS)*. Accessed May 1, 2022. Available: https://www.mindgarden.com/346-pandemic-experiences-perceptions-survey

45. Zhao JL, Jiang WT, Wang X, Cai ZD, Liu ZH, Liu GR. Exercise, brain plasticity, and depression. *CNS Neurosci Ther*. 2020 Sep;26(9):885–895. doi: 10.1111/cns.13385. Epub 2020 Jun 3. PMID: 32491278

46. Davis P. *Beating Burnout at Work: Why Teams Hold the Secret to Well-Being and Resilience*. Philadelphia, PA: Wharton School Press; 2021.

47. Pope-Ruark R. *Unraveling Faculty Burnout: Pathways to Reckoning and Renewal*. Baltimore, MD: Johns Hopkins Press; 2022.

48. Hodkinson A, Zhou A, Johnson J, Geraghty K, Riley R, Zhou A, Panagopoulou E, Chew-Graham CA, Peters D, Esmail A, Panagioti M. Associations of physician burnout with career engagement and quality of patient care: systematic review and meta-analysis. *BMJ*. 2022 Sep 14;378:e070442. doi: 10.1136/bmj-2022–070442.

49. Davis CM. The "difficult" elderly patient: stressful effects on the therapist. *Top Geri Rehab*. 1988; 3:74–84.

50. American Psychological Association. *Stress in America: Paying with our Health, 2015*. Accessed December 2019. Available: https://www.apa.org/news/press/releases/stress/2014/financial-stress

51. Abramson A. *Burnout and Stress are Everywhere*. January 2022. American Psychological Association. Accessed September 2022. Available: https://www.apa.org/monitor/2022/01/special-burnout-stress

52. American Psychological Association. *High Stress Levels During the Pandemic Are Making Even Everyday Choices Difficult to Navigate: Decision-Making Has Been Particularly Tough For Young Adults, Parents, and People of Color.* June 1, 2022. Accessed July 3, 2023. Available: https://www.apa.org/monitor/2022/06/news-pandemic-stress-decision-making

53. American Psychological Association. *Stress in America: On Second COVID-19 Anniversary, Money, Inflation, War Pile on to Nation Stuck in Survival Mode.* March 2022. Accessed May 1, 2023. Available: https://www.apa.org/news/press/releases/stress/2022/march-2022-survival-mode

54. American Psychological Association. *Stress in America, Money, Inflation, War, Pile on to Nation Stuck in CoVID 19 Survival Mode, 2022.* Accessed September 2022. Available: https://www.apa.org/news/press/releases/2022/03/inflation-war-stress

55. Smith A, Ellison J, Bogardus J, Gleeson P. Reliability and validity of the student version of the Oldenburg Burnout Inventory in physical therapist students. *J Phys Ther Educ.* 2022;36(3):205–209. doi: 10.1097/JTE.000000000000022.

56. Smith A, Ellison J, Bogardus J, Gleeson P. Development of burnout in physical therapist students and associated factors: a study during CoVID-19. *J Phys Ther Educ.* 2022;36(3):210–216. doi: 10.1097/JTE.0000000000000239.

57. Venturini E, Ugolini A, Bianchi L, Di Bari M, Paci M. Prevalence of burnout among physiotherapists: a systematic review and meta-analysis. *Physiotherapy.* 2024 Feb 1;124:164–179. doi: 10.1016/j.physio.2024.01.007.

58. Piemonte N. *Cultivating the Habits at the Heart of Patient Care: Compassion, Vulnerability, and Imagination.* Geneva Johnson Keynote Address, APTA Educational Leadership Conference, Atlanta, GA, October 2021.

59. Wellons J. *All That Moves Us: A Pediatric Neurosurgeon, His Young Patients, and Their Stories of Grace and Resilience.* New York, NY: Random House; 2022.

60. Kaplan, J. *She Knows You Are Coming.* In: National Academy of Medicine's Expressions of Clinician Well-Being: An Art Exhibition. Accessed May 1, 2022. Available: https://nam.edu/expressclinicianwellbeing/#/artwork/257

61. American Board of Internal Medicine (ABIM), *Advancing Medical Professionals to Improve Healthcare,* Accessed March 1, 2022. Available: http://www.choosingwisely.org/

62. APTA *Preventing Fraud, Abuse and Waste and the Choosing Wisely Campaign,* Accessed May 1, 2022. Available: https://www.apta.org/your-practice/ethics-and-professionalism/preventing-fraud-abuse-and-waste

63. APTA *Navigating the Regulatory Environment: Ensuring Compliance While Promoting Professional Integrity.* Available: https://learningcenter.apta.org Accessed November 23, 2024.

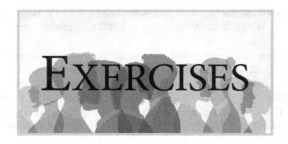

# EXERCISE 1: RECOGNIZING PROFESSIONAL STRESS

1.  I realize I am stressed when:


    Which makes me feel:


    And I react by:


    Afterwards, thinking about it calmly and quietly, I realize and tell myself next time I may choose to:


2.  Signs and symptoms of burnout for me:
    a.


    b.


    c.


    d.

3.  Coping mechanisms that I use now within my environment:

    a.

    b.

    c.

    d.

4.  Three things I did last week to take care of myself:

    a.

    b.

    c.

5.  Take a moment to consider this poem excerpt from a HCP during the Covid-19 pandemic:[60]

*Burnout comes from loss of connection to our patients, to ourselves, and to those we love. Too often in health care today we focus on tasks—on doing the appropriate tests and making the right diagnosis, when what our patients want and what we truly crave is to feel connected. —She Knows You Are Coming, Jay Kaplan, MD*

Now that you are more aware of how stress impacts health care, and why it is so important to discover and implement ways to manage your stress, visit, peruse and decompress with the online resource entitled *Expressions of Clinician Well-Being*,[60] created with the National Academies of Practice, collecting artistic insights in a variety of formats, directly from clinicians, patients, loved ones, and organizations working to prevent burnout and promote well-being. Available: https://nam.edu/expressclinicianwellbeing/#/

Journal about your feelings from these reflections.

## EXERCISE 2: MAJOR SOURCES OF STRESS IN STUDENTS

Haddad, Doherty, and Purtillo[2] noted three major sources of anxiety for students:

1.   Am I good enough? (basically)

2.   Do I have what it takes? (physically, emotionally)

3.   Can I pay?

First, do you agree that these are stressors for you? What would you add to this list? Are there life issues that cause you stress (e.g., developing identity and finding a life partner)? Is the task of breaking away from your home and parents a major stressor for you? Are you concerned that you may have chosen the wrong profession? Do you have a habit of procrastination that gets you into trouble rather consistently? Make a personal list of stressors and prioritize them. Assign relative stress points to each item.

Now, *journal* about how those stressors affect you each day physically, emotionally, mentally, and spiritually. For each stressor, list any actions you might be able and willing to take right now to minimize their negative influence and learn to put away anxiety about things you have no control over. Carrying a list of constant worries around in your mind or on your back makes it difficult to be present to the world and to people. Develop the habit of taking a regular inventory of what you are worried about, what you can do about it right now, and what you must "offer up" and get off your mind. Make it a goal regularly to flush your mind and your heart of anxieties that are not appropriate or welcome. You will feel lighter if you do. Consider this quote as you commence journaling your reflections related to your learning in this chapter:

*Students, in the course of their formation, must let the gritty reality of this world into their lives, so they can learn to feel it, think about it critically, respond to its suffering, and engage it constructively. —Rev. Peter-Hans Kolvenbach, S.J.*

## EXERCISE 3: HOW TO THINK IN A HEALTHIER WAY

Recognizing unhelpful negative thoughts is the first step to stopping them. The best way to change your thinking is to write negative thoughts down and produce alternatives. The key is to recognize, through negative feelings, that you are thinking negative thoughts and then change those thoughts and reach for the better thought to pull you up on the emotional scale toward positivity.

Track your thoughts.

Situation: Late for class. Lost track of time. Traffic was unforgiving. No place to park.

| FEELINGS/BODY RESPONSES | NEGATIVE THOUGHT | ALTERNATIVE THOUGHT |
| --- | --- | --- |
| Sick to my stomach, down on myself, anxious that I will be embarrassed in front of the group. | I'm not good enough. I'll never be successful. I can't be trusted. | I'm under a lot of stress. I'm making too much of this one incident. |

Now it is your turn. Track your thoughts.

Situation:

| FEELINGS/BODY RESPONSES | NEGATIVE THOUGHT | ALTERNATIVE THOUGHT |
| --- | --- | --- |
|  |  |  |

## *Journal Reflections*

As I reflect on my responses to the above questions, what did I learn about myself? How will I take responsibility for myself to prevent the cumulative effects of stress that lead to burnout?

# EXERCISE 4: INTEGRITY IN PRACTICE

Review the resources and links for the American Board of Internal Medicine (ABIM) Foundation (abimfoundation. org) *Advancing Medical Professionals to Improve Healthcare*[61] and Choosing Wisely Initiative (www.choosingwisely.org).

Locate your profession utilizing the clinicians' tab and review the related recommendations. Peruse the remaining website, jot down three things that you learned, three things that surprised you, and three things you are still questioning or want to know more about. Be prepared to discuss with your peers.

*Choosing Wisely …*

| WHAT I LEARNED MORE ABOUT | WHAT I WAS SURPRISED ABOUT | QUESTIONING OR WANT TO KNOW |
|---|---|---|
| 1. | 1. | 1. |
| 2. | 2. | 2. |
| 3. | 3. | 3. |

APTA Student members are highly encouraged to complete the online course for *Navigating the Regulatory Environment: Ensuring Compliance while Promoting Professional Integrity,*[63] through the APTA PT Learning Center; available via: https://learningcenter.apta.org.

The modules are particularly helpful in distinguishing perceived gray areas in health care practice.

Course instructors include: Dr. Shantanu Agrawal MD; Dr. Anthony Delitto PT, PhD, FAPTA; Katherine Karker-Jennings, JD, MS; Ellen R. Strunk, PT, MS, GCS; Becky Clearwater, PT, MS, DPT. This two-part module provides expert guidance and strategies to prevent fraud and abuse in practice. Part 1 consists of a moderated audio roundtable covering laws and regulations related to health care fraud and abuse, the government's efforts to find and address fraud and abuse, and a discussion of a mock case scenario. Part 2 provides five case vignettes drawn from real-world situations that illustrate some of the types of fraud or abuse involving physical therapist services. Interactive questions and answers guide the learner through each situation.

Be prepared to discuss your learning, insights, and feelings based upon the campaign and learning modules for promoting professional integrity.

These exercises are also available online at www.routledge.com/9781638220039.

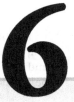

# THERAPEUTIC PRESENCE

## THE NATURE OF EFFECTIVE HELPING FOR THERAPEUTIC ALLIANCES

*Gina Maria Musolino and Carol M. Davis*

## OBJECTIVES

*The learner should be able to*:

- Justify the ideal overall aim of helping.
- Explore the behaviors that interfere with effective helping.
- Distinguish between sympathy, pity, identification, self-transposal, and empathy.
- Describe the characteristics of helping communication.
- Discover characteristics of effective helpers.
- Apply effective listening abilities.

When someone needs help, no matter what the nature of the help needed, we can assume that something is not right, that something is interfering with day-to-day function and growth. Those of us in the healing professions have devoted our lives, for the most part, to working with those who need help in understanding and overcoming illness or disability. Some of us, however, are more concerned with working with people who are essentially well but need help in becoming fitter, or in preventing illness or injury. Whatever the problem, health professionals have devoted their professional lives to helping people overcome whatever is blocking them from living fully functional, useful, and productive lives. Let's start by examining a case scenario:

Ariel, the supervisor in occupational therapy, was also the clinical/field work instructor for Erin, a student in her last clinical education experience before graduating. For the most part, Erin was independent in her patient care but occasionally would ask for Ariel's help in solving a clinical problem. At the end of one day, Erin asked

DOI: 10.4324/9781003525554-6

Ariel for the answer to a question that Ariel felt Erin should know by now. She was tempted to tell her, "Go look that up! You should know the answer to that by now." But it was late in the day, and both were tired. Ariel gave in and told her the answer to her question but then gave her a dirty look, as if to let her know she was not happy to be asked that question. Erin was confused about why she seemed unhappy.

**What should the overall aim of helping be?** When we were small and needed help, we searched out whomever we felt could fix the problem and make us feel better. As children, we lacked the skills to solve our own problems, and so we depended on our mothers and fathers or some capable adult to take charge. Unlike children, adults require a different sort of helping, because when someone constantly tries to "fix it," we often become resentful and angry, and feel helpless and dependent. It is an important sign of maturity when we prefer to complete tasks, solve problems ourselves, and take pride in our individual accomplishments.

There are times, however, when we feel particularly alone and helpless, and we may appreciate that "fixing" kind of attention and help offered by a friend. As adults, we need to acknowledge the more enduring need to feel self-sufficient and capable of identifying and solving our own problems. The same holds true for our patients and clients; we must facilitate their independence, not dependence on us as health care professionals (HCPs).

**The overall aim of mature helping always is to make the "helpee" self-sufficient, to assist the "helpee" in achieving a more effective relationship between self and others, and between self and the world.**

We have discovered in previous chapters that our behavior is an expression of our values and our beliefs. Those who believe that they are called to help others, whether they want help or not, can become annoying at the least, and obstructive to others' development at the worst. Not all help is helpful. Many of us have laughed at the turmoil that can occur when a well-meaning person tries to open a door for us and actually blocks our way. At the other end of the continuum, however, is the well-meaning friend or parent who takes great care in telling us what to do, in a given situation, and then abandons us with indifference, refusing to support us until we comply with the advice given. "You asked me. I told you. You did what you wanted. Now I will have nothing to do with you." Not extremely helpful. Imagine if we adopted that attitude with our patients and clients who are sometimes not compliant with our advisement. Now that would not be appropriate either.

As was pointed out in Chapter 2, helpers who had to develop parenting skills too early bring immature ideas about the nature of effective help into adulthood. A few familiar characteristics of unhelpful helpers, include too much concern with matters that are none of their business, a need to be told how helpful—indeed, how irreplaceable—they are to the functioning of a group, and a need to have others depend on them as if their very self-worth revolved totally around their ability to fix others' problems; *sadly*, it often does.

The important *truth*, in this matter, is that no person can take total personal responsibility for another person. **We can only take responsibility for ourselves**. Exceptions exist, of course, with children and with people who, for whatever reason, have lost the ability to be adequately in charge of their own lives—those with certain mental illnesses, those with brain dysfunction. But, for most of us, the world exists for us the way we see it, the way we think about it. No one outside of us can make us happy or unhappy unless we allow it. Circumstances exist the way they are, but we have a choice as to how we think about them.

Effective helping usually has, as a primary component, a problem identification and problem-solving process. As health professionals, we learn important knowledge, skills, and values that we offer to assist those needing help, to understand the nature of their problem(s) and to act in ways so that the problem is solved and a return to normal function and quality living is facilitated. **Our goal must always be to help the "helpee" become *self-sufficient* once again**. We must provide the conditions for our patients to identify their own goals, around their own health problems, and provide the knowledge and skill to advise them on the wisdom of their desires and then to help them get their needs met. Later in this textbook, we will discuss considerations of where one is in the ability to change (Chapter 16); for now, we shall stay focused on the nature of effective helping.

Patients may come to us with or without a medical diagnosis; however, contrary to widespread practice in most medical environments, the medical diagnosis serves as little more than a place to start in the helping process. The key questions remain: What are the problems from the *patient's or client's perspective*? And what are the *patient's goals* in the healing process? In fact, contemporary practice necessitates evidence-based practice (EBP), which first and foremost includes the patient's values, beliefs, and preferences. If these are not at the forefront, the therapeutic relationship shall almost certainly fail. David Sackett, MD, clinical epidemiologist, internist and EBP pioneer, defined EBP as "the integration of best research evidence with clinical expertise and patient values and beliefs."[1,2]

Effective helping includes not merely a provision of information and therapeutic procedures but must involve helping the patient or client with the discovery of personal meaning as well, or what good does illness or efforts toward optimal wellness serve?

Consider if the sentiments of this quote hold true today for the health care professional and why:

*It is one of the beautiful compensations in this life that no one can sincerely try to help another without helping himself.*

—Ralph Waldo Emerson

# THERAPEUTIC USE OF SELF

Central to this perspective on helping is therapeutic communication and the therapeutic use of one's self. How you view yourself will markedly affect your communication. Remember that the self-concept acts as a screen through which we view the world. Most of us have felt the discomfort of interacting with a person who continually apologizes for themselves, who distorts what we say out of feelings of insecurity, who responds with negativity and self-contempt. Each of us holds many varied opinions and ideas about ourselves, but our essential self-worth forms the core around which those ideas merge, and negative self-worth is one of the most crucial factors that needs to be changed in order to communicate from a healing perspective.

Earlier chapters focused on the development of the ideas about the self and how our feelings of self-worth evolve. This chapter focuses on the nature of effective communication in the helping process.

# THERAPEUTIC COMMUNICATION

Certain identifiable elements characterize therapeutic or healing communication. In the patient–practitioner interaction (PPI), the practitioner:

- **Speaks**—Communicates not just with an expression of ideas, but with the ability to *translate those ideas* from an inner conviction to an outer clarity. Self-awareness enables the speaker to voice articulately, and with sensitivity to the response of the other person, well-thought-out ideas regarding the patient's role in the healing process.

- **Is fully present**—Is *totally* focused on the patient or client and that individual's ideas about the problem. Does not get lost in memories of patients past or potential future problems. Allows the interaction with the patient to command undivided, focused attention by the HCP.

- **Listens**—Listens with the whole self, with the "third ear," to ascertain the patient's or client's meanings and goals. Clarifies interpretations of what is heard. Resists categorizing or projecting personal beliefs and values. Resists giving quick advice, telling the patient what to do (see Chapter 13), remains open to possibilities.

- **Develops trust**—Resists trying to influence the patient or client; instead, asks questions to ascertain the truth about the problem, as the patient or client perceives the problem. Communicates that the patient or client is worth listening to, with valuable information to add to the process. Resists assuming a priestly or paternalistic role, which conveys that the patient or client is unwise, and the HCP is smart. At the same time, however, conveys the values of expertise and confidentiality, and never neglects the opportunity for *informed consent*, so that the patient feels that trust has been appropriately placed.

- **Carefully considers, with cultural humility**—The patient's *values, beliefs, and preferences* in the development of mutually agreeable, person-centered goals and expectations.[1–4]

Thus, the art of professional helping, in the healing professions, centers around the therapeutic use of oneself, by way of a style of humanistic communication that places the patient in a position of informed, equal, and inevitably responsible for any positive outcomes in the helping process.

Health professionals:

- Listen, clarify, ask, never assume, or make quick judgments
- Identify problems with the patient, examine and evaluate
- Hypothesize causes, avoiding premature closure
- Treat through therapeutic measures and education
- Reevaluate
- Readjust to the changed states and begin again until goals are reached

Through this process of therapeutic communication, one establishes mutual trust and respect for the collaborative, professional relationship with one's patients and clients. The state of having one's whole self, present with the patient/client to optimize the patient/practitioner interaction is referred to as **therapeutic presence**.[5,6] The trust being established is one of the most valuable communication concepts, as trust relates directly to effective, therapeutic communication, a vital determining factor for patient/client satisfaction.[7] Through being fully receptive and attuned to your patients and clients through therapeutic presence establishes collaborative trust and impacts therapeutic outcomes through a reduction of anxiety and stress, thereby improving safety and recovery potentials.[7]

# A Closer Look at Interpersonal Interaction Processes

At the heart of listening with the third ear is the process of self-transposal, which is often confused with empathy.[3] *Empathy* (Figure 6.1) is very often used interchangeably with several other interaction terms. Each term has a unique meaning, and it is helpful to understand and be able to distinguish between them. The terms most commonly used interchangeably with empathy include *sympathy*, *pity*, *identification*, and *self-transposal*. Of these, pity and identification often are not appropriate to the healing process. Let's take a closer look at each of these interactive processes.

When I sympathize (Figure 6.2) with you, I feel similar feelings about something outside of us, along with you. I can feel joyful about your success, or I can feel sadness about the bad news that my patient received today. This is sympathy, or "fellow feeling." It is very commonly felt in health care, and it is totally appropriate in the healing relationship with patients.[3]

Pity (see Figure 6.2), on the other hand, rarely, if ever, is appropriate. When I pity my patient, I feel sympathy **with condescension**. "You poor thing" conveys an inappropriate inequality between myself and the other person. I lift myself up to be better than the other, and in that process I demean the personhood of the other. Granted, pity may draw us to help others, but to help with condescension gives the message to the patient that you are judging the person to be pitiful.[3]

Identification (see Figure 6.2) can interfere with healing communication as well. When I identify with my patient, I begin to feel at one with the patient; and in that process, I often lose sight of the differences between us. For example, just because we both have the same last name or we both come from similar backgrounds, I may forget the patient might have values that differ from mine. I may assume that my patient feels as I do about wanting to know everything there is to know about a disease or disorder, or I may project that my patient is best in the morning and schedule to treat them before noon. I forget to ask, to clarify. As a result, I confuse my meanings and values with those of my patient; I make assumptions and I project my values onto the patient and act in ways that make the patient less important, less relevant to the healing process. In addition, as I identify or become one with the patient, I risk losing my own perspective, which weakens my therapeutic objectivity, and I often become very subjective in the information I convey. Identification with patients often leads to being overly friendly with them and an inappropriate sharing of personal information that can interfere with the therapeutic nature of the relationship. We will expand on this more before the end of this chapter.

Self-transposal is a cognitive thinking of myself into the position of the other. It is the process most often confused with empathy, putting myself in the other person's place, or more commonly, "walking a mile in another person's shoes." In his earlier writings, Carl Rogers[4] referred to this as empathy, but in truth, self-transposal merely sets the stage for empathy to occur. In self-transposal, I listen carefully and try to imagine what it must be like for the patient to be experiencing what they are describing.[8]

# Empathy as Unique Among All Interactive Processes

The process of empathy was first fully described by Edith Stein.[8] In her scholarly work, published in the 1930s, Stein characterized empathy as absolutely unique from all other forms of interactions, distinguishable from other intersubjective processes, first by the fact that we never empathize; empathy happens to us. It catches us. It is given to us much like true forgiveness; when it finally comes, it seems to be given to us. We can want to forgive and try to forgive, but when the forgiveness finally comes, there is a sense that we have not done a thing except allowed it to happen.

Empathy takes place in three overlapping stages (see Figure 6.1). The first stage is the *cognitive attending* to the other, or self-transposal, as described previously. We listen carefully in an attempt to put ourselves in the place of the other. The second stage, following just a millisecond after, is, by far, the most significant; the *crossing over/identification* stage of empathy (emotional), wherein we feel ourselves crossing over for a moment into the frame of reference

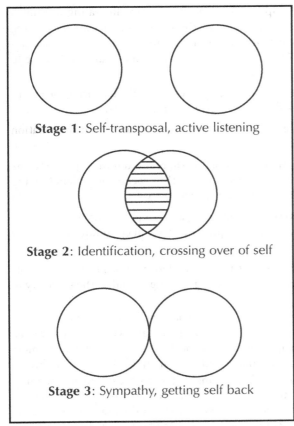

**Stage 1:** Self-transposal, active listening

**Stage 2:** Identification, crossing over of self

**Stage 3:** Sympathy, getting self back

**Figure 6.1** Three stages of empathy as described by Stein.[8]

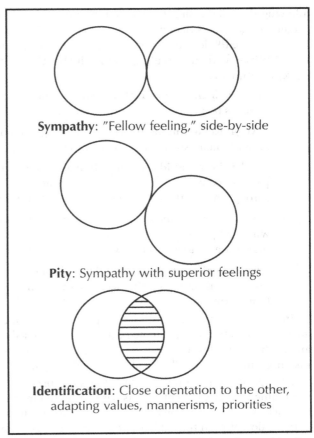

**Sympathy:** "Fellow feeling," side-by-side

**Pity:** Sympathy with superior feelings

**Identification:** Close orientation to the other, adapting values, mannerisms, priorities

**Figure 6.2** Graphic representation of three intersubjective processes.

or the lived world of the other person. We feel so at one with the other that we momentarily forget that we are two separate beings and identify completely with the other person. This only occurs if we open ourselves to the possibility.

The third stage *resolves the temporary confusion*, often referred to as *resolution*, as we come back into our own skin and feel a special alignment with the other after having experienced the crossing over.[8] This third stage resembles sympathy, a concern for others or fellow feeling, that of being *compassionate*. Thus, empathy can be described as a momentary merging with another person in a unique moment of shared meaning.[8]

When empathy occurs, helping professionals need not lose their therapeutic objectivity, as so many fear, in getting too close to their patients. Instead, what is experienced is a kind of holistic listening that can *unite* the therapist with the patient yet allows the patient and therapist to remain fully separate in the healing process. It is in identification alone that we lose our objectivity and become destructively fused with the patient, as described earlier. Thus, empathy is the intersubjective process that, among other things, empowers us to *listen with the third ear*, to communicate humanistically and therapeutically with patients, thus contributing to beneficial helping as compassionate care providers.

Jamison[9] reminds us that "empathy" is from the Greek derivative *empatheia–em* (into) and *pathos* (feeling) to share with; hence, you are traveling on a journey into the other person's situation and/or feelings. Jamison, a standardized patient, who also drew from her own experiences of pain, illness, injury, and suffering, described empathy this way: "Empathy isn't just listening, it's asking questions, that require deep listening. Empathy requires inquiry as much as imagination. Empathy requires knowing you may not know."[9]

# SETTING APPROPRIATE BOUNDARIES WITH PATIENTS/CLIENTS

The challenge, then, is for the health professional to be in a therapeutic relationship with patients yet maintain the helper–helpee relationship. It is imperative that this relationship remain functional, always serving the purpose of healing. How does the clinician reveal just enough about oneself to maintain the trust and collegiality without allowing the relationship to change into a more involved friendship or intimate relationship? Revealing too much might confuse the patient by seeming to convey that you are willing to give more than is appropriate for the helping process. Powell[10] described five different levels of communication that one can use as guidelines for communicating effectively without revealing too much about oneself. These levels lie on a continuum from near indifference to extreme intimacy.

- Level 5: **Clichéd conversation**. No genuine human sharing takes place. "How are you?" "It's nice to see you." Protects people from each other and prevents the likelihood of meaningful communication.
- Level 4: **Reporting facts**. Almost nothing personal is revealed. Some sharing takes place about information such as diagnostic data or the weather.
- Level 3: **Personal ideas and judgments**. Some information about oneself is shared, often in response to the patient's conversation. Topics talked about often relate to the patient's illness or the process the patient is going through, and if the patient looks bored or confused, conversation reverts back to level 4.
- Level 2: **Feelings and emotions**. A deep trust is required to share at this level, and if a person fears judgment it will be impossible to relate at this level. True friendship and caring require this level of communication. Each person wants to be deeply known and accepted just as they are.
- Level 1: **Peak communication**. Mutual complete openness, honesty, respect, and love are required to communicate at this level. An all-encompassing intimacy is shared, often involving relating sexually. The minority of human interactions take place at this level.

In therapeutic communication with patients, it is important for the professional to have a clear idea about appropriate boundaries that will facilitate healing. Once crossed over, interaction beyond this boundary will confuse patients, and the health professional will appear to be offering more to the helper–helpee relationship than is facilitative. In most instances, interaction will take place at levels 5, 4, and 3 with an occasional interchange at level 2, but never at level 1.

New professionals often confuse the appropriate boundaries and find themselves caring too much, spending more time with one patient than is wise, or telling inappropriate stories or jokes in an attempt to make the patient or themselves feel at ease. The reverse often occurs when the patient feels compelled to help put the practitioner at ease. Patients do not need this added anxiety; they need to relax and trust that the HCP has the best interest of the patient at heart and can manage the healing interaction free of awkwardness or threats to confidentiality and trust. As HCPs we need to meet the patient where they are, bringing the patient into healthy and collaborative therapeutic interactions to promote wholeness and healing.

# BELIEFS OF EFFECTIVE HELPERS

Combs and Gonzalez[11] conducted research on the characteristics of effective helpers and concluded:

> *Good helpers are not born, nor are they made in the sense of being taught. ... Becoming a helper is a time-consuming process. It is not simply a matter of learning methods or of acquiring gadgets and gimmicks. It is a deeply personal process of exploration and discovery, the growth of unique individuals learning over a period of time how to use themselves effectively for helping other people.*

Helpers were evaluated for their effectiveness, and the most effective responded to specific questions about their beliefs in six major categories. The results are summarized in Table 6.1. These beliefs are all developed in a growth process that is very much influenced by the way the lenses we talked about in earlier chapters are set. The key to becoming an effective helper is to allow oneself to grow, to mature, to become more aware of feelings as well as thoughts, to be able to identify those beliefs that lead to behaviors that facilitate healing, and to grow beyond defensive behaviors that result in negativity and fragmentation.

Corey and Corey[12] outline the picture of a helper who makes a significant difference:

- Is aware of personal strengths and weaknesses.
- Recognizes that "who you are as a person is the most important instrument you possess."
- Has a basic curiosity and openness to new learning.
- Possesses the interpersonal skills needed to establish good contact with others.
- Genuinely cares for people.
- Willing and able to see the world through the eyes of the "helpee."

| TABLE 6.1 |
| --- |

## SUMMARY OF THE BELIEFS OF "EFFECTIVE" HELPERS

Combs and Gonzalez[11] describe commonly held beliefs and perceptions of effective helpers in six categories.

### 1. Subject or Discipline

One is committed to knowing one's discipline well, but mere knowledge is not enough. Knowledge about one's discipline is so personally integrated and meaningful as to have the quality of belief. Effective helpers are committed to discovering the personal meaning of knowledge and converting it to belief.

### 2. Helpers' Frame of Reference

Effective helpers tend to favor an internal frame of reference emphasizing the importance of people's attitudes, feelings, and values that are uniquely human over an external frame of reference that emphasizes facts, things, organization, money, etc.

### 3. Beliefs About People

Effective helpers believe that people are essentially:
○ Able to understand and deal with their own problems given sufficient time and information.
○ Basically friendly and well intentioned.
○ Worthy and have great value; they possess dignity and integrity that must be maintained.
○ Essentially internally motivated, maturing from within and striving to grow and help themselves.
○ A source of satisfaction in professional work rather than a source of suspicion and frustration.

### 4. Helpers' Self-Concept

Effective helpers must have a clear sense of self and their own personal boundaries before they enter into relationships with others. They feel basically fulfilled and adequate, so self-discipline is well practiced. Therapeutic presence for the other is made possible by a strong sense of self, of personal fulfillment, and of personal adequacy.

### 5. Helpers' Purposes

Effective helpers believe that their purpose is to facilitate and assist rather than control people. They favor responding to the larger issues, the broader perspective, rather than the minute details in life. They tend to be willing to be themselves, to be self-revealing. Their purpose includes honesty, acknowledging personal inadequacies, and need for growth. Another purpose is to be involved and committed to the helping process. They are process oriented and committed to working out solutions rather than working toward preconceived goals or notions. They see themselves as altruistic, oriented toward assisting people rather than simply responding to selfish needs.

### 6. Beliefs About Appropriate Methods or Approaches to the Task

Effective helpers are more oriented toward people than toward rules and regulations or things. They are more concerned with people's perceptions than with the objective framework within which they practice. In helping people, the most effective approach is to discover how the world seems to that person. Self-concept is at the heart of the way one views the world, and so working with self-concept is imperative. Helpers have to be committed to gaining the trust of helpees so that self-control can be relearned in a positive way. The helping relationship makes this growth possible.

Adapted from Combs AW, Gonzalez, DM. *Helping Relationships: Basic Concepts for the Helping Professions*, 4th ed. Boston, MA: Allyn & Bacon; 1993.

- Able to challenge clients to dream. Is aware that you "cannot inspire clients to do in their lives what you are unwilling to do in your own."
- Willing to use multiple resources to assist.
- Willing to adapt approach and techniques to the patient/client's situation.
- Respects differences in the patient/client and does not expect them to fit into a preconceived mold.
- Takes care of self physically, mentally, emotionally, and spiritually. Deals with personal problems.
- Willing to examine and challenge personal beliefs and values. Recognizes that your philosophy of life has been personally developed and not imposed on you.
- Able to and has established meaningful relationships with at least a few others.
- Has a healthy sense of self-love and pride but is not self-absorbed.

# THE PURPOSE OF HELPING

Health care professionals will act according to what they believe their purpose is in the therapeutic relationship. The purpose of the mature healing professional is to listen carefully, with the "third ear"; to evaluate; to assist; to support; to help problem solve alternatives that lead to healing; to apply therapeutic measures, aimed at alleviating pain and dysfunction; to teach; to help others discover how to maneuver successfully in the world; and to solve their own problems that interfere with the highest and deepest functioning possible.

Carl Rogers[4] suggested seven key questions that lead to a form of self-examination that will help us evaluate the quality of one's helping:

1. **Can I behave in some way that will be perceived by the other person as trustworthy, as dependable, or consistent in some deep sense?** Here congruence is the key factor. Whatever feeling or attitude is being experienced must be matched by an awareness of that attitude, and actions must match feelings.

2. **Can I be expressive enough as a person that what I am will be communicated unambiguously?** The difficulty here is to be fully aware of who one truly is. Rogers[4] said this: "if I can form a helping relationship to myself—if I can be sensitively aware of and acceptant toward my own feelings—then the likelihood is great that I can form a helping relationship toward another."

3. **Can I let myself experience positive attitudes toward this other person—attitudes of warmth, caring, liking, interest, respect?** This often engenders the fear that if we allow ourselves to openly express these feelings, the "helpee" might misinterpret our intentions, and the therapeutic distance might be blurred. The key here is to remain in our professional identities and yet still relate in a caring way to the other person.

4. **Can I be strong enough as a person to be separate from the other?** This question speaks to avoiding identification. I must be ever aware of my own feelings and express them as mine, totally separate from the feelings I may perceive that the "helpee" is experiencing. Likewise, I must be strong in my otherness to avoid becoming depressed, when my patient is depressed, or fearful in the face of my patient's fear, or destroyed by their anger.

5. **Can I let myself enter fully into the world of my patient's feelings and personal meanings and see these as they do?** The key effort here is to avoid judging the patient's/client's perspectives, but instead allowing empathy to occur. In this way, once the world of the other is more fully experienced, the help that is offered can be based on this holistic level of knowing made possible by empathy. Meanings can be confronted with acceptance and modified to work toward healing. Judgment and criticism of meanings place a barrier between the helper and the "helpee."

6. **Can I act with sufficient sensitivity in the relationship that my behavior will not be perceived as a threat?** A patient who feels free of external fear or threat feels free to examine behavior and change it. Patient care can be threatening in and of itself. Whatever we can do to lower anxiety will assist the effectiveness of our helping.

7. **Can I meet this other individual as a person who is in the process of becoming, or will I be bound by their past and by my past?** Buber and Rogers used the phrase "confirming the other." This means accepting the whole potentiality of the other, the person one was created to become.[13] People will act the way we relate to them.

Let's now begin to consider the specific way or manner in which HCPs communicate effectively, through the non-verbal aspects of presence, as described by Geller[6]:

- Prosody (rhythm) in voice
- Soft facial expression
- Soft and direct eye gaze
- Open and forward leaning body posture
- Visual focus and attention toward the patient/clients

Research[14–19] supports these nonverbal elements of communication to promote safety in the clinical encounter. They help the patients to feel that the HCP is being empathically aware and setting the stage for therapeutic presence. In contrast, clinicians who exhibit such features as: monotone voices with little to no inflection; shifty eyes; contorted faces; crossed arms and legs; and diverting attention away from the patient result in patients feeling distance and discord with the HCP.

Geller[6] reminds us that HCPs must learn to "regulate to relate," suggesting that by practicing using the PRESENCE acronym that follows, HCPs can reflect on the qualities needed for therapeutic presence. Practice is essential. Practicing the PRESENCE suggestions will enhance your efforts toward establishing therapeutic presence.

## *Practicing makes PRESENCE[6]*

- **Pause** (put aside what you are doing to just rest in this moment).
- **Relax** into this moment (soften your facial and body muscles).
- **Enhance** awareness of your breath (take three deep inhalations and exhalations).
- **Sense** your inner body (bring awareness to what you are feeling in your physical and emotional body).
- **Expand** sensory awareness outwards (seeing, listening, touching, sensing what is around you).
- **Notice** what is true in this moment (both within you and around you, without judgment).
- **Center** and ground (feel your feet on the ground and the center of your body).
- **Extend** and make contact (open your eyes and ready yourself to approach the next moment while staying connected to your self and your breath).

By revisiting the suggestions from "practicing makes PRESENCE" prior to your patient–practitioner interactions, you will continue to progress in establishing effective therapeutic presence. HCPs' commitment to engage in the work of presence and working with barriers to presence is an ongoing life process.[5–6,14–19]

Therapeutic presence is a necessary component for creating safety, building stronger therapeutic alliances, and increasing the effectiveness of therapy in collaboration with patients and clients.[5–6,14–19] The more one fully comprehends the importance of the nature of the helping interaction, the more one will become committed to the growth required for consistent therapeutic use of self. Yes, our professional knowledge and skill are critical to our effectiveness, but without the ability to interact in healing ways, we sabotage most efforts.

You might be wondering by now how all this has changed when it comes to HCPs' online presence with telehealth. Indeed, it is not the same, yet with training and practice one can achieve a telepresence. Telepresence reflects that the therapist essentially "forgets" about being in an online context, feels absorbed in the interaction, and interacts with the patient/client as if they were in the same space, while gaining some insight into the patient/clients' lived experiences in alternative environments. It is essential to emphasize that the concept of telepresence is *different* from therapeutic presence yet is often complementary. Telepresence is a variable involved in the communication process between patients and HCPs in the creation and development of therapeutic connections in online PPI.[14,15,20–22] The feeling of presence is facilitated by the quality of the exchanges.[21] When being tele present, it is felt by both the HCP and the patient/client, as if they essentially no longer realize that they are not physically together, and the therapeutic bond can be established as if they were face to face.[20–22]

That is not to say that telehealth is not without barriers, which may prohibit achievements of telepresence. For example, patients/clients may be in their home environment with the very people they are having issues with that prohibit progress (e.g., telling them something different from your advisement). Patients and clients can be distracted in online environments by surroundings, pets, noises, competing media and events, etc. Additionally, therapists have technological challenges and report feeling more tired and experiencing professional self-doubt and loss of confidence working in this new way.[23] The Covid-19 pandemic resulted in additional challenges. Many therapists have also had to cope with their own personal anxiety, grief, and trauma related to the pandemic while supporting their clients to do the same.[5,6,20–22] We will further delve into aspects of telehealth challenges, benefits, and associated supports in Chapter 20.

Therapeutic presence provides the platform for HCPs' capacities, especially for those in pain, to provide emotional support, through empathic communication, with rapport building; facilitating treatment goals and promoting honesty and transparency in collaboration with our patients and clients.[24] No one is able to achieve all these helping characteristics and mannerisms immediately as a new graduate professional. Many of these behaviors and attitudes develop over time, with years of experience and history of working with all kinds of people in all situations. The queries and lists are offered to you as a benchmark, of sorts, to aspire to and as a personal self-evaluation tool as you grow along your way to becoming an effective helper; as you work to transform yourself into a responsive HCP who is person-centered, attentive, open, a listener (*third-ear*), a validator, and generally positive in your approach to care.[25] A responsive HCP underpins an "ethic of caring" that entails being oriented to care; being integrative of knowledge sources; striving for competence; being responsive for your patients and their families/caregivers; being reflective for, in and on practice; being communicative in a variety of ways, both nonverbal and verbal, through therapeutic touch and presence; and striving for acumen with clinical reasoning.[26] As you will discover in upcoming chapters, this ethic of care requires "passion to do the right thing with a balance of the technical competence with the relational dimensions of practice,"[25] (1–2) often referred to as coupling of the art of practice alongside the science.

Revisiting PPI throughout your professional growth and development as a HCP, while striving for best practice through effective therapeutic communication, will serve you well as you continue your journey and are influenced by your mentors, patients, and clients. As you gain your own first-hand experiences in your new and changed role as a HCP you shall have an opportunity for new and refreshed learning re-visiting the chapters and exercises with the new lens of experience. Upcoming in Chapter 10, you shall be further guided in your skills and abilities for self-assessment.

## AWARENESS THROUGH ACTION

The exercises that follow are aimed at helping you discover your currently held ideas about the nature of helping and why you are interested in becoming a health professional. Your **beliefs** about your self are explored, and you are given the opportunity to practice one of the major factors of effective helping: **active listening**. You will be surprised how difficult it is to really hear what someone else is saying.

## REFERENCES

1. Sackett D et al. *Evidence-Based Medicine: How to Practice and Teach EBM*, 2nd ed. Edinburgh, Scotland: Churchill Livingstone; 2000:1.
2. Law, ME, MacDermid, J. *Evidence-Based Rehabilitation: A Guide to Practice*, 3rd ed. Slack; 2013.
3. Davis CM. *A Phenomenological Description of Empathy as It Occurs Within Physical Therapists for Their Patients* [dissertation]. Boston, MA: Boston University; 1982.
4. Rogers C. The characteristics of a helping relationship. In: Rogers C, ed. *On Becoming a Person*. Boston, MA: Houghton Mifflin; 1961.
5. Geller SM, Greenberg, LS. *Therapeutic Presence: A Mindful Approach to Effective Relationships*, 2nd ed. Washington, DC: American Psychological Association; 2022.
6. Geller, SM. Cultivating therapeutic presence: strengthening your clinical heart, mind, and practice. *Transformance: The AEDP Journal*. 2020;8(10): 1.
7. Ellison DL, Meyer CK. Presence and therapeutic listening. *Nurs Clin North Am*. 2020 Dec;55(4):457–465.
8. Stein E. *On the Problem of Empathy*, 2nd ed. The Hague, The Netherlands: Martinus Nijhoff; 1970.
9. Jamison, L. *The Empathy Exams: Essays*. Minneapolis, MN: Graywolf Press; 2014.
10. Powell J. *Why Am I Afraid to Tell You Who I Am?* Niles, IL: Argus Communications; 1969.
11. Combs AW, Gonzalez, DM. *Helping Relationships—Basic Concepts for the Health Professions*, 4th ed. Boston, MA: Allyn & Bacon; 1993.
12. Corey, MS, Corey G. *Becoming a Helper*, 8th ed. Independence, KY: Engage Learning; 2021.
13. Anderson R, Cissna KN. *The Martin Buber-Carl Rogers Dialogue: A New Transcript with Commentary*. Albany, NY: SUNY Press; 1997.
14. Geller SM, Porges SW. Therapeutic presence: neurophysiological mechanisms mediating feeling safe in therapeutic relationships. *J Psychother Integration*. 2014;24(3):178–192.

15. Geller SM. Therapeutic presence: the foundation for effective emotion-focused therapy. In: Greenberg LS, Goldman RN, eds. *Clinical Handbook of Emotion-focused Therapy*. Washington, DC: American Psychological Association. 2019; 129–145.

16. Laukka P, Linnman C, Åhs F, Pissiota A, Frans Ö, Faria V, Michelgård Å, Appel L, Fredrikson M, Furmark T. In a nervous voice: acoustic analysis and perception of anxiety in social phobics' speech. *J Nonverbal Behav*. 2008;32(4):195–214.

17. Ramseyer F, Tschacher W. Nonverbal synchrony of head-and body-movement in psychotherapy: different signals have different associations with outcome. *Frontiers Psych*. 2014;5(979):1–9.

18. Vlemincx E, Abelson, JL, Lehrer PM, Davenport PW, Van Diest I, Van den Bergh O. (2013). Respiratory variability and sighing: a psychophysiological reset model. *Bio Psych*. 2013; 24–32. doi: 10.1016/j.biopsycho.2012.12.001.

19. Stellar JE, Cohen A, Oveis C, Keltner D. Affective and physiological responses to the suffering of others: compassion and vagal activity. *J Person & Soc Psych*. 2015;108(4):572–585.

20. Rathenau S, Sousa D, Vaz A, Geller, S. The effect of attitudes toward online therapy and the difficulties perceived in online therapeutic presence. *J Psychother Integration*. 2021;32(1):19–33.

21. Geller S. Cultivating online therapeutic presence: strengthening therapeutic relationships in teletherapy sessions. *Couns Psych Quart*. 2021;34(3–4):687–703.

22. Norwood C, Moghaddam NG, Malins S, Sabin-Farrell R. Working alliance and outcome effectiveness in videoconferencing psychotherapy: a systematic review and noninferiority meta-analysis. *Clin Psychology & Psychother*. 2018;25(6):797–808. doi: 10.1002/cpp.2315.

23. Aafjes-van Doorn K, Békés V, Prou TA. Grappling with our therapeutic relationship and professional self-doubt during COVID-19: will we use video therapy again? *Counsel Psych Quart*. 2020;34(3–4): 473–484. doi: 10.1080/09515070.2020.1773404.

24. Chapman CR, Woo NT, Maluf KS. Preferred communication strategies used by physical therapists in chronic pain rehabilitation: a qualitative systematic review and meta-synthesis. *Phys Ther*. 2022 Sep 4;102(9):pzac081. doi: 10.1093/ptj/pzac081.

25. Kleiner MJ, Kinsella EA, Miciak M, Teachman G, Walton DM. "Passion to do the right thing": searching for the "good" in physiotherapist practice. *Physiother Theory Pract*. 2024 Feb;40(2):288–303.

26. Kleiner MJ, Kinsella EA, Miciak M, Teachman G, McCabe E, Walton DM. An integrative review of the qualities of a "good" physiotherapist. *Physiother Theory Pract*. 2023 Jan;39(1):89–116.

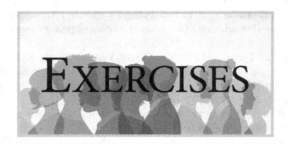

# EXERCISE 1: SELF-AWARENESS—WHY DO I WANT TO HELP?

Respond to the following questions. Discuss with two or three others in small groups. Note the variety of reasons why people are drawn to the helping professions and note the responses most of you share in common.

1. Why do I want to be a helping professional?

2. Whom do I most want to help?

3. What specific rewards do I get from helping people?

4. How do I want to be perceived by those I intend to help?

5. Do I believe people are essentially lazy and will want to have me do all the work for them, or do I believe people most of the time want to help themselves? Is there a category of patients/clients whom I believe are mostly lazy? How did I decide this?

6. I feel most anxious when I'm helping—when?

7. Those who require the most help from others are—who?

8. Answering these questions made me feel—what?

## Journal Reflections

As I reflect on my response to the above questions, what did I learn about myself? Who am I becoming?

# EXERCISE 2: BELIEFS ABOUT SELF

Complete the following self-awareness continuum. Place a mark on the line that reflects your current belief about yourself. Be as honest as possible, rather than responding as you think you should respond.

## *What I Believe About Myself Today*

### 1. Personal Strengths and Weaknesses

I feel unsure about what I am good at. Often not aware of weakness until someone else points it out.

I know myself rather well. Am clear about strengths and weaknesses. Recognize that who I am as a person is the most important instrument that I possess.

### 2. Basic Curiosity and Openness to New Learning

Most of what I am learning is not that interesting. Seems like old stuff that is just rehashed.

My learning at this stage is new and I recognize it as important to my patient care skills. I am open to most of it.

### 3. Seeing Through the Eyes of the Helpee

I have difficulty taking the view of the other. I just cannot seem to understand the point of view of the other person most of the time.

I am willing and able to put myself in the place of the other person that I am helping, even if their opinion is very different from mine.

### 4. Able to Challenge Clients to Dream

It is important for me to have the right answer, and I want to encourage my patients to do as I ask them to, without adding their own ideas.

I want to inspire my patients to be able to do what they dream they can do in their lives, and I try to also live up to my dreams.

## 5. Areas of Need and Function

I take pretty good care of myself physically and intellectually, but my feelings and my spiritual needs don't get much attention.

I deal with my personal problems right away. I take care of the needs in all areas—physical, mental, emotional, and spiritual.

## 6. Adaptability

I have studied long and hard to be able to be an effective helper. I expect my patients to be willing to follow my instructions the way I have decided is best for them.

I recognize that each patient or client brings their unique situation to me for my help and I am willing to adapt my approach and techniques to the client's situation.

## 7. Personal Beliefs and Values

My personal beliefs and values have been thought about and refined over time and are a composite of the best that my family and religious beliefs can offer.

My philosophy of life and beliefs and values have been personally developed and are my own, not imposed on me by anyone else, and I am willing to examine and challenge them.

## 8. Relationships With Others

I look forward to being able to find friends and colleagues with whom I can establish healthy relationships. So far most of my friendships have been pretty superficial.

I am blessed with good friends, and I take pride in the fact that I have established some very meaningful relationships with a few colleagues, friends, and family.

## 9. Has a Healthy Sense of Self-Love and Pride, but Is Not Self-Absorbed

I am very proud of my accomplishments, which I have to say I pretty much have done on my own. I know I am good, and I have to look out for myself. No one else can really be counted on.

I am very proud of my accomplishments. I try to live a life that I can be proud of and I like myself, but I recognize that I have achieved what I have with the help of others, and I am very grateful.

(Adapted from Corey, MS, Corey G. *Becoming a Helper*, 8th ed. Independence, KY: Cengage Learning; 2021.)

# EXERCISE 3: EFFECTIVE LISTENING

According to Rogers,[4] good listening involves the following:

- Not only hearing the words of the speaker but also hearing the feelings behind the words.
- Putting oneself in the place of the other, or self-transposal; feeling the other's feelings and seeing the world through the speaker's eyes.
- Suspending one's own value judgments in order to understand the speaker's thoughts and feelings as they experience them.

Really listening is difficult and takes practice, especially if you disagree with what is being said. Most normal conversations involve talking at one another, rather than with one another. We must reframe our communication as HCPs.

Divide into groups of three. One person serves as monitor, the other two as discussants. The monitor helps the discussants find a topic of mutual interest, but one on which they fundamentally disagree. For example, one person believes that people should have the right to assisted suicide and the other believes that life is sacred and only God can determine when it begins and ends.

The first discussant states their position. In a typical discussion, we are so concerned with what we are going to say next, or so involved with planning our response, that we often tune out or miss the full meaning of what is being said.

In this exercise, before any discussant offers a point of view, one must first **summarize the essence of the previous speaker's statement so that the previous speaker honestly feels that their statement has been understood**. It is the monitor's role to see that this process takes place with each exchange.

Discussion takes place for 10 minutes, with the monitor assuming the responsibility of ensuring that the procedure described above is followed. At the end of 10 minutes, discussants give each other feedback about how well they feel they had been heard, understood, and responded to, during the time frame allotted.

The process is repeated with the monitor assuming the role of discussant and one of the discussants becoming the monitor.

**One more note**: The role of the monitor is critical to the success of this exercise. The monitor **must insist** that each person summarize the other's statement before speaking. This is difficult to do but essential to the success of the exercise. Be insistent and be brave!

---

**These exercises are also available online at www.routledge.com/9781638220039.**

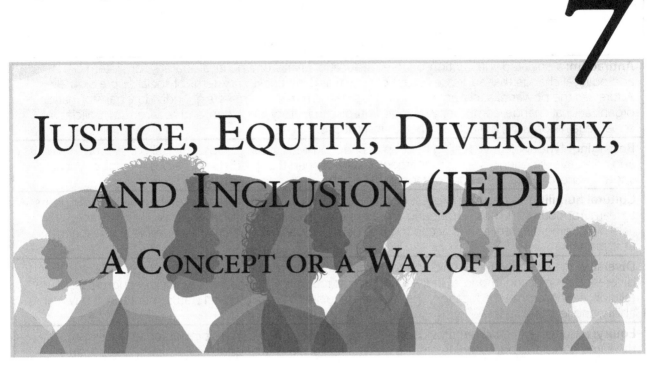

# Justice, Equity, Diversity, and Inclusion (JEDI)

## A Concept or a Way of Life

*Mica Mitchell and Gina Maria Musolino*

## OBJECTIVES

*The learner should be able to*:

- Be cognizant of the elements of diversity.

- Identify ways to implement inclusion and equity for patient–practitioner interactions.

- Discover the impact of words, actions, and policies on marginalized and underrepresented groups with respect to micro- and macroaggressions.

- Explore ways to facilitate discussions for Justice, Equity, Diversity, and Inclusion (JEDI), belonging, and antiracism.

- Recognize key indicators of victims of injustice and suggested communications.

- Apply JEDI, belonging, antiracism and cultural humility learning perspectives through reflection activities.

## INTRODUCTION

Think about a time when you first met someone, or after multiple times meeting, you pronounced their name incorrectly. Consider how the mispronunciation made you feel, and how it made the other person feel. For example, to introduce myself, my name is Mica (Mee-kuh), Mitchell, I am a cisgender Black woman, and my pronouns are she/her/hers. The inclusion of the phonetic pronunciation of my first name, (Mee-kuh), represents how you *say* my name, and assists others who may not always know the correct way to verbally state my name. Providing guidance for name pronunciations helps to decrease any awkward or embarrassing moments for yourself and others with mispronunciations. Phonetic guidance also assists others in avoiding pronouncing someone's name incorrectly.

DOI: 10.4324/9781003525554-7

| TABLE 7.1 |
|---|
| **JEDI AND RELATED DEFINITIONS**[3–5] |
| **Antiracism:** associated with "action-oriented, educational and/or a political strategy for systemic and political change that addresses issues of racism and interlocking systems of social oppression."[3] Addresses the power of social agency and can present in many formats, e.g., "individual transformation, organizational change, community change, anti-discriminatory legislation, and racial equity policies in social, legal, economic, political and health institutions."[3] |
| **Belonging:** "The subjective feeling of deep connection with social groups, physical places, and individual and collective experiences—is a fundamental human need that predicts numerous mental, physical, social, economic, and behavioral outcomes."[4] |
| **Cultural humility:** an ongoing process of self-exploration and self-critique combined with a willingness to learn from others. It means honoring another person's beliefs, customs, and values as well as acknowledging differences and accepting that person for who they are with a humble and respectful attitude.[5] |
| **Diversity:** the myriad ways in which people differ, including the psychological, physical, and social differences that occur among all individuals, such as race, ethnicity, nationality, socioeconomic status, religion, economic class, education, age, gender, sexual orientation, marital status, mental and physical ability, and learning styles.[5] |
| **Equity:** ensures individuals are provided the resources they need to have proportionate access to the same rights and opportunities, as the general population. State or quality of being just, impartial, and fair.[5] |
| **Inclusion:** the quality of welcoming, respecting, valuing, and providing opportunities for full participation for all individuals and groups. Inclusion builds a culture of belonging by actively inviting the contribution and participation of all people.[3–5] |
| **Inclusivity:** authentically bringing traditionally excluded individuals and/or groups into process, activities, and decision/policy making in a way that shares power. The practice or policy of providing equal access to opportunities and resources for people who might otherwise be excluded or marginalized, such as those having physical or mental disabilities or who have historically been excluded because of their race, gender, sexuality, or ability. Inclusion focuses on creating spaces in which diverse opinions and persons are valued and are given an equal voice, providing for a sense of belonging, coupled with respect.[5] |
| **Inclusion and inclusivity are terms associated with a sense of belonging, and feelings of being valued, coupled with respect.**[3–5] |
| **Justice:** addressing hinderances that cause inequality and supporting systems that facilitate solutions. The quality, practice, and action of being just, impartial, or fair and from a legal perspective the establishment or determination of rights according to law or equity.[5] |
| **Marginalized:** the process by which minority groups/cultures are excluded, ignored, or relegated to the outer edge of a group/society/community.[5] |
| **Minoritized:** the uncontrollable and systematically oppressive force of being in a minority group, with respect to race, religion, or other aspects of identity.[5] |
| **Racism:** specifically refers to individual, cultural, institutional, and systemic ways by which differential consequences are created for different racial groups. Often refers to "beliefs, attitudes, institutional arrangements, and acts that tend to denigrate individuals or groups because of phenotypic characteristics or ethnic group affiliation."[5] |

When we meet new people, including our patients and clients, it is important to take the time to learn how to properly pronounce their names and acknowledge their preferences. My race and gender are included in my introduction to provide context to who is presenting this information to you, and offers the beginnings of insight into my lived experiences. The acknowledgment of my being cisgender (gender identity and birth sex) normalizes discussing gender expression terms. I provide my type of gender identity to be inclusive of all genders and sexualities and in allyship to all. Allyship is a supportive association with others. Allyship is often a lifelong process of building relationships with a basis of trust, along with consistency and accountability for uniting with marginalized individuals and/or groups of people.

To encompass the entire spectrum of gender fluidity and sexual identities, the inclusive term for persons identifying as lesbian, gay, bisexual, trans, transgender, transsexual, questioning or queer, intersex, asexual, or other identities (e.g., agender, demisexual, gender fluid, gray sexual, nonbinary, pansexual, polyamorous, sapiosexual, and two-spirit) is commonly represented by the abbreviation LGBTQIA2S. A term used by Native Americans to describe a third gender for *two-spirit* (2S) is utilized in the main abbreviation as LGBTQIA2S+. Members of the LGBTQIA2S+ communities are at risk of being ignored, marginalized, and discriminated against.[1] Using an individual's preferred pronouns and offering them the opportunity to share their gender identity and sexuality shows respect, builds the patient–practitioner and colleague relationship, while promoting social justice. Relationship building strengthens the patient–practitioner alliance for better collaboration, establishing trust, and leading to improved outcomes.

This chapter is designed to guide you through a thought process, with actions that may be helpful in your interpersonal interactions with your patients. As we discuss Justice, Equity, Diversity, and Inclusion (JEDI) (see Table 7.1), the hope is that you gain an enhanced understanding of the importance of avoiding discrimination and building relationships at an individual level, to allow you to identify ways to provide equitable care and considerations for your patients, colleagues, community partners, society, and other relationships not named.[2] As we begin, let us consider the meaning of this adage in relation to contemporary society and how it applies to health care in particular:

*Not everything that is faced can be changed, but nothing can be changed until it is faced.* —James Baldwin

# DIVERSITY AND DISCRIMINATION

Originally coined by diversity advocate Verna Myers, "Diversity is being invited to the party; Inclusion is being asked to dance." While many believe this to be an oversimplification of these issues, it does provide context regarding how we can begin to understand and address these issues in health care. Throughout all facets of health care, race/ethnicity, gender, sexual orientation, immigration status, physical disability status, and socioeconomic level all play a role in representation, acceptance, and progress both within and outside of the health care setting.

Discrimination is expressed as actions and statements that are: sexist, racist, homophobic, xenophobic, classist, ageist, and/or ableist. Discrimination is an expression of violence in the lives of the victims. As we build relationships it is important not to impose harm in our interactions and understand the vulnerabilities with the individuals we will be working with for long-lasting, positive relationships.[2] Take the time to pay attention to name pronunciations and preferences of your patients and clients. Use pronouns properly. Being respectful in all patient–practitioner interactions is an important aspect to build strong, therapeutic alliances. Health care professionals often meet new people daily. When meeting new people, people different from you, do not be afraid to make a mistake during your interaction. Mistakes happen. You may mispronounce someone's name, you may misgender someone. Forgive yourself and commit to doing better with your next interaction.

Despite making an error, we should strive to keep trying to get it correct, apologize, accept any correction provided and intend to avoid repeating that same mistake. If you are unsure, seek clarifications. Immediately practicing and applying the correct information helps to reinforce the appropriate and preferred pronunciations and/or pronouns along with their importance. Learning and applying the information in this chapter is often process-oriented. Allow yourself grace and kindness on this journey.

With respect to JEDI, belonging, and antiracism, one of your goals should be to form a therapeutic alliance, to grow a strong patient–practitioner relationship, which starts with your first interaction. Before you attempt to rename, provide a nickname, or continue to mispronounce someone's name, after being provided with their correct pronunciation, remember Dale Carnegie's insights: "A person's name is to that person, the sweetest, most important sound in any language,"[6] a crucial step in relationship building.

What is JEDI and why does it matter? JEDI provides a framework to promote equitable and inclusive environments. Simply put, justice is equality, and all deserve to be treated with respect and fairness. Diversity is our differences, equity is the support an individual needs to eliminate disadvantages; while inclusion attempts to involve groups or individuals who have been excluded, due to systemic or individual barriers, and opportunities to be involved and/or engaged. The Merriam-Webster Dictionary defines diversity as:

> *the condition of having or being composed of differing elements; especially the inclusion of people of different races, cultures, etc. in a group or organization; and an instance of being composed of differing elements or qualities: an instance of being diverse.*[7]

Every individual has differences, even in the case of identical visual similarities there can be differences in thought/s or experiences. We should celebrate differences and learn from each other. However, there are differences that put individuals at risk of harm and/or exclusion. Awareness of the potential for harm allows the practitioner to identify needs and make recommendations for support or resources to improve the patient–practitioner interactions.[8]

A healthy relationship can occur despite differences. Having differences can sometimes be the very thing we have in common with another individual. We are all different, and getting to know what makes each of us unique can bring people together. Establishing healthy relationships through the implementation of JEDI can eliminate the trauma of another negative experience for our patients. Your opportunity to demonstrate your commitment to JEDI occurs within the first few minutes of your initial interactions. You must be attentive to see the individual in front of you.

Every human should be able to exist and thrive without discrimination. Increasing diversity has been shown to increase productivity and improve relationships.[9] Diversifying your friend group gives you different perspectives. Having nonjudgmental conversations with people with different lived experiences from yours will add diversity to your thoughts and actions to progress the therapeutic alliance. Equitable treatment (antiracist) of all individuals does not always occur. Marginalized individuals or groups who are treated as if they do not matter are most at risk for unfair treatment. Our patients and colleagues can be marginalized individuals or members of historically marginalized groups that often do not have a sense of belonging. It is human nature to treat people differently, without intention to be inclusive. Our biases can cause harm to vulnerable or marginalized individuals and groups, continuing the harm they experience. When more than one perspective is considered with your thoughts and actions, biases are checked, and stereotypes can be avoided for more inclusive experiences.

Diversity includes many elements, including characteristics that are both seen and unseen; as well as known and unknown.[8] There are elements of diversity that can change through life's circumstance, and factors that do not change. The primary elements of diversity, that may or may not change, which can put people at risk of experiencing discrimination and being minoritized (less representation than your own) include race/ethnicity, age, gender, national origin, sexual orientation, and mental/physical ability.[8] The primary elements of diversity develop our self-view and our world view[8] while aiding in determining what we value, hence our perceptions of what we observe and experience. The primary elements of diversity assist in forming our priorities and lived experiences.[8] All elements of diversity exist within individuals, communities, and society; the combination may have positive, neutral, or negative impacts with our relationships.[2,8] Our primary elements of diversity (see Figure 7.1) influence how we interact with individuals, our community, and society.

The secondary elements of diversity—an individual's work experience, education, political belief, family, organizational role, communication/language skills, income, religion, appearance—are the elements of diversity that can change for an individual over time.[8] The secondary elements of diversity add depth to our individual experiences.[8] An individual can have an overlap of marginalized elements of diversity, which increases their risk for discrimination and further marginalization.

The representation of diversity in our interpersonal, intrapersonal, community, and societal relationships helps practitioners consider other perspectives which may aid in minimizing prejudices and discrimination due to stereotypes. Our experiences are the essence of who we are as humans; each primary and secondary element of diversity helps develop the complex human that we present to the world (see Figure 7.2).[8]

Two individuals can have the same race but living in different socioeconomic levels can vary their lived experience; no two people are the same, and getting to know people at an individual level helps with understanding their perspective. As a health care professional (HCP), understanding a patient's perspective aids the practitioner to best support the patient to meet their goals while enhancing the patient–practitioner alliance.

# EQUITY AND INCLUSION

Have you ever felt out of place in a room? Can you identify what made you feel out of place? Could it be that no one looked like you? Was there a difference in knowledge or experience? Feeling out of place and not being received because you are different is being "othered." Being "othered" is often a continual experience for minoritized

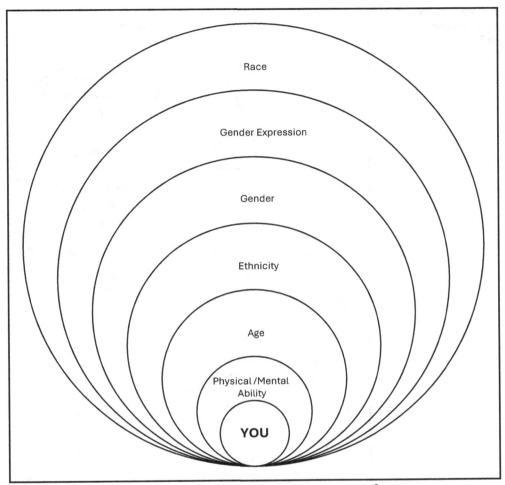

**Figure 7.1** Elements of diversity that affect our self and world views. Based on Loden.[8]

individuals in spaces with individuals and groups of majority representation, or for "other" reasons, unbeknownst to the person being subjected to being "othered." At some point in time, it is possible that you have felt uncomfortable due to a difference between you and another. That feeling of uneasiness and/or discomfort is a constant for some minoritized individuals. Not knowing the intentions of an individual from a majority group as it pertains to safety can cause worry, and the effects of toxic environments may, and frequently do, lead to chronic stress which is often a contributing factor for many chronic diseases and/or illnesses.[10,11] The acknowledgment of individuals' lived experiences, an awareness of possible previous and current trauma, along with the implementation of strategies to uplift and support assist in improving patient outcomes and patient–practitioner interactions.[12,13]

# REPRESENTATION AND JUSTICE

Diversity, equity, and inclusion need the implementation of representation and justice for the considerations of the needs of vulnerable individuals and groups to be addressed. Representation is including an individual from an underrepresented minority group. If their presence is not an option, their needs should be represented by the decision-makers that are present. The allegorical representation of Lady Justice is how we should implement justice. Her eyes are masked to illustrate her impartiality (objectivity without bias or prejudice) with scales in one hand to weigh the pro and cons of situations and a sword for often swift decisions. We need to be fair and reasonable while always ready to defend the underrepresented and most vulnerable. Increasing diversity has been shown to increase productivity and improve relationships.[9] The HCP should frequently reflect and make changes as needed to interact and provide care without discrimination. Candid discussions with a trusted colleague may also aid in identifying any challenges to facilitate needed change.

**Figure 7.2** Elements of diversity impact how we experience life. Based on Loden.[8]

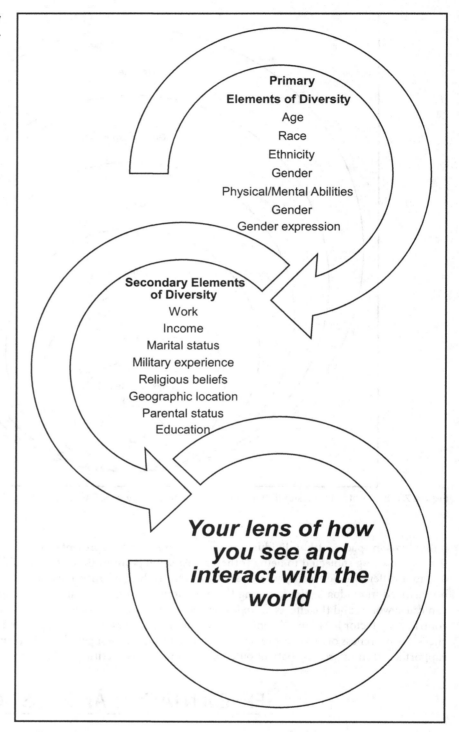

**Primary Elements of Diversity**
Age
Race
Ethnicity
Gender
Physical/Mental Abilities
Gender
Gender expression

**Secondary Elements of Diversity**
Work
Income
Marital status
Military experience
Religious beliefs
Geographic location
Parental status
Education

*Your lens of how you see and interact with the world*

# FOSTERING JEDI AWARENESS

The HCP needs to be aware of microaggressions and macroaggressions while collaborating with individuals who are at risk of being marginalized.[14–16] Microaggression consists of "brief and commonplace daily, verbal, behavioral, and environmental indignities, whether intentional or unintentional, which communicate hostile, derogatory, or negative slights, invalidations, and insults to an individual or group because of their marginalized status in society."[16(64)] Examples of microaggressions are statements that are ableist, ageist, racist, sexist, homophobic, classist, and/or xenophobic. Asking a person where they are from, not accepting their first answer, and insisting that they tell you their nation of origin is an example of a microaggression. Telling someone from a minority group that they are articulate, with notable "surprise" from how you might have expected them to speak, is a microaggression. The attacks can be delivered through words and/or actions, and the wounds that are caused can have a lasting negative and compounding effect. The prefix of micro- does not refer to the impact on the individual on the receiving end, because the effects can vary from minimal to maximal impact on the victim. Micro is used to describe the type of aggression, as a comparison with a macroaggression which is a hate crime.[15,16] Berk[16] defines macroaggression as:

> *overt, conscious, intentional hate acts and crimes. Explicit, conscious, and deliberate verbal and non-verbal attacks intended to hurt the victim. Can include intentional hate prejudice, racism, classism, sexism, homophobia, ableism, bias, and discrimination.*

Micro in microaggression also can refer to how the aggressor perceives the magnitude of the aggression.[16] The impact of a microaggression can feel macro to the aggresse.

In my youth, I have heard, and I have said, the colloquial phrase "sticks and stones may break my bones, but words will never hurt me," and that could not be further from the truth. The harm of words can include, but is not limited to, a lack of engagement and participation, as well as withdrawal and isolation, with the potential for negative health effects.[15-17] If you think you have not experienced a microaggression, imagine how it feels getting a paper cut. Think about how annoying the occurrence is, someone may have observed what happened, yet it is not always apparent that you have *actually* cut yourself. The first experience with a microaggression is annoying but possibly not enough of a disturbance to ruin your day. If you continue to get paper cuts, the compounding effects can cause increased pain with each occurrence. What would your emotional or verbal response be after even ten paper cuts per day? Then the hundredth paper cut in a day? Continued exposure to microaggressions can affect your attitude, your perception of others, and your willingness to engage, to name a few consequences.[15-19] The compounding effects of constant micro-aggressions may be a lack of engagement, or slowness to engage based on past trauma.[14,16] When a microaggression is brought to your attention, either witnessed or reported, it needs to be acknowledged, and a plan should be established to maintain open and healthy relationships. Upcoming in Chapters 8 and 9 we will further address effective communication strategies and appropriate assertiveness skills for conflict resolution.

Ignoring or minimizing individuals' experiences with microaggressions is gaslighting.[20] Gaslighting represents the "ways in which an individuals' experiences are manipulated to be an imagined experience further creating a disconnect and harm."[20] Continued gaslighting perpetuates harm. An individual may appear to have things under control in a positive way on the surface, while under the surface there are or may be a multitude of negative factors and experiences from dealing with microaggressions, as illustrated in the Microaggression Iceberg (Figure 7.3). You may not know about someone's experiences with microaggressions until they feel safe to share these experiences with you. If they share with you, be respectful and consider it an honor that they feel safe or in a place in their healing that they can talk about their experiences.

When an individual encounters a microaggression, either by being the aggresse or an observer, efforts to think about ways to recognize and react to microaggressions are important to consider.[21,22] Asking a series of questions, while considering matters of personal or psychological safety, guides what if any actions need to be taken:[18]

- Did this person intend to insult me?
- Should I respond?
- How should I respond?
- What would happen if I said something?
- Is it worth the trouble?
- Am I making a big deal about nothing?

When deciding to respond to a microaggression, remember to "Open The Front Door" while avoiding anger and accusation.[22] It is important to observe what has occurred, think about how the comment was interpreted, how the comment made the recipient feel, and the desired outcome from addressing the microaggression.[22] Here is an example of how to respond to a microaggression:[16,22]

> *You said _____, it made me think that you _____. I feel concerned about this because _____, and I would like us to discuss this further so we can come to an understanding.*

Identifying how you will respond prior to being in a situation where you have experienced racist, sexist, homophobic, xenophobic, ageist, classist comment(s) can help prepare you to address your concerns: alerting the individuals involved that there has been an offense, creating future safety through a plan, and encouraging an environment that is available for brave future conversations as needed.

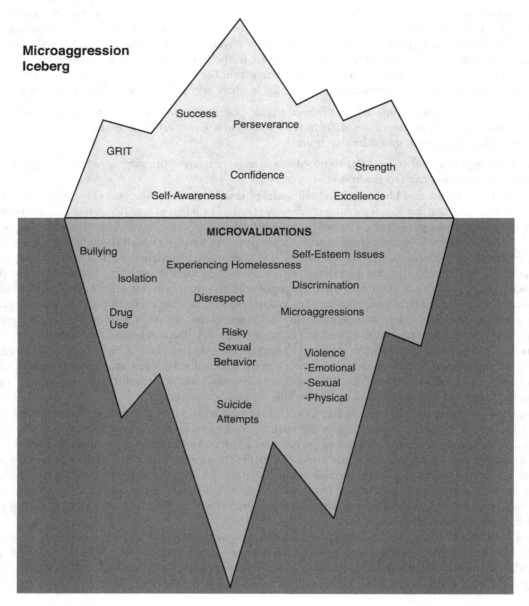

**Figure 7.3** Microaggression Iceberg.[15–16]

The harm and negativity that occur from microaggressions can seem overwhelming. Micro-affirmations provide the support needed to combat negative consequences of microaggressions.[23] Micro-affirmations are "tiny acts of opening doors to opportunity, gestures of inclusion, caring, and graceful acts of listening".[23(p 46)] Being generous with our time, using kind words, giving people their credit, and providing comfort when people are in distress can counteract the harm and violence experienced by individuals from minoritized groups. The compounding effects of genuine consistent micro-affirmations will help build relationships.[23]

Dr. Martin Luther King, Jr. in 1963 expounded on matters of injustice, proclaiming that "injustice anywhere is a threat to justice everywhere. We are caught in an inescapable network of mutuality. Whatever affects one directly, affects all indirectly." As HCPs we must be aware and watchful for signs of victims of injustice in our patient–practitioner interactions and communities of practices. Recognizing key indicators[24] of physical and mental abuse, or human trafficking[24] and smuggling, is the first step in identifying the victims of these egregious injustices and can help save a life. Table 7.2 provides some common indicators to help recognize signs and symptoms of human trafficking, human smuggling, physical, mental, and sexual abuses, and neglect.[24]

| TABLE 7.2 |
| --- |
| ## INDICATORS OF HUMAN TRAFFICKING, SMUGGLING, PHYSICAL, MENTAL, SEXUAL ABUSES, AND NEGLECT |

○ Does the person have unexplained bruises, fractures, burns, lacerations without appropriate care?

○ Does the person have consistent hunger needs, poor hygiene, lice, a distended stomach, or an emaciated appearance?

○ Does the person appear disconnected from family, friends, community organizations, or houses of worship?

○ Has a child stopped attending school?

○ Does the person present with speech disorders or delayed physical development?

○ Has the person had a sudden or dramatic change in behavior?

○ Is a juvenile engaged in commercial sex acts?

○ Does the person have torn, stained, or bloody underclothing?

○ Does the person have frequent yeast or urinary tract infections?

○ Does the person present with speech disorders or delayed physical development?

○ Is the person disoriented or confused, or showing signs of mental or physical abuse?

○ Does the person have bruises in various stages of healing?

○ Is the person fearful, timid, or submissive?

○ Does the person show signs of having been denied food, water, sleep, or medical care?

○ Is the person often in the company of someone to whom they defer? Or someone who seems to be in control of the situation, e.g., where they go or who they talk to?

○ Does the person appear to be coached on what to say?

○ Is the person living in unsuitable conditions?

○ Does the person lack personal possessions and appear not to have a stable living situation?

○ Does the person have freedom of movement? Can the person freely leave where they live? Are there unreasonable security measures?

**Physical Signs and Symptoms[24]**

○ Bruising; old, healing, or new lacerations; hematomas; signs of acute or chronic head trauma or a headache; missing hair or bald spots.

○ Trouble hearing; damage to the auditory canal or eardrum; signs of trauma to the oropharynx such as lacerations or burns, blood in the mouth, ulcerations, tooth decay, broken teeth, gingival irritation, tongue abnormalities; signs of anemia or dehydration in the oral mucosa.

○ Visual defects, sudden or gradual onset; tattoos or brands in the hairline or on the neck; signs of strangulation such as bruising.

○ Signs of chest trauma, murmurs; cigarette burns; tattoos that imply ownership; bruising in various stages of healing; signs of stress-related cardiovascular issues such as arrhythmias or high blood pressure.

○ Respiratory issues that would indicate inhalation injuries from chemical exposure, toxic fume exposure, asbestos exposure, or mold exposure.

○ Signs of tuberculosis such as night sweats, coughing up blood, fever, and weight loss.

○ Signs of stress-related respiratory or gastrointestinal problems.

○ Damage to lung tissue due to prolonged exposure to chemicals or pesticides, aspiration pneumonia or other inhalation injuries; meth lab exposure can produce burning to the eyes, nose, and mouth, chest pain, cough, lack of coordination, nausea, and dizziness.

○ Hypothermia or hyperthermia from environmental exposure from working in damp, cool, poorly insulated factories, or buildings; mold exposure signs/symptoms.

○ Signs of gastrointestinal issues such as nausea, vomiting, diarrhea, constipation, or abdomen pain; rectal pain, itching, trauma or bleeding; parasites in the feces or signs of abdominal trauma.

*(continued)*

| TABLE 7.2 (CONTINUED) |
|---|
| **INDICATORS OF HUMAN TRAFFICKING, SMUGGLING, PHYSICAL, MENTAL, SEXUAL ABUSES, AND NEGLECT** |

- Bruising to the back or scarring; tattoos that imply advertisement, ownership, or are sexually explicit in the pubic hair.
- Obstetrical and gynecological complaints such as sexually transmitted infections (STI) or recurrent STIs. An STI, especially if recurrent, in a minor may be the first and only sign of sexual abuse; repeated unwanted or unplanned pregnancies or forced abortions; anogenital trauma; evidence of retained foreign bodies such as in the vagina from packing during menstruation, vaginal bleeding, discharge, rashes, itching, signs of injury or forced sex.
- Number of sexual partners; condom use; genitourinary symptoms present such as burning, frequency, odor, dark urine, or history of frequent urinary tract infections.
- Signs of bruising or lower back scarring from repeated beatings; musculoskeletal issues such as signs of repetitive trauma; work-related injuries or injuries such as back problems from wearing heels for hours walking the streets or neck and jaw problems from frequent, forced oral sex.
- Fractures, old or new, any contractures. Cigarette or scald burns. Ligature marks/scars around ankles or wrists. Signs of scabies, infestations (scalp or body). Impetigo. Fungal infections.
- Signs of nutritional deficits such as Vitamin D deficiencies from lack of exposure to sunlight, anemia, or mineral deficiencies; brittle or fine hair.
- Signs of anorexia, bulimia, loss of appetite, malnutrition, and severe electrolyte abnormalities.
- Growth and development abnormalities in children, dental cavities, or misaligned poorly formed teeth.
- Neurological issues such as seizures, pseudo-seizures, numbness or tingling, migraines, inability to concentrate, vertigo, unexplained memory loss, and seizures.
- Insomnia, nightmares, waking up frequently.
- Signs of opioid or other addiction.

**Further Information on Reporting, Resources, Support, and Awareness Training**

- Human trafficking: www.dhs.gov/blue-campaign
- National Human Trafficking hotline: www.state.gov/humantrafficking/
- National Domestic hotline: www.thehotline.org
- National Child Abuse hotline: https://childhelphotline.org/
- National Mental Health hotline: https://mentalhealthhotline.org/
- National Elder Fraud hotline: https://ovc.ojp.gov/program/elder-fraud-abuse/national-elder-fraud-hotline
- National Human Trafficking Hotline (24/7) 1 (888) 373–7888
    Text "HELP" to 233733
    Live chat at humantraffickinghotline.org
    Email help@humantraffickinghotline.org
    If you, or any you are aware of, need immediate assistance:
    Dial 911 for emergency or immediate danger
    Dial 988 for Crisis Lifeline
- Report Online or Access Resources and Referrals: www.traffickingresourcecenter.org
    - Email: nhtrc@polarisproject.org. Live chat: www.traffickingresourcecenter.org

**Suggested Messaging from the U.S. Department of Health & Human Services**

1. We are here to help you, and our priority is your safety. We can keep you safe and protected.
2. We can provide you with the medical care you need as well as find you a place to stay.
3. Everyone has the right to live without being abused or hurt, and that includes you.
4. You deserve a chance to live on your own and take care of yourself, be independent, and make your own choices. We can help you with that.
5. We can get you help to protect your family and your children.
6. You have rights and deserve to be treated according to those rights.

| TABLE 7.2 (CONTINUED) |
|---|
| **INDICATORS OF HUMAN TRAFFICKING, SMUGGLING, PHYSICAL, MENTAL, SEXUAL ABUSES, AND NEGLECT** |
| 7. You can trust me. I will do everything in my power to help you. Assistance is available for you under the law, and special visas allow you to live safely in this country. |
| 8. No one should have to be afraid all the time. We can help. |
| 9. Help us, so this does not happen to anyone else. |
| 10. You can decide what is best for you but let me provide you with a number to call for help 24 hours a day. You do not even have to tell them your name if you do not want to. They are there to help you anytime day or night. The National Human Trafficking Resource Center hotline number is 1.888.373.7888. |

To continue to spread awareness of the signs and indicators of human trafficking, select from the following videos provided by the U.S. Department of Homeland Security (DHS): Awareness Videos | Homeland Security (dhs.gov) www.dhs.gov/blue-campaign/videos

# BELONGING, CULTURAL HUMILITY, AND MINDFULNESS MOVING FORWARD

The goals of a HCP for justice, equity, diversity, and inclusion should be representation and fairness for the underrepresented and marginalized. The HCP should be a consistent champion for JEDI with and for our patients, colleagues, profession, and the society we serve.[25] Choose to support and uplift others, to counter a lived experience of harm with individuals and minorities. In demonstrating your commitment to establishing a healthy patient–practitioner interaction, show your patients and colleagues a commitment to them and their success. Core to what makes one a human being, *belongingness*[26] consists of an integrative framework of dynamic and ongoing social interconnection of four key components, which may support positive life outcomes:

1. Competencies for belonging (skills and abilities)
2. Opportunities to belong (enablers, removal/reduction of barriers)
3. Motivations to belong (inner drive)
4. Perceptions of belonging (cognitions, attributions, and feedback mechanisms—positive or negative experiences when connecting)

Consider where you feel you belong and why. Can you identify the four components of the integrative framework that contribute to your sense of belongingness? Are all equally represented? Now consider, where do you not feel you belong and why? Can you identify which of the four components contribute to your lack of belongingness? Do you believe that if you wanted to "belong" that you would be able to effect a change for yourself and/or others? What might be a reason/s for not seeking belongingness? How can you aid others in a sense of belongingness within your sphere of influence? Take a moment to write down your journal reflections on these four components of belongingness and the queries that follow below on cultural humility.

To facilitate belongingness, one must exercise cultural humility. Through exercising cultural humility in your everyday encounters, you will improve your patient–practitioner interactions. Only through this ongoing process of self-exploration and self-critique, combined with a willingness to learn from others, will we honor another person's beliefs, customs, and values, as well as acknowledge differences and accept that person for who they are.[26–28] Jacobs[27] expounds on the need for this continual renewal of self:

> *An awareness of the self is central to the notion of* **cultural humility**—*who a person is informs how they see another. Awareness may stem from self-reflective questions such as:*
>
> - *Which parts of my identity am I aware of? Which are most salient?*
> - *Which parts of my identity are privileged and/or marginalized?*
> - *How does my sense of identity shift based on context and settings?*

- *What are the parts onto which people project? And which parts are received well, by whom?*
- *What might be my own short-sightedness and biases?*

*With this awareness, a provider can ask questions about how they receive the patient:*

- *Who is this person, and how do I make sense of them?*
- *What knowledge and awareness do I have about their culture?*
- *What thoughts and feelings emerge from me about them?*

An objective HCP, who exercises cultural humility, understands the complexities of being human. Implementation of inclusion and equity is an intentional process. Be kind to yourself and those around you along the way. Be mindful to consider an individual's lived experience as you interact and advocate for your patients. Utilizing a biopsychosocial approach to care provides the platform for providing inclusive care.[29] HCPs have both a professional and moral obligation to provide care that is individualized, welcoming, and inclusive for all.[29] Be watchful to look beneath the surface in your patient–practitioner interactions, especially noticing nonverbal cues; awareness of injustices may help to save someone's life.

# REFERENCES

1. Hill F, Condran C, Pluss A, Fons L, Bell KA. *Introduction to LGBTQ+ Competency: Handbook for Physical Therapy.* PT Proud. Available: https://cdn.ymaws.com/www.aptahpa.org/resource/resmgr/csm_2019/csm_2019_handouts/Full_Handout_LGBTQIA-doc_1_1.pdf Accessed January 15, 2023.
2. Dahlberg LL, Krug EG. Violence: a global public health problem. *Ciencia e Saude Coletiva.* 2006;11(2):277–292. doi: 10.1590/S1413-81232006000200007.
3. Calliste AM, Dei GJS. *Power, Knowledge and Anti-Racism Education: A Critical Reader.* Halifax, NS, Canada: Fernwood; 2000.
4. Allen KA, Gray DL, Baumeister RF, Leary MR. The need to belong: a deep dive into the origins, implications, and future of a foundational construct. *Educ Psychol Rev.* 2022;34(2):1133–1156.
5. University of Washington Department of Epidemiology Equity, Diversity, and Inclusion Committee. Glossary of Equity, Diversity, and Inclusion Terms. 2019. Available: https://sph.washington.edu/about/diversity Accessed January 15, 2023.
6. Carnegie D. *How to Win Friends and Influence People: Updated for the Next Generation of Leaders.* New York, NY: Simon & Schuster; 2022.
7. Diversity Definition & Meaning—Merriam-Webster. https://www.merriam-webster.com/dictionary/diversity Accessed August 25, 2023.
8. Loden M, Rosener JB. *Workforce America: Managing Employee Diversity as a Vital Resource.* Homewood, IL: Business One Irwin; 1991.
9. Gomez LE, Bernet P. Diversity improves performance and outcomes. *J Natl Med Assoc.* 2019;111(4):383–392. doi: 10.1016/j.jnma.2019.01.006.
10. Felitti VJ, Anda RF, Nordenberg D, et al. Relationship of childhood abuse and household dysfunction to many of the leading causes of death in adults: the adverse childhood experiences (ACE) study. *Am J Prev Med.* 1998;14(4):245–258.
11. Anda RF, Felitti VJ, Bremner JD, et al. The enduring effects of abuse and related adverse experiences in childhood: a convergence of evidence from neurobiology and epidemiology. *Eur Arch Psychiatry Clin Neurosci.* 2006;256(3):174–186. doi: 10.1007/s00406-005-0624-4.
12. Oral R, Ramirez M, Coohey C, et al. Adverse childhood experiences and trauma informed care: the future of health care. *Pediatr Res.* 2016;79(1–2):227–233. doi: 10.1038/pr.2015.197.
13. Boullier M, Blair M. Adverse childhood experiences. *Paediatr Child Health.* 2018;28(3):132–137. doi: 10.1016/J.PAED.2017.12.008.
14. Sue DW. *Microaggressions and Marginality: Manifestation, Dynamics, and Impact.* New York: Wiley; 2010.
15. Wells C. Microaggressions in the context of academic communities. *Seattle Journal for Social Justice.* 2013;12.
16. Berk RA. Microaggressions trilogy: Part 1. Why do microaggressions matter? *J Fac Dev.* 2017;31(1):63–73.
17. Sue DW. *Microaggressions in Everyday Life: Race, Gender, and Sexual Orientation.* Hoboken, NJ: Wiley; 2010.
18. Berk RA. Microaggressions trilogy: Part 2. Microaggressions in the academic workplace. *J Fac Dev.* 2017;31(2):69–83.
19. Berk RA. Microaggressions trilogy: Part 3. Microaggressions in the classroom. *J Fac Dev.* 2017;31(3):95–110.
20. Sweet PL. The sociology of gaslighting. *Am Sociol Rev.* 2019;84(5):851–875. doi: 10.1177/0003122419874843.
21. Torres MB, Salles A, Cochran A. Recognizing and reacting to microaggressions in medicine and surgery. *JAMA Surg.* Published online July 10, 2019.
22. Ganote C, Cheung F, Souza T. *Don't Remain Silent!: Strategies for Supporting Yourself and Your Colleagues via Microresistances and Ally Development*; POD Diversity Committee White Paper; 2015.
23. Rowe M. Micro-affirmations & micro-inequities. *Journal of the International Ombudsman Association.* 2008;1(1):45–48.

24. Toney-Butler TJ, Ladd M, Mittel O. Human Trafficking. In: *StatPearls* [Internet]. Treasure Island, FL: StatPearls Publishing; 2023 Jan 29. PMID: 28613660.
25. Nordstrom T, Jensen GM, Altenburger P, Blackinton M, Deusinger S, Hack L, Patel RM, Tschoepe B, VanHoose L. Crises as the crucible for change in physical therapist education. *Phys Ther.* 2022 Jul 4;102(7):pzac055.
26. Allen KA, Kern ML, Rozek CS, McInereney D, Slavich GM. Belonging: a review of conceptual issues, an integrative framework, and directions for future research. *Aust J Psychol.* 2021 Mar 10;73(1):87–102.
27. Jacobs K. Cultural humility. *Work.* 2022;73(4):1089–1090.
28. Richey CE, Ryder P, Bilodeau A, Schultz M. Use of an online game to evaluate health professions students' attitudes toward people in poverty. *Am J Pharm Educ,* 2016 Oct. 25;80(8):139.
29. Aird, M, Walters, JL, Ker, A, Ross, MH. Transgender, Gender-Diverse and Nonbinary experiences in physical therapy. *Phys Ther.* 2024; pzae086. doi:10.1093/ptj/pzae086.

# SUGGESTED READINGS

Aird M, Walters JL, Ker A, Ross MH. Transgender, Gender-Diverse and Nonbinary experiences in physical therapy. *Phys Ther.* 2024; pzae086. doi:10.1093/ptj/pzae086. https://pmc.ncbi.nlm.nih.gov/articles/PMC11524892/

Felter CE, Ciccone J, Mathis L, Smith DL. Identifying and addressing social determinants of learning during the COVID-19 pandemic. *Phys Ther.* 2021 Nov.;101(11): pzab210. doi: 10.1093/ptj/pzab210. https://pmc.ncbi.nlm.nih.gov/articles/PMC8499936/

Jensen GM. Time to shine the light. *Phys Ther.* 2022 March;102(3): pzab257. doi: 10.1093/ptj/pzab257. https://academic.oup.com/ptj/article/102/3/pzab257/6540028?login=true

Hoffman MC, Mulligan NF, Bell KA, Condran C, Scarince HJ, Gulick E, He V, Hill F, Wolff E, Jensen G. LGBTQIA+ Cultural competence in physical therapy: an exploratory qualitative study from the clinicians' perspective. *Phys Ther.* 2024 Feb.;104(4): pzae010. doi: 10.1093/ptj/pzae010. https://academic.oup.com/ptj/article/104/4/pzae010/7596261?login=true

Matthews ND, Rowley KM, Dusing SC, Krause L, Yamaguchi N, Gordon J. Beyond a statement of support: changing the culture of equity, diversity, and inclusion in physical therapy. *Phys Ther.* 2021 Dec.;101(12): pzab212. doi: 10.1093/ptj/pzab212. https://academic.oup.com/ptj/article/101/12/pzab212/6362882?login=true

Ross MH, Hammond J, Bezner J, Brown D, Wright A, Chipchase L, Miciak M, Whittaker JL, Setchell J. An exploration of the experiences of physical therapists who identify as LGBTQIA+: navigating sexual orientation and gender identity in clinical, academic, and professional roles. *Phys Ther.* 2022 March;102(3): pzab280. doi: 10.1093/ptj/pzab280. https://academic.oup.com/ptj/article/102/3/pzab280/6478874?login=true

Snyder CR, Frogner BK, Skillman SM. Facilitating racial and ethnic diversity in the health workforce. *J Allied Health.* 2018 Spring;47(1):58–65. PMID: 29504021. https://pubmed.ncbi.nlm.nih.gov/29504021/

Stanford FC. The importance of diversity and inclusion in the healthcare workforce. *J Natl Med Assoc.* 2020;112(3):247-249. doi:10.1016/j.jnma.2020.03.014. https://pubmed.ncbi.nlm.nih.gov/32336480/

Twardzik E, Guralnik JM, Falvey JR. Community mobility among older adults who are socioeconomically disadvantaged: addressing the poverty penalty, *Phys Ther.* 2023: pzad182. https://doi.org/10.1093/ptj/pzad182

# SUGGESTED RESOURCES

**https://healthleadsusa.org/** Health Leads is an organization that provides resources for people, health systems, and clinics to address racial inequity. You can find tools and resources on this site to identify and address social determinants of health.

**https://kirwaninstitute.osu.edu/implicit-bias-module-series** Implicit Bias Module Series© (osu.edu) The Ohio State University, Kirwan Institute for the Study of Race and Ethnicity provides a five-module Implicit Bias Training opportunity from national expert leaders on implicit bias with numerous video-enhanced lessons within each module, followed by a certificate opportunity in response to 20 questions.

**https://psychology.unc.edu/justice-equity-diversity-inclusion-jedi-education-resources/** This toolkit has resources and can help you identify ways you can provide support to improve justice, equity, diversity, and inclusion (JEDI). This toolkit will give you guidance no matter where you are on your JEDI journey. The toolkit provides opportunities for action, reflection education, discussion, and practice.

**www.ptlearninginstitute.com** The Physical Therapy Learning Institute (PTLI) provides useful DEI resources and links for students and practitioners. PTLI also provides contemporary JEDI focused videos of the annual Lynda D. Woodruff, PT, PhD Lecture Series for review and discussion of national speakers Greg Hicks, PT, PhD, FAPTA (2020), Charlene Portee, PT, PhD, FAAPT (2021), and Lisa VanHoose, PT, PhD, MPH, FAPTA, FAAPT (2022) available on the following drop-down menu websites: www.ptlearninginstitute.com/lynda-d-woodruff

**www.racialequitytools.org/glossary** Review definitions and language that will help support you in your conversations on the topics of diversity, equity, and inclusion with the racial equity tools glossary.

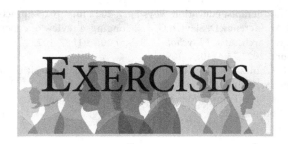

## EXERCISE 1: IDENTIFYING YOUR BIAS

Are you always truthful about the thoughts that come to mind? Sometimes we are not truthful because of embarrassment, or we are not willing to be truthful. Other times we are not honest, but we do not know that we are hiding the truth.

Self-work activity: Implicit Association Test (IAT) measures attitudes and beliefs that individuals may be unwilling or unable to report. This test can give an individual some insight into any unconscious bias they may have.

**Step 1**: Visit: https://implicit.harvard.edu/implicit/takeatest.html

**Step 2**: There are a variety of IAT tests that you can choose to take, pick two to four tests

**Step 3**: After taking those IAT tests, journal on your thoughts about the experience and answer the following questions

1.  How did the results make you feel?

2.  What is your perception of yourself after receiving your preference results?

3.  Do your results explain your preferences and actions that you take with individuals that identify with the options evaluated?

4.  How and why will this experience impact your future interactions?

# EXERCISE 2: INFLUENCES OF THE SOCIAL DETERMINANTS OF HEALTH

To further increase your understanding of the influences of the Social Determinants of Health, you are being asked to complete an online simulation of persons experiencing poverty for educational purposes only. In this online simulation of poverty, you are to survive on $1,000 a month, simulating the working, poor, single-parent family with an income between 100% and 133% of the Federal Poverty Level.[28] You are asked to make a series of decisions regarding how you may make ends meet in the simulation of life. Poverty impacts more than 15% of the U.S. population.[28] Through this simulation you will gain a better understanding of persons living in poverty and the challenges faced with respect to the Social Determinants of Health.

Please note you are *not* required to make a donation. Let's begin—complete the Poverty Simulation Game,[28] click on the *continue to spent* arrow via https://playspent.org

Post-completion of the simulation, please consider the following queries:

1.  How has this exercise changed your comfort level with interacting with persons experiencing poverty? Why?

2.  How has this exercise changed your attitudes about programs for those experiencing poverty?

3.  Compare how your attitudes about equal opportunity, basic health care rights, and having enough food to eat have been impacted because of your participation in the simulation?

4.  Discuss how the simulation made you feel and/or, if you have experienced or are experiencing poverty yourself, how you were impacted by the simulation.

# EXERCISE 3: DIVERSITY WITHIN YOUR NETWORK

**Self-work activity:** This exercise provides the opportunity for you to reflect on your individual identity, diversity in your social and professional groups, and goals for inclusion. Just as we define terms—let us define who you are:

**Step 1**: Write a *detailed* statement of how you identify, including your **elements of diversity** descriptors.

**Example:** *I am a Black cis gender woman, my pronouns are she/her/hers, I am a Christian, living in the Southeast U.S., with a doctorate degree.*

**Who you are? Diversity Elements Statement:**

**Step 2**: Describe the elements of diversity composition of your close social/professional group (the information that you know about your closest associates). Consider the following guiding questions in your response:

o   Is there homogeneity or heterogeneity of the people in your friend group to each other and/or yourself? Identify the need to increase the diversity within your social/professional group.

o   What elements of diversity are not represented in your social/professional group?

o   Is increasing diversity in your peer group something you are able and willing to do? Why/Why not?

o   What is your ability to deal with opposing opinions that can occur from diversifying your social/professional interactions?

o   Are there individual(s) in your social/professional group who have opposite views and opinions to yourself?

o   How do you facilitate conversation and resolve resolutions with this individual?

**Your Response—Peer Group Elements of JEDI and Ability to Impact:**

# EXERCISE 4: MAXIMIZE YOUR IMPACT

The awareness of elements of antiracism, belongingness, diversity, equity, and inclusion are not enough; change comes from developing a specific plan for positive change, in both your environment and communities of practice. Refer to Figures 7.1 and 7.2 to assess your environment based on the diversity elements (climate scan) for this exercise. Consider how the components of belongingness impact you.

Respond to the following stepwise queries:

**Step I: Describe how the four components of belongingness impact you:**

1. Competencies for belonging (skills and abilities)

2. Opportunities to belong (enablers, removal/reduction of barriers)

3. Motivations to belong (inner drive)

4. Perceptions of belonging (cognitions, attributions, and feedback mechanisms—positive or negative experiences when connecting)

**Step II: Environment Assessment—In what ways can your environment be more diverse?**

What are the barriers limiting inclusion?

What are the champions for inclusion?

**Step III: Goal Setting**—Create one goal that you will enthusiastically implement in your preferred future to improve your capacities and skills for JEDI, belongingness, antiracism and cultural humility within your environment and/or communities of practice. Write your goal utilizing the SMART (Specific, Measurable, Attainable, Realistic, Timely) format:

**Next:** Identify an accountability partner/individuals/organization to assist you until your goal is achieved.

**Step IV: Resource Identification**—After you have identified barriers and the goal you would like to work on, visit one or more of the following JEDI website resources, or other national website resources:

- https://healthleadsusa.org/
- https://psychology.unc.edu/justice-equity-diversity-inclusion-jedi-education-resources/
- https://clinicians.org/programs/justice-equity-diversity-inclusion/
- https://hsabc.org/node/11739

Identify three total resources that assist you in creating representation and justice and share what you have learned.

**Step V: Representation and Justice Plan**—Now that you have written a SMART goal and identified resources to assist you to meet your goal, what are three things that you are committed to doing? Share your three things in your plan with your accountability partner to see that change you desire and assure your own cultural humility in the process.

1.

2.

3.

Example:

- In the health care clinic where I am working, there are not many ethnic minority health care professionals who are treating an ethnically diverse patient population.
- The barriers limiting inclusion are some of the health care professionals do not take the time to build relationships with the patients that look different from them. The patients do not feel included in their plan of care and do not feel connected to their provider.
- A champion to inclusion is one of the health care professionals who has done their self-work and research and identified that they need to be more intentional with all their patients to build the patient–practitioner alliance and address previous trauma from experiences in health care to help improve their patients' outcomes.
- My SMART Goal: I will commit to researching different topics related to justice and belonging found in the JEDI resources and present to my colleagues in two months. I will ask my supervisor to be my accountability partner to make sure I accomplish this goal.

I want to encourage more of the practitioners to join this journey with me, so we can work on increasing a sense of belonging in the clinic. Once the barriers were brought to the attention of the practitioners at the clinic, they committed to alternating topics for monthly in-services for the next year to discuss the resources found in the JEDI Toolkit (Begin, Reflect, Do, Act, Educate, and Discuss) for things we can all do with our patients for better outcomes and patient–practitioner alliance. I will use self and peer assessment, using the belongingness competencies to address my capacities; along with using the Jacobs queries for cultural humility pre-, during, and post-patient encounters, to assure my cultural humility for myself and my patients.

# EXERCISE 5: UPSTANDER ACTIVITY

"**How will you respond?**" Please review the three discriminatory scenarios. Think about what you would do if you were the person being discriminated against and what you would do if you observed this interaction. Use **ACTION**[19] elements to help you practice how you can be an upstander for someone being victimized and to guide you in proceeding with your response, as follows:

- **A**sk clarifying questions
- **C**ome from curiosity, not judgment
- **T**ell what you observed in a factual manner
- **I**mpact exploration—discuss the impact of the statement
- **O**wn your own thoughts and feelings around the situation
- Consider the **N**ext steps

When you encounter someone being victimized, always check in with them to make sure they are safe and ask if they want you to speak up on their behalf. It is okay if ACTION is not implemented immediately. With practice, you will have the words and strategies needed when you need to address discrimination.

## *Step 1*

**Read the scenarios below, then formulate your ACTION elements individually before moving on to Step 2.**

**Scenario A:** A patient hears a racist comment from a provider. The patient arrived less than 10 minutes late due to a terrible accident on the way to their appointment. The provider is overheard saying they do not believe that story because people of the same race as the patient are always late.

**ACTION:**

**Scenario B:** While a student is providing care for their patient, they are approached by another health care provider who tells them their accent is a problem, which is why their patients cannot understand them and do not want to work with them.

**ACTION:**

**Scenario C:** During a treatment session, a patient is sharing with others in the clinic space a homophobic joke; many individuals, patients, and practitioners become visibly uncomfortable.

**ACTION:**

**Scenario D:** You are a student on your clinical/fieldwork experience in a faith-based hospital institution. You and your clinical faculty member enter the patient's hospital room and you begin to introduce yourselves to the patient. The patient asks you, the student, directly "Are you one of us?" referring to the predominant religion of the hospital.

**ACTION:**

## Step 2

Now, share your exercise responses with a partner and see if you have new insight into how you can address these scenarios. Take turns practicing talking out the six elements of ACTION for each scenario. With practice, your skills will improve. Provide feedback to each other on your ACTION efforts.

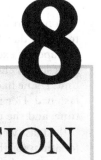

# EFFECTIVE COMMUNICATION

## PROBLEM IDENTIFICATION AND HELPFUL RESPONSES

*Gina Maria Musolino and Carol M. Davis*

## OBJECTIVES

*The learner should be able to:*

- Construct communication strategies for interactions that are confused and/or emotion laden.
- Examine one's own congruence or lack of congruence.
- Deliver effective, therapeutic communication with challenging patient practitioner vignettes.
- Critique therapeutic presence and communication utilizing the *PPI* checklist.
- Justify the importance of thoughts and feelings in communication.
- Compare the risks and rewards of communicating clearly in the presence of intense feelings.

Very often, the bulk of our communication throughout the day is quite superficial. Rarely do we communicate with the express purpose of trying to understand in order to be helpful. Even when we make a greater-than-usual attempt to listen carefully because we care and are concerned, it is rare that our interaction might be said to be truly helpful. **Therapeutic communication requires learning a new skill, but more than that, it requires unlearning habitual, nonhelpful ways of interacting.**

Building upon prior chapter learnings, this chapter provides opportunities for the skill development components so vital for effective patient–practitioner interaction (PPI). This chapter is devoted to teaching therapeutic methods of communicating with the express purpose of developing your abilities to use communication as an integral aspect of your therapeutic presence with patients and clients. The remaining chapters are problem oriented and will help you apply skill-based solutions with particularly demanding situations, not uncommon in health care. Let's begin with a case example.

DOI: 10.4324/9781003525554-8

Jonathan was enjoying the seventh month of his first position as a physical therapist in a rehabilitation center. Each day, he was experiencing more confidence in his skills in evaluation and treatment, especially using therapeutic exercise for patients with spinal cord and brain injury. One of his favorite patients was a 14-year-old high school cheerleader, who had been referred to him two months ago while still in a coma in the intensive care unit. Diane had gone through the front windshield of her mother's car, a consequence of not having her seatbelt fastened. Her mother escaped injury but was feeling tremendous guilt. She and Diane had been arguing at the time, and she mistakenly ran a stoplight that resulted in the accident.

Just last week, Diane began to respond to light and sound, and yesterday, she opened her eyes and looked at Jonathan for the first time after he had transferred her to a chair at the bedside. He was feeling elated and was very hopeful that soon she would be responding to verbal commands.

Diane's mother, Ms. Graham, visited every day and often was present while Jonathan treated Diane. Today, Ms. Graham seemed particularly discouraged. Although Diane was showing obvious signs of recovery from her coma, she was still unable to move. When Jonathan came to treat Diane, Ms. Graham left the room but returned as he finished and told him she wanted to speak to him. As they walked out into the hallway, Ms. Graham turned to Jonathan and shouted, "You're not helping her! No one is helping her recover. I asked around and found out you're a new therapist and you can't know what you're doing, or my daughter would have been well long before this! I want you to stop seeing her. I want a therapist with experience to treat my daughter. I never want you to set foot in her room again!"

This is an example of an emotion-laden interaction, similar to many that take place daily in hospitals and health care facilities. If you were Jonathan, how would you have responded? What would you have felt? Would you have quickly defended yourself? Would you have argued that Diane was showing remarkable signs of improvement? Would you have shouted, "Nobody speaks to me like that!"?

When people are ill and injured, emotions run high on the part of the ill, their families, and those caring for them. Illness and injury stir up feelings of vulnerability and fear. People generally feel out of control and must give over control of their lives to strangers, often in institutions that seem like strange, impersonal, frightening cultures all their own. This aspect of people "giving over control" for their loved ones needing health care was exponentially heightened when Covid-19 pandemic restrictions often led to complete isolation from ill patients in many health care settings.

At the root of every emotion-laden interaction is a problem. **What, exactly, is the problem in this situation, and whose problem is it?** Ms. Graham would say that the problem is that her daughter is being treated by an inexperienced physical therapist and is not recovering because of this fact. Therefore, Jonathan and his inexperience are the problem. Jonathan might say that the problem is that Ms. Graham is feeling helpless and responsible for her daughter's pain and injury and lashed out at him in her frustration. Another analysis might offer that the problem is that Diane did not have her seatbelt on and, if she had, she would not be in a coma. **Again, oftentimes sources of all conflicts are missed expectations. Effective communication provides the opportunity for clarity of expectations.**

# THE IMPORTANCE OF IDENTIFYING THE PROBLEM UNDER THE EMOTION

Now we are going to focus on identifying problems and clarifying problem ownership in interchanges that are characterized by intense emotions. Amid an interchange like the one between Jonathan and Ms. Graham, it is often difficult to sort out what is happening and what might be appropriate responses to help resolve the situation. Our reflex response is to defend ourselves from attack, which tends to just heighten the emotion and further obscure the problem. As a health care professional (HCP), one of the new attitudes that will be helpful to learn is that it is often not the most important thing to be right in a situation. Solving the problem, separate from assigning blame or assigning who is right and wrong, becomes critically important. Different skills are required depending on the nature of the problem and who "owns" the problem.

Hence, the theme for helpful responses in effective communication is the following: **Communicating in ways that help to solve problems, while at the same time respecting and honoring human beings, will facilitate the healing**

**process**. Because we collaborate with people who are ill and disabled, it is not enough to make the correct diagnosis and give the most appropriate treatment. Something more is expected of us. That something more includes helping the patient understand their illness or disability to the extent that patients and clients can make choices with regard to treatment and modifying lifestyle, to prevent further problems, and to live successfully with the problems that are not going to be resolved.

# LEARNING NEW COMMUNICATION SKILLS

Each of us enters the helping professions having communicated all our lives. Little patient care experience is needed to quickly learn that the communication skills that served us quite adequately in our private lives often fall short of helping us to relate adequately to patients, families, caregivers, and colleagues in day-to-day patient care. As Dr. Eric Cassell[1] wrote in his book, *Talking With Patients*, without effective communication, we are unable to acquire objective and subjective information in order to make decisions that are in the best interests of the patient, and, more important, we are unable to use the relationship between HCP and patient for therapeutic ends. Communication is even further challenged when utilizing the barriers of personal protective equipment (PPE) for safety and infection control, which is often necessary in health care settings, especially and in times of pandemics/endemics. Keep this in mind as we consider effective methods for communication. This chapter focuses on sorting out emotion-laden communication to help patients identify and solve their own problems. Chapter 9 extends this theme in teaching you the skills of assertiveness, and Chapter 14 instructs you in conducting a helping interview.

# EMOTION-LADEN INTERCHANGES

Communication connects us to the world. Humans are essentially social and need to feel a connection to others. Getting our basic needs met, more often than not, requires some form of communication.

Barriers to the effectiveness of communication might include the use of a foreign language (or the use of jargon), carelessness in choosing the words that convey exact meaning, and/or an inability or unwillingness to listen to each other carefully (e.g., hearing deficit, distraction by environmental noise, masks and other PPE interfering or blocking normal body language and speech sounds, unwillingness to concentrate, multitasking, defensiveness, etc.). Many of us are rather unaware of how effective (or ineffective) we are in day-to-day communication. It is difficult to come outside of ourselves and watch ourselves interact with others, reflecting on our feelings and the way in which we react to others.

Some of us have been given direct feedback about our communication. Statements such as, "I appreciate the way you listen so intently to what I say and wait until I'm finished before you respond" vs. "I wish you would hear me out instead of mentally practicing a quick comeback!" give us clear information about how we are doing as we communicate in that moment.

Social media has encouraged video communication, yet much of it has been a one-way display, rather than interactive with others. In addition, in many instances social media has encouraged quick retorts or tweets, with escalating taunts, rather than reflective, active communication and meaningful dialogue. Limited attention spans and word capacities, along with lack of respect for justice, equity, diversity, and inclusion (JEDI), as discussed in Chapter 7, have further reduced meaningful messaging and effective communication on many platforms.

# DIFFICULTIES INTRODUCED WITH TEXTING, SOCIAL MEDIA, AND DIGITAL TECHNOLOGIES

The fundamentals of communication consist of a sender, a message, a receiver, and an environment. In an emotion-laden interchange, the message is obscured by the fact that someone is upset and unable to identify clearly what the heart of the problem is and how to best go about solving the problem. Communication is difficult enough when the conversation is face to face or by phone. The introduction of email, texting, and other means of communication through social media platforms and digital technologies presents an entirely new set of considerations and problems.[2]

It was 8:00 a.m. Jason was waiting for his patient to arrive and decided to check his emails on his phone in the staff room. At 8:05 a.m., his patient arrived, and the receptionist announced this to him, but it was 8:15 a.m. before he came out to greet his patient, who was quite upset for having to wait for 10 minutes and told him so in front of his clinical instructor.

Jason bit his tongue and apologized. Later, when he opened his emails at home, he found a note from his clinical instructor telling him that he needed to be more prompt in greeting his patients. Jason was furious. He fired off a response to his clinical instructor indicating that he was waiting for his patient to arrive at 8:00 a.m., and when he was not yet there by 8:05 a.m., he went back to the staff room for just a minute or so to check his emails.

Furthermore, Jason wrote, he resented his clinical instructor calling him on this and not giving him the benefit of the doubt when she herself checked her emails several times each day. He took this opportunity to also write that he resented her picking on him and felt that because he was not a student from the school from which she had graduated, he could do nothing right.

Suffice it to say that had that exchange occurred in person, rather than via email or text, it would likely have been different. Up to 75% of communication is conveyed nonverbally, and when you take away all the nonverbals (see Chapters 12 and 20) and have only the written word, there is a lot of room for miscommunication. Likewise, "speaking" (i.e., texting, via gaming) on a device allows one to not have to pay attention to how one's words are being received; and meanings can be misunderstood, blown out of proportion, or taken out of context. Improved technologies with visual platforms (Zoom, MSTeams, FaceTime) with some limited visual complements do help some with electronic communications, yet are still not the same as face to face (F2F), as with physical, first-hand interaction. Initially, the use of telehealth was more out of access necessity prior to the Covid-19 pandemic but became a primary method during the height of pandemic restrictions. Today, telehealth is becoming more of a viable alternative based upon convenience, preferences, or necessity.

No matter the means of communication, effective communication remains requisite for HCPs' successful communication. For example, in a qualitative study[3] exploring how stakeholders (physical therapists, telephone coaches, and patients) experienced, and made sense of, being involved in an integrated program of physical therapist–supervised exercise and telephone coaching for people with knee osteoarthritis, the necessity for effective communication was re-iterated as needing to be patient-centered, collaborative, and consistent; even though different views were expressed about the preferred medium of communication (including F2F, email, and via the Web-based protocol).[3]

Once again, as mentioned in prior chapters, we will address additional considerations of telehealth more in Chapter 20. Yet for now keep technology-based formats of communication in mind as you consider the elements of effective communication in this chapter. Growing up digitally you may be more comfortable interacting in digital formats, rather than F2F; your patients/clients may or may not be digitally savvy. The exercises in this chapter will assist you in practicing effective F2F interactions for emotion-laden communication. If this is not your typical form of communication, you may wish to repeat practice with others outside of the classroom opportunities, remembering, in preparation for effective communication, to **practice therapeutic presence**, as you learned in Chapter 6.

What is most important now is that you realize that the luxury of simply spontaneously reacting to others, in digital formats, which you experienced as a private citizen before you made a commitment to becoming a HCP, must now be replaced by a commitment to use effective, emotion-laden communication (even when you feel personally attacked) as an opportunity to practice your therapeutic effectiveness. Furthermore, as you become a HCP and think about your future career, you may want to rethink your social media activities and digital presentation. We shall discuss this more in Chapter 12.

# LESS-THAN-HELPFUL RESPONSES

The most unhelpful response is indifference. To fail to listen is indicative of an inability, or unwillingness, to be therapeutically present to the one in need of help. Next would be anger or defensiveness, which can soon escalate emotion to rage, which further buries the original problem (see Chapter 9, Figures 9.4 and 9.5). Other less-than-helpful techniques include the following:[4]

- **Offering reassurances**. Statements such as "Oh, it can't be all that bad" or "If you think you have it bad, you should just look around you" do little but signal an unwillingness to listen to patients' perceptions of their problems. At the heart of this reply is a HCP who is not aware of their own feelings about the topic or who pretends to offer more time and attention than there is to give and is trying to get away as rapidly as possible.

- **Offering judgmental responses**. Judgmental responses include those that convey approval or disapproval, verbally or nonverbally, at an inappropriate moment; those that convey advice at a time when it is more important for the patient to make their own decision; and those that are stereotypical: "Adults should know better than to act like children."
- **Defensiveness**. When we feel threat to the ego, we respond defensively. Defensiveness indicates a personalization and a refusal to listen carefully to what the patient is saying. A response such as "You're always late. I've got better things to do than wait for you, you know" may be true but does little to solve the patient's tardiness problem.

# Values That Underlie Therapeutic Responses

Nonhelpful responses are often impulsive and reactive and do not reflect value-based behavior. The values that underlie therapeutic responses were described in Chapter 3. Attitudes such as caring, warmth, respect, compassion, and empathy will help interrupt an immature, impulsive response to an emotion-laden communication.

Acceptance of the other person as doing the best that they can in the moment and acceptance of the responsibility to be therapeutic in the midst of a chaotic situation are signs of a mature HCP. These responses emanate from the essential self, not the ego or persona. Remember, the goal of rehabilitation is to help the patient regain control over their life such that independent function at the highest and deepest levels is restored. The role of the HCP in emotion-laden communication is to ascertain **what the problem is, as well as whose problem it is.**

# Identifying Problem Ownership

Learning to send clear messages and receive accurate messages in intense situations requires identifying who owns the problem.[5] Different skills are required for each. For the sake of learning this skill, the rule that applies in every case is that **the person exhibiting the intense emotion is the owner of the problem, even if they are trying desperately to inform you that the problem is really yours.**

For example, if the patient is upset with you for being late and shouts at you as you enter the clinic, "You're late!", you do not have a problem. You just walked into the clinic. The patient who is upset has a problem, even though they might be trying to convince you that you are their problem.

In this new process that you are learning—identifying problem ownership—the person with the emotion owns the problem. The first step to resolving the issue is to realize the different skills required depending on who owns the problem. Figure 8.1 illustrates the two sets of skills required: active listening and "I" statements.

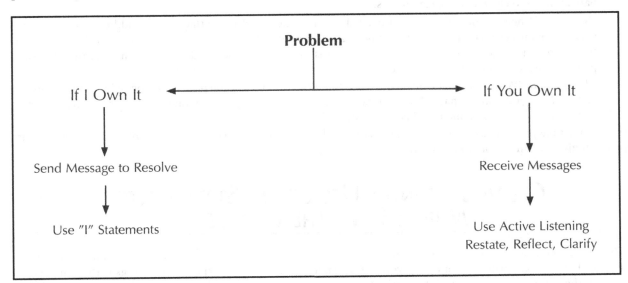

**Figure 8.1** Identifying problem ownership.

Emotion-laden exchanges are cluttered with intense feelings, derogatory remarks, apologies, illustrations, etc. To sort out the problem, special listening skills are needed to defuse the emotion and get at the problem. Critical to this method is resistance to the desire for the unhelpful response of wanting to fix it right away to get rid of the anger or conflict. The alternative is to listen by resisting the quick advice or the defensive reply ("pause for the cause").

## ACTIVE LISTENING—WHEN THE OTHER HAS THE PROBLEM

*Active listening* is a form of therapeutic listening that helps the agitated person with the problem clearly hear what they are trying to say. It involves **paraphrasing the speaker's words rather than reacting to them to clarify if you have caught the intended meaning**. You must suspend your thoughts and attend exclusively to the words of the other person. Paraphrasing is not easy and requires development as a new skill. In a sense, it requires self-transposal, where you work to put yourself in the other person's shoes, to understand rather than judge or defend against. For some, it will require significant effort to resist responding with a suggestion of what to do because the desire to fix it for others is so habitual.

Active listening is made up of three different processes:[5]

1.  **Restatement:** Repeating the words of the speaker as you have heard them.

    *Example*: "I get so frustrated that I never have a day free from my back pain."

    *Restatement*: "You're frustrated because the back pain never leaves you?"

    Restatement can be annoying if not timed appropriately. When done well, it assures the patient that you have indeed heard the content of what they are saying. The main purpose of restatement is to help the person continue speaking and should only be used in the initial phases of active listening. Once you have reassured the patient that you are hearing their words, reflection and clarification become more useful responses.

2.  **Reflection:** Verbalizing the content and the implied feelings of the sender.

    *Example*: "This pain has been going on for months. I just can't go on any longer."

    *Reflection*: "You're exhausted and feeling defeated from the constant pain?"

    The purpose of reflection is to express in words the feelings and attitudes sensed behind the words of the sender. This aspect of listening indicates you're hearing more than just the words; you're hearing the emotion behind them. Sometimes we guess incorrectly, but this gives the sender the chance to clarify for us and for themselves exactly what they are feeling. Awareness of feelings is critical to identifying the real problem. When the listener wants to help the sender to examine more extensively both thoughts and feelings, or to focus thoughts and feelings, clarification is used.

3.  **Clarification:** Summarizing or simplifying the sender's thoughts and feelings and resolving confused verbalizations into clear, concise statements.

    *Example*: "When the doctor told me I needed physical therapy, I knew that you would be the person who would help me get rid of my pain. But it's been 2 weeks now and the pain just keeps coming back. I am afraid that I'll have this pain forever. I'm not sure what it is that I'm supposed to do. Do I just have to live with this pain, or will somebody please help me?"

    *Clarification*: "When you first came to physical therapy, you thought the pain would be relieved more immediately. Now you realize that ridding yourself of the pain is going to take longer than you expected and is more than a matter of somebody just fixing it?"

These skills take practice, as does resisting the answer that tends toward fixing it. The exercises at the end of the chapter will give you an opportunity to practice.

## CLEAR SENDING—USE OF "I" STATEMENTS WHEN I OWN THE PROBLEM

When I feel the emotion and want to communicate to another person that I am upset, clear communication is facilitated when I am congruent. That is, my words clearly match my feelings. I express my feelings with "I" messages rather than the commonly used editorial "they," "you," or "everyone." First, let's look at congruence.

## *Congruence*

*Congruence* is a term that indicates that the words and the music match. Congruence is present **when what I say matches what I do and what I feel**.[5] Incongruence appears ingenuine and dishonest and does not ring true. How often have we been caught in incongruence when someone asks for a compliment: "Well, do you like my new haircut or not?" "Yes, it's okay I guess." What was felt was less than okay, but no one likes to appear rude. When a person is congruent, they appear open, honest, genuine, and authentic. Nonverbal cues and tone of voice are consistent with the words spoken.

Congruence requires reflection. Before speaking, you must realize feelings and thoughts and reconcile such pulls as not wanting to be hurtful yet wanting to be honest. A congruent response to the requested compliment might be: "You know, I noticed you had a new haircut, but I believe I liked it better the old way." With this response, the person realizes that you value honesty and are willing to be honest and can avoid being rude. The message rings true, and you feel better. More important, the person knows you will resist responses aimed at trying to please others.

Congruence is best conveyed when it is communicated with sensitivity and thought. Congruent communication should never be used as a rationalization for insensitive and rude honesty.

## *"I" Messages*

*"I" messages* are necessary when you feel emotion, you own the problem, and you want to get the problem solved. Our tendency is to blame when we feel uncomfortable. An example might be, "You always leave the dirty dishes in the sink! I'm getting sick and tired of cleaning up after you."

What is the problem, and whose problem is it?

Well, I'm upset, so the problem is mine and requires a clearer message than that if I want to get it solved in a helpful way. Using an "I" message is the way I would proceed: "I'm feeling very frustrated. This is the third night in a row that I've found dirty dishes in the sink, and I'm tired of doing them for you. Let's talk about this."

With "I" messages, I clearly own my frustration. Then, it's up to the other person to respond, hopefully with concern, perhaps even with active listening. Please note, however, that **use of an "I" statement does not guarantee that the other person will respond in a helpful way. What it does guarantee is that your own feelings will be expressed, and you will take responsibility for your being upset, rather than blaming someone else.** Another person might never get upset over dirty dishes in the sink!

Using "I" statements involves taking a risk: I speak in the first person, and I own my feelings rather than ignore, disclaim, or minimize them. It takes reflective thought to decide what it is that I'm feeling and how it is I can express that. Sending "I" messages tells the other person that you are owning your upset and that you and they are each worthy and capable of solving this problem with appropriate, clear, respectful discussion. The exercises at the end of the chapter will help you practice this important skill.

Remember Jason in the earlier example. Emails are never an effective way to communicate any sort of emotion (emojis are insufficient and can be misinterpreted too!) so I would recommend that Jason respond to his clinical instructor with a neutral message: "I understand that you are disappointed in my behavior. I would like to make an appointment to discuss this with you before we start tomorrow morning, say about 7:45 a.m.? Will that work for you?"

Jason needs to own his frustration, F2F, and hopefully his clinical instructor will use active listening skills to respond. In the interim, he may conclude that his clinical instructor had every right to mention his lateness to him: "I feel frustrated that I was late with my patient because I got distracted with my emails when the patient did not arrive on time at 8:00 a.m. I apologize and will work to not let it happen again. But I must also comment that my frustration is in part due to my perception that I feel I may be being singled out by you. Is that the case?"

# CONCLUSION

Communication that is helpful resists the need to impulsively respond, become defensive, or offer quick advice or a quick solution to a problem. Instead, therapeutic communication strives to clarify the problem and assist the person with the problem to solve it for themselves. When we were children, we needed adults to "fix it" for us, to put a bandage on our bruised knees or our bruised egos. As mature health HCPs, we must unlearn the natural tendency to help by giving advice. We must respect and value the communication process as one more tool in our repertoire of therapeutic responses, where we help the other person help themself, "facilitating opportunities for the other person to express their own reasons for change (change talk)".[6] As Singh et al.[6] reiterated: "Communication within a *patient-centered* framework aims to change the power dynamic from one in which health care providers instruct patients to one in which health care providers and patients share information and *engage collaboratively* in decision-making" (our emphasis).

Let's return to the case example at the beginning of the chapter. Jonathan and Ms. Graham are standing in the hallway outside Diane's room, and Ms. Graham has just let Jonathan have it. What is the problem and whose problem is it?

Clearly, it is Ms. Graham's problem. Jonathan has practiced his effective therapeutic communication skills and, instead of defending himself, he responds with, "Ms. Graham, you are obviously upset and frustrated at the apparent lack of progress on Diane's part, and you believe that is due to my inexperience."

Ms. Graham says yes and goes on for another few minutes while Jonathan keeps up with her with active listening responses. Soon she calms down and, feeling really listened to, she looks at Jonathan and admits that the real problem is that she feels that this is all her fault, and she feels so helpless. Jonathan explores with Ms. Graham. Jonathan discusses what he believes her choices and opportunities for support are in dealing with the guilt that she feels. Jonathan then then offers to include Ms. Graham in the therapy sessions to a greater extent so that she can provide minor aspects of treatment in the evenings. Ms. Graham shakes his hand, thanks him, and agrees to see a counselor to work on her feelings of guilt.

Not all communications will end this amicably, but the majority will end far less amicably if the HCP responds impulsively or simply reacts. Therapeutic communication is the most useful way to ensure a helping response to emotion-laden communication. Managing one's stress, as discussed in Chapter 5, will assist you as a HCP in being able to effectively provide best practice with therapeutic communications as you collaborate with your patients/clients and their families, significant others, friends, and/or caregivers.

# REFERENCES

1.  Cassell EJ. *Talking With Patients: Vol 1. The Theory of Doctor-Patient Communication*. Cambridge, MA: MIT Press; 1985.
2.  Goleman D. Email is easy to write (and to misread). *New York Times*. October 7, 2007.
3.  Hinman RS, Delany CM, Campbell PK, Gale J, Bennell KL. Physical therapists, telephone coaches, and patients with knee osteoarthritis: qualitative study about working together to promote exercise adherence. *Phys Ther*. 2016;96(4): 479–483. doi: 10.2522/ptj.20150260.
4.  Berman A, Snyder S, Frandsen G. *Koizer & Erb Fundamentals of Nursing: Concepts and Procedures*, 11th ed. Boston, MA: Pearson; 2021.
5.  Munson PJ, Johnson RB. *Humanizing Instruction, Or Helping Your Students Up the Up Staircase*. Chapel Hill, NC: Johnson Self-Instructional Package; 1972.
6.  Singh S, Orlando JM, Alghamdi ZS, Franklin KA, Lobo MA. Reframing clinical paradigms: strategies for improving patient care relationships. *Phys Ther*. 2021;101(7): pzab095. doi: 10.1093/ptj/pzab095.

# SUGGESTED READINGS

Clancy C. *Critical Conversations in Healthcare Scripts & Techniques for Effective Interprofessional & Patient Communication*. Indianapolis, IN: Sigma Theta Tau International; 2014.

Crisp DH. *Anatomy of Medical Errors: The Patient in Room 2*. Indianapolis, IN: Sigma Theta Tau International; 2016.

Scholl I, Zill JM, Härter M, Dirmaier J. An integrative model of patient-centeredness—a systematic review and concept analysis. *PLoS One*. 2014;9(9):e107828. doi: 10.1371/journal.pone.0107828. PMID: 25229640; PMCID: PMC4168256.

Singh S, Orlando JM, Alghamdi ZS, Franklin KA, Lobo MA. Reframing clinical paradigms: strategies for improving patient care relationships. *Phys Ther*. 2021;101(7): pzab095. https://academic.oup.com/ptj/article/101/7/pzab095/6178887.

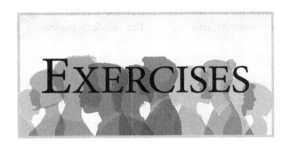

# EXERCISE 1: CURRENT PATTERNS

1.  Think of a recent situation in which you felt emotionally upset or frustrated. Describe the situation briefly.

2.  Whose problem was it? If you were upset, it was your problem. How did you communicate? Did you communicate at all, or did you swallow it and hope it would go away or at least change so that it was no longer a problem?

3.  What did you communicate, exactly?

4.  How would you change that now, using "I" statements or active listening? Do you think the outcome would have changed if you had used "I" messages or active listening?

5.  Write an "I" statement designed to communicate you're upset.

# EXERCISE 2: ACTIVE LISTENING AND "I" MESSAGES

Active listening involves restatement (of the words of the sender), reflection (of the words and underlying feelings of the sender), and clarification (summarizes and focuses the sender's message). Practice writing all three types of responses.

- *Restatement*
- *Reflection*
- *Clarification*

## Restatement

| SENDER | RESPONSE FROM YOU |
|---|---|
| I'm very worried about my shortness of breath. | You are worried about your shortness of breath? |
| I used to be able to jog for a whole hour, but now my joints start to ache. | |
| I wish I could swim for 100 laps without getting so tired. | |

## Reflection

| SENDER | RESPONSE FROM YOU |
|---|---|
| This pain has been going on for months now. I just wish someone would fix it for me or someone would help. | Your pain just drags on and you wish to relieve it. Perhaps you are concerned that it will never go away? |
| Yesterday was a good day, but today I feel the same old way. | |
| It's hard remembering to do my exercises. | |
| I want to get better, but it's hard. | |

## Clarification

| SENDER | RESPONSE FROM YOU |
|---|---|
| I wish someone would tell me what's going on with my knees. When I get up in the morning they're fine, but by noon they're swollen and feel tired. I'm too young to be suffering with joint problems. Is this arthritis or what? Do I have to live with this forever? | You're worried that your knee problem might be arthritis, and that you'll never be rid of it? |
| So, when the chiropractor told me I had a curved spine and I had to keep coming back for more adjustments every day, I felt that surely there must be something I could do for myself. I got a little frustrated by having so little to do to help myself. | |
| I almost didn't make it here. I got a horrible headache as I was driving here. The traffic is so stressful in this city. Will it ever end? New cars every day on the road. I don't know if I can keep up driving with these headaches. Is there anything you can do for me? | |

Now, read each situation and the "you" message (blaming response) and then write an "I" message in the third column.

| SITUATION | "YOU" MESSAGE | "I" MESSAGE |
|---|---|---|
| The aide has neglected to clean the whirlpool for 3 days in a row. | What's the matter with you? Are you getting lazy or what? | I'm confused and frustrated. For three days the whirlpool hasn't been cleaned. What's the problem? |
| Your patient has arrived late and set your schedule back by a half-hour all day. | You're late again! Now I'm going to be a half-hour behind for the last three treatment sessions. | |
| The patient seems depressed and has been reluctant to speak up for several days. | You're so quiet lately. Did I do something to make you mad? | |

# EXERCISE 3: PATIENT—PRACTITIONER INTERACTIONS

A series of vignettes follows, and as notable in the quote by Benjamin Franklin, you will now have the opportunity to practice your PPI skills for your enhanced learning.

> *Tell me and I'll forget. Show me and I may remember. Involve me and I may learn.* —Benjamin Franklin

In fact, you may find that repeating the vignettes, playing different roles, further develops your PPI skills.

Now, divide into groups of three, where one person is the HCP, one is the patient, and one is the observer.

Role-play the first vignette for 5 minutes or so or until an appropriate place to stop occurs. The observer should have in hand a copy of the **PPI Checklist** (located at the end of the exercise vignettes). At the conclusion of the vignette, the observer asks the patient how they are feeling and then asks the HCP the same question. The observer then gives the HCP feedback, as recorded on the checklist. At the end of the first round (approximately 15 minutes), remain in the same group of three but exchange roles and repeat the same vignette. After all three of you have role-played the HCP, discuss the experience among yourselves. Take a risk and give each other helpful feedback, areas to improve, and areas not in need of improvement (strengths), both negative and positive, about your communication skills. Do not shy away from constructive feedback. The gift of constructive feedback assists in your continued professional formation as an effective, therapeutic communicator.

Journal about the experience, focusing on what it felt like to be the HCP, the patient, and the observer giving constructive feedback to a classmate or colleague.

## *Vignettes*

Each person playing a role should see the description for that role only. Read the brief description and then act out the part as you would if it were happening to you. These vignettes are written for the role of physical therapist, but feel free to alter the descriptions to make them more applicable to the role that you are preparing for in your education if it is not physical therapy.

### VIGNETTE 1

#### *Physical Therapist*

You've been working with this patient, who uses a wheelchair, for 4 months. The past 3 weeks, the two of you have focused on the patient's discharge home. The patient seems pleased to be returning home but also anxious. You notice lately that the patient is short tempered and cuts people off who try to help. You hate conflict and want to avoid it at all costs.

#### *Patient*

You must use a wheelchair to get about and have been working in physical therapy for 4 months with the same therapist. The past 3 weeks, the two of you have focused on your discharge home. You've begun to be very anxious about separating from the rehabilitation center and are experiencing intermittent episodes of chest pain. You're afraid to tell anyone about this because you fear that they will discount your symptoms and label you as overly dependent, and you're actually afraid that they might be right. You're exhausted because you haven't slept more than 1 or 2 hours for the past 3 nights. You decide to confide your fears in your physical therapist, but you're feeling exhausted and defensive. You decide to just blurt it all out and hope that your therapist will understand.

### VIGNETTE 2

#### *Physical Therapist*

You are the therapist for a program for children with cerebral palsy. One mother brings her child three times a week to your center and stays and watches you treat her daughter along with the other children. This child is Black, and children of several races and ethnicities are represented at the center. You are White. This center is the only place where children with cerebral palsy can get treatment in this small town.

#### *Patient's Mother*

You are the mother of a child with cerebral palsy. You bring your child to physical therapy at the rehabilitation center in your small town three times each week and wait while she receives treatment. You notice that the physical therapist seems to spend less time with your daughter than she spends with two other children. You are Black and the others are White, as is the physical therapist. You've decided to confront the therapist with your suspicions. You're angry and hurt, but you fear that if you say the wrong thing, your daughter will be treated even less than before. This is the only center in town that offers treatment for your child. This is not the first time you've felt that you and your family were being discriminated against because of your race.

## VIGNETTE 3

### Physical Therapist

Your patient, who is 20 years old, had minor knee surgery 2 days ago and is still complaining of pain. He keeps his knee elevated with ice, hates to do exercises, screams with pain, and uses his crutches only with assistance and only to go to the bathroom. The surgeon is anxious to discharge the patient home, but you're convinced that he is not ready and will surely fall. He has ten stairs to climb just to get from the sidewalk to the front door of his house. You're subconsciously afraid that your lack of experience in caring for patients with knee surgery has contributed to his poor postoperative adjustment, so you're feeling guilty.

### Patient

You just had knee surgery 2 days ago and are experiencing a lot of postoperative pain. You're protecting your knee, keeping it very still so it will heal faster and hurt less. Your physical therapist seems to think you should be discharged home today and is frustrated with your oversensitivity to the pain. You've never had surgery before, and no one really prepared you for this experience. You're afraid you'll be discharged suddenly, and you feel very shaky with your crutches. You have no idea how you'll climb up the 10 steps to your front porch, let alone the 15 to your bedroom. You're upset with yourself for being afraid, you hurt, and you're fearful of being thrown out in the cold with no help. You decide to talk to your therapist before physical therapy today. You feel angry at her for putting you in this position.

## VIGNETTE 4

### Physical Therapist

You are with a private practice assigned to cover the patient care needs at a nursing home and, although you love the patients and enjoy the interaction with them, you realize that much of their functional activity must be supervised by the nursing staff when you are not there. The nurses love the patients also, but they are understaffed. They are constantly asking you to help them with nursing functions while you are doing therapy, and you cooperate but are becoming increasingly frustrated. You decide to talk to the head nurse about this after you discuss one of your patients who needs to be ambulated three times a shift to build endurance. You approach the nurse as she is making out her daily census report.

### Nurse

You are in charge of a unit of elderly patients, and you are understaffed. The administrator has been criticizing you for inefficiency, and you feel that she is being unrealistic in her demands on you. Secretly, you fear that if one more thing goes wrong, you are likely to lose your job. The physical therapist has asked to see you, and you are angry at her because she seems to make more work for your nurses so that their nursing tasks do not get completed. The physical therapist is always asking the nurses to dangle patients to help ambulate them; you think they should hire another therapist and let your nurses do nursing care.

## VIGNETTE 5

### Physical Therapist

You are working with a football player who is the star quarterback of his college team. He has had a tear of his adductor tendon in his right leg and is receiving physical therapy so that he can heal quickly and return to playing. You have a lot of pressure on you to help him return to the game as soon as possible, and so he has been assigned to rehab 2 hours in the morning and 2 hours each afternoon after his classes. He is an extremely popular person on Twitter, and each time you try to collaborate with him, he delays his treatment several times so that he can tweet his fans.

*Patient—Star Football Player*

You are recovering from a groin injury sustained during a football game and are assigned to come to rehab 4 hours a day—2 hours in the morning and 2 hours after classes in the afternoon. You are so bummed about not being able to play, and you are afraid that your fans will abandon you and forget about you, so your one hope is to hold onto them by Tweeting a moment-by-moment description of what rehab for a groin injury is like. It is especially important for you to be able to maintain their attention so that you can count on their support when you return to playing.

## Patient–Practitioner Interaction Checklist

The observer in the triad responds to these questions during each role-play situation and then uses this information to give feedback to the HCP about their therapeutic communication.

How well did the HCP:

1.  Attend to and address the patient's (or nurse's) emotional state and feelings?

2.  Identify what the problem was and who had the problem?

3.  Use reflection and clarifying responses during active listening and use "I" statements when he or she owned the problem?

4.  Use open-ended questions and statements to encourage the patient to talk more?

5.  Remain silent when appropriate?

6.  Respond to the patient with signs of sympathy and self-transposal?

7.  Avoid judging, defensive, or blaming statements?

8.  How could the therapist improve communication next time?

Now go back and repeat a selected vignette to communicate utilizing PPE and digital communication instead of F2F. Consider the query critiques above and then consider: How were things different? What was more or less challenging?

# JOURNALING

At the conclusion of the exercises, journal your feelings about this new form of communicating. How do you feel about its usefulness? Do you believe that you will be able to develop skill in using "I" statements? Are you willing to practice at home? How about active listening skills? Make a commitment to practice using these skills at least once each day until you believe that you've developed some skill and remember that this form of communication is now a choice for you in any situation.

---

**These exercises are also available online at www.routledge.com/9781638220039.**

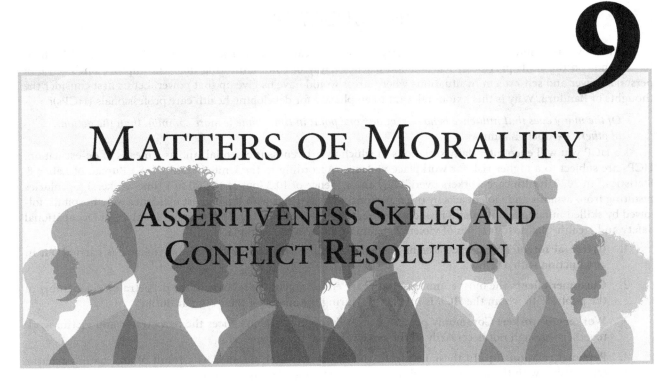

# MATTERS OF MORALITY

## ASSERTIVENESS SKILLS AND CONFLICT RESOLUTION

*Gina Maria Musolino and Carol M. Davis*

## OBJECTIVES

*The learner should be able to*:

- Appreciate the importance of using assertive communication in healing interactions.
- Differentiate between nonassertive, assertive, and aggressive communication.
- Identify the rights we all share as human beings.
- Discover situations in which each person tends to give up personal power.
- Demonstrate how to defuse a hostile, angry reaction.
- Define bullying and moral integrity, moral dilemma, moral problem, moral distress, moral uncertainty, moral injury, and moral courage.
- Describe bullying behaviors and threats to moral integrity in the workplace.
- Codify challenges to moral integrity and matters of moral injury and burnout for health care professionals (HCPs).
- Construct appropriate assertive communication responses for clinical vignettes.
- Role-play and critique applied assertive communication with clinical scenarios.
- Propose the opportunity to contract for changing negative, reactive behavior to positive, assertive behavior.
- Appraise one's assertiveness and conflict management style as a developing HCP.

DOI: 10.4324/9781003525554-9

# INTRODUCTION

In the previous chapter, we learned a new way of communicating in intense or emotional moments. This chapter expands on the skills previously learned and teaches a way of communicating that will improve one's sense of personal power and self-esteem in situations where stress would have us give up that power. Let us first consider the thoughts of Bandura. Why is this axiom relevant to emphasize for developing health care professionals (HCPs)?

> *Of the many cues that influence behavior, at any one point in time, none is more common than the actions of others.* —Albert Bandura

As a HCP you will encounter daily situations in which assertiveness is essential, and as a means of de-escalation. HCPs are subject to a higher risk for workplace violence. According to the United States (U.S.) Bureau of Labor & Statistics,[1] in 2020, health care workers overall had an incidence of 10.3 (out of 10,000 full-time workers) for injuries resulting from assaults and violent acts by other persons; work settings with the highest incidence were hospitals, followed by skilled nursing facilities and residential care, then private industry. The National Institute of Occupational Safety and Health[2] define four types of violence that may occur in the workplace:

1. **Criminal intent:** The perpetrator has no relationship with the victim, and the violence is carried out in conjunction with a crime.

2. **Customer/client:** The most common health care environment-based assault, the perpetrator is a member of the public with whom the HCP is interacting during the course of their regular duties.

3. **Worker-on-worker:** Commonly perceived as bullying, in these instances the perpetrator and victim work together—though not necessarily in the same role or at the same level.

4. **Personal relationship:** In these incidents, the victim has been targeted as a result of an existing exterior relationship with the perpetrator, with the violence taking place in the workplace.

Let's consider a worker-on-worker example:

Sheila Lester, registered nurse, was standing at the nurses' station reading her patient's chart before going into the patient's room to give her treatment. The patient's physician came to the station and was searching for the chart. When he saw that Sheila was reading it, he turned to her and said, "Give me the chart, Honey. That's my patient and I have to see her now." Sheila felt as if she were being treated in a nonprofessional way, to say the least. She felt her heart begin to race, she knew she was blushing, and she realized that she felt degraded and humiliated. Before she could stop herself, she turned to the physician and shouted, "My name is not Honey, and this is my patient as well!" The physician looked up with amusement and returned, "Well, well. What is your name then, Honey?" Sheila felt as if the battle were lost and put the chart down and walked away in anger.

# ASSERTIVENESS TRAINING

Assertiveness training has become well known in the past decade, and many people claim its benefits as a communication skill, but it also carries a negative connotation in some circles. Images of the "uppity" woman or the aggressive man come to mind. These images result from our socialization, from the messages we heard from our parents as we grew up. As rambunctious children, many of us were taught that we should "know our place" and practice humility. As we grew older, we heard other messages: "Children should be seen and not heard!" "Go to your room until you can come out with a smile on your face!" "If you can't say something nice, don't say anything at all!" Certainly, Traditionalists and Baby Boomers and families from strong ethnic cultural backgrounds heard, "Women belong in the supportive role to their husbands." More recently, we hear phrases such as, "Don't worry, be happy!" and "Don't sweat the small stuff!" and "Chill out!" and "Shake it off!" and "Keep calm and carry on."

The accumulative effect, especially on all those who suffer from low self-esteem and those who feel disempowered in the community, can result in communication that is not healthy or healing in nature. Following rules that do not encourage genuine and appropriate expression of feelings results in multiple unhealthy behaviors. These can include the bottling up of genuine emotion and the repression of feelings over time that often results in stress-related illness, passive-aggressive silence or manipulation, and inappropriate outbursts of anger, rage, defensiveness, and frustration. At the extreme, we see the rampage killings at schools and public gathering places often committed by adolescents and teens who were enraged by bullies or psychological manipulation ("gaslighting") and felt powerless to communicate their feelings to others. Unfortunately, instances of microaggressions[3] are rampant today; bullying and gaslighting have become a greater issue in the workplace. In 2021, 30% of adult Americans were bullied at work, with 43% of remote workers also experiencing bullying; just over 61% were bullied by the same gender, with an overall impact of 76.3 million workers.[4] HCPs, as healers, need to be a part of the solution.

# BULLYING DEFINED IN THE WORKPLACE

The Workplace Bullying Institute[4] defines workplace bullying as "repeated, health-harming mistreatment of one or more persons (the targets) by one or more perpetrators. It is **abusive conduct** that is:

- Threatening, humiliating, or intimidating; or
- Work interference—sabotage—that prevents work from getting done; or
- Verbal abuse."

The bully's behavior is deliberate and targeted to a specific victim, occurring frequently and with a level of intensity over a period of time. Bullying behaviors are overt and covert, which often make it difficult for the victim to recognize, identify, respond to, and report bullying. Being bullied at work has also been said to resemble the first-hand experience of a battered spouse. The Workplace Bullying Institute states that "not calling bullying 'bullying,' to avoid offending the sensibilities of those who made the bullying possible, is a disservice to bullied individuals whose jobs, careers, and health have been threatened as the result."[4] Raynor and Hoel[5] identified five categories of bullying behaviors (Figure 9.1).

The American Nurses Association (ANA) maintains a position statement, "Incivility, Bullying, and Workplace Violence,"[6] to combat workplace abuse and harassment of nurses. The ANA[6] provides recommendations for action to proactively reduce the growing problem of workplace abuse, harassment, and bullying of nurses and to explore collaborative solutions with other disciplines and organizations to leverage resources for research and education. The ANA[6] also provides resources for reporting and to support a culture of reporting abuses in the workplace. Although your professions code of ethics may address the topic in a general manner, bullying today is very specific in that it is directed toward control and clear destabilization of another person within the workplace (see Figure 9.1) and the need to create safer workplaces has become increasingly evident, with an even more significant need due to the Covid-19 pandemic personal protective equipment (PPE) crises and HCP shortages.

Several aspects of bullying have occurred in the workplace, including aggression, emotional abuse, intimidation, gaslighting, harassment, victimization, emotional abuse, intentional isolation, and psychological mistreatment. Let us be clear that HCPs setting high work standards, having differences of opinion, and/or providing constructive feedback are *not* aspects of bullying.

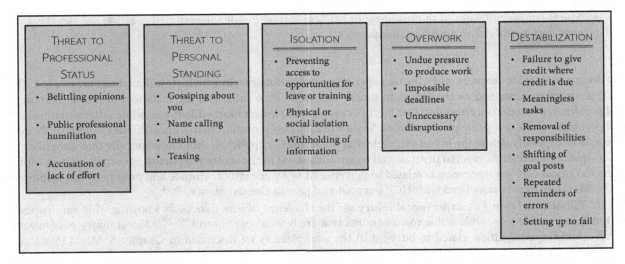

**Figure 9.1** Raynor and Hoel's five categories of bullying behaviors. (Adapted from Raynor C, Hoel H. A summary review of literature relating to workplace bullying. *J Community Appl Soc Psych*. 1997;7:181–191.)

The Joint Commission[7] proclaimed its intolerance of intimidating and disruptive behaviors in the document "Behaviors That Undermine a Culture of Safety." This document includes 11 suggested actions to ensure compliance; a Leadership Standard (LD.03.01.01) that addresses disruptive and inappropriate behaviors in two of its elements of performance, which requires reporting systems, as part of the Environment of Care and Human Resource Standards, to address prevention and post-incident strategies, training, and education to decrease workplace violence:[7]

> *Element of Performance 4: The hospital/organization has a code of conduct that defines acceptable and disruptive and inappropriate behaviors; and*
> *Element of Performance 5: Leaders create and implement a process for managing disruptive and inappropriate behaviors.*

Work remains to be done with respect to making workplaces safer and more civilized; bullying has no place in health care and confronting bullying remains a matter of safety for all. The Healthy Workplace Bill,[8] which provides protection from bullying to employees and employers, was initiated in 2001. As of mid-2024 (with efforts slowed due to the pandemic), 32 U.S. states have introduced the bill and in 2020 Puerto Rico enacted the bill into law. Training-only mandates for all employers have been instituted in California and for state-only employers in Utah. As President Maltby of the National Workrights Institute stated, "Bullying is the sexual harassment of 20 years ago; everybody knows about it, but nobody wants to admit it."[9] (Title VI of the Civil Rights Act currently covers sexual harassment and discrimination.)

# HEALTH CARE PROFESSIONALS' MORAL MATTERS

Recall in Chapter 4 we explored moral dilemmas. Let's look more closely now at some additional important ethical terms:[10,11]

- **Moral integrity:** Virtue composed of veracity, fidelity, benevolence, wisdom, and moral courage.
- **Moral problem:** Competing moral claim or principle; one principle is clearly dominant.
- **Moral dilemma:** Situation in which two or more ethically plausible principles are in opposition to each other and only one may be chosen.
- **Moral distress:** Internal response that occurs when a health care provider believes they inherently know the correct ethical action that is needed but cannot act on that knowledge.
- **Moral injury:** The challenge of simultaneously knowing what care patients need but being unable to provide it due to constraints that are beyond our control.
- **Moral uncertainty:** Internal conflict that arises when the person cannot define what moral principles apply but has a strong feeling that something is not right.
- **Moral courage:** Relates to the readiness of being able to willingly take purposive action for moral reasons despite the risk of adverse consequences.

As discussed in prior chapters, as HCPs we experience many situations in which ethical analyses are needed. The situations are often described as challenges to moral integrity. Often situations are instances of moral dilemmas, moral problems, or moral uncertainties. Conflicts between principles are moral dilemmas, while other situations are moral problems where one principle dominates. Some situations also result in moral uncertainties, where HCPs may not be able to explicitly define the moral principle that is specifically applicable, but know morally that something is just not right. Moral distress is when institutional constraints stand in the way of the pursuit of correct actions. Moral distress in critical care environments is related to perceptions of a poor ethical climate and poor personal empowerment.[12] Moral distress is associated with HCP burnout and patient care avoidance.[12–14]

Dean, Talbot, and Dean[11] describe **moral injury** as "the challenge of simultaneously knowing what care patients need but being unable to provide it due to constraints that are beyond our control."[(p 401)] Moral injury goes beyond the individual responsibilities related to burnout in the workplace as we discussed in Chapter 5. Moral injury is a war-related term that was first described regarding patient care for those who were nonresponsive to typical therapies for post-traumatic stress disorder (PTSD) in the Vietnam War.[13] HCPs are often forced to consider the "demands of other stakeholders—the electronic medical record (EMR), the insurers, the hospital, administration, the health care system, seeking sufficient patient and care delivery resources, even our own financial security—before the needs of our patients."[11(p 400)] Moral injury describes the conundrum of today's HCPs as knowing how to best care for patients but often being impeded from doing so by systemic barriers related to the business side of health care.[11,14] Certainly not all burnout is caused by moral injury, yet moral injury (violating one's/professional core values) can certainly lead to burnout.

Moral injury re-emerged in the health care discussions quite recently because of the difficulties and challenges health care workers and health care systems faced in the context, and many unfortunate realities, of the Covid-19 pandemic. Dale et al.[15] discovered HCPs were consistently experiencing both burnout and moral injury at high rates associated with specific morally distressing health care experiences, Covid-19 work impacts, Covid-19 protection concerns, and leadership support. Burnout predictors included self-moral injury, Covid-19 work impacts, depression symptoms, and leadership support; while moral injury was related to prior adversities, HCP roles, Covid-19 health worries and Covid-19 diagnosis.[15] Health care administration and supervisors should be cognizant of these needs for HCPs and pro-actively offer support to maintain a healthy and productive workforce. Dale et al.[13,15–16] considered threats to HCPs' moral integrity and aspects of moral distress, morally distressing events, and moral injury:

> *Moral distress is present when one is aware of the right thing to do but is unable to do so because of occupational constraints. In the context of the COVID-19 pandemic, HCPs may be experiencing what we term as **healthcare morally distressing events**, such as being unable to provide frequent enough care, conduct necessary procedures or assessments, and refer patients for necessary procedures or specialists. Additional stressors may be present for providers doing telemedicine, such as discomfort with the use of telemedicine or belief that they are providing inadequate care. These events may lead to **moral injury**, a construct well studied within military populations but less investigated among HCPs. **Moral injury** occurs when one's deeply held moral beliefs have been transgressed by perpetrating, failing to prevent, or witnessing what are considered by the individual to be immoral acts, thus producing a lasting psychological, biological, spiritual, behavioral, and social impact. Individuals experiencing **moral injury** may feel shame and guilt, emotional distress, weakened trust, reduced self-forgiveness, view of self as immoral/irredeemable in an unjust world, and suicidality. **Moral injury** can have tragic consequences and has been implicated in the increased rates of suicide among HCPs, especially when making life-and-death decisions about which patients to treat and where to allocate the limited resources.*

If you or anyone you know are experiencing thoughts of suicide or in crisis, you are not alone, please call or text to **988** National Suicide Prevention & Crisis Hotline for support or https://988lifeline.org/. For further information: www.nimh.nih.gov/health/topics/suicide-prevention.

A scoping review was conducted by Čartolovni et al.[17] and reiterated that moral injury involves a "deep, emotional wound and is unique to those who bear witness to intense human suffering and cruelty with a strong relationship to moral distress, with a feeling of 'not doing enough' overtime, circumstances and contexts, leading to moral injury."[(p 590)] Take a moment to consider Figure 9.2, which details the challenges to HCPs' moral integrity and the commonalities and differences of moral injury and distress.[17] Čartolovni et al.[17] also further cautioned that moral injury leads to severe consequences, with need for further investigations, especially following the pandemic.

Dean et al.[11] summarized: "Every time we are forced to make a decision that contravenes our patients' best interests, we feel a sting of moral injustice. Over time, these repetitive insults amass into moral injury".[(p 400)] HCPs who step up with moral courage often call upon moral creativity to resolve and reframe challenges while attempting changed methods and solutions. A nonthreatening, generative discussion and brainstorming session with peers is helpful for solutions-oriented efforts. The crises of conscience that occur challenge HCPs' moral courage daily and we will be talking about ways to advocate for change in Chapter 11. Yet, before we embark on leadership and advocacy, we need to realize the importance of using assertive communication in individual healing interactions with patients and colleagues.

# THE CHALLENGE OF COMMUNICATING WISELY IN HEALTH CARE

As HCPs move away from traditional assistive roles and toward more prominent primary care responsibilities, such as in the clinical doctoral degree programs for physical therapists (DPT), occupational therapists (OTD), and nurse practitioners (DNP), more appropriately assertive communication styles are required to be effective as a HCP

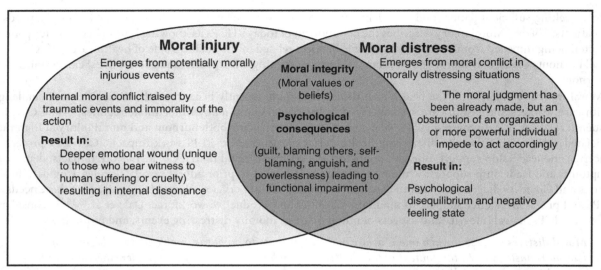

**Figure 9.2** Interplay between moral injury and moral distress. (Adapted from Čartolovni A, Stolt M, Scott PA, Suhonen R. Moral injury in healthcare professionals: A scoping review and discussion. *Nurs Ethics*. 2021 Aug;28(5):590–602.)

collaborating with patients as part of interprofessional health care delivery. These skills do not come automatically with the conferring of the degree.[18] In addition, health care calls for a concerted practice when dealing with fellow HCPs who are often working under stress and when dealing with patients and their families who are feeling intensely vulnerable. Emotional communication, including anger, is very prevalent in the practice of health care. Many situations occur daily in which a person is stimulated to react, either in anger or in giving up personal power and feeling helpless.

# GENDER DIFFERENCES

We live in an evolving society that has been historically male dominated and patriarchal. The culture of the West has very gradually moved toward equality, although the reality of the need for balance is well established in all cultures. Historically, nurses, who are predominantly women, feel especially affected by disparate power structure in the health care systems. In a study conducted by Friedman[19] on nurse–physician relationships, nurses reported that they had to deal with the following: condescending attitudes, lack of respect as either a person or a professional, humiliation, temper tantrums, blaming, disregard for professional input, and/or public disparagement. The continuum of insensitive behavior, issuing from people in power to those in less powerful positions, can run from poor taste and bad manners to outright sexist abuse, bullying, and harassment. The sources of verbal abuse to nurses described in Friedman's[19] article were primarily physicians, then patients' families, and lastly the nurse supervisor. Although it is true that part of the power struggle in health care has to do with the difficulties in our culture of people relating equally with each other, it is not as simple as that.

As much as all children are alike, developmentalists have shown us that children are different in the way they are treated by adults, their goals and ideals, the way they see their place in the world, and the way they make decisions about right and wrong, despite efforts today for gender neutrality. But, all people have a genderless essential self, a core identity that is good, that underlies the public self or persona and the ego. All people have the natural desire to become more, to grow, to learn, to increase self-esteem, to have influence, and to feel capable and able to facilitate change for the better. For the most part, people in health care want to help others, to change conditions of illness and pain or the inability to function fully as a human being in the world. To help in healing ways, one must exercise personal and professional power for the good. The goal must be to mature beyond the need for the ego to defend itself and to reach down to the essential self, where we are confident of our personal rights and assured of our equality and from where we can communicate with empathy and understanding.

# CULTURAL DIFFERENCES

As the United States becomes increasingly diverse in population, health care professionals' classrooms reflect this broad diversity. As you will learn in Chapter 13, some cultures emphasize the inappropriateness of asserting oneself in a leadership role, deeming assertive behavior as rude or selfish, and emphasize more passive ways of achieving goals that would not be effective in the health care system in our country. These behaviors, such as not making eye contact or speaking in an exceptionally low tone of voice, would seem out of place and weak to colleagues and patients and would be ineffective as healing behaviors in the United States and other Western countries.[20]

# EXERCISING OUR PERSONAL POWER

In previous chapters, we learned that how we feel about ourselves has everything to do with how we view the world and how we view other people. How we feel about our own self-worth is directly connected to how much personal power we feel we have and how we use that power. *Webster's Dictionary* defines power as a possession of control, authority, or influence over another; the ability to act or produce an effect; legal or official authority, capacity, or right; physical might; or political control or influence.[21] Notice that power is a neutral term, having neither positive nor negative value connotations. If we want to facilitate change to make the world better, we must learn how to exercise power.

Historically, women in our society have been taught to play a role secondary to, or supportive of, men. Men have been taught to seek out and expect the support of women. But we are all born equal. **We learn to give up our power.** Some beliefs we develop that result in a giving up of personal power include the following:

- I am not as important as the other person (often the physician or supervisor).
- I am lucky to be treated with respect by others (those in authority).
- I have years of training and experience, but they still do not compare to medicine.
- I must act in ways that indicate I know my place so that I can keep my job, keep referrals coming, and keep peace for others' sake.
- When criticized by a superior, I must not respond but agree to save face and avoid further criticism.
- My needs are not as important as those of others.

Some situations seem inherently more apt to stimulate stress than others; thus, we can predict that we might be tempted to give up power, or respond defensively with anger, when we find ourselves required to respond. Ten such situations that may cause stress for some or all of us include the following:

1. Command—Someone orders us to do something
2. Anger—Includes name calling, using obscenities, shouting
3. Negative criticism—Someone judges us as being less than adequate, without suggestions for improvement
4. Unresponsiveness—Indifference to us or to our request
5. Depression—A feeling of gloom in another, extreme sadness
6. Impulsivity—Someone becomes extremely angry, acts crazy
7. Affection—Someone expresses love and affection or asks us for it
8. Making mistakes—Fear that you cannot make a mistake; feeling as if you must always have the right answer
9. Sexual content—Someone makes an overt or covert sexual comment or sexual advance
10. Pain—Feelings of wanting to flee in the face of pain

# PERSONAL RIGHTS

When we hear terrifying stories of people's inhumanity to each other, we are often moved to righteous indignation. For example, none of us can hear recounting from Holocaust victims without cringing with horror. Likewise, prisoner of war stories and inhumane treatments revealed from the War on Ukraine, the Iraq War, and Guantanamo, and Islamic State of Iraq and Syria human rights abuses, terrorists' actions, and war crimes move us to anger and outrage. Human beings deserve to be treated in certain ways, simply because we are human. What rights do all people have as human beings? What does each human being deserve, simply by virtue of the fact that they are a person alive on this Earth? Make a list of the basic rights of all human beings. Do you act in ways that are consistent with your beliefs about your rights? Are there certain rights that you fail to claim for yourself? If so, why is that? How does this list change when a human being becomes ill or disabled?

Thoughts or beliefs we develop even before we can talk lead to feelings (rational or not), which then lead to behaviors or reactions. It is a universal right that every person is entitled to act assertively and to express honest thoughts, feelings, and beliefs. Assertiveness training teaches us that we have a choice of communicating in a way that allows us to convey our thoughts and feelings with tact and respect for others and honor for ourselves. As human beings, each one of us has the right to the following:[22]

- Being treated with respect.

- Having needs and having those needs be as important as other people's needs. We have the right to ask (not demand) that other people respond to our needs and to decide whether we want to respond to others' needs.

- Having feelings and expressing those feelings in ways that do not violate the dignity of others.

- Changing our minds.

- Determining our own priorities.

- Asking for what we want.

- Refusing without making excuses.

- Forming our own opinions and expressing them or having no opinion at all on a certain topic.

- Giving and receiving information as fellow health care professionals.

- Acting in the best interests of the patient.

When we allow our rights to be overlooked, we assume a dependent role, which lowers self-esteem and fosters nonassertive behavior. Recognizing that we have rights is the first step in the cognitive retraining that is essential to assertiveness.

# ASSERTIVENESS

What exactly is assertiveness? The concept of assertive behavior can best be described in comparison with what it is not—nonassertive (passive) and aggressive behavior.

## Nonassertive Behavior

- Failing to get your point across by remaining quiet or passive. Perceived by others to be weak, easily taken advantage of, or manipulated.

- Key message conveyed: I do not count. My feelings are not as important as yours.

## Aggressive Behavior

- Getting your point across but perceived by others as hostile, angry, offensive, sarcastic, or humiliating.

- Key message conveyed: This is what is true. Any reasonable person would agree. You are stupid to disagree. What I want is most important; what you want, feel, or think does not matter.

## Assertive Behavior

- Getting your point across without offending others. Direct, congruent expression of thoughts, feelings, beliefs, and opinions in a non-offensive way.

- Key message conveyed: This is how I view the situation. This is what I think and feel at this moment.

Alberti and Emmons[23] noted ten key elements to assertive behavior:

1. Self-expressive

2. Respectful of the rights of others

3. Honest

4. Direct and firm

5. Equalizing, benefiting self and relationship

6. Verbally appropriate, including the content of the message (feelings, rights, facts, opinions, requests, limits)

7. Nonverbally appropriate, including the style of the message (eye contact, voice posture, facial expression, gestures, distance, timing, fluency, listening)

8. Appropriate for the person and the situation, not universal

9. Socially responsible

10. Learned, not inborn

# EXAMPLES OF ASSERTIVE RESPONSES

Many of us have found ourselves in the situation when, dining out, we order our meal, and something happens to make it less acceptable than we had expected. We find ourselves in a situation where we feel that it is necessary to speak up to enjoy the meal that we've requested. Let's say that the dinner is completely cold. What are our choices in this situation?

- Passive—Say nothing at all. When the server asks, "How's your dinner?" you respond, "Fine." (The person you're dining with, however, receives the brunt of your hostility all evening.)

- Aggressive—Stand up, shout for the server, and say in a loud and angry voice, "This meal is ice cold. I'm willing to pay good money for a good dinner, but you have the nerve to bring me a meal that has been sitting around for half an hour, and I resent it. Take this meal back immediately and bring me some hot food."

- Assertive—Motion for the waiter, state calmly that your food has become cold, and request that it be heated and brought back to you as quickly as possible.

Upon comparison, it is easy to value assertive communication as superior to nonassertive and aggressive modes. Difficulty in acting assertively in appropriate situations with any consistency stems from the real or perceived threat of rejection, anger, or disapproval. Often, this reluctance to be assertive is based more on habit and subconscious fears that we learned long ago and that now guide our responses in an automatic way. Assertiveness helps us realize that we have a real choice to stand up for ourselves and to hold on to our power in demanding situations. Why in the world would anyone sit and eat a cold dinner while not enjoying it and be willing to pay for it? What is the fear behind speaking up to ask for your rights? For many of us it is simply a matter of overlearning the dictate, "Don't make waves, don't cause a fuss, and don't do anything that will bring attention to yourself." Behind this admonition is the basic feeling that others' rights are more important than mine—that I don't count.

Likewise, why would someone stand up and shout at a waiter in anger for something that is easily remedied? Usually, this kind of behavior is acting out anger or frustration with something not related to the meal at all. Or the customer carries a sense of entitlement and feels that it is their responsibility to teach others the right behavior.

# TYPES OF ASSERTIVE RESPONSES

There are eight types of assertive responses that can benefit us in the practice of health care and in our day-to-day interactions:[23]

1. Being confrontational

2. Saying no

3. Making requests

4. Expressing opinions

5. Initiating conversation

6. Disclosing self

7. Expressing affection

8. Entering a room of strangers and being willing to get to know others and allowing ourselves to be known

The first two areas can be described as assertive responses that express what commonly appear to be negative emotions; the next three responses are emotionally neutral responses that are task specific; and the last three responses call for expressing positive emotions. In the exercises at the end of the chapter, you will be given the opportunity to draft assertive, passive, and aggressive responses to each situation.

# ATTRIBUTION AND THE DESIRE TO ACT ASSERTIVELY

A person can be quite knowledgeable about assertiveness but may not think to use these skills for any number of reasons. For example, if one believes that no matter what is done the attempt will end in failure, assertiveness does not seem important. This problematic way of thinking illustrates one aspect of behavior, which can partially be explained by attribution theory.[24] The exercise in Figure 9.3 will help you discover the nature of your attributions, or how your lenses are set today. Chart your numbers in the grid at the bottom of the figure.

Note the differences in your perceptions of the causes of success and failure. If you are like most people, you tend to attribute success to causes that are different in nature from those to which we attribute failure.

Attribution theory provides a framework to understand the ways that a person's lenses are set. An attribution is what we feel or think caused an outcome we have experienced.[25] How we view outcomes, as successful or failing, is critical in determining our expectations and our future actions. The three dimensions of the causes to which we attribute success or failure are the *locus* (due to something inside or outside of me), *stability* (lasting or temporary), and *controllability* (to what extent I can control this) dimensions.

Attributions that we assign to outcomes have a great deal to do with how we think about ourselves or relate directly to how our lenses are set regarding our self-esteem. If we have good self-esteem, we are likely to attribute the cause of our successes to something inside of ourselves, something that is stable or controllable. If we have low self-esteem, we are likely to see our successes as due to forces outside of ourselves that are unstable and uncontrollable, such as luck or the difficulty of the task. In contrast with failure, a person who indicates a cause that is internal, unstable (changeable), and controllable, such as the amount of effort we expended or the strategy we chose, will be more likely to expect success in the future by increasing effort or changing the ineffective strategy.[24]

**In other words, with high self-esteem, we choose to believe that we are going to succeed directly because of our actions, and if we fail, it is not because of a fixed internal trait (we have low ability or a poor personality) but because of circumstances that can change if we apply a different, more successful strategy to the task.**

In summary, when failure is attributed to stable, external, and uncontrollable events, there is little we can do to effect change and we are unlikely to use assertiveness or any other strategy to get the job done. This is a loser's or victim's "script."

It is important to describe the nature of success and failure in ways that allow success to be judged realistically and over the long term.[25] The most adaptive attributions occur when success is defined in other than all-or-nothing terms, are realistic in the circumstances, and are attributed to one's personal ability, effort, or good judgment.[26] In health care, many frustrating situations are unlikely to change, but we can change how we think about them and how we deal with them to experience success over the long term. If success is seen as having all patients be discharged from our services after being carefully cured or having Medicare pay for 100% of treatment in 100% of eligible cases, few HCPs would ever feel as if they succeeded. Compromise, realistic expectations, and acceptance of long-term strategies are necessary, along with avoiding dualistic right–wrong judgments.

In sum, we must change the way we define failure and think about the causes of failure for assertiveness to be useful and successful. If we believe that failure is attributed to external events that are uncontrollable and stable, we will be unlikely to use assertiveness. But, if we reframe our thoughts, decide that our goal might have been a little too unrealistic, and decide to use another strategy to work for success, assertiveness can be a useful tool to solve problems.

# LEARNING TO ACT ASSERTIVELY

The skill of assertive behavior is not inborn; to develop it requires learning five new behaviors:[23]

1. **Recognize situations in which you are tempted to become passive or aggressive in your communication**. Develop the skill of observing yourself. Be conscious of situations where you automatically give up your power, have irrational thoughts that do not relate to the present moment, or feel the necessity to put the other person down.

2. **Recognize when you are tempted to attribute failure to forces that are uncontrollable and stable, such as a powerful person's unpleasant personality traits or a medical system that fails to acknowledge patient needs**. Challenge yourself to think of a strategy to replace feelings of hopelessness or negativity.

Put yourself in a time when you've done a project that was highly praised. What did you do? Who praised you? How did you feel? How did this influence future activity? Write down one major cause of your success.

1. IS THE CAUSE DUE TO SOMETHING ABOUT YOU OR DUE TO SOMETHING OUTSIDE OF YOU?

Internal         1         2         3         4         5         6         7         External
(Inside you)                                                                      (Other resources)

2. IS THE CAUSE SOMETHING THAT WILL REMAIN STABLE OR BE ONLY TEMPORARY?

Lasting         1         2         3         4         5         6         7         Temporary
(Stable)                                                                           (Unstable)
(Constant [IQ])                                                                    (Changing [weather])

3. DO YOU SEE THIS CAUSE AS SOMETHING YOU CAN CONTROL OR IS THIS BEYOND YOUR CONTROL?

Controllable  1         2         3         4         5         6         7         Uncontrollable
(Whether I study or not)                                                           (Other person's mood)

4. HOW LIKELY ARE YOU TO EXPERIENCE THE SAME OUTCOME IN THE FUTURE?

Highly likely  1         2         3         4         5         6         7         Unlikely

Now, think of a time when you have experienced a failure, for example, given an important talk and the audience reacts negatively or cooked a meal that no one liked. Write down one major cause.

5. IS THE CAUSE DUE TO SOMETHING ABOUT YOU OR SOMETHING OUTSIDE OF YOU?

Internal         1         2         3         4         5         6         7         External

6. IS THE CAUSE SOMETHING THAT WILL REMAIN STABLE OR BE ONLY TEMPORARY OR CHANGING?

Lasting         1         2         3         4         5         6         7         Temporary
(Stable)                                                                           (Unstable)

7. DO YOU SEE THIS CAUSE AS SOMETHING YOU CAN CONTROL OR IS THIS BEYOND YOUR CONTROL?

Controllable  1         2         3         4         5         6         7         Uncontrollable

8. HOW LIKELY ARE YOU TO EXPERIENCE THE SAME OUTCOME IN THE FUTURE?

Highly likely  1         2         3         4         5         6         7         Unlikely

Now chart your numbers on this grid:

|                              | *SUCCESS* | *FAILURE* |
| ---------------------------- | --------- | --------- |
| Internal/External            |           |           |
| Stable/Unstable              |           |           |
| Controllable/Uncontrollable  |           |           |

**Figure 9.3** Attribution exercise.[26]

3. **Replace these old thought patterns with different, more positive, and powerful thoughts.** Cognitively interrupt the old thought patterns of "You're right, I'm no good" or "How dare you attack me, you arrogant fool?" or "It's no use!" Alone or with another trusted person, do the following:

   ○ Discuss the nature of the situation that aroused the emotion

   ○ Confront the tendency to react passively or aggressively

   ○ Identify the belief that lies behind your reaction

   ○ Replace the erroneous belief with a counteracting right

   ○ Identify a more positive thought that will bring more confident feelings

4. **Practice thinking new thoughts as a first step in changing the feelings that go with the old thoughts, thus deflating the energy behind the old reaction.** You will know that you are on the right track when the new thoughts make you feel positive and hopeful.

5. **Practice the new behavior that goes along with the ownership of the right.** Be assertive. Count your blessings and feel good about your ability to make a positive difference in the world.

How might Sheila, the nurse in the example at the beginning of the chapter, communicate assertively? Chapter 8 taught one aspect of assertive communication, the use of "I" statements. This mode of communicating transforms an aggressive, blaming, or accusatory response to an assertive, responsible, and clear expression of feeling, essentially telling the other person what effect their behavior has on you. In many cases, an "I" statement alone initially is sufficient to get your assertive message across. The situation Sheila found herself in calls for a confrontational assertion. Sheila feels diminished, less than a colleague. Her feeling response is anger at being treated so poorly, and her initial reaction is to be angry. When her anger does not get her what she wants, the messages in her head revert to "See. You're just not as good as the physician. Your rights are not important here." She gives up and walks away in frustration. What she hoped for was a collegial relationship with the physician because both fulfill clinical responsibilities with patients. This calls for a confrontational response aimed at helping her avoid becoming aggressive in anger and avoid passively giving up her power to silently comply with the physician's rude request.

First, Sheila must be aware of her feelings in the situation and her tendency to react in anger and give up her power. She must be aware of what causes she attributes the outcomes in this situation to. Next, she must pay attention to the messages she gives herself and challenge the negative thoughts with more affirming, positive thoughts that confirm her rights as a human being. Then she is ready to respond with an assertive reply aimed at exercising her right to express her honest thoughts, feelings, and beliefs around this situation. One format for an effective response is through the **describe, express, specify, and consequences (DESC) approach** of framing your response.

# DESC RESPONSE AS A FORMAT FOR ASSERTIVE COMMUNICATION

The DESC format described by Bower and Bower[27] incorporates "I" statements but expands them and is useful when a more detailed interaction is required to get the other person's attention to your point of view. DESC is an acronym for:

- **Describe** the situation.

- **Express** your feelings about the situation: "I feel ..."

- **Specify** the change you want: "I'd like for you to ..."

- **Consequences.** Identify the results that will occur: "In that way ..."

Let's compose a DESC response for Sheila in the situation outlined at the beginning of the chapter:

**D**—"Yes, Dr. Dutton, I realize that this is your patient. She's my patient as well; I'm her nurse."

**E**—"My name is Sheila Lester. When you call me 'Honey,' it demeans me, and I do not appreciate it."

**S**—"I'd like you to call me Sheila or Ms. Lester because I'd like to discuss this patient with you as a colleague would, and I would like you to treat me as a colleague."

**C**—"In that way, I feel the patient will receive better care because we are collaborating with her in a more respectful and collegial way."

Sheila took a significant risk with this physician by speaking up to tell him how his behavior made her feel. She must have trusted that this was a risk worth taking. We would hope that the physician would respond in a mature way and treat her request with respect. Assertive communication does not guarantee this, however, as we'll discuss in a moment.

Sometimes you know that the risk is not well placed. An alternative to the DESC confrontation is the **describe, indicate, specify, and consequences (DISC) confrontation**, which is used when you are confronting a person who will not care what you feel, so you eliminate the expression of feeling and substitute I for "indicate," indicating the problem the behavior is causing. DESC and DISC are just amplifications of the effective "I" statement, but using them in a practiced, disciplined way provides an opportunity to erase an old, ineffective way of responding by replacing it with an assertive response.

An illustration of the DISC response for a physical therapist would be a powerful physician who refers a patient with low back pain to you, a physical therapist, and specifically orders the following: evaluate and treat with heat and massage and no exercise, no mobilization. Upon evaluation, you realize that this back pain is the result of an acute muscle spasm that occurred recently and was facilitated by poor body mechanics and weak flexor and shortened extensor muscles. Your professional knowledge requires that you treat with ice and teach exercises to relax the current problem and prevent recurrence.

Your DISC confrontation might go something like this:

D—"I'd like to talk with you about Mr. Doughty's back problem. I appreciate the opportunity to provide physical therapy."

I—"Your physical therapy referral is for heat and massage. However, my physical therapy examination reveals this to be an acute spasm, which evidence and clinical practice guidelines indicate responds faster and more effectively to mobilization, therapeutic exercise, and ice. The patient presents with poor body mechanics, weak abdominal muscles, with his back extensors in spasm, with shortened hamstring muscle length. The patient needs gentle relaxation exercise to reduce the spasm and eventual instruction in proper body mechanics."

S—"I'd like for you to approve my plan to evaluate and treat the patient utilizing my professional clinical judgment. If you and the patient agree, I plan to treat with therapeutic exercise, ice, mobilization, and teach him stretching and strengthening exercises and proper body mechanics and posture to prevent recurrence."

C—"That way, perhaps we can help him recover and get him strong enough and wise enough to keep him from reinjuring himself."

Organizing your thoughts will be more difficult at first, so the exercises for this chapter will provide practice following this four-step method by writing out your response to a past situation that was particularly difficult for you. The key to your success will be paying attention to the way you feel. When you feel negative feelings, reach for a more positive thought. Thoughts are highly creative, and we have a built-in indicator of how well we are doing with moving in a positive and growing direction. Good thoughts feel good. It's as simple as that.

You are probably wondering how you will learn to respond quickly and on the spot with such a detailed DISC or DESC format when an assertive response is indicated. At first, you will not be so organized. The most you can hope for is to recognize your feelings, avoid giving up your power angrily or passively, and buy time before responding at all. Eventually, however, it will become second nature to speak up with an "I" statement or a DESC/DISC response.

# ASSERTIVELY DEALING WITH ANGER

Occasionally, you will have to deal with an angry, defensive person. Feeling trapped in another's lashing out usually stimulates a fight-or-flight response or passive or aggressive behavior. The ego is stimulated into defending itself, or the ego caves into fear and wants to run away. In Chapter 8, we learned to use active listening when the other person has the emotional outburst; this continues to be the most effective response in an assertive mode. Using active listening skills to help the person defuse the energy behind the outburst, which is most often secondary to fear, allows you then to use "I" statements to offer your assertive response. Utilizing **restatement, reflection**, and **clarification** provides the platform for de-escalation.[28]

# HOSTILITY CURVE

A hostile, angry person will use a predictable pattern when raging[29] that looks somewhat like what is shown in Figure 9.4.

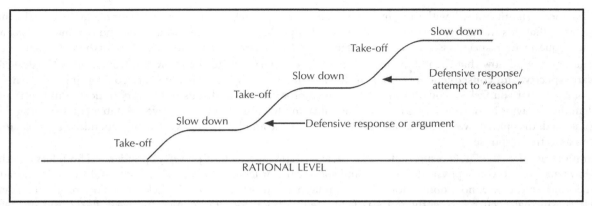

**Figure 9.4** Hostility/rage pattern of escalation. (Adapted from Allaire B, McNeil R. *Teaching Patient Relations in Hospitals—The Hows and Whys.* Chicago, IL: American Hospital Association; 1983.)

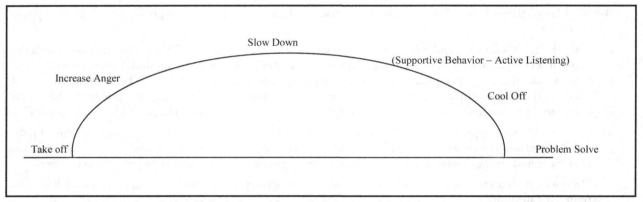

**Figure 9.5** Hostility curve handled skillfully. (Adapted from Allaire B, McNeil R. *Teaching Patient Relations in Hospitals—The Hows and Whys.* Chicago, IL: American Hospital Association; 1983.)

When you argue or respond defensively with someone who is raging, this will only fuel their fire and produce another take-off, escalating the argument to higher levels. Likewise, if you interrupt the hostile person and appeal to them to "be reasonable," a similar response will result. One person just keeps setting off the other, and no problem is identified, let alone solved.

Skillful handling[29] of a person who is raging (Figure 9.5) involves the active listening skills we practiced in Chapter 8.

During the raging person's irrational phase, it is best to simply wait and listen carefully but not say anything. Wait for the moment when the angry person seems to run out of steam and then demonstrate that you have been listening and say something supportive, such as "If the same thing had happened to me, no doubt I would be angry too" or "I know this has been a very difficult experience for you."

Being supportive does not require your agreeing with the person but simply hearing them out. This eventually will serve to defuse the increasing emotion, and the person will begin to cool off. Very often the person will apologize for losing composure. At this point, it is important to help the angry person save face. Lead the person to a private area, where you can sit down and use your neurolinguistic psychology *match, pace* and *lead* skills that you will learn in Chapter 12 to establish rapport.

What people are asking for most is recognition and understanding. Active listening gives you the chance to stand still and offer a therapeutic response, which will increase the chances for a positive outcome to the interchange. Once emotions have dissipated, offer your assertive point of view, and offer to work together to solve the problem.[27] It is important that you vent your own feelings with a trusted friend after the incident is over, and keep in mind these important and impacting words from Mother Teresa:

> *People are often unreasonable, irrational, and self-centered. Forgive them anyway. If you are kind, people may accuse you of selfish, ulterior motives. Be kind anyway. ... The good you do today will often be forgotten. Give your best anyway. In the final analysis, it is between you and God. It was never between you and them anyway.*

# BENEFITS OF ASSERTIVENESS

In a study with nursing and medical students, students' assertiveness, and self-esteem at post-test and one-month follow-up measurements of the experimental group after training were significantly increased compared with the pretest measurement.[30] There are several benefits to using assertive behavior:

- It is our ethical and healing responsibility
- It increases our self-respect
- It increases our self-control
- It improves self-confidence
- It helps us develop more emotionally satisfying relationships with others
- It increases the likelihood that everyone's needs will be met
- It helps to prevent burnout
- It allows us to exercise our personal rights without denying the rights of others

To exercise our personal rights relates to competency as a citizen, a consumer, a member of an organization or school or work group, and a participant in public events to express opinions, work for change, or respond to violations of one's own rights or those of others.[23] In the health professions, we must work side by side with colleagues, helping our patients regain their feelings of confidence and ability to function independently in the world. To make sure this happens, everyone's rights are important, and the exercise of those rights is critical to the healing process.

# COMMON MYTHS ABOUT ASSERTIVENESS

As valuable as assertive communication is, there are some common myths that accompany this process:

**If I speak up with assertiveness, others will like what I say and do what I ask.** Using assertive communication is no guarantee for anything, except that you have expressed yourself with dignity, honesty, and regard for others. How others respond to you is always a question and has much to do with the other person. Most important, you never have the right to violate another person's rights, even when you use assertiveness.

**All I must do is say the assertive words and I will be perceived as being assertive.** Assertive words are critical to an assertive message. But assertive words spoken passively or aggressively destroy the basic message of assertiveness. The posture of assertiveness is an appropriate tone of voice, a steady voice, open posture, and good eye contact.

**Once I learn assertiveness skills, I must use them all the time in every situation that tends to make me feel powerless.** There are times when the best assertive response is to simply walk away and say nothing. One good example is deciding not to retaliate to an aggressive person. Then it is best to say nothing. Always remember, you are free to choose not to assert yourself in a situation. Ask yourself:

- How important is this situation to me?
- How am I likely to feel afterward if I don't assert myself?
- What do I gain by being assertive? What do I lose?
- What do I gain by not being assertive? What do I lose?

**One assertive reply is all that is needed.** The first assertive response is the easiest. It is the comeback response that is more difficult. People will argue with your assertive response and try to get you to give up your power despite your effectiveness. For example, saying no when you mean no often takes several repeats of the no, and you may decide to end the conversation with "Don't try to make me feel guilty. I told you I care about you, but I will not say yes this time. I said no. I mean no. End of discussion."

# PRACTICE LEADS TO ACTION

As discussed in the beginning of the chapter, bullying has been defined[4,5] and specifically linked with resultant medical errors in patient care within a variety of health care enviornments.[6-8] Bullying in health care settings has been identified as an international problem,[31–42] with guidelines to address bullying now being provided by professional societies to address and assist in mitigating the problem.[6–8,42] In a qualitative study of eight final-year physiotherapy students in the United Kingdom, only one of the eight subjects reported experiencing a specific incident of abusive bullying on clinical internship.[40] In the United Kingdom study, four main themes were identified by the researchers:[40]

> *(1) external and situational influences of bullying; (2) students' reactions to the experience of bullying; (3) inability to reveal the experience; and (4) overcoming problems. Bullying had a range of adverse effects on the students, with many expressing self-doubt in their competence and viewing their supervisor as unapproachable and unsupportive. Five students were not initially able to recognize the experience as bullying. In addition, students did not feel able to report the experience and use the support mechanisms in place. This may have been a result of having concerns that the problem would escalate if they reported the experience and, as a consequence, have a negative effect on their grade. Students were keen to offer a range of strategies for clinical practice in order to prevent bullying for future generations of students.*

The authors concluded, "students' health, security, and confidence in their ability as a physiotherapist can be at great risk from bullying. Support is needed to ensure students are better protected from bullying and feel able to address bullying behavior during clinicals."[40]

Through reading this chapter on appropriate assertive behavior, you now have the tools to confront bullying and stop it before it becomes an insurmountable concern. You will also realize the importance of assertive communication as a means for stress management to impede burnout and alleviate challenges to moral integrity and promote a culture of safety, so that we don't become complicit, provide suboptimal care, and potentially cause harm.[43] Encouraging yourself, supervisors, and organizations to support rest, recovery, and refuge is a measure to assert to defend HCPs' moral integrity.[43–46] Utilize your newly acquired DISC and DESC assertive behavior skills to confront potentially abusive behaviors in an appropriately assertive manner.

A student recently contacted me regarding some "mild" concerns that her clinical instructor might be being a bit inappropriate. She was not sure, and was reaching out for support. In her description, she relayed that her instructor had made her uncomfortable with some of his statements on several occasions. I asked her to describe the statements. She revealed that the instructor said, "Your hair looks better brown than blonde" when he was examining her identification badge with respect to her current hair color. Then, a few days later, after walking through an area of construction within the hospital grounds, he said, "You look hot in that construction hat." Finally, while walking to the parking garage together, he said, "Let's have dinner together sometime and we can discuss your cases."

After debriefing, the student felt that, overall, the clinical experience was going well and she was learning a lot from the instructor with the patient encounters, but she was beginning to become quite concerned and rather uncomfortable at times regarding the instructor's comments. He was a married man with children, and she felt the comments were completely inappropriate. She was correct and was instructed to implement her DESC response of assertive communication. She practiced the response with me and successfully relayed her concerns to the clinical instructor. The clinical instructor responded appropriately and received the constructive critique in the manner intended. The clinical instructor immediately adjusted his behavior and communication and apologized to the student, without further interventions required. In follow-up, the student no longer felt uncomfortable and had no further issues or matters of concern. She did have lunch in the hospital cafeteria with her clinical instructor to debrief following her midterm review, in an area that was not within earshot of others but was within eyesight of others. She successfully completed her internship, met all learning goals, and accomplished additional abilities in her forthright and appropriate assertive communication with her supervising instructor. Imagine if the student had not elected to report and take appropriate action.

Bullying has been described as the sexual harassment of this era.[4] Do not be one who allows any type of bullying to thrive. Trust yourself that you have the ability to address bullying behavior, whether it is your being subject to inappropriate language (cussing, foul language) by someone ranting and raving or your being purposefully embarrassed in front of others by those charged to provide constructive feedback. You should no longer just ignore bullying behavior, yet appropriately confront the abuse or potentially abusive behavior so that it does not escalate, and the workplace is healthier for you, the rehab team, and the patients/clients we serve. Remember that, as a student, you are in a partnership with the clinical affiliate and the university or school, and you should seek support in the process for the important conversations that need to occur in a professional manner. Seek additional counseling and support services and security measures to be taken, if needed.

The following exercises begin with self-awareness about your own tendencies to respond passively or aggressively in certain situations. The exercises proceed into opportunities for you to practice assertive communication with your classmates in role-playing situations.

Don't forget to journal about the impact that the readings and exercises have on you. How does all of this make you feel? For some of you, at first your new behavior will feel awkward and disingenuous. For many of us, we have overlearned the feelings that accompany low self-esteem and need to dramatically break up harmful, reactive behaviors to false beliefs, so assertive communication may be particularly challenging for you. Practice. Ideally, we could all experience the necessary inner transformations quickly and congruently. Life is a bit more complex, so start the process from outside-in rather than from inside-out. The goal is the same. The outer behavior, as inauthentic as it feels—for example, to be equal to a physician or experienced colleague—is still in everyone's best interest. Function as if you have every one of those rights, and eventually you will accept it as the truth. Act as you believe someone you admire would act in this situation. Soon you will feel the inner confidence needed to ensure authentic assertive and kind behavior under the greatest of stress. Believe in yourself; imagine your success and it will come quickly.

# REFERENCES

1. United States Bureau of Labor & Statistics. *Injuries, Illness & Fatalities.* 2020. Available: https://www.bls.gov/iif/oshwc/osh/case/ostb4760.pdf Accessed May 1, 2021.
2. National Institute of Occupational Safety and Health, Centers for Disease Control. *Occupational Violence.* August 2021. https://www.cdc.gov/niosh/violence/about/?CDC_AAref_Val=https://www.cdc.gov/niosh/topics/violence/default.html Accessed October 30, 2024.
3. Jana T, Baran M. *Subtle Acts of Exclusion: How to Understand, Identify, and Stop Microaggressions.* Oakland, CA: Berrett Koehler Publishers; 2020.
4. The Workplace Bullying Institute. *The WBI Definition of Workplace Bullying.* https://workplacebullying.org/. Accessed June 15, 2015.
5. Raynor C, Hoel H. A summary review of literature relating to workplace bullying. *J Community Appl Soc Psych.* 1997;7:181–191.
6. American Nurses Association (ANA). Violence, Incivility, & Bullying in the Work Environment. 2019. https://www.nursingworld.org/practice-policy/nursing-excellence/official-position-statements/id/incivility-bullying-and-workplace-violence/. Accessed May 15, 2022.
7. The Joint Commission. Behaviors that undermine a culture of safety. *Sentinel Event Alert,* Issue 40. June 2021. https://www.jointcommission.org/-/media/tjc/documents/resources/patient-safety-topics/sentinel-event/sea-40-intimidating-disruptive-behaviors-final2.pdf. Accessed June 21, 2021.
8. Healthy Workplace Bill. https://healthyworkplacebill.org/. Accessed May 1, 2021.
9. Daniel TA. Bullies in the workplace: a focus on the "abusive disrespect" of employees. https://thepeoplegroup.com/wp-content/uploads/2008/04/article-bullies-in-the-workplace1.pdf. Accessed March 1, 2021.
10. Vaughn L. *Bioethics Principles, Issues and Cases,* 4th ed. New York: Oxford University Press; 2019.
11. Dean W, Talbot S, Dean A. Reframing clinician distress: moral injury not burnout. *Fed Pract.* 2019 Sep;36(9):400–402. Erratum in: *Fed Pract.* 2019 Oct;36(10):447. PMID: 31571807; PMCID: PMC6752815.
12. Altaker KW, Howie-Esquivel J, Cataldo JK. Relationships among palliative care, ethical climate, empowerment, and moral distress in intensive care unit nurses. *Am J Crit Care.* 2018 Jul;27(4):295–302. doi: 10.4037/ajcc2018252. PMID: 29961665.
13. Shay J. Moral injury. *Psychoanal Psych.* 2014;31(2):182–191.
14. Al Jazeera Media Network. Wener J, Dean W. *Burned Out Doctors or Broken Healthcare System.* February 20, 2020. Available: https://www.aljazeera.com/program/the-stream/2020/2/20/burned-out-doctors-or-broken-healthcare-system. Accessed March 1, 2020.
15. Dale LP, Cuffe SP, Sambuco N, Guastello AD, Leon KG, Nunez LV, Bhullar A, Allen BR, Mathews CA. Morally Distressing Experiences, Moral Injury, and Burnout in Florida Healthcare Providers during the COVID-19 Pandemic. *Int J Env Res and Pub Health.* 2021;18(23):12319. doi: 10.3390/ijerph182312319.
16. Litz BT, Stein N, Delaney E, Lebowitz L, Nash WP, Silva, C, Maguen S. Moral injury and moral repair in war veterans: a preliminary model and intervention strategy. *Clin Psychol Rev.* 2009;29:695–706.
17. Čartolovni A, Stolt M, Scott PA, Suhonen R. Moral injury in healthcare professionals: a scoping review and discussion. *Nurs Ethics.* 2021 Aug;28(5):590–602.
18. Timmins F, McCabe C. Nurses' and midwives' assertive behaviour in the workplace. *J Adv Nurs.* 2005;51(1):38–45.
19. Friedman FB. A nurse's guide to the care and handling of MDs. *RN.* 1982;45(3):39–43,118–120.
20. Bosher S, Smalkoski K. From needs analysis to curriculum development: designing a course in health care communication for immigrant students in the USA. *English for Specific Purposes.* 2002;21:59–79.
21. Merriam-Webster Online Dictionary, 2022. www.merriam-webster.com. Accessed May 1, 2022.
22. Chenevert M. *STAT: Special Techniques in Assertiveness Training for Women in Health Professions,* 4th ed. St. Louis, MO: CV Mosby; 1993.
23. Alberti RE, Emmons ML. *Your Perfect Right,* 9th ed. San Luis Obispo, CA: Impact Publishers; 2008.
24. Anderson C, Jennings DL. When experiences of failure promote expectations of success: the impact of attributing failure to ineffective strategies. *J Pers.* 1980;48(3):393–407.

25. Weiner B. Attribution theory and attributional therapy: some theoretical observations and suggestions. *Br J Clin Psychol.* 1988;27(pt 1):93–104.

26. Curtis K. Altering beliefs about the importance of strategy: an attributional intervention. *J Appl Soc Psychol.* 1992;22(12):953–972.

27. Bower SA, Bower GH. *Asserting Yourself: A Practical Guide for Positive Change.* Boston, MA: DeCapo Press; 2004.

28. Silber M. Managing confrontations: once more into the breach. *Nurs Manage.* 1984;15(4):54–58.

29. Allaire B, McNeil R. *Teaching Patient Relations in Hospitals: The Hows and Whys.* Chicago, IL: American Hospital Association; 1983.

30. Lin YR, Shiah IS, Chang YC, Lai TJ, Want KY, Chou KR. Evaluation of an assertiveness training program on nursing and medical students' assertiveness, self-esteem and interpersonal communication. *Nurse Educ Today.* 2004;24(8):656–665.

31. Stubbs B, Soundy A. Physiotherapy students' experiences of bullying on clinical internships: an exploratory study. *Physiotherapy.* 2013;99(2):178–180.

32. Askew DA, Schluter PJ, Dick ML, Régo PM, Turner C, Wilkinson D. Bullying in the Australian medical workforce: cross-sectional data from an Australian e-Cohort study. *Aust Health Rev.* 2012;36:197–204.

33. Crutcher RA, Szafran O, Woloschuk W, Chatur F, Hansen C. Family medicine graduates' perceptions of intimidation, harassment, and discrimination during residency training. *BMC Med Educ.* 2011;11:88.

34. Bairy KL, Thirumalaikolundusubramanian P, Sivagnanam G, Saraswathi S, Sachidananda A, Shalini A. Bullying among trainee doctors in Southern India: a questionnaire study. *J Postgrad Med.* 2007;53:87–90.

35. Frank E, Carrera JS, Stratton T, Bickel J, Nora LM. Experiences of belittlement and harassment and their correlates among medical students in the United States: longitudinal survey. *BMJ.* 2006;333:682.

36. Ahmer SYA, Bhutto N, Alam S, Sarangzai AK, Iqbal A. Bullying medical students in Pakistan: a cross-sectional questionnaire survey. *PLoS One.* 2008;3:e3889.

37. Mukhtar F, Daud S, Manzoor I, et al. Bullying of medical students. *J Coll Physicians Surg.* 2010;20:814–818.

38. Department of Health. *Bullying of Staff within the National Health Services Trust.* London: Department of Health; 2008.

39. Cheema S, Ahmad K, Giri SK, Kaliaperumal VK, Naqvi SA. Bullying of junior doctors prevails in Irish health system: a bitter reality. *Irish Med J.* 2005;98:274–275.

40. Whiteside D, Stubbs B, Soundy A. Physiotherapy students' experiences of bullying on clinical internships: a qualitative study. *Physiotherapy.* 2014;100(1):41–46.

41. Ross MH, Hammond J, Bezner J, Brown D, Wright A, Chipchase L, Miciak M, Whittaker JL, Setchell J. An exploration of the experiences of physical therapists who identify as LGBTQIA+: navigating sexual orientation and gender identity in clinical, academic, and professional roles. *Phys Ther.* 2022;102(3): pzab280. doi: 10.1093/ptj/pzab280.

42. Chartered Society of Physiotherapy. *Dealing with Bullying: A Guide for Physiotherapy Students on Clinical Placement.* London: Chartered Society of Physiotherapy; 2010.

43. Archer CA. Expanding moral injury: why resilience training won't fix it. *JAMA.* 2022;328(12):1199–1200. doi: 10.1001/jama.2022.15721.

44. Best J. Undermined and undervalued: how the pandemic exacerbated moral injury and burnout in the NHS. *BMJ.* 2021; 374:n1858. doi: 10.1136/bmj.n1858.

45. Pathman DE, Sonis J, Rauner TE, et al. Moral distress among clinicians working in US safety net practices during the COVID-19 pandemic: a mixed methods study. *BMJ Open.* 2022;12:e061369. doi: 10.1136/bmjopen-2022-061369.

46. Dean W. *If I Betray There Words: Moral Injury In Medicine And Why It's So Hard for Clinicians To Put Patients First.* Lebanon, NH: Steerforth Press; 2024.

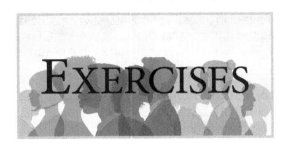

# EXERCISE 1: SELF-AWARENESS: ASSERTIVENESS INVENTORY

Complete the Assertiveness Inventory from Alberti and Emmons's *Your Perfect Right*.[23] As directed at the bottom of the survey, circle the three statements that most often result in your giving up your power and becoming passive or so angry that you become aggressive.

1. Look at your responses to questions 1, 2, 4, 5, 6, 7, 9, 10, 11, 12, 14, 15, 16, 17, 18, 19, 21, 22, 24, 25, 27, 28, 30, and 35. These questions are oriented toward nonassertive behavior. Are you rarely speaking up for yourself? Or is there one situation that gives you more trouble than the others? If so, journal about it starting with the earliest memories you have about that incident.

2. Look at your responses to questions 3, 8, 13, 20, 23, 26, 29, 31, 32, 33, and 34. These questions are oriented toward aggressive behavior. Are you pushing others around more than you realized? Does one question give you more trouble than the others? Again, journal about it.

3. Few people are assertive, aggressive, or passive all the time. The situation often dictates the response. On rereading your total responses, do you see a pattern? Do you favor one way of responding over the others? Draw some conclusions about yourself from the inventory and journal about them. Which situations cause you the most trouble? Which situations do you handle with no trouble at all? Why is that?

4. Can you identify obstacles that stand in the way of asserting yourself confidently? What beliefs do you hold about yourself and the world that make it difficult or easy to assert yourself? What is the worst thing that could happen? Journal about your learning.

5. Ask family members and trusted friends to give you honest and specific feedback about their observations of your behavior under stress. Do you show patterns of passivity or aggressiveness? Ask them to illustrate their points with examples. Resist the natural desire to defend yourself as they respond. Just listen and take notes, then journal about what you learned and about your feelings.

# ASSERTIVENESS INVENTORY

The following questions will be helpful in assessing your assertiveness. Be honest in your responses. All you have to do is draw a circle around the number that describes you best. For some questions, the assertive end of the scale is at 0, for others at 4. Key: 0=no or never, 1=somewhat or sometimes, 2=average, 3=usually or a good deal, 4=practically always or entirely.

1.  When a person is highly unfair, do you call it to their attention?.................................................0  1  2  3  4
2.  Do you find it difficult to make decisions?.....................................................................................0  1  2  3  4
3.  Are you openly critical of others' ideas, opinions, behavior?....................................................0  1  2  3  4
4.  Do you speak out in protest when someone takes your place in line?.....................................0  1  2  3  4
5.  Do you often avoid people or situations for fear of embarrassment?.....................................0  1  2  3  4
6.  Do you usually have confidence in your own judgment?.............................................................0  1  2  3  4
7.  Do you insist that your spouse or roommate take on a fair share of household chores?.........0  1  2  3  4
8.  Are you prone to "fly off the handle"?.............................................................................................0  1  2  3  4
9.  When a salesperson makes an effort, do you find it hard to say "no" even though the merchandise is not really what you want?.....................................................................................0  1  2  3  4
10. When a latecomer is waited on before you are, do you call attention to the situation?............0  1  2  3  4
11. Are you reluctant to speak up in a discussion or debate?...........................................................0  1  2  3  4
12. If a person has borrowed money or a book/garment/thing of value and is overdue in returning it, do you mention it?.................................................................................................0  1  2  3  4
13. Do you continue to pursue an argument after the other person has had enough?...................0  1  2  3  4
14. Do you generally express what you feel?.........................................................................................0  1  2  3  4
15. Are you disturbed if someone watches you at work?...................................................................0  1  2  3  4
16. If someone seems to be kicking or bumping your chair in a movie or a lecture, do you ask the person to stop?.........................................................................................................................0  1  2  3  4
17. Do you find it difficult to keep eye contact when talking to another person?.........................0  1  2  3  4
18. In a good restaurant, when your meal is improperly prepared or served, do you ask the waiter/waitress to correct the situation?...............................................................................0  1  2  3  4
19. When you discover merchandise is faulty, do you return it for an adjustment?.......................0  1  2  3  4
20. Do you show your anger by name-calling or obscenities?..........................................................0  1  2  3  4
21. Do you try to be a wallflower or a piece of the furniture in social situations?........................0  1  2  3  4
22. Do you insist that your landlord/mechanic/repairperson make repairs, adjustments, or replacements that are their responsibility?.......................................................................................0  1  2  3  4
23. Do you often step in and make decisions for others?..................................................................0  1  2  3  4
24. Are you able to openly express love and affection?.....................................................................0  1  2  3  4
25. Are you able to ask your friends for small favors or help?..........................................................0  1  2  3  4
26. Do you think you always have the right answer?...........................................................................0  1  2  3  4
27. When you differ with a person you respect, are you able to speak up for your own viewpoint?...0  1  2  3  4
28. Are you able to refuse unreasonable requests made by friends?..............................................0  1  2  3  4
29. Do you have difficulty complimenting or praising others?..........................................................0  1  2  3  4
30. If you are disturbed by someone smoking near you, can you say so?.......................................0  1  2  3  4
31. Do you shout or use bullying tactics to get others to do as you wish?.....................................0  1  2  3  4
32. Do you finish other people's sentences for them?.......................................................................0  1  2  3  4
33. Do you get into physical fights with others, especially with strangers?...................................0  1  2  3  4
34. At family meals, do you control the conversation?.......................................................................0  1  2  3  4
35. When you meet a stranger, are you the first to introduce yourself and begin a conversation?...0  1  2  3  4

Now go back and circle the 3 statements that most often result in you giving up your powers and becoming passive or that anger you so much you become aggressive.

(Reprinted with permission from Alberti RE, Emmons ML. *Your Perfect Right*. 2nd ed. San Luis Obispo, CA: Impact Publishers; 1974.)

# EXERCISE 2: ASSERTIVE, AGGRESSIVE, AND PASSIVE RESPONSES

Practice making responses to the following situations. The first situation is done for you as an example.

## *Saying No*

The head nurse stops you on the floor as you are just about to evaluate a new patient. "Mr. Johnson needs to be supervised in the use of his walker as he goes to the bathroom, and none of us have time. I wonder if you'd mind walking with him right now."

1. Passive: "Well, I'm very busy, but if he has to go right now, I suppose I can help."

2. Aggressive: "Look, I taught him how to use that walker. It's your job to supervise him in bathroom activity. I've got a patient to evaluate, and I don't appreciate your inconsiderate views of the value of my time."

3. Assertive: "No, I can't do that right now. Mrs. Adams is able to help him, as can his family members. I have a new evaluation that can't wait."

## *Making Requests*

It's the end of the day and you have three more patients to evaluate before leaving. You're going to need some help or you'll be working very late. How do you ask for it?

1. Passive:

2. Aggressive:

3. Assertive:

## *Expressing Opinions*

An edict comes down from above that all staff must treat at least four "units" of patient care per hour. You feel that this is unreasonable and interferes with establishing a therapeutic presence with your patients. How do you respond?

1. Passive:

2. Aggressive:

3. Assertive:

## *Initiating Conversation*

You're attending a workshop and you've always wanted to talk with the speaker about a topic of great interest to you. You feel shy and somewhat intimidated by the speaker and his reputation.

1. Passive:

2. Aggressive:

3. Assertive:

## Self-Disclosing

Your parents are amid a year-long divorce battle that has brought great grief to your younger brother. Last night, he called you and spoke of thoughts of suicide. They live far away, and you feel frightened and helpless. At work, you seem distracted and upset. A friend asks, "Is there anything wrong? You seem preoccupied today."

1. Passive:

2. Aggressive:

3. Assertive:

## Expressing Affection

A patient who you have been working with is being discharged. You go to the room, and his family is there packing to help him move back home. He asks to speak to you privately and takes your hand and thanks you for everything you've done for him and gives you a warm hug.

1. Passive:

2. Aggressive:

3. Assertive:

## Entering a Room of Strangers

You've just moved to a new city to begin your first position after graduating. A new colleague invites you over for a party. You walk into the apartment and you realize you do not know one person in the room except the host. Everyone else seems to have known each other for years. No one is dressed the way you are.

1. Passive:

2. Aggressive:

3. Assertive:

Reflect in your journal which of these situations was easiest for you to envision handling assertively and which was most difficult. Which responses were easiest to come up with? Do you find that how you might respond has very much to do with your perception of the stress inherent in the situation?

Now, for further insights, appraise your style or approach to conflict by completing the Conflict Management Style Assessment, via: www.blake-group.com/sites/default/files/assessments/Conflict_Management_Styles_Assessment.pdf.

# EXERCISE 3: ASSERTIVE COMMUNICATION

In this chapter, you learned about DISC and DESC communication. Now you have a chance to role-play various assertive responses to the following vignettes. Before role-playing, however, you are asked to write the DISC or DESC response. The HCP or student is in the assertive response position; the other person should use this opportunity to practice the active listening skills learned in Chapter 8. A third person serves as the observer, giving feedback at the end of the dialogue on the effectiveness of the communication. Use the Observer Response Guidance that follows to jot down your observations as they occur. Each person should choose an appropriate vignette and write a DISC or DESC statement before breaking up into groups of three. For each vignette, write a DESC response and then role-play practicing the DESC/DISC communication.

## Vignette 1

You are a student on your first of two final clinical assignments. The clinical facility is very high-powered, with a superior reputation. You feel that, no matter what you do, you could never achieve the level that is expected of the staff. You truly feel that you're doing your best, but you are under constant stress to prove yourself. You are to be checked out on a knee evaluation, but you've forgotten some of the basic steps, and you've asked for help from the orthopedic star of the staff, who always says, "Yes, but I'm too busy. Catch me tomorrow." Your clinical instructor stops you as you are ready to go home and relax at the end of the day and says, "I've let you off the hook long enough. You should be proficient in that knee evaluation by now. Come with me and let me check you out."

## Vignette 2

You are a clinical instructor. You've observed your student for three weeks and feel that she may be weak in evaluation skills, and you feel that she is not taking the assignment seriously. When you suggest a check-off session, your student always asks for more time. Yet all you hear is talk about lots of parties and after-hours fun, and you notice a real reluctance to read or show initiative in looking things up or asking for help. You think she might be trying to squeeze through without the appropriate amount of responsibility. You've decided to confront your student and ask for check-off on a knee evaluation.

## Vignette 3

You've just accepted a position at a health care facility that also has an active student program. The staff seems to ignore the dress regulations, and everyone wears what they wish, so you decide you will wear what you wish as well and come to work in comfortable clothes: hip-huggers and a tunic top. Your supervisor tells you to go home and change your clothes and come back in the "regulation uniform." You decide to confront them.

## Vignette 4

In the middle of a treatment, your patient, a young and rather seductive member grabs your arm and tells you that they have very strong sexual feelings for you and wonders if you might meet privately at the end of the day.

## Vignette 5

You are a professional on the staff for more than a year. You still lack skill in one treatment technique that an aide knows how to do flawlessly. In front of the patient, the aide comes up to you and chastises you for not knowing how to do even the simplest procedures. You are embarrassed and decide to confront the aide.

## Vignette 6

Your colleague, who always takes advantage of others, comes up to you in front of a patient and asks you to cover for them because they must make an important phone call. Your colleague then disappears and does not return for 2 hours. When they return, you decide to confront them.

# Vignette 7

You are instructing a woman in pelvic stabilization exercises, and the patient is having difficulty recruiting her lower abdominals and pelvic floor. Suddenly, the patient begins to cry, saying that her back hurts so much that she and her partner have not been able to be intimate for 6 months and she feels as if her partner no longer desires her. How do you respond? (Hint: Resist the common desire to fix patient's problems and remember active listening skills.)

# Vignette 8

Your supervisor notices that you are taking longer than is common for a patient treatment with one of your patients who had a stroke. Your supervisor suggests you delegate the care of this patient to an assistant. You believe the patient requires the attention of a professional. What do you say?

# Vignette 9

## KYLE

Chuck has been your clinical instructor/fieldwork supervisor for the past 4 weeks on your final clinical education internship and has already identified you as a potential for some opportunities at the hospital in the future. Chuck is easy to work with and has given you a great deal of autonomy. You feel comfortable making your own decisions and are quite satisfied with your style of patient care management. You are happy to be entering practice in a few months.

## CHUCK

You are Kyle's instructor, and you are pleased with Kyle's overall progress and patient care. However, lately you have noticed that Kyle has been letting his long hair and facial hair become excessive. Even though he pulls his hair back in a ponytail for patient care, you noticed it getting caught up in the patient's underarm when he was instructing the patient with crutch training and again when he was doing shoulder mobilizations. Kyle's beard has grown out excessively, and some of your coworkers say he is looking "criminal." How can you, as his clinical instructor, confront Kyle using the DESC/DISC method to assure that he understands not only the safety and hygiene factors but also the consequences in terms of his professionalism ratings?

# Vignette 10

Your student, LaTonya, has just decided to poke the patient in intermediate care with her long fingernails to check for pain sensation. You recommend to your student that she use monofilaments for testing sensory status. The recommendation was not accepted. Later, after lunch, you overhear LaTonya gossiping about another staff member in a negative light to other students in a disrespectful manner. Use the DESC/DISC to confront the student and effect a change.

# Vignette 11

While ambulating and conducting balance training with a patient with Parkinson's Disease that is at risk for falls, your clinical instructor (licensed supervisor) does not want you (student) to utilize a gait belt in order to simulate real-time environments. You recommend that you think you should utilize a gait belt due to associated fall risks, claims data, and to assure you are challenging the patient to their greatest abilities while keeping them safe. Use the DESC/DISC to address your position with your clinical instructor to effect a change and potential compromise.

# Vignette 12

Review your responses from the Assertiveness Inventory in Exercise 1. Create a vignette that typifies a situation that is predictably problematic for you. Teach your partner how to act in a way that is sure to elicit passive or aggressive behavior from you. Then write a DISC or DESC response and role-play.

## Observer Response Guidance

As an observer, your role is to facilitate a dialogue that has an adequate assertive response. The dialogue may begin with the aggressor making the statement that requires the assertive response, or it may begin with time having elapsed since the incident and the assertive response is occurring now. Keep track of time and keep the interchange to 2 or 3 minutes. At the conclusion, ask the assertive responder how they feel and then ask the other partner the same. Proceed to give feedback to both on these various aspects of their communication.

1.  How well did the assertive communicator:

    a.  Communicate using "I" statements and DISC or DESC responses?

    b.  Stay nonaggressive, nonjudgmental, and nonaccusatory?

    c.  Listen and respond in an assertive way to the other's response?

2.  How well did the aggressor use active listening skills and still stay in character?

3.  How would you suggest each could improve their communication?

## EXERCISE 4: REFLECTIVE RUMINATIONS

Take a moment now to review the following website for new learning related to moral injury: www.fixmoralinjury.org Next, share with a partner what you discovered, then exchange your favorite app for coping with stress.

**These exercises are also available online at www.routledge.com/9781638220039.**

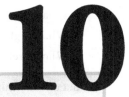

# READINESS FOR REFLECTIVE PRACTICE

## PEER AND SELF-ASSESSMENT

*Gina Maria Musolino*

## OBJECTIVES

*The learner should be able to*:

- Discover the concept of self-assessment (SA) and reflective practice (RP) theories.

- Apply and practice self-assessment and peer assessment (PA) to facilitate RP.

- Contrast the barriers, challenges, and support for peer and self-assessment.

- Explore students' awareness and perceptions of reflective practice, self-assessment, and peer assessment cap-abilities as determinants for development as a health care professional (HCP).

- Appreciate the professional responsibilities and gifts of peer and self-assessment, along with potential impacts for patient care and development toward expertise in practice.

- Consider career development and lifelong learning opportunities, in relation to peer and self-assessment, including the role of clinical education instruction.

## YOUR THOUGHTS AND ASSUMPTIONS

Let's start by considering if you agree or disagree, and why or why not, with this statement by a Greek philosopher who is often considered the founding father of Western philosophy:

*An unexamined life is not worth living. —Socrates*

Now, thinking about peer and self-assessment, jot down or share your thoughts and assumptions for the following queries:

- What is self-assessment? Peer assessment?

- Why should you consider doing self-assessment? Peer assessment?

DOI: 10.4324/9781003525554-10

- What might be some of the challenges and barriers to doing self-assessment? Peer assessment?
- What might be some of the support and rewards for doing self-assessment? Peer assessment?
- What is reflective practice?

What does a health care professional (HCP) need to know about reflective practice (RP) to develop one? Is any HCP able to be a reflective practitioner? How can merely reflecting on one's work improve practice? How does the theory of RP relate to the profession's values and professional codes of ethics, which you learned about in Chapter 3?

# REFLECTIVE PRACTICE: CONCEPTS

When the concept of RP is first encountered, many wonder why it is of value or worth taking the time and energy to complete. Initially, you may find this novel, foreign, esoteric, or just plain peculiar or strange. The concepts of self-assessment and tenets of RP theories do not necessarily match with how you think you should be taught or learn. Many think that being a clinician is all about knowing skills and applying techniques.

Certainly, appropriate skill levels and proper techniques are needed and required elements for professional practice; however, how we arrive at the best choices for our evidence-based practice skills and become more proficient with our techniques are what distinguish us from nonprofessionals. To become the best health care professional, this is a matter of RP. Try to be open-minded because becoming less reliant on traditional, passive teaching as an emerging HCP and enhancing your self-assessment abilities as a developing reflective HCP will lead to expertise in practice sooner rather than later for the willing health care professional. Reflective practice leads to improved academic performance and enhanced metacognitive skills for a novice health care professional, which benefits your patients' clinical outcomes.[1–7]

Remember to be journaling along the way as you develop your RP abilities as a new HCP. In relation to RP, cogitate on the key words of Sir William Osler (1849–1919), Canadian medical physician and founder of Johns Hopkins Hospital, who stated that when education is done right, the learner "begins with the patient, continues with the patient, and ends with the patient," reiterating the need, today, for evidence-informed practice with the patient at the center of collaborative care. How can we develop as reflective practitioners striving for expertise?

Let's look more closely at the concepts and tenets of self-assessment and examine the theories of RP. Osterman and Kottkamp[8] defined the purpose of reflection as twofold: "(1) to initiate a behavioral change, and (2) to realize an improvement in professional practice." Kirby and Teddlie[9] defined a reflective practitioner as one who has:

> the ability to integrate research with practice in response to uncertainty and complexity that, citing, according to Russell and Spafford,[10] qualifies the practitioner for professional status. This theory is vital to occupations where theory is incomplete or where multiple, even conflicting theories confront the practitioner.

Does the definition of a reflective practitioner match up with your profession? The theory and tenets of RP have been examined and continue to be studied in the professions of architecture, art, teaching, law, medicine, nursing, physical and occupational therapy, pharmacy, dentistry, etc. According to Brookfield,[11] the concept of RP is defined as:

> Rooted in the Enlightenment idea that we can stand outside of ourselves and come to a clearer understanding of what we do and who we are by freeing ourselves of distorted ways of reasoning and acting. There are also elements of constructivist phenomenology in the understanding that identity and experience are culturally and personally sculpted, rather than existing in some kind of objectively discoverable limbo.

Hence, RP is not a passive process but an active one that challenges us to see ourselves as others see us. As reflective practitioners, we are challenged to think about what we do and how we act, to consider alternatives and reason through the possibilities, and to consider options while simultaneously noting environmental and cultural influences.

Dewey,[12] an American philosopher, psychologist, and educational and social reformist, purported reflection as a cognitive activity that begins in perplexity and "forked-road" situations but is an active, persistent, and careful consideration of any belief or knowledge. Dewey[12] first identified reflection as a cognitive activity with five stages of reflective thought:

1. Perplexity, confusion, doubt
2. Attentive interpretation of the given elements
3. Examination, exploration, and analysis to define and clarify the problem
4. Elaboration of the tentative hypothesis
5. Testing the hypothesis by doing something overtly to bring about anticipated results

The cognitive activity of reflection includes a responsibility for future consequences and is retrospective and progressive. Osterman and Kottkamp[8] shared six key assumptions for RP:

1. Everyone, regardless of age, stage, or attitude, needs professional growth opportunities

2. All professionals have a natural desire to want to improve

3. All professionals want to learn

4. All professionals are capable of assuming responsibility for their own professional growth and development

5. All people need and want information about their performance

6. Collaboration with other professionals enriches one's professional development

Kolb[13] advanced reflection a step further and noted that reflection should be to take action to a new and changed behavior. Kolb detailed this concept in the experiential learning profile, where a learner flows through a cycle of **experiencing, reflecting, thinking**, and **acting** (formerly categorized as learning style preferences of concrete experiences, reflective observation, abstract conceptualization, and active experimentation). Kolb's[13] experiential learning profile (KELP) approach provides the opportunity for input and processing of information, from each learner's unique perspective. Kolb described how learners reflect on experiences, learn from these experiences, then try out what they have learned and cycle through again on subsequent practice attempts, leading to enhanced metacognition through reflection activities. Oftentimes, we may get hung up in one aspect of the cycle, and need to further adapt, and that is where it is of benefit to consult with colleagues or those who think differently from our preferred style or approach to learning (see Chapter 11 resources for links to learning preferences and style).

# REFLECTIVE PRACTICE: METHODS AND MODELS

Why is this critical reflection so important? Brookfield[11] asserted that it helps professionals to make informed decisions and take informed actions and to develop a rationale for practice. Brookfield[11] believed that it "helps professionals avoid self-laceration, serves for emotional grounds, enlivens professional practices, and increases democratic trust." The importance was elaborated on by Donald Schön,[14,15] an influential thinker who developed the theory of RP for professional learning in the twentieth century. He asserted that managing the complexity is the challenge for the reflective practitioner.[14,15] He also maintained that a reflective practitioner has an unprecedented requirement for adaptability and is cognizant of the tension between theory and practice.[15] Schön alluded to the balance of the art and science in the health professions.[14,15] Schön[14,15] believed in the RP concepts of *reflection-in-action, knowing-in-action, reflection-on-action*, and *recognizing surprise* in terms of professional work interactions. These frameworks serve us effectively to foster RP abilities. We can reflect within these frameworks and ask ourselves guiding questions to facilitate our abilities in RP using the tenets of theory as a guide (e.g., "How do you think that went while you were performing the technique?").

- **Reflection-in-action**: As you performed the grade I to grade II mobilizations, you realized, based on prior experience with mobilization and on the patient's response and joint movement perceived, that you could proceed with the next level of mobilization and moved readily to grade III without hesitation.

How did you know that you would get the expected result from the technique?

- **Knowing-in-action**: As you performed rhythmic stabilization with the patient, how did you know that the technique would illicit the outcome you expected?

How do you think you did? Did you get the outcomes you were hoping for with the techniques? What could you have done differently? Is there another approach?

- **Reflection-on-action**: Over the weekend, while taking your morning swim, you are thinking back about the patient you worked with last Thursday. You realized that you could likely have reached her better by using a visual approach to her learning when instructing her in the home exercise program and that you may have overloaded her with too much written information. You forgot to ask her about her preferred learning style in her history, but you recalled how well she responded when you first demonstrated proper lifting techniques, first showing her, and then allowing her to repeat-demonstrate to you the proper technique.

How could you have done better? What is going well? How can you progress from here?

Schön[15] stated that "good practice generates new knowledge." He looked critically at how a professional readjusts in day-to-day practice as key for development.[14,15] Hatcher and Bringle[16] echoed Schön's[14,15] sentiments, with clear linkages to self-assessment. They noted that reflection activities develop self-assessment skills, as a lifelong learner, and explore and clarify values that can lead to civic responsibility. They believed reflection activities serve to "engage students in the intentional consideration of their experiences in light of particular learning objectives and provide an opportunity for students to do the following:

- Gain further understanding of the course content and discipline;
- Gain further understanding of the service experience;
- Develop self-assessment skills, as a life-long learner; and
- Explore and clarify values that can lead to civic responsibility."

The reflection activities incorporate learning from experiences in society, such as through clinical and fieldwork education, in the health professions, and service-learning activities that meet objectives for those served and the learners. Eyler et al.[17] considered the "4 Cs of reflection" as viable activities for the development of RP, including the following:

1. Continuous reflection
2. Connected reflection
3. Challenging reflection
4. Conceptualized reflection

Likewise, Williams and Driscoll[18] proposed the following guidelines for facilitating reflection: "Structured as ongoing aspects of a course (or clinical), offered in multiple forms, included in assessment, modeled by the instructor, connected to the course content, and supported by class context." Not surprisingly, RP was favored by medical interns as a self-assessment and critical evaluation process; through deep analyses of events, with an aim to learn from experiences, and ultimately make changes in their perceptions or behaviors.[19] RP focuses on lifelong learning of the developing practitioner and development of professional identity through reflection. Reflection is utilized to inform education, clinical practice, and professional growth.[20]

Hatcher and Bringle[16] offered the following examples of reflection activities: personal journals, directed readings and writings, case studies with guiding questions, portfolios with self-assessments, rubrics with self-assessment techniques, experiential research, service-learning with opportunities for reflection, and personal narratives. Dressler et al.[21] also discovered that utilizing Tweet-style (HIPAA compliant) reflective writing aided learners in surgical clerkships to reflect on both positive and challenging patient–practitioner interactions, education, teams, and future careers potentials. Boyd et al.[22] also discovered that dialogic discussion and critically reflective writing further promote RP with interprofessional groups of student learners in medicine, speech-language pathology, and occupational therapy.

Osterman and Kottkamp[8] defined RP as a "professional development strategy designed to enable professionals to change their behavior, thereby improving the quality of their performance." They contended that RP is neither a solitary nor a relaxed meditative process; rather, it is a demanding practice that is most often successful in a **collaborative mode**.[8] Reflective practice exposes the discrepancy between theory and practice and creates a self-awareness of the unacceptable outcomes and drives toward a new behavioral change for development. Hence, RP is not only an active and collaborative process, but also one of maturation as a HCP and peer colleague. Provided in appropriate contexts, as a peer colleague, peer assessment provides an invaluable gift for professional growth.

May et al.[23] identified that students in physical therapy, according to clinical instructors and clinical coordinators of clinical education, need to be able to demonstrate the ability to **self-assess, self-correct, and self-direct** in their commitment to learning as shared in the developed professional behaviors abilities instrument. The Professional Behaviors Assessment Tool (PBAT) will be further examined in Chapter 12 (see Table 12.1 and Chapter 20, Appendix). The American Physical Therapy Association (APTA) Clinical Performance Instrument[24] (APTA CPI) and American Occupational Therapy Association (AOTA) Fieldwork Performance Evaluation Form[25] require that students in clinical education or fieldwork experiences self-assess their abilities in terms of performance criteria for professional development and professional practice management, along with the clinical instructor's or fieldwork instructor's assessment. Learners who do not develop requisite professionalism are more likely to be deficient in terms of the critical professional behaviors and interpersonal skills that are foundational elements for practice and essential to professional competence within the professions.[23] The evaluative tools require quantitative ratings and narrative statements with respect to self-assessments.

The APTA and AOTA national professional member associations provide the opportunity for licensed practitioners to use tools for self-assessment of their clinical/fieldwork instructor abilities. To assist new and experienced clinical instructors, both national associations offer basic and advanced training for the instructors through the AOTA

Fieldwork Educators Certificate Workshop[26] and the APTA Credentialed Clinical Instructor Programs (CCIP)[27]—Level 1 and Level 2 to address identified needs from the self-assessment for continuing competency to enhance clinical educators' skills, abilities, and development of clinical education programs. Many of the skills are translatable to administration, management, and supervision of support staff, as well as enhanced patient/client management, especially in terms of education and conflict negotiation. The AOTA and APTA trainings, to credential clinical and field work instructors, incorporate peer and self-assessment. Although the time may seem far away when you are deeply immersed in your professional education, as an early career HCP, you should consider the credentialing training in your career pathway to further develop your RP skills and abilities and to continue the opportunity to pay it forward as a future clinical or fieldwork instructor. We will discuss early career pathways in Chapter 20.

Once you are a licensed health care professional, assessments for continuing competence entail various formats of self-assessment and often incorporate peer assessment for maintaining contemporary knowledge and licensure; hence, fostering RP capabilities remains relevant throughout your career and for pursuing advanced specializations. Self-assessment remains an appropriate means to evaluate HCPs' clinical competencies and identify needs for additional training as both developing and practicing clinicians.[28] As a HCP, one must strive to become a self-regulated learner to become adaptive, staying curious and striving to be more efficient and effective, in the provision of health care in the ever-changing health care environment.[29]

Today, over 75,000 physical therapists and physical therapist assistants are APTA Credentialed Clinical Instructors. Musolino et al.[30] examined why more than 300 licensed health care professionals in the state of Florida sought the APTA CCIP credential status and determined their learning goals and outcomes post course. They discovered that the participants overwhelmingly would recommend the continuing competency course to a colleague.[30] Musolino et al.[30] reported that CCIP participants readily achieved learning outcomes that facilitated the subject's RP skills as a clinical instructor, especially in the areas of communication, feedback and assessment methods, teaching and learning styles, goal setting, and goal-writing skills for clinical education instruction, along with formative feedback methods for the student's learning and progression as a reflective practitioner.

Let's now consider RP statements, modified from Kirby and Teddlie's[9] reflective teaching instrument. As you reflect on each statement, please consider your level of agreement in your own practice or in your observations of other health care professionals:

- I feel that it is important for me to integrate theory and research into my health care professional practice.
- It is incumbent upon me as a good HCP to be familiar with current research in my profession.
- I often revise my practice methods after trying them with a patient.
- I want my patients to question my way of looking at things.
- I often think about the hidden agenda (i.e., does my practice help my patients adopt the values and attitudes I want them to acquire for their health?).
- I sometimes find myself changing practice strategies in the middle of a treatment session.
- If I can't get through to a particular patient, I experiment with different approaches.
- If my patients are having trouble in the health care setting, it is up to me to find a solution.
- I have a great deal of influence on the personality and attitudes of my patients.
- I can make the least motivated patient like therapy.
- If my patients do poorly in therapy, I blame myself.
- I'm responsible for the behavior of the patients under my care.
- In my practice setting, I should have the final decision in determining what is to be done and how.

While considering each of these statements, you likely had varying levels of agreement based on your own experiences, or those of observing others, or the amount of accountability and responsibility you may consider to be in or out of your control as a health care professional. You also likely acknowledged the need for problem-solving capacities and clinical decision-making skills as hallmarks for reflective professional practice.[31-33] You probably also noted aspects of personal causation within the reflective practice statements relative to the HCP's ability to influence the patient and practice settings. As a health care professional, one cannot be totally personally responsible for all aspects of care, yet one can work to influence and change the multifactorial impacts of care. True reflection and experience are parallel to achieving action and a new and changed behavior with reflective practice,[13-15,23] and, as you will soon learn, the environment also has a substantial impact on our abilities to peer and self-assess.

| TABLE 10.1 |
|---|
| ## DATA MODEL |
| **Describe:** Identify and specify the situation at hand in detail, reflecting on the whole context and the setting; describe what has occurred and answer the following queries:<br><br>*What is going on in this situation? Who is involved? What is the context? What happened?* |
| **Analyze:** Examine the "why" as a central focus; examine your own and others' beliefs, assumptions, biases, and preconceived notions. Consider practical questions:<br><br>*How can I solve this dilemma? What is the best way to deal with the situation? Why are things going the way they are going? What are my assumptions and beliefs in this situation? What are/were your feelings and emotional responses? What was good? Bad?* |
| **Theorize:** Practical theory or practice-based reasoning addressing questions such as:<br><br>*What do I believe is needed? Why is this solution better than other potential solutions? What has worked before and how well? Is there relevant literature to indicate this option is better than others? What sense can you make of the situation, and what resources might you need?* |
| **Act:** Determine the theoretically best solution to address the situation. Answer the following queries:<br><br>*What are you going to do about it specifically? What is the developed plan of action? What steps are needed? What will you do differently in the future? What is your plan of action now?* |
| Adapted from Smith FL, Barlow PB, Peters JM, Skolits GJ. Demystifying reflective practice: using the DATA model to enhance evaluators' professional activities. *Eval Program Planning*. 2015;52:142–147. |

Schön's[15] work describes RP as the "ability to critically and deliberately think about the things that happen in daily practice in order to learn from them, in action, as well as after the events happen." Peters[33] built upon Schön's works and offered the following:

> *Reflective practice involves more than simply thinking about what one is doing and what one should do next. It involves identifying one's assumptions and feelings associated with practice, theorizing about how these assumptions and feelings are functionally or dysfunctionally associated with practice, and acting on the basis of the resulting theory of practice.*

Smith et al.[34] devised a method to assist in simplifying one's abilities to introduce reflective practice through the *Describe, Analyze, Theorize, and Act (DATA) model*. Although this framework is simple, it helps promote the novice's ability to begin the concept of RP through self-assessment and adaptation through action. Each step in the Model[34] is interrelated to the others. The DATA model makes the RP steps straightforward and overlaps with some of the thought processes while practically bridging theory into real-world practice. An adapted summary of the DATA model is shown in Table 10[34] we shall revisit it with the chapter exercises. You will likely find it helpful when applied to problem-solving with patient/client cases and when your self-assessment may be incongruent with others' assessment of you and/or in conflicting situations in relations with others.

# REFLECTIVE PRACTICE: PEER AND SELF-ASSESSMENT

So, what is self-assessment exactly? At the beginning of the chapter, you were asked to consider how you defined self-assessment (SA), what you believed were barriers or challenges to self-assessment, and why you might want to do this thing called self-assessment.

Practice in peer and self-assessment shall assist you in developing as a mature health care professional. Musolino[35] stated that self-assessment skills are not only essential for health care professionals but also crucial to becoming a reflective practitioner[14,35,36] and highly relevant for moving along the professional development continuum from novice to expert practice.[2–8,11,30,31,33,35,37] Musolino[35] reported, in her qualitative research study of self-assessment abilities, that to foster self-assessment for RP, physical therapy students and new graduates required professionalism, reflection, time management, support, and change management. Musolino[35] discovered self-assessment was improved and promoted through a variety of self-starting, self-steering, self-directed, and self-pacing activities with subjects' motivation for professional competence and self-improvement. Related to practice effects, the greatest barriers to self-assessment, noted by the research subjects, were time, complacency, negativity, self-esteem, and lack of objectivity. However, the greatest support for self-assessment included taking the time, seeking feedback, being honest and objective, creating a safe environment for feedback, setting goals, having supportive peers and faculty, and using the guides for written and oral assessments. Musolino's[35] study findings paralleled not only Schön's[14,36] concept of RP but also supported Bandura's[38-41] social learning theory in the resulting developed, conceptual model of self-assessment (Figure 10.1).

Albert Bandura,[38] an innovative scholar who did pioneering work in social cognitive theory, related that people's level of motivation, affective states, and actions are based more on what they believe than on objectivity, and that human behavior can only be understood in terms of a reciprocal interaction between external stimuli and internal cognition. Bandura[38-41] proposed that a fundamental way humans acquire skills and behaviors is by observing the behavior of others. The learner must be able to reproduce the behavior that has been observed. Sometimes the reproducible behavior stems from a lack of requisite cognitive or motor skills but often reflects the learner's lack of

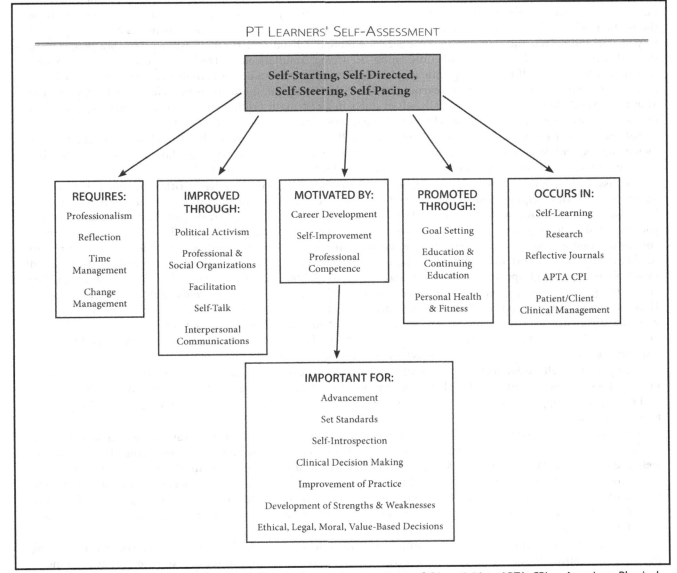

**Figure 10.1** Conceptual model of physical therapy learners' perceptions of SA activities. APTA CPI = American Physical Therapy Association Clinical Performance Institute; PT = physical therapy. (Reprinted with permission from Musolino GM. Fostering reflective practice: self-assessment abilities of physical therapy students and entry-level graduates. *J Allied Health.* 2006;35(1):37.)

feedback about what the learner is actually trying to accomplish. Bandura[41] called this "reciprocal determinism": the world and a person's behavior cause each other, or one's environment causes behavior and behavior causes the environment. Converting RP didactic skills into actual clinical abilities likely requires a transformative process for novice clinicians.

As HCP educators, we see the transformation from novice to more experienced reflective practitioner and on to expertise, when students take self-assessment and RP seriously. Students work from initial unconscious incompetence toward more conscious competence in their professional development and practice management skills and abilities through self-assessment. Self-assessment assures you are able to identify gaps in your learning and seek support to address, pro-actively. Initially you will not know exactly what you do not know because you have never before been asked to be the professional you are becoming, and your clinical or fieldwork instructor is your guide on the side, facilitating your abilities and providing you with benchmarks and guidance. Your Directors of Clinical Education and faculty may ask you to complete RP activities in both formative (along the way) and summative (mid-points, endpoints) assessments to assist you in becoming more consciously competent. As you progress in your abilities with RP, you shall become more enlightened, progress in your conscious competence, and ultimately realize how much more there is yet to know, even once you know what you do and do not know in practice!

An often-cited barrier to self-assessment abilities is time. Frankly, self-assessment does not take a lot of time. Certainly, there are recesses when contemplating your navel and letting your mind wander are welcome reprieves from the hectic world we live in today. Self-assessment does not demand hours, but frequent moments and the opportunity to stop and reflect, and thus eventually it becomes more of a habit or natural occurrence. Notably, people learn through experience and training, with unlearning occurring simultaneously. Deliberate efforts to learn involve action, reflection, and self-monitoring with adaptations. Learning to learn becomes more of an awareness of self and active examination of what happens as learning occurs. Self-assessment, therefore, is not a laissez-faire approach to awarding the self, but the ability to critically self-evaluate in a systematic fashion. The heart of the learning process is developing the awareness and capacities for effective self-monitoring and active reflection.

**Self-assessment is the ability to assess one's own skills, identify one's own educational needs, evaluate one's own progress, and determine one's performance.**[42] Self-assessment is "not merely one who minimally qualifies, but one who seeks an ever more perfect understanding and performance of one's work."[43]

Peer assessment is essentially self-assessment, but it involves being constructively critical of your peers' performance and abilities, helping them to see themselves as you do, usually in relation to a set of standards or criteria. Peer assessment also improves your own metacognitive skills and abilities to provide constructive feedback, which you also need to do for your patients. Peer assessment also supports enhancing your own listening, interprofessional communication, and visual appraisal skills. The peer assessment process correspondingly provides the opportunity to further reflect on your work in a comparative manner, to standards, as well. Peer and self-assessment may be initiated by simply asking thought-provoking questions verbally or in a guided journal reflection: *What went well? It would be even better if? The next step would be? How could you approach differently? What else could be the problem or going on? How did you incorporate your findings with your decision making along the way? Thinking back now, how might you approach differently? Thinking back, what additional information, if any, would you like to have gathered that you may have missed? Where in the learning do you think you might have been challenged? What resources are needed to adapt?* Explain your thought process in your approach before, during, and after the encounters.

Your peer and self-assessment should be substantive and not just simple, easy comments, but deeper assessment providing a true, meaningful gift of feedback for improvement and reinforcement. Do not just gloss over the feedback and introspection opportunities. Be hard on the problems or areas for improvement, not the person. Guide yourself and your peers.

A method of fast-formative feedback for clinical education is the **2-Minute Clinical Instructor activity**. The HCP student learner and the clinical instructor share with each other, **in 2 minutes' time, two things they are doing well and two things they need to work on, along with what resources might be helpful** and then reverse roles the next time. The 2-Minute Clinical Instructor–Student learner exchange provides a platform for self-assessment and becoming more consciously competent of where you are, or are not, on the learning curve for your clinical/fieldwork education and, voilà, it only takes 2 minutes! This rapid reflection also leads to enhanced abilities for deeper reflections for learning.

Try it out! Have a 2-minute conversation with a peer. The brief time-out for fostering self-assessment is reassuring for you as the learner to receive feedback and insights, and for your instructor to see that you are initiative-taking in your learning processes. The 2-Minute Clinical Instructor is a formative feedback opportunity and is likely positive because it is meant to be informal, constructive, and transformative. Through the 2-Minute Clinical Instructor activity, you are provided with the gift of constructive feedback about your self-assessment and abilities to progress toward RP and of achieving your clinical learning goals for patient care.

Once you have graduated, unless you have a strong mentor or colleague, which we hope you will, you will need to be more self-reliant on your abilities for self-assessment, and ultimately RP, for the benefit of your patients and clients. The formative work of self-assessment, as you continue your professional development, shall guide you to achieving more understanding and insight into the performance of your work as a HCP as you progress in your capabilities as an autonomous practitioner for your patients and society. Peer and faculty assessment can also be followed up by showing a peer what you were to improve, explaining or demonstrating how you have improved, and then asking for their additional feedback. Deep reflection is needed for all learning stages for adaptation, and aids not only in exploring the emotions associated with learning and in supporting HCP well-being in the process but also in removing barriers to learning[44] and moving needed adaptations along the learning and teaching continuum.

Time was mentioned previously as a perceived barrier to self-assessment, and additional barriers to self-assessment were discovered by Musolino,[35] which were also sometimes perceived as potentials for self-assessment support (Table 10.2). Being aware of the potential barriers and/or supports for self-assessment shall assist you in overcoming barriers and assuring you have the needed support for progressive self-assessment. Furthermore, self-assessment is fundamental to critical reflection that promotes deep exploration of assumptions and alternative assumptions, whilst developing emotional insights, informing action and changing it over time while also shaping safety in real-world practice.[45]

Let's consider some reflective quotes from those who have gone before you in their professional development. For example, self-talk reflections of a new graduate clearly demonstrate tenets of Schön's[14,15] theory of RP, noted in parentheses:[35]

> *I look at what I'm doing and what I've done and try to decide if it's the right thing, the wrong thing, how I can change, how I can make it better … am I prepared to treat this person, was I prepared to handle this situation (**recognizing surprise**), this new person that came in, this returning person that … what do I need to know … what did I do good (**knowing-in-action**) … what should I have done differently, what would have helped for the future … I think about this during the situation (**reflection-in-action**), at the end of the day, driving home in the car (**reflection-on-action**), it spans everything from treatment sessions to time management or administration of care … reviewing step-by-step how to improve to be ready for the next morning.*

| TABLE 10.2 | | |
|---|---|---|
| **SUMMARY OF BARRIERS AND SUPPORT FOR SELF-ASSESSMENT** | | |
| **SUPPORT** | **BARRIERS** | **BARRIER AND/OR SUPPORT** |
| Honesty | Awareness/complacency | Time |
| Observation/comparing | Dishonesty | Feedback/networking |
| Self-focus/self-talk | Unsafe environments | Peers and teamwork |
| Goal setting | Lack of goals | Faculty feedback or not |
| Objectivity | Pressure | |
| Written and oral SA | Negativity | |
| Cases/patients/projects | Payer demands | |
| Clinical faculty queries and debriefing | Lack of cultural competence | |
| Clinical performance instruments | Incongruent philosophy | |
| Portfolios and reflective journals | Low self-esteem | |
| Family | Ambiguity | |
| Positive self-esteem | | |
| Ambiguity in practice | | |
| Safe/supportive environment | | |
| Reprinted with permission from Musolino GM. Fostering reflective practice: self-assessment abilities of physical therapy students and entry-level graduates. *J Allied Health.* 2006;35(1):30–42. | | |

> *I think as far as ethics, values, and morals, it is important too because if you don't reflect on those things you can make bad decisions or sometimes not necessarily bad, but not as good as they could be for the patient, or the best for your company or coworkers.*

Reflecting on these thoughts and potential barriers and/or support aspects of self-assessment will assist you on your journey to becoming a reflective practitioner and being present and capable of best serving your patients/clients and supporting your peers and colleagues in the process of self-assessment for best practice. Now, let's consider the reflective thoughts of a few professional students immersed in training regarding their support and/or barriers to doing self-assessment in the classroom or laboratory:[35]

> *Sometimes people are afraid to give constructive criticism and this might hurt another when actually it is helpful when done correctly, but there has to be time and people can't say "that's a bunch of BS" or it is immediately stifled or they might say, "Just hurry up and get it over with" … the time crunch factor.*
>
> *In labs it can be kind of embarrassing, I don't like to admit that I'm really weak in this area, I compare myself to others and this can be a barrier because you may gain strengths and weaknesses and it's really hard to catch my own weaknesses … but if I have a video of myself that helps a lot to see a vision of yourself as a whole person and be able to break things down … especially with low self-esteem or someone who is joking around or making culturally derogatory statements that might be supposed to be in fun, but it is a big barrier.*
>
> *Sometimes you are lazy and just don't want to do it, it is a matter of putting forth the effort and taking the fifteen minutes during the day or night before I go to sleep, on the long drives on the commute home to just think and not letting others discourage you from doing self-assessment because it is important and can make a difference. … I ask what have I learned, what do I need to learn, where do I need to go now to learn.*

Are you able to identify Schön's RP concepts in the above reflections? Let's also contemplate the importance of educators in the role of facilitating self-assessment from the learner's perspective:[35]

> *When I am "forced" to write down my peer and self-assessment or if others ask me that is helpful to self-assessment, when faculty pushes it and group interactions help too.*
>
> *It is the obligation of educators to make sure that they are not sending out people who are only going to be good for the next 6 months, but for the duration of their careers. And that's much like patient education, I can train someone how to walk with crutches down the busy hall, but if I don't educate them how to fall and other safety related issues, then I have not done them much justice either. Just like our patient, we need to think about what we are doing, how we are doing it, and what might need to change physically and behaviorally … constantly considering the changing environment.*

Some authors[2,11,35,37,46,47] have noted the influence of critical thought and reflective action through the process of self-assessment and the need for guided feedback to affect a change toward what Epstein[46] refers to as mindful practice. The novice learners and new graduates echoed the sentiments that professional education will be overshadowed by "unreflective doing"[46] if self-assessment does not remain at the forefront of day-to-day educational processes through the "teachable moments"[46,47] in clinics and classrooms. Students do not begin to learn until asking questions of themselves.[1] Much of what future clinicians may need to know for practice is not even known today and, consequently, cannot necessarily be taught. Hence, the importance in education lies in being able to teach learners how to acquire knowledge and to critically assess. Learners must master how to do self-assessment and adapt in relation to contemporary expectations and meeting the needs and responsibilities of patients and clients.[42–50]

As a novice practitioner, you may be more stressed by the fast-paced clinical environment; therefore, practice may, unfortunately, be more routine than reflective.[37] Similar to Orest's[51] findings with practicing physical therapist clinicians, Musolino[35] discovered that learners in physical therapy and recent graduates were motivated to perform self-assessment through the desire for self-improvement, through career development, and through efforts for clinical and professional competence. These processes included advancement efforts; setting or achievement of practice standards; self-introspection efforts; clinical decision making; development of strengths and weaknesses; and ethical-, legal-, moral-, and value-based decision making. Learners believed that self-assessment is improved through self-talk, interpersonal communications, and mentoring in professional and social networks, and, in some cases, that it may lead to or be fostered through political activism.[35]

In Figure 10.1, the developed conceptual model for self-assessment is summarized.[35] **Consider how the conceptual model agrees or disagrees with your thoughts and assumptions regarding self-assessment from the beginning of the chapter**. The conceptual model of physical therapy learners' self-assessment may assist you in becoming increasingly sophisticated in your abilities to actively assess your own performance and that of your peers and enhance your lifelong learning through conscious and genuine efforts along your learning continuum for RP.[35] To enhance your self-assessment abilities, several recommendations should be considered, including the following: videotaping, with reviews[47]; experiential guides and workbooks, such as the *Patient Practitioner Interaction* one you are using; learning style (e.g., Kolb Experiential Learning Style Inventory-KELP[52]) and personality inventories (e.g., Myers-Briggs Type Indicator-MBTI[53]); self-assessment with clinical education evaluative instruments; facilitation of active training for teaching and learning; provision of time to complete self-assessment; guided reflective journals; guided debriefing inquiries; and practice sessions with immediate feedback, such as from standardized patients, the 2-Minute Clinical Instructor activity, and peer and self-assessment, along with instructor feedback.[54] Effective peer and self-assessment capabilities provide the foundation for progression to sound clinical reasoning abilities, which are expected of the doctoring professions.[54–58]

# CONCLUSION

We have now considered the concept of self-assessment and theories of RP. Shortly, we will provide the opportunity for you to practice peer and self-assessment and to facilitate your abilities specifically. However, as you have noted from considering the pithy quotes of professional learners who have gone before you and the related research, it is important to not only be positive in the effort to enhance self-assessment, but also be mindful of your own impact on the learning and teaching environment to support peer and self-assessment. The influence of the learning environment is key for peer and self-assessment success as evidenced through Bandura's social learning theory.[40]

You have had the opportunity to explore, change, and/or adapt your perspectives and considerations for self-assessment and are now cognizant of the gifts of peer and self-assessment for best RP and the concordance with expertise, for those we serve in health care. Our hope for you is that you are able to continue to translate your newly acquired knowledge for your progression of learning in the affective, cognitive, psychomotor, and spiritual domains (see Chapter 3, Appendix, and Chapter 15) as you continue your professional development journey toward reflective practice because your patients and clients are counting on you! The work of self-assessment is challenging, yet the rewards are worth the time and effort. Self-assessment is a viable process, and you shall ultimately have greater learning gains in this mode of active learning with serious thought and considerations than with more passive learning methods; the process of self-assessment shall promote your continuous learning.

It is time now for you to try thinking on your feet (reflection-in-action), working to make sense of your experiences after they occur (reflection-on-action) to learn more deeply, and scaffolding your learning (knowing-in-action) for RP.[14,15,35,36,54] We want you to now challenge your assumptions as learners; ask new questions; make sense of your experiences; not be afraid to admit errors and make course corrections (recognize surprise) and stay curious through self-assessment and feedback; put what you are learning into deeper memory as active, engaged learners; and assist your peers and colleagues in the process.[14,15,35,36,54] Make it a point to thrive on constructive feedback and gently provide the gift of peer assessment for others to succeed. Self-regulated learning, through peer and self-assessment, promotes collaborative learning and will continue to aid you in your professional formation by helping to answer the "why" question[59,60] for the gaps in your cognitive learning, affective behaviors, and/or clinical performance for patient-centered learning. Seeking insights from your HCP educators on your self-assessments as a developing HCP will guide you and facilitate your learning. Perhaps Bandura[38–41] said it best: "Of the many cues that influence behavior, at any one point in time, none is more common than the actions of others."

As you transition from classroom to clinics and hospitals, you may find it helpful to complete guided self-assessment in relation to specific aspects of your patient–practitioner interactions. Gremigni et al.,[61,62] Italian researchers, were interested in both clinicians' and patients' perceptions of patient-centered care. They investigated how HCPs self-evaluate their ability to relate to patients in day-to-day practice from a patient-centered perspective. Gremigni et al.[61] evaluated the psychometric properties of a developed instrument called the Provider-Patient Relationship Questionnaire (PPRQ). They studied 50 nurses from a sample of 600 in eight hospitals (six in northern Italy and two in southern Italy) and determined good reliability and validity of the 16-item PPRQ instrument, rating each statement using a scale from 1 to 5, where 1 = not at all and 5 = very much. The study examined HCPs' communication, interest in their patients, empathy, and care involvement from a self-assessment standpoint. The PPRQ reports on 16 common considerations when working with patients in a hospital setting. Consider the PPRQ's 16 items, provided here, as you transition to patient-centered care and use the framework to facilitate your self-assessment of your patient–provider interactions in these specific areas:

1. I provided clear information.

2. I was interested in what the patient feels about their current health status.

3. I turned to the patient in a calm and quiet tone.

4. I understood the emotions that the patient may have.

5. I was interested in what the patient knows about the disease/prognosis.

6. I respected the patient as a person.

7. I was interested in what the patient wants from care.

8. I was able to listen.

9. I was paying attention to what the patient said.

10. I was able to put myself in the patients' shoes.

11. I gave the patient time to ask and to talk about the disease.

12. I inspired confidence and security when touching the patient and being nearby.

13. I asked questions that allowed the patient to express their view.

14. I was interested in what the patient expects from care.

15. I gave the patient encouragement and transmitted optimism.

16. I offered the patient the opportunity to discuss and decide together the things to do.

Take a moment to journal on the important PPI considerations following your patient interactions or role-plays to complete a self-assessment and reflect upon areas for improvement.

# REFERENCES

1. West KM. The case against teaching. *J Med Educ.* 1966;41(8):776–771.
2. Jensen GM, Gwyer J, Shepard KF. Expert practice in physical therapy. *Phys Ther.* 2000;80:(1):28–43.
3. Jensen GM, Shepard KF, Hack LM. The novice versus the experienced clinician: insights into the work of the physical therapist. *Phys Ther.* 1990;70(5):314–323.
4. Shepard KF, Hack LM, Gwyer J, Jensen GM. Grounded theory approach to describing the phenomenon of expert practice in physical therapy. *Qual Health Res.* 1999;9(6):746–758.
5. Jensen GM, Shepard KF, Gwyer J, Hack LM. Attribute dimensions that distinguish master and novice physical therapy clinicians in orthopedic settings. *Phys Ther.* 1992;72(10):711–722.
6. Yusfuff KB. Does self-reflection and peer-assessment improve Saudi pharmacy students' academic performance and metacognitive skills? *Saudi Pharm J.* 2015;23(3):266–275.
7. May BJ, Dennis JK. Expert decision making in physical therapy—a survey of practitioners. *Phys Ther.* 1991;71(3):190–202.
8. Osterman KF, Kottkamp RB. *Reflective Practice for Educators: Professional Development to Improve Student Learning*, 2nd ed. Thousand Oaks, CA: Corwin Press; 2004.
9. Kirby PC, Teddlie C. Development of the reflective teaching instrument. *J Rsch Dev Educ.* 1989;22(4):45–51.
10. Russell TL, Spafford C. *Teachers as reflective practitioners in peer clinical supervision.* Paper presented at AERA; April 1986; San Francisco, CA.
11. Brookfield S. *Becoming a Critically Reflective Teacher.* San Francisco, CA: Jossey-Bass; 1995.
12. Dewey J. *How We Think.* Boston, MA: Heath; 1933.
13. Kolb DA. *Experiential Learning: Experience as the Sources of Learning and Development.* Englewood Cliffs, NJ: Prentice Hall; 1984.
14. Schön DA. The theory of inquiry: Dewey's legacy to education. *Curriculum Inquiry.* 1992;22(2):119–139.
15. Schön DA. *The Reflective Practitioner: How Professionals Think in Action.* New York, NY: Basic Books; 1983.
16. Hatcher JA, Bringle RG. Reflection: Bridging the gap between service and learning. *College Teaching.* 1996;45(4):153–158.
17. Eyler J, Giles DW, Schmeide L. The impact of a college community service lab on students' personal, social and cognitive outcomes. *J Adolescence.* 1994;17:327–329.
18. Williams D, Driscoll A. Connecting curriculum content with community service: guidelines for student reflection. *J Public Service Outreach.* 1997;2(1):33–42.
19. Panda S, Das A, Das R, Shullai WK, Sharma N, Sarma A. Teaching and learning medical professionalism: an input from experienced faculty and young graduates in a tertiary care institute. *Maedica (Bucur).* 2022 Jun;17(2):371–379. doi: 10.26574/maedica.2022.17.2.371.
20. Ziebart C, MacDermid JC. Reflective practice in physical therapy: a scoping review. *Phys Ther.* 2019 Aug 1;99(8):1056–1068. doi: 10.1093/ptj/pzz049.
21. Dressler JA, Ryder BA, Connolly M, Blais MD, Miner TJ, Harrington DT. "Tweet"-format writing is an effective tool for medical student reflection. *J Surg Educ.* 2018 Sept–Oct;75(5):1206–1210. doi: 10.1016/j.jsurg.2018.03.002.
22. Boyd VA, Woods NN, Kumagai AK, Kawamura AA, Orsino A, Ng SL. Examining the impact of dialogic learning on critically reflective practice. *Acad Med.* 2022 Aug 9. doi: 10.1097/ACM.0000000000004916.

23. May WW, Morgan BJ, Lemke JC, Karst GM, Stone HL. Model for ability-based assessment in physical therapy education. *J Phys Ther Educ*. 1995;9(1):3–6.

24. American Physical Therapy Association. Clinical Performance Instrument, 2023 Alexandria, VA: American Physical Therapy Association. https://www.apta.org/for-educators/assessments/pt-cpi Accessed May 1, 2023.

25. American Occupational Therapy Association. Understanding the OT/OTA fieldwork performance evaluations. https://www.aota.org/education/fieldwork/fieldwork-performance-evaluation Accessed May 1, 2024.

26. The American Occupational Therapy Association. Fieldwork Educators Certificate Workshop. https://www.aota.org/education/fieldwork/fieldwork-educators-certification-workshop Accessed May 1, 2024.

27. American Physical Therapy Association. Credentialed Clinical Instructor Program (CCIP). http://www.apta.org/CCIP/. Accessed May 1, 2024.

28. Taylor I, Bing-Jonsson P, Wangensteen S, Finnbakk E, Sandvik L, McCormack B, Fagerström L. The self-assessment of clinical competence and the need for further training: a cross-sectional survey of advanced practice nursing students. *J Clin Nurs*. 2020 Feb;29(3–4):545–555. doi: 10.1111/jocn.15095.

29. Stringer JK, Gruppen LD, Ryan MS, et al. Measuring the master adaptive learner: development and internal structure validity evidence for a new instrument. *Med Sci Educ*. 2022;32:183–193. doi: 10.1007/s40670-021-01491-9.

30. Musolino GM, van Duijn J, Noonan AC, Eargle LK, Gray DL. Reasons identified for seeking the American Physical Therapy Association-Credentialed Clinical Instructor Program (CCIP) in Florida. *J Allied Health*. 2013;42(3):e51–e60.

31. Alspach JG. *The Educational Process in Nursing Staff Development*. St. Louis, MO: Mosby; 1995.

32. Bridges EM, Hallinger P. Using problem-based learning to prepare educational leaders. *Peabody J Educ*. 2002;72(2): 131–146.

33. Peters JM. Strategies for reflective practice. *New Directions for Adult and Continuing Educ*. 1991;51:89–96.

34. Smith FL, Barlow PB, Peters JM, Skolits GJ. Demystifying reflective practice: using the DATA model to enhance evaluators' professional activities. *Eval Program Planning*. 2015;52:142–147.

35. Musolino GM. Fostering reflective practice: self-assessment abilities of physical therapy students and entry-level graduates. *J Allied Health*. 2006;35(1):30–42.

36. Schön DA. *Educating the Reflective Practitioner: Toward a New Design for Teaching and Learning in the Professions*. San Francisco, CA: Jossey-Bass; 1987.

37. Jensen G, Denton B. Teaching physical therapy students to reflect: a suggestion for clinical education. *J Phys Ther Educ*. 1991;5:33–38.

38. Bandura A. *Self-Efficacy: The Exercise of Control*. New York, NY: W.H. Freeman; 1997.

39. Bandura A. Self-efficacy: toward a unifying theory of behavioral change. *Psychol Rev*. 1997;84(2):191–215.

40. Bandura A. *Social Learning Theory*. Englewood Cliffs, NJ: Prentice-Hall; 1977.

41. Bandura A. The self-system in reciprocal determinism. *Am Psychologist*. 1978;33(4):344–358.

42. Watts NT. *Handbook of Clinical Teaching: Exercises and Guidelines for Health Professionals Who Teach Patients, Train Staff or Supervise Students*. New York, NY: Churchill Livingston; 1990.

43. Jonsen A. *The New Medicine and the Old Ethics*. Cambridge, MA: Harvard University Press; 1992.

44. Campbell F, Rogers H. Through the looking glass: a review of the literature surrounding reflective practice in dentistry. *Br Dent J*. 2022 May;232(10):729–734. doi: 10.1038/s41415-022-3993-4. Erratum in: *Br Dent J*. 2022 Aug;233(3):226. PMID: 35624264

45. Sarraf-Yazdi, Shiva MD, MEHP. Perks, processes, and pitfalls of reflective practice. *Acad Med*. 2021 May;96(5):769. doi: 10.1097/ACM.0000000000003864.

46. Epstein RM. Mindful practice. *JAMA*. 1999;282(9):833–839.

47. Seif GA, Brown D. Video-recorded simulated patient interactions: can they help develop clinical and communication skills in today's learning environment? *J Allied Health*. 2013;42(2):e37–e44.

48. Barrows HS. *Practice-Based Learning: Problem-Based Learning Applied to Medical Education*. Springfield, IL: Southern Illinois University School of Medicine; 1994.

49. Barrows HS. *What Your Tutor May Never Tell You: A Medical Student's Guide to Problem-Based Learning*. Springfield, IL: Southern Illinois University School of Medicine; 1996.

50. Jensen GM, Shepherd KF, Gwyer J, Hack LM. Attribute dimensions that distinguish master and novice physical therapy clinicians in orthopedic settings. *Phys Ther*. 1994;72(10):711–722.

51. Orest M. Clinicians' perceptions of self-assessment in clinical practice. *Phys Ther*. 1995;75(9):824–829.

52. Kolb D, Kolb A. *Kolb Experiential Learning Profile*. Institute for Experiential Learning. Available: https://experientiallearninginstitute.org/the-kolb-experiential-learning-profile-kelp/ Accessed May 1, 2024.

53. Briggs KC, Myers IB. *Myers-Briggs Type Indicator (MBTI)*. The Myers & Briggs Foundation. www.mbtionline.com Accessed May 1, 2022.

54. Musolino GM, Mostrom E. Reflection and the scholarship of teaching, learning, and assessment. *J Phys Ther Educ*. 2005;19(3): 52–66.

55. Dreyfus HL, Dreyfus SL. The relationship of theory and practice in the acquisition of skill. In: Benner P, Tanner CA, Chalsa CA, eds. *Expertise in Nursing Practice*, 2nd ed. New York, NY: Springer; 2009:1–24.

56. Dreyfus SE, Dreyfus HL. *A five-stage model of the mental activities involved in directed skill acquisition*. Berkeley Operations Research Center, University of California, Berkeley; 1980. doi: 10.21236/ADA084551.

57. Furze J, Black L, Hoffman J, Barr JB, Cochran TM, Jensen GM. Exploration of students' clinical reasoning development in professional physical therapy education. *J Phys Ther Educ.* 2015;29(3):22–33.

58. Furze J, Gale JR, Black L, Cochran TM, Jensen GM. Clinical reasoning: development of a grading rubric for student assessment. *J Phys Ther Educ.* 2015;29(3):34–45.

59. Ginzburg SB, Santen SA, Schwartzstein RM. Self-directed Learning: a New Look at an Old Concept. *Med Sci Educ.* 2020 Oct 20;31(1):229–230. doi: 10.1007/s40670-020-01121-w. PMID: 34457877; PMCID: PMC8368943.

60. Regan L, Hopson LR, Gisondi MA, Branzetti J. Creating a better learning environment: a qualitative study uncovering the experiences of Master Adaptive Learners in residency. *BMC Med Educ.* 2022 Mar 4;22(1):141. doi: 10.1186/s12909-022-03200-5.

61. Gremigni P, Casu G, Sommaruga M. Dealing with patients in healthcare: a self-assessment tool. *Patient Educ Couns.* 2016 Jun;99(6):1046–1053. doi: 10.1016/j.pec.2016.01.015.

62. Casu G, Gremigni G, Sommaruga M. The Patient-Professional Interaction Questionnaire (PPIQ) to assess patient centered care from the patient's perspective. *Patient Educ Couns.* 2019;102(1):126–133. doi: 10.1016/j.pec.2018.08.006.

# SUGGESTED RESOURCES

## *Examples of Narrative Self-Assessment on the APTA Clinical Performance Instrument*

**Professional Practice—Safety:** *I consistently attempt to establish a safe working environment prior to each patient session. I put down mats in cases where patients will be swinging and will need to land on cushioned ground. I remain vigilant of changes in patient conditions by asking them about their pain using pain scales, in addition to observation of physiological changes, such as skin color or respiratory rate. In cases where a patient may have a shunt, I ensure that I do not perform activities where a patient would be placed in an upside-down position. When I feel uncomfortable performing an intervention due to lack of experience, I ask for assistance from my clinical instructor to ensure the patient remains safe. I consistently utilize proper body mechanics in order to protect myself and my patients. I am well versed in the facility's safety procedures as well. I am continuously learning about how to keep pediatric patients safe and that it requires constant vigilance on my part. Over the next few weeks, I will continue to expand my safety skills by efficiently learning where to keep my hands so they can be ready in case a patient has an outburst or movement alteration that could make them a fall risk.*

**Professional Practice—Communication:** *When working with a complex patient, I seek communication from my clinical instructor during that patient's session to ensure I am being safe and my reasoning with treatment is logical. When I feel uncomfortable or unsure of the quality of my service, I can communicate this to my clinical instructor immediately and efficiently with verbal cues. I consistently actively listen to my patients and their parents and commonly review what they have stated to me to ensure all parties are on the same page. My verbal and nonverbal messages are consistent, and I strive to have the tone in my voice match what I am asking a patient to perform. When a patient performs a task correctly, I utilize a positive, encouraging tone. My clinical instructor has educated me on what tones and level of wordiness are appropriate for different diagnoses, and I have since applied this on a more consistent basis. I still require further practice using a more authoritative voice with a patient whose behavior is inappropriate. When communicating with a patient and parent about what the home exercise program consists of, I commonly perform the exercises with them in the clinic. I also offer pictures and take-home worksheets to help the patient visualize the exercises and give them a way to remember and replicate the exercises I am asking them to perform at home. In cases where a patient may not be able to verbalize their needs, I utilize nonverbal signs, such as crying or parental cuddles to determine what the patient needs. In some cases, I also utilize sign language, as demonstrated by speech therapists on staff.*

**Patient Management—Clinical Reasoning:** *I offer a logical rationale for my clinical decisions. If a patient has sensory deficits, I will be sure to include some aspect of sensory input into that day's session. If a patient exhibits trunk and lower extremity weakness, I will include fun muscle-building activities in the session. I select my interventions based on results from pediatric examination tools and patient preferences. For a patient who has a fear of therapy balls, I avoid interventions that utilize transitioning or stretching on the ball. I consistently integrate patient needs, such as being able to ride a bike or jump to play with friends, into their plan of care. When an intervention is ineffective for a child, I am able to recognize this and implement a new variation of the intervention instead. I consistently and efficiently utilize peer-reviewed articles, textbooks, parents, medical records, and other members of the therapy staff to formulate plans of care and make clinical decisions for patients.*

After reviewing these examples, remember to journal about your thoughts on RP.

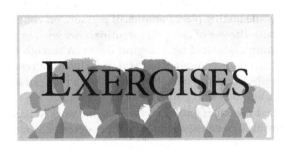

# EXERCISE 1: WARMING UP WITH PEER AND SELF-ASSESSMENT— CHECK YOURSELF BEFORE YOU WRECK YOURSELF

All health care professionals work to maintain good body mechanics throughout all our work activities and in daily living. We also educate our patients in proper postural alignment for good musculoskeletal health and their work, recreational, and daily activities. The environment does not allow us to always maintain proper body mechanics, yet maintaining strength and flexibility provides the ability to adjust to the demands of gravity and challenges with body mechanics on a daily basis. Many students initially struggle with maintaining their own safety when first entering a practice setting due to the competing demands and being novices. So, let's check your posture and your peer and self-assessment abilities for the psychomotor skills of good posture and body mechanics as a warm-up self-assessment activity.

## Part A

Find a partner and ask your partner to lift a readily available item (chair, books, backpack, trash can, or similar) from the floor to the table and back down again. While the lifting trial is being completed, review the checklist, answer yes or no, and make notations. When your partner is finished with the lifting trial, have your partner/s complete a self-assessment using the ratings, and then you should compare your responses and discuss. Then reverse roles and complete it again.

### BODY MECHANICS LIFTING TRIAL—PEER AND SELF-ASSESSMENT

| | | | | |
|---|---|---|---|---|
| 1. | Overall good postural body alignment throughout the activity: | Yes | No | Note: |
| | a. Maintains slight cervical lordosis | Yes | No | Note: |
| | b. Maintains slight thoracic kyphosis | Yes | No | Note: |
| | c. Maintains slight lumbar lordosis | Yes | No | Note: |
| 2. | Appropriate base of support: | Yes | No | Note: |
| | a. Too wide | Yes | No | Note: |
| | b. Too narrow | Yes | No | Note: |
| 3. | Carries the load close to the body within the base of support | Yes | No | Note: |
| 4. | Avoids twisting of the trunk | Yes | No | Note: |
| 5. | Avoids bending from the waist | Yes | No | Note: |

Now, consider if mobile devices are wreaking havoc on your body? Heads up—are you developing text neck?

# *Part B*

The person evaluating first in Part A should now be the one to initiate the activity while the partner evaluates. As you are likely aware, poor posture while texting places pounds of pressure on your neck. Just as we teach our patients regarding proper body mechanics with the use of computer terminals, we wish to avoid having degenerative cervical spine problems and the corresponding associated neurological issues. Although overuse injuries are also causative factors associated with prolonged texting or computer use with poor posture repeatedly over time, we can work to prevent musculoskeletal imbalances by checking ourselves before we wreck ourselves. Poor posture causes tension headaches, neck, and shoulder pain, and breathing difficulties.

Ask your partner to send a few text messages and/or complete some work at their laptop, notebook, iPad, or other mobile electronic device. After they have been engaged for a while, describe what is good or not so good regarding their posture (you need not limit yourself to just the cervical spine). Complete your visual assessment, asking your partner to complete their self-assessment, and then debrief and later reverse roles (when they don't think you are watching) and provide your recommendations.

Posture while using an electronic mobile device:

- Good:



- Not So Good:



- Recommendations:

# EXERCISE 2: PONDERING FOR PRACTICE: GUIDED REFLECTION ALONG THE WAY

Consider a recent concrete experience in your learning, classroom or clinical. Reflect on your experience and respond to the following queries:

1. What was the muddiest point in your learning experience?

2. What percentage of mud was due to the following:

    a. Unclear presentation?

    b. Lack of the opportunity to ask questions?

    c. Your lack of preparation?

    d. Your lack of participation?

    e. Your lack of setting a specific goal?

3. What theories or concepts did you draw upon or discover from the experience?

4. How could you have been more present and available for the learning experience?

5. Who are you becoming as a professional?

(Adapted from Musolino GM, Mostrom E. Reflection and the scholarship of teaching, learning, and assessment. *J Phys Ther Educ.* 2005;19[3]:52–66.)

# EXERCISE 3: DATA-DRIVEN MODEL—REFLECTION

Recall the DATA model.[34] Refer to the DATA steps. Recall a specific interaction—classroom, practical, or clinical—and apply the model.

- **Describe—the situation:**

- **Analyze—examine the why:**

- **Theorize—practice-based reasoning:**

- **Act—the best solution:**

# EXERCISE 4: REFLECTIVE JOURNALS—APPLYING SCHÖN'S REFLECTIVE PRACTITIONER THEORY

The following are sample reflective journal entries in response to Schön's queries of recognizing surprise and reflecting-on-action, which also contains an element of surprise. As you continue your learning journal, the next time you are surprised, take a moment to respond to the queries.

## Part 1

### RECOGNIZING SURPRISE

Reflect on a recent patient interaction or learning encounter and share your biggest surprise and how you adapted.

**Example A**: *"I also believe that I have adapted and changed in the way I approach every patient interaction. When I first began this program, I approached each clinical mentoring, exam, standardized patient encounter, and practical as a pressure situation and a memorization exercise. As I have progressed in this program, I have learned that this is not the case and that building trust and having compassion is just as important as stating facts. It is more important to go with the flow of each evaluation and interaction."*

**Example B**: *"Recently, I have had the opportunity to work with a stroke survivor in his early sixties with significant left-side neglect and weakness. I interact with not only this patient daily, but also his son. During my session with him, my biggest surprise was to see how much my patient and his son trusted me and my knowledge base while collaborating with him. I know that I have studied, prepared, and worked hard to get to this point, but I don't think I had actually put into perspective how much my patients appreciate my help. It was an eye opener for me and extremely rewarding to be able to work with this patient daily and see how he progresses and how I can challenge myself to be a better clinician for him and his functional progress."*

**Example C**: *"We recently had a patient who did not want to be evaluated or observed by a student. I respectfully understood her opinion and left the evaluation room while my clinical instructor performed the evaluation. This was a massive surprise to me because I have never encountered this with any patient in my clinicals. I asked the other physical therapists if they wanted any help with their patients and worked with two other patients that hour."*

**Example D**: *"Yesterday, I had a new outpatient evaluation with a patient status post stroke. The patient had global aphasia, which made the entire evaluation difficult to complete because the patient was unable to provide the information I needed to successfully complete it. I surprised myself by my ability to adapt to this situation. I used simple steps, first by remembering to take his baseline vitals and repeating them during the exam, and then by using one-step commands and tactile cues to complete the majority of the evaluation. After 20 minutes, while he was in a rest mode, I noticed that he was becoming more unresponsive, was flushed, and began sweating. I quickly went to the patient and assisted him to hook-lying with the assistance of my clinical instructor. We rechecked his vitals, the paramedics were called, and the patient was transferred to the hospital for further workup. I surprised myself again by my ability to remain calm, help calm the patient's spouse, and act quickly to ensure the patient had the care he required."*

**Example E**: *"In the past few weeks, I saw a patient whom my clinical instructor had evaluated and deemed as difficult due to his prescription drug-seeking behaviors and multiple inappropriate comments during his evaluation. When I treated him, I was extremely nervous as to how he would act toward me as a student. Surprisingly, he acted appropriately, with only some signs of symptom magnification that we were able to work through. This instance helped me to learn that it is always important to go into treating each patient with an open mind and to be nonjudgmental, despite anything I may have heard about the patient. By being friendly and treating the patient as I would have despite my clinical instructor's warnings, I was able to have a productive and appropriate treatment session with him."*

Now it's your turn. Reflect on a recent patient interaction or learning encounter and share your biggest surprise and how you adapted.

# *Part 2*

## REFLECTION-ON-ACTION

Consider a recent patient or personal encounter that did not go the way you had anticipated. Reflecting on the encounter, describe the following:

- What happened?
- What were you thinking/feeling?
- What sense did you make of the situation?
- What else could you have done?
- What was good and bad about the experience?
- If the same were to arise again, what would you do?

## EXAMPLE

**What happened?** *"A patient was admitted for continued management of respiratory failure with multiple comorbidities, had an extensive past medical history, and was being evaluated for physical and occupational therapies. Upon chart review, I imagined the patient as needing total assist with extremely poor functional mobility. When I got in the room, the patient was able to roll in bed with minimal assistance and could even perform a stand pivot transfer with moderate assist of two people. This was contradictory to what I had imagined the patient interaction would be during the initial encounter."*

**What were you thinking/feeling?** *"I felt as though I had overlooked something in the chart. I knew the patient's prior level of function was good, but the recent change in medical status led my mind to imagine a patient who would present in far worse condition from a functional perspective. I felt a bit embarrassed, thinking back now."*

**What sense did you make of the situation?** *"I just went with it and acted as if I had expected the patient to perform this well all along. After the encounter, it made me realize that, in the long-term/acute care setting, the patient's status can change drastically in 24 hours or less and that I should only rely on the documentation for clarification. Also, this situation taught me to never get so focused on a mental image; it's good to have going in, but it's never the same image you imagined once you leave the room. Whether it's better or worse than you originally imagined, it's always impacted by the patient encounter."*

**What else could you have done?** *"I could have allowed the patient to do more at the beginning of the encounter, rather than acting as if the patient were dependent with everything. After the evaluation, I felt as though I was too cautious and that the patient might have been capable of more than I allowed him to do on his own; the session could have been maximized more in terms of progression."*

**What was good and bad about the experience?** *"The patient felt comfortable and performed better than I expected. I wish I would have acted as if the patient were completely independent or much more capable, rather than initially acting as if he were dependent with everything."*

**If the same were to arise again, what would you do?** *"I would not allow my chart review prior to the patient interaction to cloud my judgment of how I perceive the patient's functional capabilities. Also, going into the room, I would first see what the patient could perform on his or her own rather than being quick to assist with everything."*

Now it's your turn. Consider a recent patient or personal encounter that did not go the way you had anticipated. Reflecting on the encounter, describe the following:

- What happened?



- What were you thinking/feeling?



- What sense did you make of the situation?

- What else could you have done?


- What was good and bad about the experience?


- If the same were to arise again, what would you do?


A final note: Remember that taking the time to write down your reflections makes your self-assessment explicit and observable to you for any improvements for the future and also self-recognition of areas of strength. Keep cultivating your skills and abilities with self- and peer- assessment as you continue your professional development. Collaborate with your peers and instructors to effect changes and address any gaps, explicitly addressing your learning needs identified through self-assessment and peer-assessment.

**These exercises are also available online at www.routledge.com/9781638220039.**

# 11

# LEADERSHIP AND ADVOCACY FOR HEALTH CARE

*Gina Maria Musolino*

## OBJECTIVES

*The learner should be able to*:

- Discover the value of incorporating leadership concepts for patient/client health care.
- Value Covey's *7 Habits of Highly Effective People: Powerful Lessons in Personal Change*.[1]
- Proactively investigate one's own leadership queries for personal and professional changemaking for leadership development and professional formation.
- Respect the benefits of every person's ability to lead and follow.
- Examine and reflect upon leadership principles and leaders.
- Foster high-functioning interprofessional teamwork.
- Discover leadership resources to explore and develop as interprofessional leaders.
- Advocate for the health care needs of society.
- Value the need to exercise empathy through voluntary advocacy action for those we serve.

Most people want to make a difference in this world, whether it is through teaching others, scrubbing floors, changing bandages or diapers, or herding cattle—most people want to do an excellent job and make a difference. Everyone has the opportunity to be a leader in life to create an even grander difference.

## IGNITING YOUR THOUGHTS ON LEADERSHIP

Let's first consider the words of the American diplomat and sixth U.S. President, and think about how you are a leader in everyday life.

> *If your actions inspire others to dream more, to learn more, to do more, and to become more, you are a leader.*
>
> —John Quincy Adams

DOI: 10.4324/9781003525554-11

209

Now take a moment to reflect on your future leadership potentials:

- Describe the kind of leader you want to be.
- As a leader, what do you want to be able to achieve?

While visiting the Smithsonian National Museum of American History in Washington, DC, I was pleasantly surprised to see an entire display dedicated to the First Ladies of the United States (FLOTUS), exploring the unofficial, yet ever important and often influential, position of the FLOTUS. The displays included many of their first inaugural ballgowns (the oldest displayed is Martha Washington's), lovely portraits, and how FLOTUS contributed to the work of the nation during the presidential administrations' of her husband. The role of the FLOTUS is not specifically defined, is an unofficial title, and carries no specific official duties; however, FLOTUS have contributed in meaningful ways leading a specific, focused agenda/s (Eleanor Roosevelt and Louisa Adams, women's rights; Martha Washington, Abigail Adams, Edith Roosevelt, and Dolley Madison, sociopolitical influencers; Laura Bush, education and 911 relief fund efforts; Lady Bird Johnson, highway beautification; Betty Ford, women's reproductive rights and alcoholism treatment center; Rosalyn Carter, mental health; Jackie Kennedy, interior design, fine arts, and fashion; Grace Coolidge, Red Cross; Lou Hoover, Girl Scouts of America; Barbara Bush, children's literacy, reproductive and civil rights, along with AIDS awareness; Nancy Reagan, drug awareness; Michelle Obama, *Let's Move*-focused on childhood obesity; Melania Trump, *BE BEST* focused on three pillars; well-being, online safety, and opioid abuse; and expanded to helping  teach the importance of social, emotional, and physical health, including bullying prevention and online safety, to protect the most vulnerable. FLOTUS are much more than spouses, dresses, or adornments; they served the nation with specific, intentional leadership agendas (humanitarian efforts, environmental protection, volunteerism, substance abuse, mental health, literacy, health care, obesity, cyberbullying awareness, military families, etc.) often not completely uncovered until they were in the history ("herstory") books.

Leadership is not necessarily a formal position or role; one does not need an official position of leadership to be a leader. Leadership is action to guide and direct. Every day leaders are changemakers. Each one of us with a growth mindset has the capacity to be what Budak[2] has described as a "changemaker one who takes action, leading positive change from where they are."[(p 22)] Budak considers changemaking a process, with an ongoing dedication and commitment, just as one makes a commitment to personal fitness, by taking daily actions to regular training, hard work, and dedication to health. Leading, as a changemaker, is a journey, not a destination.[3] Leadership takes courage and resilience. As a resilient professional leader, you focus on where you are capable of effecting change, yet also realize the need to accept the things you cannot. As we have discussed in prior Chapters 5, 9, and 10, health care professionals (HCPs) are bombarded with threats to our well-being, yet we also find ways to tune in to the good, so as not to be swallowed up by the negative.

Every day, we provide guidance for our patients, families, and caregivers to direct their abilities for movement and function. Leadership remains an important aspect of every health care team and is a foundational skill for the development of HCPs who lead their patients and families/caregivers. Incorporating the concepts of leadership throughout didactic and clinical education is important for fostering leadership skills in novice HCPs. Every HCP, at one time or another, shall be called upon to lead in everyday patient care encounters for the management of patient care. Our profession's futures shall be positive or dismayingly inadequate, depending on our abilities to serve as everyday leaders in health care. In a moment, we are going to begin with a pre-exercise that allows adult learners to explore leadership concepts and skills through a proactive leadership[4] reading, reflection, and writing. The activity is a catalyst for personal change and a primer for professional adaptation for HCPs. Through this priming exercise, you will, as Covey[1] stated, "begin with the end in mind."

Initially in this chapter, we are going to reverse our approach and thinking now that we are diving into the second half of *Patient Practitioner Interaction* (PPI). We are going to apply the leadership constructs of *Leading With Soul: An Uncommon Journey of Spirit*[5] and, through social influence, begin to proactively work toward supporting future patient health care needs, examine our abilities to collaborate in health care teams, and thrive through application of evidence-based and evidence-informed practice[6] leadership concepts and frameworks.[7,8] We are going to explore some of the classic and contemporary theories of leadership, including Bolman and Deal's[7] leadership frameworks, Kouzes and Posner's[9] leadership challenges, and Covey's[1] *The 7 Habits of Highly Effective People: Powerful Lessons in Personal Change* as you begin to examine your foundational capacities for everyday leadership.

Bolman and Deal,[5] in *Leading With Soul: An Uncommon Journey of Spirit*, ask the reader to consider Jesus's words when thinking about the direction of a true leader, paraphrasing: "What do we profit if we gain the whole world, but lose our own soul in the process?" (Matthew 16:26). Bolman and Deal[5] reminded us not to lose our heart and soul in the process of our work as leaders. We consider these concepts at the outset of the chapter to benefit from the leadership insights from their lifetime of work as educational leaders and researchers. In the often challenging yet highly rewarding works as HCPs, it remains relevant for you to not lose sight of the emotional side of leadership nor compromise professional values (as discussed in Chapter 4). Staying in touch with your affective domain (Chapter 3, Appendix) and the emotional aspect of care allows for a strong leader to be sensitive to the rhythms of the people we lead and influence, be it patients, clients, and/or peers. We shall further address aspects of spirituality related to patient care in Chapter 15; however, we will touch upon it briefly here with respect to leadership.

Mitroff and Denton[10] conducted a landmark study examining spirituality in the workplace. The researchers defined spirituality as "the basic feeling of being connected with one's complete self, others, and the entire universe." Mitroff and Denton[10] discovered that

> *people do not want to compartmentalize or fragment their lives. The search, meaning, purposes, wholeness, and integration is a constant, never-ending task. To confine this search to one day a week or after hours violates people's basic sense of integrity, of being whole people. In short, the soul is not something one leaves at home.*

An example shared from a research participant's interview was when a chemical worker awoke one morning and decided his work was wounding his soul because he could not reconcile the fact that the chemicals he was using to manufacture and treat furniture were highly toxic and very lethal to the environment.[10] The worker's spirit could no longer cope with the mismatch of his occupation with his own self-concept (reminding us of moral injury, moral distress, and moral integrity discussed in Chapter 9). The chemical worker's moral compass helped him to make a judgment between his beliefs of right and wrong—which impacted his soul in his everyday leadership. His moral compass allowed him to consider and act upon the greater good.

More than likely, you elected to pursue your dream to become a HCP because the professional career allows you to marry your soul with a higher calling to provide for others in the service of health care delivery. Thus, you can give of yourself more fully as a health care leader, sharing your genuine spirit while helping to transform others' lives through helping others. Consider these selected quotes from Bolman and Deal's[5] *Leading With Soul: An Uncommon Journey of Spirit*:

> *Perhaps we lost our way when we forgot that the heart of leadership lies in the hearts of leaders. We fooled ourselves, thinking that sheer bravado or sophisticated analytic techniques could respond to our deepest concerns. We lost touch with a most precious human gift—our soul. If you show people you don't care, they'll return the favor. Show them you care about them, they'll reciprocate. When people know that **someone really cares, you can see it**. It's there in their faces. And in their actions. Love really is the gift that keeps on giving. The essence of leadership is not giving things or even providing visions. It is **offering oneself and one's spirit**.*

- How do these perspectives relate to your school, health care institution(s), and home environment?
- Do you think the concepts could apply to any situation? Why or why not?
- Do you think the concept of spirituality belongs in health care? Why or why not?

Now that you have warmed up to the idea of leadership, let's consider the habits of those who are highly effective through Pre-Exercise 1.

# PRE-EXERCISE 1: PROACTIVE READING, REFLECTION, AND WRITING—*THE 7 HABITS OF HIGHLY EFFECTIVE PEOPLE: POWERFUL LESSONS IN PERSONAL CHANGE*

As Covey[1] stated, we are going to "begin with the end in mind" and start with a proactive pre-exercise related to leadership and engaging your developing self-assessment and peer-assessment skills, which you gained from Chapter 10. You will need to obtain a copy of the internationally popular text, *The 7 Habits of Highly Effective People: Powerful Lessons in Personal Change*, a seminal work on the universal and timeless habits for the foundations of leadership, written by Stephen R. Covey (1957–2012). If you have had the pleasure of previously reading it, it is worth revisiting. However, if you have read it within the last year or so, you may wish to select another contemporary leadership text for the proactive reading and reflection (resourced at the end of the chapter); however, you should revisit Covey's book as a refresher because we shall be discussing the impact of the habits related to you as a developing, adaptive HCP. Most learners find *The 7 Habits of Highly Effective People: Powerful Lessons in Personal Change* a timeless text that provides for new learning at any point along life's journey.

Once you have obtained a copy of *The 7 Habits of Highly Effective People: Powerful Lessons in Personal Change*, you are going to complete what is called proactive reading, reflection, and writing. Reading proactively is a skill I learned while working on my Doctor of Education degree in my leadership coursework and subsequently used successfully over the past decade with my own and HCPs' leadership learning.[4] Proactively reading—*reading actively with questions in mind*—is an important skill to develop now. It serves to remain current in contemporary literature, which may be helpful to your work as a HCP. Yet, you may not always have the time to delve deeply into the popular readings and helpful contemporary texts; hence, you can read them proactively.

Similar to being an effective HCP, an effective, proactive reader is able to look at the big picture of the text (as you do with the whole-to-part considerations with your patient examinations) and then consider questions to search for answers in the reading (similar to how we conduct a focused history with our patients), subsequently scanning the covers, front matter, back matter, prologue, table of contents, and index (as you would with screening a patient). Then, begin to actively search for answers, diving into the content (your more focused exam components with your patient, discovering answers and problem solving to affirm and support your clinical decisions), learning as you go how the findings apply to your leadership capabilities and abilities.

As a real-world HCP, one cannot possibly keep current on all evolving concepts in leadership and management; the proactive reading and writing is one approach to facilitate your critical thinking while consuming contemporary media that may or may not be viable for practice. What do you want to get out of the resource text? What's most important for you to learn right now (i.e., you won't be able to conduct every test in the book with your patients either)? The method involves first posing critical questions from your preview, then proactively reviewing the contemporary text, looking for crucial responses and supporting with pithy quotes and concepts from the text, fostering currency in contemporary leadership principles, all in an efficient manner. HCP students enjoy this exercise because it gives them the opportunity to learn about *The 7 Habits of Highly Effective People*, learn how to proactively read, and incorporate the lessons learned for their current and preferred futures, while experiencing the opportunity to critically perform peer and self-assessment of drafts, and then develop and revise the writing until satisfied with the final product.[4]

## *Proactive Reading, Writing, and Reflection Steps to Follow*

First, **preview** the information about the text and the author. Then, based on the preliminary information about the book and author, reflect on this information.

Second (**query**), **write down three specific questions** that you are interested in learning more about regarding the perspectives the author is presenting. One question should relate to you **personally** for **personal change**, one should be about your own **professional adaptation and development** along the journey, and the third should be about your own **preferred future**; the final question may relate to your personal and professional future but must include consideration about your preferred professional future.

Third (**review and write**), review the text proactively, skimming for answers with your three questions in mind related to personal development, professional development, and preferred future (which may include personal perspectives and must include professional perspectives). Then, write out your well-considered responses based upon the author's guidance. Do not copy long quotes from the text; rather, incorporate key concepts from the author and synthesize with your thoughts to respond to your query. The responses should <u>not</u> read like a book report but should be a thoughtful and meaningful discussion incorporating what you have learned from the book in a proactive manner from posing a query first, then searching the text for how it is guiding you for your personal and professional growth and development, and your preferred future query. Your initiative-taking, reflective writing should not exceed five to seven pages in total. Be certain to cite any notable quotes or unique ideas attributable to the author and include a reference page (including any other text you may have referenced).

Finally (**assess**), prepare your self-assessment and plan for peer and faculty assessment. Once you have completed your proactive reading, writing, and reflection, complete your own self-assessment using the proactive assessment form (Figure 11.1). Be prepared to exchange and peer review, and consider the learning shared by your peers. Be prepared to debrief regarding the book and leadership lessons in class discussions. Based upon peer feedback, you will most certainly wish to revise your proactive writing before seeking final instructor review of your last draft.

Once you have completed Pre-Exercise 1, with your first draft of the proactive reading, reflection, and writing and self-assessment completed, continue reading Chapter 11.

<u>**Proactive Reading, Reflection & Writing Assessment Feedback Rating**</u>

1. **Name/Date** ☐ Included? Comments:

2. Includes **3 Questions** (underlined) with Responses ☐Included? Comments:

3. **Underline major headings:** Introduction *(1-2 paragraphs)*, Questions and Response, Conclusion, References *(1 page)*
   ☐ Included? Compliance? Comments:

4. **Length:** Excluding the reference page, the Proactive Reading & Writing should fall between 5-7 pages *(double spaced, 11-12 pt font)*
   ☐ Compliance? Comments:

5. Paper includes all **inclusion items**, as indicated above Yes ☐ No ☐ Comments:

6. <u>**Substantive Content Review**</u>: *Each question (Q) response has sufficient **breadth** (wide range) and **depth** (complexity and reflective) of **personal thought** to answer the question & **provides substantive support** from the **text** within the response; consider each Q response individually:*

    a) Q 1 Yes ☐ No ☐ <u>**Provide your rationale /guidance-**</u> **Why or Why not?**

    b) Q 2 Yes ☐ No ☐ <u>**Provide your rationale/guidance** </u>**-Why or Why not?**

    c) Q 3 Yes ☐ No ☐ <u>**Provide your rationale/guidance** </u>**-Why or Why not?**

7. Appropriate reference citations are utilized where needed and direct quotes when required to provide appropriate citation format (AMA) include any additional references that you may cite or reference in addition to Covey; does not rely on long quotes, per directions; form and style also includes spelling, grammar, punctuation, capitalization, et al. **Form & Style Compliance:** Yes ☐ No ☐ Comments:

**Signature of Peer Reviewer, Faculty Reviewer or Self-Assessment:**_____

**Figure 11.1** Proactive reading, reflection, and writing assessment feedback rating.

# TIME AND COMPETENCY FOR LEADERSHIP HABITS

As a HCP, you must demonstrate competency and proficiency with technical standards, ensure you have time to devote your full attention to your patients, and not be too distracted by technology and social media to focus on your studies and patient care. Technology may be used as an asset for health care, such as with telehealth; however, it can also be a barrier. Many HCP learners incorporate decreased social media as a personal behavior change goal (which you will soon have the opportunity to formulate in Chapter 16) because they quickly realize, with the demands of professional school and adjustments needed to dedicate themselves to becoming the type of adaptive learner and professional they hope to become, a personal change is needed. With a few setbacks along the way, most HCP learners are able to achieve their goals to decrease their social media use, be device-free in the clinic, utilize technology in responsible ways for health care, and make improvements in time management.

As a developing leader in health care, you will need to be able to lead and model the way[9] when it comes to reducing the non-health care-oriented use of technology in your practice and learning environment while assuring that you are actively present and engaged so as not to miss firsthand learning application opportunities. When HCP students transition from classroom to clinical education/fieldwork environments, physical challenges will present in time management too. For example, even though developing HCPs are advised to begin a regular walking, endurance program prior to initiating clinical/fieldwork, many do not heed the advisement. Hence, during the early weeks of clinicals, developing HCPs quickly become physically tired (sitting in the classroom and periodic workouts do not prepare one for the physical demands of hands-on health care practice); students have challenges acclimating to many of the environmental demands of the clinical setting requirements (time management, responsible or device-free use, physical endurance, safety awareness for self and others, multitask management, prioritization, etc.). Consider which of Covey's[1] Quadrants are in play for your time management matrices and where you should be spending your time.

Covey[1] provided important lessons for change that lend to the required skill sets that translate for clinical practice success. We must shift to deeper learning and reduce distractions for learning.

Your education, right now, is your investment in your future and that of society. Your future patients/clients and colleagues are counting on you, and the value for your monetary investment is only as good as the work you put behind the effort. Make certain you have time for learning. Do not allow others to hinder or sabotage your learning through negativity or by distracting your time needed to learn and develop, or by hovering too closely, and allow yourself the opportunity to develop competency to be a leader.[1,5,8–12] How do you intend to keep *The 7 Habits of Highly Effective People*[1] at the forefront, model the way,[9] and resist and stay out of the unproductive quadrants?

Leadership remains an important aspect of every health care team and is a foundational skill for development that you will need to demonstrate in your patient–practitioner interactions as a HCP. As you incorporate *The 7 Habits of Highly Effective People*, as well as the 4 Quadrant time management lessons regarding where you spend your time, in your daily life and as a HCP, they will become just that—helpful habits, providing a solid foundation for your success and leadership. As a reminder, habits 1 to 3 are related to **self-management**; habits 4 to 6 to **leading others and teaming**; and habit 7 to **unleashing your potentials** and **renewal of ourselves in body, heart, mind, and soul** (Table 11.1).[1] We must not only manage our time, but our energies for renewal.

| TABLE 11.1 |
| --- |
| ## COVEY'S *THE 7 HABITS OF HIGHLY EFFECTIVE PEOPLE: POWERFUL LESSONS IN PERSONAL CHANGE* |
| Habit 1: Be Proactive—The Habit of Choice |
| Habit 2: Begin With the End in Mind—The Habit of Vision |
| Habit 3: Put First Things First—The Habit of Integrity & Execution |
| Habit 4: Think Win-Win—The Habit of Mutual Benefit |
| Habit 5: Seek First to Understand, Then to Be Understood—The Habit of Mutual Understanding |
| Habit 6: Synergize—The Habit of Creative Cooperation |
| Habit 7: Sharpen the Saw—The Habit of Renewal |
| Adapted from Covey SR. *The 7 Habits of Highly Effective People: Powerful Lessons in Personal Change.* New York, NY: Simon & Schuster; 2020. |

- Think for a moment about what has energized you in the past 24 hours.
- How can you utilize Covey's[1] Habits to assure you are making positive energy for renewal a priority?
- How do Covey's[1] Habits and 4 Quadrants relate to decreasing the impacts of burnout and moral injury we discussed in Chapters 5 and 9?

# LEADERSHIP VALUES

Donald Clifton,[13] known as the Father of Strengths-Based Psychology, developed the StrengthsFinder® and, with the Gallup Group of scientists, they examined over 1 million work teams, and discovered leaders' abilities. The leaders' abilities were classified into four distinct domains of leadership strengths: **executing**, **influencing**, **relationship building**, and **strategic thinking**.[13] Leadership teams were strongest and most cohesive when all domains within the organizational leadership were represented. Within the leadership teams studied, high-performing teams exemplified the following elements:

- Conflict did not destroy the teams, teams are results-oriented; healthy debate is good
- Prioritization of organizational needs for decisioning and all moving forward—together
- Dedicated to both their personal lives and their work, "work hard, play harder"
- Diversity is embraced by strong teams
- Strong teams are magnets for talent

Furthermore, three key findings emerged from the Gallup[13] study with respect to effective characteristics of leaders:

1. Always investing in employees' strengths and therefore well-being, and organizational capacities.
2. Surrounding themselves with the right people, with all strength-based domains represented and, therefore, maximizing abilities as high-performing teams.
3. Understanding their followers' needs.

So, not surprisingly, Gallup[13] scientists wanted to know what are the followers' needs from their respective leaders? Likewise, studying over 10,000 followers, Gallup[13] scientists discovered the most influential leaders exhibited the following characteristics that led to greater work engagement: **trust** (*honesty, integrity, respect*); **compassion** (*caring, friendship, happiness, love*); **stability** (*security, strength, support, peace*); and **hope** (*direction, faith, guidance*). Take a moment to look back now to Chapter 3, "Exercise 1. Values Priority" and compare the followers' expectations of their leaders with your personal prioritized values.

# LEADERSHIP QUALITIES AND CHALLENGES: MANAGERS, LEADERS, AND SERVANT LEADERSHIP

Real leaders, with a strong moral compass, genuinely care about the success of others and are open to innovative ideas, not just their own. True leaders appreciate others and do not steal credit; they genuinely and openly credit others in public ways. True leaders are humble, have appropriate self-insight, and recognize the importance of teamwork. Great leaders instill trust, connect with people, and are good listeners. Fearless leaders are not afraid to confront tough problems and do so with grace. Real leaders are never too self-important to jump in and get their hands dirty. True leaders hope their protégés exceed their own accomplishments. Most effective leaders often step in to determine function and capacities firsthand so as not to lose sight of all perspectives of those being led. Leaders know when to follow and let others lead and how to turn problems into solution-oriented opportunities. Leaders will never hesitate to improve themselves and role-model the same for their teams. Leaders are not afraid to ask for help and often utilize counseling services regularly and do not hesitate to call upon their team members for feedback and insights in a pro-active manner. Kouzes and Posner[9,14] also believe that "leaders are most often ordinary folks demonstrating extraordinary courage, skill and spirit to make a significant difference," while Bennis[15] provided clear distinctions between managers and leaders (Table 11.2). Being a good manager is not negative; however, to be a strong leader, one must be transformational. Real leaders take risks and reach across generations, working to be inclusive and collaborative, and all while encouraging and modeling authenticity.

| TABLE 11.2 | |
| --- | --- |
| **BENNIS'S DISTINGUISHING QUALITIES** | |
| **MANAGERS** | **LEADERS** |
| Administer | Innovate |
| Ask how and when | Ask what and why |
| Focus on systems | Focus on aligning people |
| Maintain | Develop and set direction |
| Rely on control | Inspire trust |
| Short-term perspectives | Long-term perspectives |
| Accept status quo | Challenge status quo |
| Have an eye on the bottom line | Have an eye on the horizon |
| Imitate | Originate |
| Emulate the classic good citizen | Are their own person |
| Copy and organize | Create strategy |
| Adapted from Bennis W. *On Becoming a Leader: The Leadership Classic.* 4th ed. New York, NY: Basic Books; 2009. | |

As a HCP, you will be called upon to be a strong manager and an innovative leader within your organization, with your patients and their families, and with coworkers. Both skills sets and activities of managers and leaders are necessary for an organization to succeed; the challenge is continuing to find the best balance of management and leadership in order to respond to be able to manage the complexities and change needed in health care environments.

You will also be asked to serve as an advocate for your patients and clients through letters of necessity; appeals for nonpayment of services; and with local, state, and federal government authorities that influence how we are able to practice and serve our patients through federal and state laws and rules. You may also take advantage of opportunities to serve in leadership roles with your membership organizations in your districts, regions, states, and nationally, and with other community-based and support groups that value your expertise and leadership capacities for health care.

Consider: What is the best leadership practice for the patients and clients our profession serves? Why?

According to Ebener:[16]

> *Leadership is an interactive process where leaders and followers influence each other to bring about change. Leaders and followers move toward a common goal. Leadership is a voluntary and interactive relationship to bring about a change in thinking, action, attitude, policies, structures, culture, and strategy.*

Leadership is very distinct from management. Ebener[16] stated that "[m]anagement is positional, while leaders can emerge from anywhere. Management can and does use authority. Leadership is not coercive. Leaders inspire, invite, and influence. When we rely solely on positional authority, we are not leading." Leaders transform self, others, organizations, and society. Maxwell[17,18] concurred, and said that the "true measure of leadership is influence—nothing more nothing less … it's about disposition, not position." Kotter[19] agreed, stating that "Most organizations are over-managed and under-led." Ebener[16] further explained that "[l]eadership is a function, not a position," lending further credence to the everyday leadership that occurs in health care by HCPs.

Leadership is about being a transformative agent of change. Leadership also requires lifelong learning, which is why the concept of self-assessment and reflective practice, discussed in Chapter 10, is central for your development as a leader. Leaders stimulate change and serve as catalysts to effect change. Leadership is constantly influenced by external and internal factors and demands. The fast-paced, multigenerational society we live in today demands that we become increasingly more flexible as leaders. Ebener[16] shared the need for teaming with leadership and said that the essence of leadership is this:

> *Leaders bring about change. They feel passionate about something that needs to change and influence others to join them in creating and carrying out a strategy to change. They realize they cannot do it by themselves. They then develop their followers into leaders, because most big things need many leaders.*

This should speak to you as a HCP today. The "big thing" is the Quadruple Aim of health care:[20] for achieving value-based care, a compass setting the direction. The Quadruple Aim framework addresses improving the individual experience of care, improving the health of populations, reducing the per capita cost of care, and enhancing the patient experience, with full consideration of the Social Determinants of Health (SDoH; see Figure 1.1 in Chapter 1), while improving the life of the HCP and the well-being of the health care team.[20] Today, one in three adults are experiencing multiple chronic conditions. Nearly 80% of health outcomes are driven by SDoH, with 30% of patients likely to be re-admitted due to lacking clear understanding of care instructions, and one in four patients reporting breakdowns in care communication between specialists and primary care providers.[20] Research has demonstrated clearly that the HCPs experience less burnout (see Chapter 9) when the social needs of their patients are adequately addressed. The Quadruple Aim will only happen through strong managers and leaders in health care working toward the quadruple aims.

Stop now and reflect a moment. Can you think of ways right this moment how you, either from your own firsthand experiences or those of others you know, might effect a change in the Quadruple Aim? Considering Bennis's[15] distinguishing qualities (see Table 11.2), what would your approach be as a manager vs. a leader in order to do the following?

- Improve health care experiences
- Reduce health care costs
- Improve the health of a population
- Enhance the patient experience while improving the life of the HCP and the well-being of the health care team

Kouzes and Posner[9,14] shared that leadership is more about behavior and inspiring others to lead and follow. Leadership qualities that are most welcome and needed in health care systems today include appropriate interpersonal skills, the ability to work on a team, strong ethics and integrity, and solid analytical/problem-solving skills. In *The Truth About Leadership*, Kouzes and Posner[21] shared that it does not matter what generation you represent in order to produce positive work attitudes; good leadership is good leadership. They noted that the context of leading may change a lot, but the content of leading changes little. The true fundamentals of leadership have not changed over the past decades. Kouzes and Posner[9,14] provided the fundamental challenges of leadership, which hold true today, to guide us in our own personal and organizational leadership development (see Table 11.3).

In addition to using Kouzes and Posner's practices and commitments as guideposts along the leadership roadmap, you will find Maxwell's[17] 360 leadership principles particularly helpful in the process steps for effective leadership. Maxwell's[17] 360 method involves multipoint influences, checks along the way, and the need for formative and summative evaluative information, considering all stakeholders' input, including the following:

- Coaching and feedback
- Developing trust and respect

| TABLE 11.3 |
|---|
| **KOUZES AND POSNER'S LEADERSHIP CHALLENGE** |

| 5 LEADERSHIP PRACTICES | 10 COMMITMENTS |
|---|---|
| **Model the way** | ○ Clarify **values**<br>○ Set the **example** |
| **Inspire a shared vision** | ○ Envision the **future**<br>○ Enlist others for a common **vision** |
| **Challenge the process** | ○ Search for opportunities for **innovation**<br>○ Experiment and take **risks** |
| **Enable others to act** | ○ Foster **collaboration**<br>○ Strengthen and develop **competence** |
| **Encourage the heart** | ○ Recognize **contributions**<br>○ Celebrate the **value** and **victories** |

Adapted from Kouzes JM, Posner BZ. *The Leadership Challenge: How to Make Extraordinary Things Happen in Organizations.* 5th ed. San Francisco, CA: Jossey-Bass; 2017.

- Inspiring and motivating others
- Building teamwork and collaboration
- Clarifying purposes (mission) and direction (vision)

Think of a leader you admire or someone whom you believe is a good leader. Can you think of leaders or leadership situations in which the preceding leadership practices have been experienced or demonstrated? What worked? What did not work? Why were the leaders effective or ineffective?

According to Blake and Mouton,[22] leadership has a dual focus that emphasizes task orientation or achieving results and developing relationships. **Servant leaders**, as first described by Greenleaf[23] and later Ebener[16] and Keith,[24] are more motivated to serve than to lead. Servant leaders are motivated by missions, visions, and core values, and their heart is at the service of the organization. Servant leaders are at the service of others and are therefore willing to share their power with others.[5,16,23,24]

Leadership is truly about change. What do you want to change as a leader? And more importantly, why? Generally speaking, only babies with wet diapers really thrive on change. As a leader, to empower change, you will need to somehow convince others *why* a change is needed. How will you facilitate change to occur as a leader? How will you incorporate the leadership qualities and characteristics to lead as a HCP more effectively?

Did you know that the best test of leadership is not how many followers you lead, but how many leaders you develop? The "Beatitudes of a Leader" are shared here for your reflection, further exemplifying the servant leader concepts:[23,24]

> *Blessed is the leader who has not sought the high places, but who has been drafted into service because of their ability and willingness to serve.*
>
> *Blessed is the leader who knows where they are going, how they are going, and how to get there.*
>
> *Blessed is the leader who knows no discouragement, who presents no alibi.*
>
> *Blessed is the leader who knows how to lead without being dictatorial; true leaders are humble.*
>
> *Blessed is the leader who seeks the best for those they serve.*
>
> *Blessed is the leader who leads for the good of the most concerned and not for the gratification of their own ideas.*
>
> *Blessed is the leader who develops leaders, while leading.*
>
> *Blessed is the leader who marches with the group and interprets correctly the signs on the pathway that leads to success.*
>
> *Blessed is the leader who has their head in the clouds, but their feet on the ground.*
>
> *Blessed is the leader who considers leadership an important opportunity for service.*

# LEADERSHIP: FRAMEWORKS AND TEAMING

In *Reframing Organizations, Artistry, Choice and Leadership*, Bolman and Deal[7] described that there are at least four frames, or ways of looking at organizations, to help make sense of the organizations within which we work. Bolman and Deal[7] said that the frames help us to see things and look at things differently from before and, therefore, people find them helpful. Typically, the four frames are in a cross shape, as in a window frame. The frames are defined as follows: (1) The **Structural Frame** is the rationale side of an organization, with a central concept of efficiency; (2) the **Human Resource Frame** is the people side of an organization, with a central concept of needs, skills, and relationships; (3) The **Political Frame** is the conflict side of an organization, with a central concept of power and competition; and (4) The **Symbolic Frame** is the cultural side of an organization, with a central concept of culture and meaning. Each frame is further described with metaphors, values with frameworks, and tools for organizing experiences within the organizations.[7] As a leading choreographer of change, you will "conduct" or work as a leader in all four frames.

Most organizations exhibit at least one, and often two, of the frames or depend upon only a few frames for daily operations and function, which are representative of the culture within the organization. A preference is shown for one or two frames; ideally no one uses only one frame all the time. The idea is that, at various times, to solve leadership challenges one may need to reframe the organization (e.g., to keep an organization heading in the right direction [Structural Frame] or to keep people involved and informed [Human Resource frame]). Bolman and Deal[7] suggested that, in order to not misread things, the correct frame needs to be identified in which to act, and in order to understand complex problems leaders need to use multiple lenses or frames. Learning to use all four frames allows leaders to be effective architects, servants, advocates, and prophets. The four-frame approach deepens the appreciation for and understanding of the organizations within which we lead or serve in health care teams.

Speaking of teams, this chapter would be lacking if we did not also consider how to differentiate how teams are working, or not, in health care. HCPs work collaboratively in interprofessional teams daily, delivering the highest quality of patient care. This is only accomplished through ongoing formal and informal communication, collaboration, and coordination. In fact, the Interprofessional Education Collaborative (IPEC)[25] has designated four core competencies to drive these best practice team efforts, which are likely incorporated within your respective professional didactic and clinical education curricula. We will further explore and apply the IPEC competencies in the end of chapter exercises. Take a moment now to familiarize yourself with these key core competencies for interprofessional collaborations.

## IPEC CORE COMPETENCIES[25]

ipecollaborative.org
- Competency 1. **Values and Ethics**: Work with team members to maintain a climate of shared values, ethical conduct, and mutual respect.
- Competency 2. **Roles and Responsibilities**: Use the knowledge of one's own role and team members' expertise to address individual and population health outcomes.
- Competency 3. **Communication**: Communicate in a responsive, responsible, respectful, and compassionate manner with team members.
- Competency 4. **Teams and Teamwork**: Apply values and principles of the science of teamwork to adapt one's own role in a variety of team settings.

Source: Interprofessional Education Collaborative (IPEC). *Core Competencies for Interprofessional Collaborative Practice: 2023 Version 3*. Washington, DC: IPEC. (Available: https://www.ipecollaborative.org/ipec-core-competencies)

Zenger et al.[26] provided excellent team evaluation instruments that you may wish to consider using in your learning and health care teams (Table 11.4) as you work with your developing professional and interprofessional learning teams. Use the instrument with your team to determine if you are helping to create a team identity, moving the team forward, or making the most of team differences. Part A considers your contributions to the team, and Part B, the teamwork. Remember to take the initiative in fostering your self and teamwork functions to yield stronger and higher performing teams through honest assessment and constructive insights bringing suggestions for improvements.

## *What Is Your Leadership Signature?*

You may be beginning to wonder about your own personal leadership style or questioning how you will be perceived as a leader. To better understand how leaders lead, West et al.[27] created a psychometric survey to measure the interrelated facets of leadership. Specifically, they did the following:

> *identified degrees of leadership in (a) a thriving "mind-set"[28] (including a sense of purpose, deep commitment to learning and conveyed sense of optimism); (b) a combination of self, social and situational awareness; and (c) essential leadership values such as performance orientation, ethical integrity, ability to collaborate and openness to change, among others.*

| TABLE 11.4 |
| --- |
| ## ZENGER-MILLER SAMPLE TEAM EVALUATION INSTRUMENTS |

Part A: Response choices:

Never (1)    Seldom (2)    Sometimes (3)    Usually (4)    Always (5)

Part A: How often do you make a conscious effort to do the following?

1. Help clarify and reinforce the overall purpose of the team.
2. Help the team set clear, achievable goals.
3. Recognize and celebrate the team's achievements.
4. Treat team members with respect while acknowledging their different motivations, values, work styles, and traditions.
5. Encourage each team member to participate fully.
6. Help the team get unstuck when differences lead to conflict.
7. Keep an open mind about new ways of doing things.
8. Encourage and reward team members who promote innovation.
9. Share new information with the team.

Part B: Response choices:

Strongly        Disagree (2)        Neither                Agree (4)        Strongly
Disagree (1)                        Disagree or Agree (3)                    Agree (5)

Part B: How well are we working together as a team?

1. The team knows exactly what it has to get done.
2. Team members get a lot of encouragement for innovative ideas.
3. Team members freely express their real views.
4. Every team member has a clear idea of the team's goals.
5. Everyone engages in the decisions we must make.
6. We tell each other how we are feeling.
7. All team members respect each other.
8. The feelings among team members tend to pull us together.
9. Everyone's opinion gets listened to.
10. There is truly little bickering among team members.

Are you satisfied or dissatisfied with the way you are working as a team? _____

Why? _____

Identify the item the team needs to work on most when examining your results compared with the team's:

_____

This item needs attention because: _____

My best idea for helping the team work better together currently is: _____

_____

Note: Teamwork is considered strong if the average score is Agree or Strongly Agree; if the average is neither Agree nor Disagree, teamwork is considered healthy, with room for improvement; if the average is Disagree or Strongly Disagree, something is getting in the way of teamwork. Whatever the score, discussing it with the team with an open mind is likely to improve teamwork.

Reprinted with permission from Zenger JH, Musselwhite E, Hurson K, Perrin C. *Leading Teams: Mastering the New Role.* Homewood, IL: Zenger-Miller, Inc, Business One Irwin, 1994. Reproduced with permission of McGraw-Hill Education.

| TABLE 11.5 |
|---|
| **THE EIGHT ARCHETYPES OF LEADERSHIP** |
| **Collaborator:** Empathetic, team building, talent-spotting, coaching-oriented |
| **Energizer:** Charismatic, inspiring, connects emotionally, provides meaning |
| **Pilot:** Strategic, visionary, adroit at managing complexity, open to input, team-oriented |
| **Provider:** Action-oriented, confident in their path or methodology, loyal to colleagues, driven to provide for others |
| **Harmonizer:** Reliable, quality-driven, execution-focused, creates positive and stable environments, inspires loyalty |
| **Forecaster:** Learning-oriented, deeply knowledgeable, visionary, cautious in decision making |
| **Producer:** Task-focused, results-oriented, linear thinker, loyal to tradition |
| **Composer:** Independent, creative, problem-solving, decisive, self-reliant |
| Adapted from West K, Stixrud E, Reger B. Assessment: what's your leadership style? *Harvard Business Review.* https://hbr.org/2015/06/assessment-whats-your-leadership-style. Published June 25, 2015. Accessed July 11, 2022. |

With more than 1,000 research participants, U.S.-based executives at companies with more than 250 employees, West et al.[27] discovered eight archetypes of leadership (Table 11.5).

West et al.[27] emphasized that there is no right or wrong in these leadership types, but recognizing a person's go-to style may be helpful, just as recognizing your own personal learning style helps you to be a better learner and teacher; knowing your type of leadership approach would benefit your own understanding of leadership and other styles and approaches that could make one a better leader in varying situations that one might encounter. You may also wish to check out your own leadership archetype results using the leadership inventories resources at the end of the chapter to determine your leadership archetype and/or leadership style. Leaders should know and be aware of their leadership style and ask how they can make the day of those they lead easier, e.g., "How can I help?".

# ADVOCACY IN ACTION

Leaders are always advocating for their employees, the strategic plan, resources, benefits, and reimbursement. Health care is rapidly evolving. Due to changes in reimbursement and decision making surrounding health care, medical necessity, and the management of care, our roles as HCPs have had to expand. This is partly due to social and economic change and partly due to having no clearly established meta-paradigm in relation to other professions. We have discovered that economic and social influences contribute to a person's health and disease. Hence, HCPs have taken on new responsibilities and skills to include much more advocacy work. If we do not act, the professions that exist today may be gone tomorrow, or they may be assumed by others who may be less expert at providing the rehabilitation care needed. We need to assist others in understanding not only what we do, but also what differences and impacts or value we have on those we serve in society. Political advocacy is the art of persuading policy makers to change policy; there is often opposition. Just like leadership, advocacy is also an influential process; your attitude toward advocacy and shared experiences can have an impact.

Our national membership organizations help us to accomplish advocacy for those we serve because advocacy is not the work of one, but of many working together to effect a change. Often, our national rehabilitation organizations work collaboratively on issues of mutual import. Most national organizations have things readily set up for you to advocate directly through the professional association resources. Take Action sites are as follows:

- American Physical Therapy Association (APTA): www.apta.org/Advocacy/
- American Occupational Therapy Association (AOTA): www.aota.org/advocacy
- American Speech-Language-Hearing Association (ASHA): www.asha.org/advocacy/

Take a look at the website that applies most directly to you or your profession and consider the issues that are part of the public policy plan that your professional organization is directly addressing currently. Consider the following:

1. What is the aim of the proposed policy or bill(s)? What outcomes are desired if the bill were to be achieved? What is the problem that is being addressed?

2. Who are the main constituents? Who are the stakeholders?

3. What are the obstacles, if any, regarding the issue? Who might be against the bill? Why?

We will revisit these websites again in the exercises. Advocacy is a key competency for HCPs to be capable of speaking up on behalf of your patients and acting on any of their unmet needs. You may also wish to collaborate with local, community-based, and national support groups.

Understand that your target audience for advocacy is your elected officials at the state and national levels. To be effective, you will need to become a constituent who has a relationship with your legislators. To promote a bill or policy change with your elected legislators, they need to know the following three things:

1. **Who?** Who you are, what you do for their constituents, and how you serve society; get to know your legislators on a personal level first! What do you have in common with them in your district?

2. **What?** What is the issue you want them to act on (bill numbers), and what are the merits of the bill, as well as the pros/cons, in brief?

3. **Why?** Share your powerful and impacting patient story of why the bill is relevant (or not) and the change the policy would make for others.

To accomplish advocacy, you need to have a practiced and polished "elevator talk" to be able to deliver your messaging in 2 minutes or less because you may not have much time, especially during the legislative sessions; if you get more time, then expand. You may be speaking with a legislative aide (LA) who also has much influence, and you should not be disappointed to speak with the LA or health LA. Reach out via phone and email, and in person when possible, participate in town halls. Unfortunately, as we will discuss in Chapter 17, policy does not change rapidly or overnight in most instances. Some legislation has taken decades. (A quick revisit to how a bill becomes a law illustrates the many steps: https://commons.wikimedia.org/wiki/File:Visualization-of-How-a-Bill-Becomes-a-Law_Mike-WIRTH.jpg) There can be many hurdles and detours in committees and subcommittees and unrelated or positive amendments that need to be renegotiated, along with political pressures and re-crafting of language. So, repeat messaging is required, too!

We need you to join the cause and help the effort for our patients! You must be appropriately persistent, and compromise will often need to occur. Money and votes speak to policy makers. Contributing to your membership's political action committee, in any amount, for the cause will help. Advocating to convince your lawmakers that a significant amount of the voting public shall benefit from, care about, and support the cause that a particular bill stands for is most relevant and part of our professional obligation in service to society today. If we don't speak up, who will? We need to develop relationships with our legislators so that we can engage with them regularly and persuade them to co-sponsor and sponsor legislation needed by our patients and in many cases to ensure that patients are able to continue to receive needed care. In my experience with advocacy, not only have I been able to expand my scope of influence and help have our patients' needs be better met, but I have also made new friends and interprofessional colleagues pulling for the same cause. Our developing HCPs regularly participate in advocacy days and events at the state and nation's capital, as well as repeatedly via the Take Action sites provided. Spread the word, assist those who cannot always help themselves, get involved today, and always keep the grassroots advocacy going in your local community. We will have the opportunity to further address this in Exercise 3.

# LEADERSHIP: TRANSFORMING SOCIETY

Through the readings and exercises in Chapters 8 and 9, we discovered and practiced effective communication and appropriate assertiveness skills. As leaders, our communication and especially listening and engagement skills are just as important. In a Harris poll of approximately 1,000 U.S. workers, the impact of communication was key when it came to pointing out where leaders fell short in being effective. Note that the communication issues that were most often cited as preventing effective leadership included not recognizing others' achievements (63%), not giving clear directions (57%), not taking time to meet with others (52%), taking credit for others' ideas (47%), not offering constructive feedback (39%), not communicating on the phone or in person (34%), and not getting to know your team players (23%).[29] According to Solomon,[29] in order to continue to connect while achieving every day, leaders can easily rectify this by simply asking or saying the following:

- Here's what I appreciate about you or your contribution...
- Thank you (personal and public)
- What do you think?
- Here's what's happening and what you can expect...
- I have some feedback for you...
- Let me tell you about something I learned the hard way...
- Hello [insert the person's name]...

Have you done any of the above lately with your peers, educators, patients and/or interprofessional colleagues? If not, begin today! Although leadership is a journey, can be hard, and influencing others is also challenging, promoting real change in others is part of what we do as HCPs. Leaders must practice these engagement skills during "normal" times so that when more challenging, turbulent times ensue, we have a solid foundation upon which to efficiently and effectively be responsive.

In more recent years, owing to the Covid-19 pandemic, many leaders have exhibited what is referred to as Turbulent Leadership.[30] Turbulence Theory[30] considers the impacts of the environment, security, and economics. It consists of four frameworks, akin to flight take-off, which may or may not be navigated by leaders during times of challenge, defined as follows:

1. Light—associated with ongoing issues, little or no disruption in the everyday working environment, and subtle signs of stress (normal)

2. Moderate—widespread awareness of issues with specific origins

3. Severe—fear for the entire enterprise, the possibility of large-scale community demonstrations, a feeling of crisis

4. Extreme—structural damage to normal operations is occurring—the collapse of reform seems likely[30]

The goal for leading during turbulent times is to make every effort to operate in the least turbulent frames possible, which entails not only leadership skills but also advocacy. During crisis leadership, leaders take the opportunity to reflect more regularly with teams, with a focus on two-way communication, repeat communication, using multiple methods, and taking care of one another, again "Leading with Soul,"[5] asking questions such as:

*What is the most important thing learned? How are we treating one another? How are you? How can I help? What are the priorities in terms of our values? What else might we try?*

The collaborative goal is to return to normal and reduce turbulence levels. Those most impacted by the "turbulence" may not have the ability to recover on their own and may require focused support for restoration. Lateral thinking is often employed with a true emphasis on self-care for all stakeholders as a priority. In health care, turbulent times will ebb and flow, yet quickly addressing and collaborating will assist in keeping the situation from becoming riskier and less safe, and help it to resolve more readily. Decision making for leaders in turbulent times must consider the "ethic of care" where moral action centers on interpersonal relationships and care or benevolence as a virtue (Chapter 4), to assure a resilient, healthier community of practice. What examples can you think of that cause turbulence for HCPs?

According to the Joint Commission, "sentinel events in healthcare include patient safety events (not primarily related to the natural course of the patient's illness or underlying condition) resulting in death, permanent harm, or severe harm."[31] In 2023, reported sentinel events persisted consistently with prior years reporting trends. Patient falls were the leading event type reviewed (48%). Patient outcomes from reported sentinel events were death (18%), permanent harm (8%), severe harm (57%), and unexpected additional care/extended stay (12%). Unfortunately, as in prior years, failures in communication, teamwork, and consistently following policies were leading causes for reported sentinel events.[31] Since 2019, the leading sentinel event indicator remained as **patient falls**. Trending upwards annually, patients falling while ambulating was the leading mechanism for falling, followed by falling from the bed and falling while toileting. Of the reported falls, all falls data increased in 2023, with 35% of falls occurring during ambulation; 25% were a result of falls from the bed; and 19% occurred while toileting.[31] Reported contributors to falls included lack of following policies (e.g., fall risk assessment), lack of competency to identify abnormal clinical signals and/or signs, inadequate staff-to-staff communication with handoff procedures and/or transitioning of care, and deficiencies in a shared understanding or mental model regarding plans of care.[31] Sentinel events that resulted in death in 2023 were most associated with patient suicide (29%), delays in treatment (23%), and patient falls (10%).[31] Events resulting in severe temporary harm were most associated with patient falls (67%).[31]

How is leadership demonstrated by the health care providers who reported? Furthermore, in the Joint Commissions investigations of the reported events, failures were discovered in "communication, teamwork and consistently following policies" as the key drivers for the incidents.[31] Clearly the data suggests the need for greater attention to these areas of individual professionalism, professional practice, and team leadership. How can movement specialists/rehabilitation professionals engage as leaders to effect a change and manage the known risks related to falls specifically? How can the health care team enact to assure better prevention and work to reduce sentinel events as leaders and through peer and self-assessment? What ethical principles, standards of practice, core values, and legal considerations guide you in proactively addressing sentinel events? Describe how you would specifically address communication, teamwork, and policy compliance in a variety of health care delivery settings to lead by example. Tip: Review the Joint Commission[31] website sentinel event information and root-cause analysis framework for sentinel events to facilitate your individual and team and actions as a health care leader and discuss with your peers. How will your generation of HCPs effect a downward trend in these preventable sentinel events?

Changing our own and others' paradigms is no easy task (we will practice more in Chapter 16). However, there is extraordinary joy in serving as a leader and guiding others to achieve. Some of the greatest leadership successes of HCPs are when we assist our patients in achieving their goals, when someone we have mentored achieves their goals, when we finally achieve a long-term battle related to advocacy action, when we have recovered from turbulence, even if temporarily, and when an organization or team that we have led accomplishes more than they thought possible—these make it all worthwhile! Most of these accomplishments involved transforming society in some manner with remarkable resilience by many. Let's look more closely now at the concept of transformation over time with respect to the Movement System.

One of the many influential leaders in our profession, Shirley Sahrmann, PT, PhD, FAPTA,[32,33] describes **movement** as the core of physical therapy and how we have evolved from technicians to professionals in the evolution of thinking about the **Movement System**. She shared how a team of leaders gathered *over decades* to continue the ideas of professional identity, integrating the concepts of movement science in professional education, leading up to the new vision for the profession and subsequent ongoing discussions regarding diagnostic dilemmas[32,34] related to the Movement System. The guiding principles in the APTA Vision Statement state that:

> *the physical therapy profession's greatest calling is to maximize function and minimize disability for all people of all ages. Movement is key to optimal living and quality of life for all people of all ages that extends beyond health to every person's ability to participate in and contribute to society.*[35,36]

The culmination of the efforts over time led to the adoption by the APTA's House of Delegates, of the APTA's Vision Statement for the Physical Therapy Profession: "Transforming society by optimizing movement to improve the human experience."[35,36] Much of the work of leadership is done through voluntary efforts.

Although this vision is specifically for the physical therapy profession, it may inspire others in society and other disciplines to promote movement and collaborate with physical therapy. I asked doctor of physical therapy (DPT) professional learners on clinical education experiences how they were serving as leaders to meet the intents of the APTA Vision Statement and its guiding principles for the profession of physical therapy. You may find the following excerpts of different students' voices inspiring as you reflect on your continued personal and professional leadership ahead, envisioning your success as a HCP.

# CLINICAL EDUCATION: TRANSFORMING SOCIETY

Following your reflections on these voices, take time to journal. Consider and answer how you will transform society by optimizing movement to improve the human experience. (You may substitute your own profession's vision or that of your organization.)

I feel that my job at the cancer center is completely transforming society and the people in it. I have patients who are postsurgery procedures from cancer (e.g., total hip and knee replacements due to bone tumor, soft tissue resections, radical mastectomies, etc.) who have many limitations. After a few days of working with a patient postoperatively, they are walking more than 150 feet with an assistive device. I love to see how much people can improve, and in such a short amount of time. At first, the patient is hesitant and scared and feels that they may not get better. But with just a few days of physical therapy and teaching them how to ambulate again, strength and mobility come back. Endurance takes much longer. I also work with many patients with leukemia who come in for bone marrow transplants. Typically, about 1 week after transplant, their white blood cell count and platelets decrease dramatically, so weakness and fatigue are quite common. I always try to remain as positive as possible and let each patient know that I am here for them and for their recovery. I actually started a new thing—making certificates for patients. I made one called the "marathoner award." It is for patients who are here for a very long time but continue to push through and work as hard as they can every day. I gave it to a man with leukemia who has been here since the day I started at the cancer hospital (about 6 weeks now). He was so happy. It gave him even more motivation to keep trying and working hard. I love seeing people transform themselves and feel better overall. Working with people who have cancer is very inspirational. Each day I go home thinking about the patients I have treated and how lucky I am to have met such amazing people who have such great attitudes, work very hard, and are overall a pleasure to work with, and I have the greatest job to lead them back to health, optimizing their movement to improve their function.

Currently, my caseload has a significant portion of patients with amputations. Every month, the patients get together for an empowerment group. They refer to this as an empowerment group, *not* a support group because that's what it is—empowering! The prosthetic empowerment group meetings are all about how patients optimize their performance in society; they reach out to each other and discuss the successes and obstacles they have encountered along their paths. Their objective is to work together to become more empowered in the community, and I am pleased to say I will be presenting at their next meeting. I am preparing a presentation on wound care for people with amputations because 75% of people with amputations experience dermatologic issues with their limb, and 65% experience these issues more than once. To further optimize movement and improve the human experience, I am reaching out to this population to further empower them on what they can expect and how they can react when these issues arise. I will be creating a brochure/handout for everyone to take home as well. I am finding out what they know in advance and planning for what new information I can share and the best format.

I am helping society through improving movement and function through building rapport with patients and their caregivers. In my view, no matter how knowledgeable someone is, if he or she cannot build a professional, friendly relationship with a patient, then that patient's optimal human experience through movement will be very difficult to obtain. The pediatric setting is where this applies most because children at young ages will not sit there and comprehend what you as a physical therapist are trying to accomplish. Building rapport, making timid kids open up, and making a majority of treatment interventions into games will help facilitate advancement toward set goals, thus optimizing the human experience via movement. Also, with parents who just see pediatric physical therapy as play, building rapport with them is even more crucial for patient success because the parents/caretakers are the ones ultimately responsible for the child's home exercise program and compliance with therapy. Education and explanation of the rationales for what you, the physical therapist, do for their daily experiences will help caretakers realize that what you're doing with their children has meaning and purpose and why home exercise compliance is so needed! For instance, the children are not just walking upstairs or putting a dinosaur magnet on a board; they are strengthening their entire lower extremity musculature, developing motor planning through the activity, and developing safety and environmental awareness through verbal and tactile cues, all while improving proprioceptive input into their ankle, knee, and hip joints to improve body function and motor control, which decreases their risk for falls and helps them become more independent. Patient/caregiver education is critical to patient success, and without building rapport with patients and their caretakers, it is pretty hard, if not impossible, to improve their livelihood. I lead toward the vision by educating and facilitating movement with children and their caregiving parents or family/support members.

I am transforming society by optimizing movement to improve the human experience by treating the whole patient, not just a body part. In orthopedics, it can be easy to get hung up on the referring diagnosis, such as hip pain, but treating just the hip is not likely going to fix the problem. Educating the patient is an important part of this plan because he or she may wonder why you are working on something such as foot posture when they came in for hip pain. I am presently doing this on my clinical education internship by performing thorough examinations, creating detailed documentation, and educating patients on all of my findings. I treat the deficits that I find and then work toward incorporating functional activities into the treatments that are meaningful to the patient's desires and goals. This mantra should be applied in any setting ("treating the patient, not the disease") because treating the disease or treating just one body part is not going to get the patient back to the functional goals for which he or she is seeking physical therapy.

We have the opportunity to serve and rehabilitate all people from society, regardless of their medical status. I have been mainly treating people within the neurological population, and with them, I am constantly reminded that every day is a gift. I help them learn how to sit, stand, walk, negotiate stairs, and perform any other functional movement—functional activities that "normal" people take for granted every day. Last week, I evaluated an older man who sustained a left-side stroke infarction that left him with right-side hemiparesis and severe expressive and receptive aphasia. He could not follow any commands during the initial evaluation period and required two people to perform a sit-to-stand transfer. However, this week, he was fully alert and oriented, only required minimal assistance of one person for sit-to-stand transfers, and now is able to ambulate approximately 60 feet with a rolling walker and minimal assistance of one person for balance and safety. I am blessed to help people rehabilitate to a life that they feel is worth living by optimizing their movement, and it is also my pleasure to be doing a lunch talk for the local Optimist Club, which meets at the hospital, to talk about what physical therapists do and how we impact society.

# REFERENCES

1. Covey SR. *The 7 Habits of Highly Effective People: Powerful Lessons in Personal Change*. New York, NY: Simon & Schuster; 2020.
2. Budak A. *Becoming a Change Maker: An Actionable Inclusive Guide to Leading Positive Change at Any Level*. New York, NY: Hachette Book Group, Grand Central Publishing; 2022.
3. Harris CA. *Lead to Win: How to Be a Powerful, Impactful, Influential Leader in Any Environment*. New York, NY: Penguin Publishing Group; 2022.
4. Musolino GM. Fostering leadership in entry-level DPT education. Abstract presented at: Annual Conference and Exposition of the APTA; June 8–11, 2011; National Harbor, MD.
5. Bolman LG, Deal TE. *Leading With Soul: An Uncommon Journey of Spirit*, 3rd ed. San Francisco, CA: Jossey-Bass; 2011.
6. Sackett DL. *Evidence-Based Medicine: How to Practice & Teach Evidence-Based Medicine*, 2nd ed. Philadelphia, PA: Elsevier Health Sciences; 2000.
7. Bolman LG, Deal TE. *Reframing Organizations: Artistry, Choice and Leadership*, 6th ed. New York, NY: Wiley; 2017.
8. Bolman LG, Deal TE. *The Wizard and the Warrior: Leading with Passion and Power*. San Francisco, CA: Jossey-Bass; 2006.
9. Kouzes JM, Posner BZ. *The Leadership Challenge: How to Make Extraordinary Things Happen in Organizations*, 6th ed. New York, NY: Wiley; 2017.
10. Mitroff II, Denton EA. A study of spirituality in the workplace. *Massachusetts Institute of Technology Sloan Management Review*. 1999;40;(4):83–92.
11. Stahl A. Five reasons why helicopter parents are sabotaging their child's career. *Forbes*. May 27, 2015. https://www.forbes.com/sites/ashleystahl/2015/05/27/5-reasons-why-helicopter-parents-are-sabotaging-their-childs-career/. Accessed September 1, 2022.
12. Vinson KE. Hovering too close: the ramifications of helicopter parenting in higher education. *Georgia State University Law Review*. 2013;29:423–451.
13. Gallup Press. *Clifton Strengths-based Leadership: Great Leaders, Teams, and Why People Follow*. Omaha, NE; 2009.
14. Kouzes JM, Posner BZ. *The Leadership Challenge Workbook*, 3rd ed. New York, NY: Wiley; 2017.
15. Bennis W. *On Becoming a Leader: The Leadership Classic*, 4th ed. New York, NY: Basic Books; 2009.
16. Ebener DR. *Blessings for Leaders: Leadership Wisdom from the Beatitudes*. Collegeville, MN: The Liturgical Press; 2012.

17. Maxwell JC. *The 360 Degree Leader*. Nashville, TN: The Thomas Nelson; 2011.
18. Maxwell JC. *The 21 Irrefutable Laws of Leadership*. New York, NY: Harper Collins Leadership; 2022.
19. Kotter JP. *Leading Change*. Cambridge, MA: Harvard Business School Press; 2012.
20. Lovén M, Pitkänen LJ, Paananen M, Torkki P. Evidence on bringing specialised care to the primary level-effects on the Quadruple Aim and cost-effectiveness: a systematic review. *BMC Health Serv Res*. 2024 Jan 2;24(1):2. doi: 10.1186/s12913-023-10159-6.
21. Kouzes JM, Posner BZ. *The Truth About Leadership: The No-Fads, Heart-of-the-Matter Facts You Need to Know*. San Francisco, CA: Jossey-Bass; 2010.
22. Blake RR, Mouton JS. *The Managerial Grid: Leadership Styles for Achieving Production Through People*. Houston, TX: Gulf Publishing; 1996.
23. Greenleaf RK. *Servant Leadership: A Journey into the Nature of Legitimate Power and Greatness*. Westfield, IN: Greenleaf Center for Servant Leadership; 2002.
24. Keith KM. *The Case for Servant Leadership*. Westfield, IN: Greenleaf Center for Servant Leadership; 2017.
25. Interprofessional Education Collaborative (IPEC). *Core Competencies for Interprofessional Collaborative Practice: 2023 Update*. Washington, DC: IPEC. https://www.ipecollaborative.org/assets/core-competencies/IPEC_Core_Competencies_Version_3_2023.pdf Accessed July 17, 2024.
26. Zenger JH, Musselwhite E, Hurson K, Perrin C. *Leading Teams: Mastering the New Role*. Homewood, IL: Irwin Professional; 1994.
27. West K, Stixrud E, Reger B. Assessment: what's your leadership style? *Harvard Business Review*. https://hbr.org/2015/06/assessment-whats-your-leadership-style. Published June 25, 2015. Accessed July 11, 2022.
28. Dweck CS. *Mindset: The New Psychology of Success*. New York, NY: Ballantine Books; 2007.
29. Solomon L. Leadership: the top complaints from employees about their leaders. *Harvard Business Review*. http://hbr.org/2015/06/the-top-complaints-from-employees-about-their-leaders. Published June 24, 2015. Accessed July 11, 2022.
30. Gross SJ. *Applying Turbulence Theory to Educational Leadership in Challenging Times: A Case-Based Approach*. New York, NY: Routledge; 2020.
31. The Joint Commission. Sentinel Event Data, 2023 Annual Review, 2024. https://www.jointcommission.org/resources/sentinel-event/ Accessed July 17, 2024.
32. Sahrmann SA. The Twenty-Ninth Mary McMillan Lecture: Moving precisely? Or taking the path of least resistance? *Phys Ther*. 1998;78(11):1208–1219.
33. Sahrmann SA. The human movement system: our professional identity. *Phys Ther*. 2014;94(7):1034–1042.
34. Stith JS, Sahrmann SA, Dixon KK, Norton BJ. Curriculum to prepare diagnosticians in physical therapy. *J Phys Ther Educ*. 1995;9(2):46–53.
35. American Physical Therapy Association. Vision, mission, and strategic plan. www.apta.org/apta-and-you/leadership-and-governance/vision-mission-and-strategic-plan Accessed July 11, 2024.
36. American Physical Therapy Association. Human movement system. www.apta.org/movementsystem/ Accessed July 11, 2024.

# SUGGESTED READINGS

Afremow J. *The Leader's Mind: How Great Leaders Prepare, Perform, and Prevail*. New York, NY: Harper Collins Leadership; 2021.

Alexander E. *Proof of Heaven: A Neurosurgeon's Journey Into the Afterlife*. New York, NY: Simon & Schuster; 2012.

Aquinas T. Vol 1–5. *The Summa Theologica of St. Thomas Aquinas* Rev ed. London: Burns, Oates and Washburne; 1920.

Binder-Macleod S. Fifty-first McMillan Lecture. What I know: The value of mentoring and leadership. *Phys Ther*. 2021;101(12):pzab199. doi: 10.1093/ptj/pzab199.

Blanchard K, Hodges P. *Lead Like Jesus: Lessons from the Greatest Role Model of All Time*. Nashville, TN: Thomas Nelson; 2008.

Buckingham M, Coffman C. *First, Break All the Rules: What the World's Greatest Managers Do Differently*. Washington, DC: Gallup Press; 2016.

Budak A. *Becoming a Change Maker: An Actionable Inclusive Guide to Leading Positive Change at Any Level*. New York, NY: Hachette Book Group, Grand Central Publishing; 2022.

Cain S. *Quiet: The Power of Introverts in a World That Can't Stop Talking*. New York, NY: Broadway Books; 2013.

Collins J. *Good to Great: Why Some Companies Make the Leap…and Others Don't*. New York, NY: Harper Business; 2001.

Craik RL. Thirty-Sixth McMillan Lecture: Never satisfied. *Phys Ther*. 2005;85:1224–1237.

Delitto A. We are what we do. *Phys Ther*. 2008;88(10):1219–1227.

Divine M. *The Way of the SEAL: Think Like an Elite Warrior to Lead and Succeed*. New York, NY: Reader's Digest; 2013.

Dowden C. *A Time to Lead: Master Yourself… So You Can Master Your World*. New York, NY: Forefront Books; 2022.

Duncan PW. One grip a little stronger. *Phys Ther*. 2003;83(11):1014–1022.

Dunwoody A. *A Higher Standard: Leadership Strategies from America's First Female Four-Star General*. Philadelphia, PA: Da Capo Press; 2015.

Elmore TA. *New Kind of Diversity: Making the Different Generations on Your Team a Competitive Advantage*. Duluth, GA: Maxwell Leadership; 2022.

Eyal, N. *Indistractable: How to Control Your Attention and Choose Your Life*. Dallas, TX: BenBella Books; 2019.

Gawande A. *The Checklist Manifesto: How to Get Things Right.* London: Picador; 2011.

Gladwell M. *Outliers: The Story of Success.* Boston, MA: Little Brown and Company; 2011.

Greenleaf RK. *The Servant-Leader Within: A Transformative Path.* Mahwah, NJ: Paulist Press; 2009.

Guccione AA. Destiny is now. *Phys Ther.* 2010;90(11):1678–1690.

Haley N. *If You Want Something Done: Leadership Lessons from Bold Women.* New York, NY: St. Martin's Publishing Group; 2022.

Haley N. *With All Due Respect: Defending America with Grit & Grace.* New York, NY: St. Martin's Publishing Group; 2020.

Harris CA. *Lead to Win: How to Be a Powerful, Impactful, Influential Leader in Any Environment.* New York, NY: Penguin Publishing Group; 2022.

Harrison, C, ed. *Leadership during Crisis: A Focus on Leadership Development.* London and New York, NY: Routledge, Taylor & Francis Group; 2024.

Hislop HJ. Tenth Mary McMillan Lecture: The not-so-impossible dream. *Phys Ther.* 1975;55(10):1069–1080.

Jensen GM. Learning: what matters most. *Phys Ther.* 2011;91(11):1674–1689.

Jette AM. 43rd Mary McMillan Lecture: Face into the storm. *Phys Ther.* 2012;92(9):1221–1229.

Johnson GR. Twentieth Mary McMillan Lecture: Great expectations: a force in growth and change. *Phys Ther.* 1985;65(11):1690–1695.

Kearns Goodwin D. *Team of Rivals: The Political Genius of Abraham Lincoln.* New York, NY: Simon & Schuster; 2006.

Kearns Goodwin D. *Leadership in Turbulent Times.* New York, NY: Simon & Schuster; 2009.

Kendall FP. Fifteenth Mary McMillan Lecture: This I believe. *Phys Ther.* 1980;60(11):1437–1443.

Kim WG, Mauborgne R. *Blue Ocean Strategy.* Boston, MA: Harvard Business Review Press; 2015.

Kounios J, Beeman M. *The Eureka Factor: Aha Moments, Creative Insight, and the Brain.* New York, NY: Random House; 2015.

Laker B, Cobb D, Trehan R. *Too Proud to Lead: How Hubris Can Destroy Effective Leadership and What to Do About It.* New York, NY: Bloomsbury USA; 2021.

Lencioni P. *Death by Meeting: A Leadership Fable About Solving the Most Painful Problem in Business.* San Francisco, CA: Jossey-Bass; 2010.

Lencioni P. *Overcoming the Five Dysfunctions of a Team: A Field Guide for Leaders, Managers, and Facilitators.* San Francisco, CA: Jossey-Bass; 2010.

Magistro CM. Twenty-Second McMillan Lecture. *Phys Ther.* 1987;67(11):1726–1732.

Markova D, McArthur A. *Collaborative Intelligence: Thinking With People Who Think Differently.* New York, NY: Spiegel & Grau; 2015.

Maxwell J. *Leading in Tough Times.* New York, NY: Center Street, Hachette Book Group; 2021.

McRaven, WM. *Make Your Bed: Little Things That Can Change Your Life … And Maybe the World.* New York, NY: Grand Central Publishing; 2017.

Michels E. Nineteenth Mary McMillan Lecture. *Phys Ther.* 1984;64(11):1697–1704.

Mittroff II, Mittroff D. *Fables and the Arts of Leadership: Applying the Wisdom of Mister Rogers to the Workplace.* New York, NY: Palgrave Macmillan; 2012.

Moffat M. Thirty-Fifth Mary McMillan Lecture: Braving new worlds: to conquer, to endure. *Phys Ther.* 2004;84(11):1056–1086.

Moss J. *The Burnout Epidemic: The Rise of Chronic Stress and How We Can Fix It.* Boston, MA: Harvard Press; 2021.

Patterson K, Grenny J, McMillan R, Switzler A, Roppe L. *Crucial Conversations: Tools for Talking When the Stakes Are High*, 3rd ed. New York, NY: McGraw Hill Education; 2021.

Phillips DT. *Lincoln on Leadership: Executive Strategies for Tough Times.* New York, NY: Warner Books; 1993.

Pope Francis. *The Church of Mercy.* Chicago, IL: Loyola Press; 2014.

Pope John Paul II. On social concerns. *Population and Development Review.* 1988;14(1):211–217.

Pronovost P, Vohr E. *Safe Patients, Smart Hospitals: How One Doctor's Checklist Can Help Us Change Health Care From the Inside Out.* New York, NY: Penguin; 2011.

Purtillo RB. Thirty-First McMillan Lecture: A time to harvest, a time to sow: ethics for a shifting landscape. *Phys Ther.* 2000;80(11):1112–1119.

Raei M, Guenther SK, Berkely LA. *Leadership at the Spiritual Edge: Emerging and Non-Western Concepts of Leadership and Spirituality.* London and New York, NY: Routledge, Taylor & Francis Group; 2024.

Rothstein JM. Thirty-Second McMillan Lecture: Journeys beyond the horizon. *Phys Ther.* 2001;81(11):1817–1829.

Schein EH, Schein PA. *Humble Leadership: The Power of Relationships, Openness and Trust.* Oakland, CA: Berrett-Koehler Publishers; 2023.

Shepard KF. Mary McMillan Lecture: Are you waving or drowning? *Phys Ther.* 2007;87(11):1543–1554.

Synder-Mackler L. Forty-sixth McMillan Lecture: Not Eureka. *Phys Ther.* 2015;95(10)1446–1456.

Treasurer B. *Two Words at a Time: Simple Truths for Leading Complicated People.* Oakland, CA: Berrett Koehler Publishers; 2022.

Weisinger H, Pawliw-Fry JP. *Performing Under Pressure: The Science of Doing Your Best When It Matters Most.* New York, NY: Crown Publishing; 2015.

Whitehurst J. *The Open Organization: Igniting Passion and Performance.* Boston, MA: Harvard Business Review Press; 2015.

Winstein CJ. The best is yet to come. *Phys Ther.* 2009;89(11):1236–1249.

Wolf SL. Thirty-third Mary McMillan Lecture: "Look forward, walk tall": exploring our "what if" questions. *Phys Ther.* 2002;82(11):1108–1119.

Wood R. Twenty-third Mary McMillan Lecture: Footprints. *Phys Ther.* 1989;69(11):975–980.

# LEARNING AND LEADERSHIP STYLES AND SIGNATURE INVENTORIES

Galford RM, Maruca RF. Your Leadership Legacy Assessment. http://www.yourleadershiplegacy.com/assessment/assessment.php

Learning Style—What's your learning style (*Visual, Auditory, Kinesthetic*)—Link to complete and discover. http://www.educationplanner.org/students/self-assessments/learning-styles

Kolb Experiential Learning Profile (KELP). Institute for Experiential Learning. https://experientiallearninginstitute.org/what-is-experiential-learning/

Kolb Learning Preferences Questionnaire—Complete Instrument to determine Kolb Learning Style. https://aim.stanford.edu/wp-content/uploads/2013/05/Kolb-Learning-Style-Inventory.pdf

Leadership Practice Inventory. www.leadershipchallenge.com/

Leadership Style: Brief assessment. https://hbr.org/2015/06/assessment-whats-your-leadership-style

West KA. What's your leadership signature? https://www.heidrick.com/en/insights/leadership-development/whats-your-leadership-signature

# ASSOCIATION RESOURCES

**American Occupational Therapy Association—Emerging Leaders Development.** Program for students and new practitioners that provides training to become leaders. For more information, visit www.aota.org

**American Physical Therapy Association—Oral Histories.** First-person recollections of leaders who have shaped or continue to shape the profession. Audio and video have been recorded since 1980, via www.apta.org (see Exercise 2).

**Leadership Development Training: APTA—Academy of Leadership & Innovation.** A specialty component offers Leadership, Administration, Management, and Professionalism Certificate Programs—The Institute for Leadership in Physical Therapy for the development of personal and professional leadership skills. For more information, visit www.aptaali.org

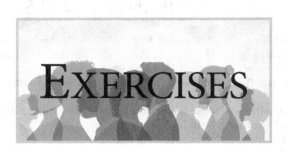

# POST-EXERCISE 1: REFLECTIONS ON *THE 7 HABITS OF HIGHLY EFFECTIVE PEOPLE: POWERFUL LESSONS IN PERSONAL CHANGE*

In Pre-Exercise 1, through your proactive reading, reflection, and writing exercise, you explored your own personal and professional leadership queries. Now, as you continue your formal and informal leadership and on into clinical education health care teams and in advocacy work for our patients served by the health care professions, you will continue to grow and develop as a leader. Because real-world HCPs cannot possibly keep current on all evolving concepts in leadership and management, proactive reading and writing is one approach to facilitate critical thinking while consuming contemporary media that may or may not be viable for practice.

Now, in Post-Exercise 1, you are asked to consider peer insights provided in Table 11.6, with excerpts from initiative-taking reflections of key learning by peers who have traveled this journey before you. In Post-Exercise 1, you are simply asked to reflect on the responses provided and link back to your leadership learning (see Pre-Exercise 1). Consider how you will continue to develop and change as a leader.

Take time now to journal about who you are becoming as a leader.

| TABLE 11.6 | |
|---|---|
| **PROACTIVE READING REFLECTION RESPONSES** | |
| **QUERY** | **SELECT RESPONSE EXCERPTS** |
| **How can I maintain my morals and continue ethical decision making in my daily life?** | *By living "proactively" as Covey[1] states, I realize that I am responsible for the choices I make. My favorite Covey[1] quote is "response-ability—the ability to choose your response." As obvious as it may be, people often forget they have a choice. Likewise, if I don't set my values, it will be difficult to make decisions with which I am happy.* |
| **How can I practice effectively to ensure I run my practice morally and ethically and challenge myself to stay current in knowledge?** | *Far too often, therapists get aggravated with patients for being lazy, but they may not realize what the patient is going through. Covey[1] related, "Breaking deeply embedded habitual tendencies such as procrastination, impatience... involves more than willpower and a few minor life changes." If I really want to change, I must work on it daily and recognize the need to stay current. Like Eartha Kitt said, "I am learning all the time; the tombstone will be my diploma."* |
| | *(Continued)* |

| Table 11.6 (continued) |
|---|

## PROACTIVE READING REFLECTION RESPONSES

| QUERY | SELECT RESPONSE EXCERPTS |
|---|---|
| **How can I be a nurturing mother, loving wife, and thriving professional?** | *To "begin with the end in mind"[1] means to approach my role as a parent, as well as my other life roles, with my values and directions clear. "First seek to understand" the needs of my patients, children, and life partner... Additional discussion on Quadrant II ("things that are not urgent, but important"[1]). One must identify the key roles and make them the priority while avoiding burnout by trying to accomplish too much, "sharpening the saw," and taking time for rest and relaxation.* |
| **How can I improve my problem-solving skills?** | *... 4-step process... "First see the problem from the other point of view. Really seek to understand"[1]... through utilizing empathic and reflective listening like we discussed in the Patient Practitioner Interaction workbook.... Fourth is "new options to achieve results." The topics I picked were based on my clinical education mentoring, and I realized I lacked most in communication in the early weeks and worked on this through the 4-step process, which motivated me to do better. The process is key, and it is good to have for future reference.* |
| **How does leadership content relate to physical therapy practice?** | *"admission to ignorance is often the first step in our education."[1] In physical therapy, we must learn to listen and acquire understanding... we must build an emotional bank account with our patients and trust is an important part of leadership... as physical therapists, we must do continuing education to improve knowledge and skills. This helps to earn the patient's trust... If you do not have trust, the patient will doubt your ability to heal and may not value what you have to offer.[5]... Covey[1] described "diagnose before you prescribe,"... which is so important for professional liability and efficiency and effectiveness[5] in practice...* |
| **How can I have a successful physical therapy business?** | *Covey[1] shed some positive light on this... unfortunately, many close acquaintances started their own businesses with purely a monetary motivation... Covey[1] described "no commitment, no involvement"; in other words, I need a shared mission statement with those I work with, and it needs to be revised regularly to change with times. There is also a necessary balance to be a manager and a leader at contrasting times.* |
| **How can I prevent becoming complacent as a physical therapist?** | *One of the worst downfalls of physical therapy is to become complacent... it is easy to get overly routine and lose interest in new techniques or learning. I have seen this happen with certain types of patients, and not individualized care. I do not want to fall into this category. "Habits are powerful factors in our lives... constantly express character and produce effectiveness or ineffectiveness."[1] Covey[1] talked about having knowledge, skill, and desire... need to fall out of "works for me, so why change?"... think of each patient as unique and always examine the evidence for best practice and continuously be open to learn...* |

Note: Excerpts shared anonymously with author permission; with special gratitude and acknowledgment to the USF SPTRS Tampa, FL, DPT classes of 2011 and 2012.

Adapted from Musolino GM. Fostering leadership in entry-level DPT education. Abstract presented at: Annual Conference and Exposition of the APTA; June 8–11, 2011; National Harbor, MD.

# EXERCISE 2: FUTURE LEADERSHIP TRANSFORMATION

The next time you encounter a leadership challenge, ask yourself these questions to assist in guiding you through your leadership challenge:

- Why is there a challenge?
- What am I trying to achieve?
- What am I doing that is working?
- How have I communicated the goal(s)?
- Have I developed and set direction?
- How am I addressing all generations with which I am working through this effort?
- Have I gathered all the information needed to inform the process?
- How am I influencing others to participate (or not)?
- What am I doing that is slowing me down?
- Where in the process did a breakdown occur?
- What can I do to change?
- Is the solution the best or are others possible?
- How can I better incorporate Covey's Habits 4 to 6?
- How can I enable others to act?
- Where is the process stuck and how can I reset the direction?
- Are there or were there missed expectations?
- Am I inspiring others to lead? What do I love about being a leader?

Alternatively:

- Interview a respected leader in your profession about their own leadership challenges and use the previous questions to guide your interview. Summarize their responses and what you learned in one to two pages.
- Review one of the APTA Mary "Mollie" McMillan Lectures. Summarize and share your learning reflections in one to two pages. See Suggested Readings in this chapter (or available via https://academic.oup.com/ptj).
- View or listen to one of the APTA Living History interviews. Available to check out with APTA information resources, www.apta.org

Interviews:

| | | | |
|---|---|---|---|
| Leon Anderson | Robert Bartlett | Otto Cordero | Rebecca Craik |
| Mary Edmonds | Vilma Evans | Helen Hislop | Geneva Johnson |
| Steven L. Wolf | Florence Kendall | Charles Magistro | Otto Payton |
| Ben Massey | Bella May | Blair Packard | Senora Simpson |
| Bob Richardson | Jan Richardson | Marilyn Moffatt | Lynda Woodruff |
| Peter Towne | Mary Toole | Nancy Watts | Helen Kaiser & Mary Clyde Singleton |

# EXERCISE 3: ADVOCACY IN ACTION

As the demand for rehabilitation services has grown, unfortunately payment for services has not. Cuts and payment differentials with Medicare have particularly impacted health care payments. The cuts have ignored the impacts and positive patient outcomes for interprofessional health care services. The Centers for Medicaid/Medicare (CMS) have reduced payment to seniors for rehab services at a time when the need has only increased. Continued cuts to payment could lead to harm for patients to access care when needed. Hence the need for advocacy at the Federal level has never been greater. What can you do? Time to *take action*!

Discover your local grassroots legislators and your national leaders in Congress; if you do not already know, you can look them up via the League of Woman Voters website (http://lwv.org/); select "Contact Your Local Officials" then "Find Your Elected Officials" by inserting your ZIP code. Or look up your elected officials via your county website. You are then provided with the contact information for those you want to reach out to regarding issues of importance for the patients we serve. You are also able to find additional information on the websites for your state and national legislators on your state and national websites.

- The US House of Representatives: www.house.gov
- The US Senate: www.senate.gov

You may also research on the Library of Congress (www.congress.gov). Through this website, you can look up any bill being considered by Congress. (Your state website offers similar opportunities.) Plug in your profession (e.g., physical therapy or occupational therapy), related health care terminology (e.g., rehabilitation), or perhaps a disease (e.g., Parkinson's, rare diseases, or stroke, etc.) and see how many bills are in process or under consideration for the current Congressional session. Why do you think these bills are important, timely, and worth consideration to become law? Try some additional related terms for current issues impacting HCPs and the patients we serve: Medicare payment differential, Medicare Fee Schedule, Telehealth, Locum Tenens, National Health Services Corps, Allied Health Workforce, Prevent Pandemics, Seniors Access to Care, Prior Authorization, Pelvic Health, etc.

Now, find out what the key legislative issues are in the current year for the public policy agenda items being considered by your profession for our patients and clients; within your district, region, state; or at the national level. Check with your national and state membership organizations to determine which bills are being worked for co-sponsorship and which are opposed. Then, do your part and advocate for the health care bills by doing any, or all, of the following:

1. Contact your national or state membership organizations (APTA, AOTA, etc.) to obtain the latest information and talking points regarding bills affecting your patients and profession. Most national organizations have things set up for you to advocate directly through the association resources. Take Action Advocacy Sites are as follows:

   - APTA: www.apta.org/advocacy
   - AOTA: www.aota.org/advocacy
   - ASHA: www.asha.org/advocacy/

2. Email your Congress persons directly, provide your reasons why they should support the bill and why it will benefit society and the patients you serve, and share your story. The national Take Action sites are all set up for you to be able to take action directly, without much effort, and you should continue with repeat messaging as the bill goes through multiple committees and until the final bill is acted upon or the session ends. (Then the process starts up all over again in the next session!) Congress listens to constituents!

3. Visit your members of Congress when they are in your district and do the same with your local state representatives. Get to know them in person as their constituent and ask them to visit your practice. Again, don't be shy; this is the time to brag about how you help your patients and how they can help you to better serve society. Have your members of Congress speak with a few of your grateful patients to share firsthand the impact of the work of the profession.

4. Follow the bill and continue to follow up with your state and national representatives. Have your patients help by showing them how to act, too! APTA offers a specific Take Action Center just for patients. Promoted positively, social media can be a tremendous help in getting messages out and building enthusiasm for the policy agenda.

5.  If you enjoy legislative advocacy, contact your state and national membership staff and elected leaders from your APTA, AOTA, ASHA, and other member associations to see how you can further assist in defending occupational therapy, physical therapy, and other health care rehabilitation needs for our patients. You may also find it helpful to partner in the advocacy efforts with local community health organizations, health care centers, and support groups. All politics remain local; hence, it is relevant to connect on the national and local levels at every opportunity. Participate in town halls and other events in your home district and share with others how your profession makes a difference!

# EXERCISE 4: CAPTURING CORE COMPETENCIES CLINICALLY

Examine the IPEC competencies via: www.ipecollaborative.org/ipec-core-competencies

Explore the four overarching competencies and the 33 sub-competency statements.

Consider the operational definitions provided and distinguish the terms: cultural competence and cultural humility.

Discuss how cultural competence and cultural humility are achievable through the IPEC competencies and how you would facilitate as a leader in health care within your clinical practice setting.

# 12

# MINDFUL MATTERS
## COMMUNICATION TO ESTABLISH RAPPORT

*Alecia Helbing Thiele, Gina Maria Musolino, and Helen L. Masin*

## OBJECTIVES

*The learner should be able to*:

- Champion developing rapport for effective communication.
- Recognize principles of neurolinguistic psychology (NLP) to assist health care professionals (HCPs) in developing effective verbal and nonverbal communication skills for professional formation.
- Compare NLP, primary representational systems, and the impact on effective communication skills.
- Interpret preferred representational system predicates.
- Distinguish generational differences in communication styles.
- Appreciate the impact of digital applications in communication.
- Discover and practice mindfulness principles to reduce HCP stress and enhance patient–practitioner interactions (PPIs).
- Model principles of positive psychology, which recognize human strengths and promote resilience and resourcefulness in ourselves and in our patients.
- Apply principles of nonverbal communication for enhancing PPIs.
- Adopt the problem-solving approach of "MYOUR" as used in NLP as a model for enhancing effective communication skills.

The importance of rapport has long been recognized in health care; it is commonly referred to as *bedside manner*. Exactly what constitutes appropriate bedside manner? A patient can easily tell you when it is present and when it is not present, although the patient may not be able to describe specifically what characteristics exemplify good PPI. If a HCP has good rapport, the patient may perceive that HCP as warm and caring. However, if the HCP has poor rapport, the patient may perceive that HCP as cold and distant. The purpose of this chapter is to help you recognize rapport and develop skills in using rapport to enhance your therapeutic presence for best practice with PPI. Communication entails expression of aspects of all three learning domains (Chapter 3, Appendix), *affective* (feelings, attitudes, emotions), *cognitive* (knowledge, perception, reasoning), and *psychomotor* (physical movement, motor skills).[1] We will be

DOI: 10.4324/9781003525554-12

considering all three domains in this chapter activities for enhancing communication to establish rapport and reduce negativity.

Stop now and think of a time when you went into a health care professional's office for the initial visit. In your mind's eye, envision this experience from beginning to end before reading this chapter.

If you felt comfortable with the HCP, you may have decided to use their services again. If you did not feel comfortable, you probably decided to find another HCP. Take a moment to list the factors that made your experience comfortable or not very comfortable. Specifically, what were some of the HCP's behaviors that you identified? What were some of your responses to those behaviors? Finally, focus on what role verbal and nonverbal communication played in your interpretation of the behaviors.

Body language remains a compelling form of nonverbal communication, imparting extremely relevant emotional information and one's intentions, at the same time. Through neuroimaging, Ferrari et al.[2] discovered the ability to infer others' emotions from their bodily movements and postures, which entails recruitment of an extended brain network encompassing both subcortical and cortical regions, finding that the cerebellum is involved in both biological motion perception and in discrimination of bodily emotional expressions. In summary, your brain controls your thoughts and expressions of both, verbally and nonverbally.

How is a connection made with communication, without communication? What does it mean to truly understand another's predicament? Let's take a moment to reflect on the wisdom imparted by a short story writer, novel writer, and photographer:

> *My continuing passion is to part a curtain, that invisible shadow that falls between people, the veil of indifference to each other's presence, each other's wonder, each other's human plight.* —Eudora Welty

To be effective, health care requires interaction with people who often are not functioning at top levels or sometimes are unable to even verbalize their challenges and concerns. Increasingly, HCPs are bombarded with information regarding the importance of effective communication skills. May et al.[3] identified ten abilities that clinicians determined were essential for success as a physical therapy professional. One was **communication** skills, or the ability to communicate effectively (speaking, body language, reading, writing, listening) utilizing all domains, for varied audiences and purposes. A second was **interpersonal** skills, including the ability to interact effectively with patients, families, colleagues, other HCPs, and the community and to deal effectively with cultural, ethnic, and diversity issues. A third was use of **constructive feedback**, which involves the ability to identify sources of feedback, seek out feedback, and effectively use and provide feedback for improving personal interactions.

Building upon May's Generic Abilities,[3] Kontney et al.[4] conducted a focus group study with all clinical education stakeholders, which resulted in the *Professional Behaviors for the 21st Century, 2009–2010* (Table 12.1) and the Professional Behaviors Assessment Tool (PBAT see Chapter 20, Appendix). Critical thinking abilities were noted as highly relevant for the doctoring profession. Communication and interpersonal skills and use of constructive feedback are clearly identified by professionals as essential professional behaviors for HCPs.[3,4] Schmoll[5] reinforced the need for responsive PPIs, stating, "Increasingly, our professional role will encompass that of an educator. If I treat you, it's for today. If I teach you, it's for a lifetime." In classical Latin, *doctor*, from "docere," means just that—**to teach**.

An essential component for success in the health care environments is to listen to the customer (patient/client).[6] By listening carefully to your customers (patients/clients), you will find that the things that satisfy them are not the costly things that you do.[6] Be sure that what you are doing has demonstrated value to your customer (patient/client). All the interactive processes are critical to the rendering of effective health care and health care education.

As discussed in Chapter 6, professional knowledge and skill are critical to HCPs' therapeutic capabilities, but we also need to be able to interact in healing ways to have therapeutic presence. Indeed, "how we approach patients, speak to them, touch them, and listen to them has as much, or more of an impact on healing, than do knowledge and skills of our professional preparation."[7] For HCPs, the ability to communicate with patients is a critical component to being successful in therapy with patients. To be successful in these therapeutic processes, we must understand the nature of communication, the nature of therapeutic relationships, and the context in which this communication takes place (see Chapter 13). As HCPs we must listen to and be fully aware of our patients, listen and be aware of our own bodies, and listen with our hearts and minds.

| TABLE 12.1 |
| --- |
| ## PROFESSIONAL BEHAVIORS FOR THE TWENTY-FIRST CENTURY |
| **Critical thinking**—The ability to question logically; identify, generate, and evaluate elements of logical argument; recognize and differentiate facts, appropriate or faulty inferences, and assumptions; and distinguish relevant from irrelevant information. The ability to appropriately utilize, analyze, and critically evaluate scientific evidence to develop a logical argument, and to identify and determine the impact of bias on the decision-making process. |
| **Communication**—The ability to communicate effectively (i.e., verbal, nonverbal, reading, writing, and listening) for varied audiences and purposes. |
| **Problem solving**—The ability to recognize and define problems, analyze data, develop and implement solutions, and evaluate outcomes. |
| **Interpersonal skills**—The ability to interact effectively with patients, families, colleagues, other HCPs, and the community in a culturally aware manner. |
| **Responsibility**—The ability to be accountable for the outcomes of personal and professional actions and to follow through on commitments that encompass the profession within the scope of work, community, and social responsibilities. |
| **Professionalism**—The ability to exhibit appropriate professional conduct and to represent the profession effectively while promoting the growth/development of the physical therapy profession. |
| **Use of constructive feedback**—The ability to seek out and identify quality sources of feedback reflect on and integrate the feedback and provide meaningful feedback to others. |
| **Effective use of time and resources**—The ability to manage time and resources effectively to obtain the maximum possible benefit. |
| **Stress management**—The ability to identify sources of stress and to develop and implement effective coping behaviors; this applies for interactions for self, patients/clients and their families, members of the health care team, and in work/life scenarios. |
| **Commitment to learning**—The ability to self-direct learning to include the identification of needs and sources of learning and to continually seek and apply new knowledge, behaviors, and skills. |
| Reprinted with permission from Kontney L, May W, Iglarsh A. *Professional Behaviors for the 21st Century, 2009–2010.* Marquette University College of Health Sciences—Physical Therapy. https://www.marquette.edu/physical-therapy/documents/professional-behaviors.pdf |

# COMMUNICATION FROM A QUANTUM PERSPECTIVE

Because so much of what we know about the process of interpersonal interaction involves nonverbal communication, or energetic vibration (we even refer to the "vibes" someone is sending), it is important to take a closer look at the concept of energy exchange as a significant process in interaction and communication. We now know that that "energy" or vibe is translatable into movement when other systems fail!

Research in quantum physics supports a view that acknowledges the importance of relationships. In the quantum world, relationships are not just interesting. To many physicists, relationships are all there is to reality.[8] The physics of our universe is revealing the primacy of relationships. As we let go of our Cartesian, linear, and mechanistic models of the world, we begin to step back and see ourselves in new ways, to appreciate our wholeness.[8] We are observing in ourselves, as well as in all living entities, boundaries that preserve us from and connect us to the infinite complexity of the outside world. Jantsch[9] stated that, "in life, the issue is not control but dynamic interconnectedness." None of us exists independent of our relationships with others. If this is true, then all of us need to develop better skills in communicating in all our relationships.

The developments in quantum physics present us with a dramatic paradigm shift regarding what we perceive as real. Newtonian physics taught us that the basic elements of nature were small, solid, indestructible objects.

However, quantum physics teaches us that atoms, the building blocks of all matter, consist of vast regions of space in which exceedingly small particles move. Depending on how these small particles are observed or considered, they may behave as particles or as waves. Given this quantum interpretation, solid objects are no longer perceived as solid. Even though our five senses tell us that we are made up of solid matter, we are probably more like a mass of energy set in constant motion. This energy is constantly breaking itself down and building itself back up. Research in psychoneuroimmunology addresses this "energy flow" as a force that responds to our own inner chemistry. Mind and body are united in a whole nurtured by the flow of vital energy, or chi.[10]

This paradigm shift is important for HCPs to understand in facilitating the healing process. Many of the integrative therapies in rehabilitation, such as reflexology, craniosacral therapy, and acupuncture, address the concept of energy flow in the therapeutic process.[10] What this chapter means to emphasize is that all interaction is, at its essence, vibrational. Therefore, sensitivity to one's own energy (vibration) and the energy of others helps a great deal to clarify and improve the effectiveness of our communication.

In quantum physics, relational holism demonstrates how whole systems are created among subatomic particles. Through this interaction of particles, parts of the whole are changed, drawn together by a process of internal connectedness. Electrons are drawn into intimate relations as their wave aspects interfere with one another, overlapping and merging; their own qualities of mass, charge, spin, position, and momentum, become indistinguishable from one another. According to Zohar,[11] it is no longer meaningful to talk of the constituent electrons' individual properties because these continually change to meet the requirements of the whole. If we apply this microcosmic model from quantum physics to the macrocosmic model of human communication, then we have a dynamic paradigm for communication that reflects the interactive processes that occur with each communication encounter.

Remember from Chapter 6 that the process of empathy as described by Stein[12] and Davis[13] includes self-transposal, followed by a "crossing over" or shared moment of meaning, followed by responsive understanding. This unique form of intersubjectivity illustrates the dynamic interactive aspect of communication and introduces this idea that energy, as meaning, can cross over and be exchanged in meaningful interaction.

## SLIGHT ADJUSTMENTS CAN MAKE LARGE DIFFERENCES

Another fascinating finding from the research in quantum physics indicates that an exceedingly small change may have an impact far beyond what could have been predicted. Until recently, observations from empirical research that fell outside the predicted, linear, hierarchical model were generally discounted or explained away. For example, we were trained to believe that small differences averaged out, that slight variances converged toward a point, and that approximations would give us a fairly accurate picture of what could happen. However, the research in chaos theory has changed these beliefs; when we view the world as a dynamic, changing system, the slightest variation can have explosive results.[8] If we were to create a difference in two values as small as rounding them off to the thirty-first decimal place after 100 iterations or repetitions of the values, the whole calculation would be skewed. Scientists now find that the exceedingly small differences at the beginning of a system's evolution may make prediction impossible, referred to as "sensitive dependence on initial conditions."[8] Iteration or repetition creates powerful and unpredictable effects in nonlinear systems. For example, in the first six months of human pregnancy, the embryo may experience a change that will significantly modify the outcome of the newborn infant, such as a cleft lip or palate, or even a tumor that will not manifest until much later in life (e.g., schwannoma, acoustic neuroma).

In complex ways that we do not understand, the system feeds back on itself, enfolding all that has happened, magnifying slight variances, and encoding it in the system's memory. In this way, prediction is prohibited. If we apply this concept to communications models, slight variations in communication patterns may produce dynamic changes in communicative interactions. As stated in Chapter 8, therapeutic communication requires learning new skills, as well as unlearning habitual, nonhelpful ways of interacting. The purpose of using effective communication is to improve one's therapeutic presence with patients. By communicating in ways that help to solve problems while simultaneously respecting and honoring the human being, practitioners can facilitate the healing process. In sum, practitioners can use the patient–practitioner relationship itself, so important in the nonlinear quantum model, for therapeutic intervention.

## NEUROLINGUISTIC PSYCHOLOGY (NLP)

The utilization of neurolinguistic psychology (NLP) has been reported to enhance communication effectiveness in health care settings.[14–16] Laborde[17] defined NLP as a discipline based on the idea that neurology, language, and behavior are interrelated and can be changed by specific interventions. The theoretical basis for NLP emerged from studies of the work of experts in several fields.[17] O'Connor and Seymour[18] defined NLP as the art and science of excellence, derived from studying how top people in different fields obtained their outstanding results. They described NLP as a practical set of models, skills, and techniques for thinking and acting effectively in the world. Bandler and Grinder[19] believed that by identifying excellence, one could analyze it, model it, and use it. Their initial work studied three outstanding communicators: Perls,[20] founder of Gestalt therapy; Satir,[21] founder of family therapy; and Erickson,[22] psychiatrist, and hypnotherapist. Grinder and Bandler[19] were also strongly influenced by the work of Bateson,[23] a British anthropologist who wrote on communication and systems theory.

The basic framework for NLP comes from the awareness that our neurological processes are sensory based and that we use linguistics, or language, to order thought and behavior and to communicate with others. In our roles as HCPs, we are constantly challenged to communicate effectively with our patients, their families, colleagues, and support staff. NLP gives us the tools and skills to assist us in enhancing our verbal and nonverbal skills. In NLP terms, the meaning of communication is based on the response that you get. As HCPs, this puts a great deal of responsibility on the provider to use forms of communication to which the patient can respond. Research conducted by Mehrabian and Ferris[24] using the word *maybe* has shown that communication has multiple aspects. Asking the listener how they interpreted what the communicator meant by *maybe*, the interpretation by the listener was 55% from body language (including posture, gesture, and eye contact), 38% from tone of voice, and 7% from the verbal content of the message. Because the study only used one word, it is difficult to generalize the findings to multiple word communications. However, the study raises awareness that the process of our communication may be even more important to the message than the content of our communication. This again reaffirms Ferrari et al.'s[2] findings that your "head" needs to be in the game, impacting not only what you think but how you act and the way that your verbalizations and nonverbalizations are presented by you and received by your patients/clients.

# THERAPEUTIC PRESENCE: COMMUNICATION WITH HEAD, HEART, AND BODY

You have learned the benefits of utilizing open-ended questions, appropriate expressions of empathy, and the need to establish collaboration for effective communication with patient–practitioner interactions. Collaboration builds rapport with your patient/client and establishes trust. Empathy assures you surrender your own perspective to view your patients/client's situation from their viewpoint, while open-ended questions facilitate for the patient/client the opportunity to fully share their history and current concerns. Open-ended queries assure no unintended leading of your patient, while you are listening with open body language that demonstrates full engagement and establishes trust. The meaningful discovery that occurs through intentionally establishing rapport and reducing negative influences is foundational for best practice in therapeutic communications.

You are also learning the importance of reflective communication, to further establish with the patient/client that you understand their concerns and to reinforce that you are listening through this crucial skill of stating or restating what the patient/client has imparted to you. Summarization is another method utilized for effective reflective listening. Summarization can be accomplished through *collecting, linking,* and *transitioning* techniques.[25] Collecting is a reinforcement of the patient/client insight, e.g., *Let me see if I understand what you have related to me so far.* Linking consists of connecting two parts or points of a discussion, e.g., *Earlier you stated that you wanted to … Maybe now we can consider trying.* Transitioning wraps up the conversation and/or interaction, e.g., *Today we have completed … and next time … before your next visit/treatment session I would like for you to … what do you think?*

Utilizing these techniques and strategies in your approach to establishing therapeutic presence assures the patient/client has confidence and trust in you and themselves. You are also forecasting their rehabilitation progress and potentials working in collaboration, while facilitating the patient/client's own abilities to change their lives, while taking responsibility in partnership with you for their health. Let's consider additional ways to establish rapport.

# RAPPORT

To effectively communicate, we must first establish rapport with our client, creating an atmosphere of trust and confidence. Rapport also helps to solidify the participation within which people can respond freely. Think back to your opening visualization at the beginning of this chapter. What were the behaviors that you identified in the scenario with the HCP that helped establish rapport? What were the behaviors that broke rapport with the HCP in the PPI?

When two people in conversation are in rapport, communication seems to flow. Body language and voice tonality flow together; bodies and words match each other. What is said can create or break rapport, but remember that verbal communication is only part of the total communication. People in rapport tend to match each other's posture, gestures, and eye contact. When rapport is established, people mirror each other, and their body language is complementary.[18] At its best, rapport flows into a focus of concentration that takes on a life of its own, and for a few moments, time is forgotten. Rapport implies a working relationship between two people.[14] The patient and practitioner recognize each other's needs, share information, and set common goals. Rapport implies mutuality, collaboration, and respect; however, rapport results from more than simply good intentions. Words and actions must be carefully and sensitively chosen in PPIs.

The presence of rapport helps to diminish illness, enhances satisfaction and compliance, and prevents malpractice litigation.[14] Egbert et al.[26] described a special therapeutic rapport that was established with an experimental group of patients undergoing elective laparotomy; these patients received extra reassurance and information. As you might expect, postoperatively, the patients needed only half as many analgesics and were discharged almost 3 days earlier than the control patients. Another study by Inui et al.[27] found that enhanced communication skills of physicians resulted in clinically significant improvement in the patients' blood pressure control.

Studies of mothers' compliance with physicians' recommendations were reported by Korsch et al.[28] and found that mothers' satisfaction and compliance with treatment depended on whether the doctor was perceived as friendly and on how well the physician conveyed information. Finally, malpractice specialists reported that poor rapport between the physician and patient might be the single most common cause of malpractice suits. The risk of litigation increases when patients experience the HCP as uncaring, when they fail to discuss or disclose, or when patients are left with unrealistic expectations.[14]

# NEUROLINGUISTIC PSYCHOLOGY AND RAPPORT

NLP provides a framework that assists HCPs in establishing rapport with their clients. The three key steps in establishing rapport are **matching**, **pacing**, and **leading**.[18] Matching a person's body language with sensitivity and respect helps to build a bridge between the practitioner and the patient's model of the world. The premise is based on the idea that when people are like each other in body language, they will be more easily connected and in sync. In a sense, the practitioner is matching the patient's explanatory model as described by Kleinman[29] through matching the patient's body language (see Chapter 13).

## Matching

Matching is quite different from mimicry. Matching involves the subtle modeling of others' movements by small hand movements, body movements, and head movements. It also involves matching distribution of body weight and basic posture. Matching breathing and voice matching are other ways to develop rapport. Matching can occur with voice tonality, speed, volume, and rhythm of speech. Vocabulary and voice matching can be used in telephone conversations as well as in face-to-face encounters.[18]

For some people, matching another initially may feel uncomfortable or unnatural. For others, it may happen naturally. Notice your reactions when you are matching or when you are being matched. If you want to establish rapport and the person has fidgety movements, you may want to crossmatch by subtly swaying your body or moving subtly without actually fidgeting yourself. It is not necessary to be exactly like the person to establish rapport. You are using this skill to better understand the person and thus develop a working relationship with them.[18] Try it with someone you have difficulty understanding. Matching their body posture and movements may help you grasp the other person's point of view. In some situations, by matching the other person's body language, you may experience what they are feeling in your own body and thus better appreciate their nonverbal communication with you.

In some cases, you may choose not to establish rapport. For example, in a situation in which the other person appears hostile, you may choose to break rapport. You can break rapport by mismatching body language, tonality, speed, volume, or rhythm of speech. If you are seated, you may stand up to indicate nonverbally that the interaction is over and/or step away and distance yourself. If you need to continue the communication later, you can suggest another time to meet once the person has had some time to calm down. You might ask the person to write down their concerns to bring to your subsequent meeting. By writing down their concerns, they may release some of the tension (de-escalating) that caused you to end the initial meeting. If you sense that you are still unable to resolve the issue at your rescheduled meeting, you may wish to ask another colleague to be present for your meeting to help mediate.

Tim and Chris were trying to decide whether to spend the evening going to a movie or studying for an exam they had coming up next week. Chris really wanted to go to the movie and was angry with Tim for "never wanting to have any fun." Chris was disappointed that Tim was not interested in going to the movie with her. However, she decided to see the situation from Tim's perspective. She matched his posture and his tone of voice and suddenly she remembered that he had barely passed the last exam and was worried that he might not pass this course. As she matched his voice and posture, she felt his fear and vulnerability and suggested that they both study alone for a while and then quiz each other later. Tim breathed a sigh of relief and suggested that if they got enough accomplished, they might go out for a while later.

A good example of a time when you would want to break rapport would be when a patient was acting inappropriately, such as in a sexual manner.

Judy, a physical therapist, was treating a man with cervical disk herniation with manual therapy while he lay supine on the treatment table. She was seated at his head, and was gently mobilizing his very tense neck muscles, when he asked her unexpectedly, "Are you turned on when you do this?" She responded, directly but not unkindly, that she was thinking about his neck pathology and that sexuality was not at all a part of her concern. Besides that, she was happily married and wanted to keep the relationship with her patients on a strictly professional level. Not to be put off, her patient replied, "Well, does your husband make you happy in bed?"

At that point, Judy knew she had to break rapport. She stood up, looked her patient in the eye and said firmly, "This treatment is over. As I said, it is especially important that we keep a professional relationship between us. If you cannot do that, I will have to refer you to another therapist. Please make a follow-up appointment for next week but recognize that I will not see you if you continue to be inappropriate with me."

## *Pacing and Leading*

Once you have established rapport with someone, you can change your behavior, and they are likely to follow you. This is referred to in NLP as *pacing and leading*, and it consists of the use of rapport, developing respect for the other person's world view, and assuming a positive intention. To pace and lead successfully, one must pay attention to the other person and be flexible enough in one's own behavior to respond to what one sees, hears, and feels.[18] Superior teachers do this intuitively. First, they establish rapport with their students, enter the students' world, and then pace the students to move into the subject or skill that is being taught; HCPs can do the same thing with practice.

Pacing or matching behavior creates the bridge through rapport and respect. When leading, you change your behavior so that the other person can follow. However, one must have rapport before one can pace and lead. When the HCP is pacing the patient, the HCP matches the patient's posture, verbal tonality, and speed of speaking to establish rapport. When the HCP recognizes that they have matched the patient's pace and that they have rapport with the patient, the HCP introduces a change in posture, verbal tonality, and speed of speaking, and the patient then follows the HCPs lead. This only occurs once the HCP has established rapport with the patient by first matching and pacing the patient on several levels of communication (e.g., posture, tonality, speed). Rapport is a critical skill in intercultural communication, as will be discussed in Chapter 13. Without rapport, intercultural communication may be doomed from the start. Because much of communication is perceived nonverbally, there is a chance to establish rapport even though there are verbal language differences.

Nonverbal communication is the language of culture. Through the development of rapport, the HCP matches the patient's body language, and the tonality, speed, volume, and rhythm of speech.[18] If the dialogue is between a low-context (individualistic) and a high-context (collectivistic) individual, the practitioner can take nonverbal cues from the patient that will assist in establishing rapport, even if the practitioner does not speak the language of the patient. The person from a low-context (individualistic) culture will generally rely heavily on the spoken word and demonstrate little gesturing or touching in the communication interaction. The person from the high-context (collectivistic) culture will generally rely less on spoken words but will use more gesturing or touch in the communication interaction.

When using a medical interpreter, the HCP can match the body language and tonality of the patient while listening to the medical interpreter. Thus, at the unconscious level, the therapist is establishing rapport nonverbally with the patient/client, while listening to the words of the medical interpreter.[30]

Pacing is especially helpful in dealing with intense emotions in communications. If someone is angry, you must first match that person's anger at a lower intensity. This will keep the anger from escalating. Once you have matched, you gradually reduce the intensity of your own behavior to lead the person to a calmer state. If someone approaches you with a sense of urgency, you can match them by speaking a little louder and quicker than usual and then pace the person to a softer and slower speed.[18] When lack of pacing and leading occurs, the PPI can escalate, or the other person may sense a lack of understanding. The nuances of PPI require much practice and attentiveness. Try videoing yourself practicing pacing and leading with the simple scenarios described above and review to learn how you are progressing. Consider each of the learning domains—affective, psychomotor, and cognitive—with replay analyses.

# PREFERRED REPRESENTATIONAL SYSTEMS—PREDICATES

As human beings, we are all capable of thinking. However, we tend to think about *what* we are thinking about rather than *how* we think. Because of this, we often believe that other people think in the same manner we do. This often causes difficulty in communications with people who have different ways of thinking. In NLP, these patterns or ways of thinking are called **representational systems**. They are another tool in NLP that may assist HCPs in communicating with patients.

Representational systems are the ways in which we take in, store, and code information in our minds through seeing, hearing, feeling, tasting, and smelling. Thought patterns have direct physical effects on the mind and body. For example, think about eating your favorite food. Although the food may be imaginary, your production of saliva is measurable. This Pavlovian conditioned reflex is a good example of the influence of the mind on the body. We use the same neurological paths to envision or represent experience inwardly, as we do to experience it outwardly or directly. These same neurons generate electrochemical charges that can be measured by electromyography readings. We use our sensory systems (sight, touch, hearing, smell, and taste) to perceive the world, and then we inwardly represent the world in our minds.[18]

According to O'Connor,[18] visual (V), auditory (A), and kinesthetic (K) systems are the primary representational systems in Western cultures. In NLP, the senses of taste and smell are often included with the kinesthetic sense. People from Western cultures generally use all three of these primary systems all the time, but they are not equally aware of them, tending to favor some over others. The visual system has external (E) representations when one is looking at the outside world (VE) and internal (I) representations when one is mentally visualizing (VI). The auditory system is divided into hearing external sounds (AE) and internal sounds (AI). The auditory system of internal sounds includes the internal voices and dialogue of the individual.[18] For example, the HCP may be hearing the patient/client say "good morning" in the external environment of the clinic and, at the same time, the HCP may be having an internal dialogue about why they got a speeding ticket on the way to work. Remember from Chapter 2 that the way we view ourselves and the world is directly influenced by the internal sounds of the voices of our parents that we have interjected or incorporated, usually not on purpose.

The kinesthetic system includes the feelings that accompany tactile sensations such as touch, temperature, and moisture (KE) and internal feelings (KI) of remembered sensations; emotions; and inner feelings of balance, body awareness, and proprioception. Human behavior is based on a mixture of these internal and external sensory experiences. If a person uses one internal sense habitually, it is called their **preferred representational system (PRS)**. The words that a person uses in conversation indicate their PRS, and thus yield important clues for establishing rapport.[18] For example, we all know some people who constantly respond, "Oh, I see," and others who reply, "I hear you."

According to Jepson,[15] the visual PRS is found in about 60% of the population. People who are organized, appearance oriented, and observant tend to fall into this category. They are good spellers and memorize in their mind's eye. They are distracted by noise but often have difficulty following verbal instructions. They prefer reading for themselves (visual) rather than hearing the words (auditory). They become distracted if they are given too much verbal information.[15] Stop and think—are you a person who will read the written instructions first before attempting to put a new purchase together out of the box? What is your preferred method to learn how to solve a problem?

People with auditory PRS account for about 30% of the population. They are experts at matching pitch, accents, timbre, and tones. When reading silently, they may move their lips. They may have a tendency to talk out loud to themselves. They are good listeners and can follow verbal instructions easily.[15] Stop and think—would you rather have someone verbally teach you a new theory than read about it?

The remaining 10% of people have a kinesthetic PRS. They enjoy hands-on experiences and prefer to learn by doing. They are generally physically oriented and physically demonstrative. They may tend to appear restless. They may live in a disorganized environment.[14] Stop and think—do you want to put that new purchase together from the box without reading the directions first?

Remember that to build rapport, the listener matches the speaker. As a HCP, one can listen for the language that a person uses to find out whether someone's PRS is visual, auditory, or kinesthetic. Because language communicates our thoughts, words will reflect the PRS that we prefer using. For example, three people with different PRSs may read the same book. The visual individual might say that they *saw eye-to-eye* with the author's premise. The auditory person might say that the author's message *sounded clear as a bell* to them. Someone who is primarily kinesthetic might say that they have a *solid grasp* of the author's premise. Although all three read the same book, they all responded differently. One was thinking in pictures (visual), one in sounds (auditory), and one tactilely (kinesthetic).

In NLP terms, these sensory-based words (verbs, adjectives, and adverbs) are called **predicates**. Understanding the use of predicates enables a HCP to match predicates with the patient as another means of gaining rapport. When working with a patient who is nonverbal, it is best practice to use a mixture of visual, auditory, and kinesthetic predicates to optimize the communication because the person's PRS cannot be elicited verbally. It is also important to use a mix of predicates when addressing a large group of people to engage all three PRS styles.[18]

# DISCOVERING PREFERRED REPRESENTATIONAL SYSTEMS: OBSERVING EYE MOVEMENTS

Another valuable tool in NLP is the observation of what is termed **eye accessing**. Neurolinguistic researchers[31] discovered visible behavioral changes that signaled neurophysiological outputs that were clues to PRSs, including eye movements made during accessing of memory, breathing changes, skin color changes, and body postural changes. Neurological studies have shown that eye movement laterally and vertically appears to be associated with activation of different parts of the brain. It is useful to observe eye movements in someone to better understand that person's experience as we are communicating with others. There appears to be some common neurological connection between eye movements and PRS because the same patterns are found worldwide (except for the Basque region of Spain).[18] When patients visualize from the past, they tend to move their eyes up and to the left. When they construct a picture or imagine something they have never seen, they tend to move their eyes up and to the right.

Defocusing the eyes or looking straight ahead is another way to know if the speaker is using visualization. The speaker will appear to be looking beyond the listener as if watching an imaginary movie picture. The eyes tend to move to the left for remembered sounds and across to the right for constructed sounds. When the eyes go down and to the right, the patient is usually accessing kinesthetic PRS. When the patient talks to themself, the observer will see the eyes go down to the left (Figure 12.1).[18]

Eye accessing cues occur quickly, so the observer needs to watch the patient closely. In some cases, the eye accessing directions may be reversed. The person observing needs to ask several questions to determine whether the patient may have a reverse eye accessing pattern. Reverse eye accessing is sometimes seen in individuals who are left-handed, but it may occur in anyone.

# POSITIVE DESCRIPTIVE STATEMENTS

The NLP tool of using positive descriptive statements is useful in communicating with patients. A **positive descriptive statement** explains the behavior that you want the patient to do, rather than the behavior that you do not want. For example, if a child is told, "Don't spill the milk," they first must visualize spilling the milk in order to not spill it. If an adult is told, "Don't cross your legs" as a hip precaution, they first visualize crossing their legs in order to not cross them. The HCP might want to instead say, "Keep your legs parallel" or "Keep your feet pointing straight ahead" so that the person can visualize only the outcome that is being recommended. The HCP is then reinforcing the preferred visual image to support the physical movement desired.

When working with children, elderly patients, or patients who are easily confused, the use of positive descriptive statements makes a substantial difference in the patient's understanding of your directions. When writing home programs for patients, using positive descriptive statements is extremely helpful in assisting the patients to understand the

**Figure 12.1** This illustration shows what you see when looking at another person.

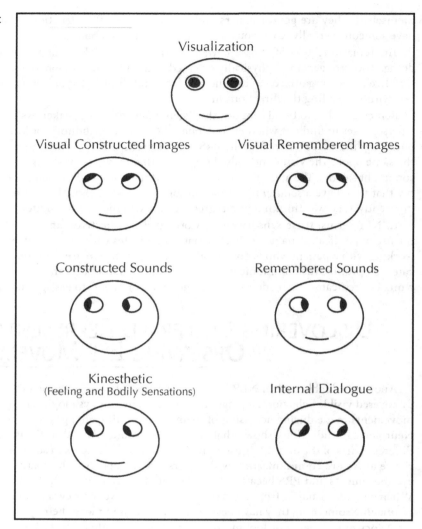

exercise you want them to practice. However, HCPs should be careful not to bombard a patient with overstimulation or redundant repetition within any PRS realm. The patient may stop listening, tune out, or be overwhelmed with too many stimuli, resulting in the opposite desired effect. Less is more in most situations and allowing time for processing is imperative for successful PPIs, especially when the movement systems are affected by disease processes.

## GENERATIONAL DIFFERENCES IN COMMUNICATION

Generational differences (see Table 2.3 in Chapter 2) may also impact communication in unexpected ways. Expectations regarding feedback in communication vary across generations. Traditionalists feel that "no news is good news." Baby Boomers feel that feedback is best once a year, whether it is needed or not. Generation Xers frequently ask, "How am I doing?" Millennials prefer feedback from a "virtual coach" at the push of button,[32] while Generation Z prefers instantaneous feedback. At present, Generation Alpha prefers hearing from and communicating with voice bots and kid-peers. Technology has impacted our communication dramatically. Computers, Internet, email, cell phones, texting, instant messaging, social media, gaming, and smart devices with voice bots have made instant communication possible, but the expectations of appropriate communication vary across the generations.

Many Traditionalists and Baby Boomers use more formal written communication and prefer that titles be used in oral and written communication. Many Gen Xers and Millennials are more informal and prefer not to use titles in oral and written communication. Because of these differences, conflicts may arise between individuals of different generations in educational settings and clinical settings. For example, a Baby Boomer faculty member may be offended by a Millennial student who not only does not use their formal title in oral or written communication but also greets them by first name. In the clinic, a Traditionalist patient may be offended by a Gen-X physical therapist who calls them by their first name instead of addressing them by title and surname. As valuable as it is to recognize and honor these important generational differences in style, the fact remains that it is important for HCPs to value and demonstrate respect for the older client or faculty member if the student or HCP wishes to build effective rapport and enhance communication across all the generations. Respect and rapport across these generations often begin with the use of a title or surname. As we discussed in Chapter 7, it remains important to know your patients' and colleagues' preferences and ask, and not make any assumptions. To assure rapport, simply ask, "How do you prefer to be addressed?"

# DIGITAL COMMUNICATION AND PROFESSIONAL BEHAVIOR

Gen Xers, Millennials, and Gen Zers have been described as "digital natives," and Traditionalists and Baby Boomers have been described as "digital immigrants."[33] Because Gen Xers, Millennials, Gen Zers, and Gen Alphas have grown up with digital communications, they are generally more comfortable with email, texting, social networking, and blogging compared with Traditionalists and Baby Boomers; however, the landscape is changing, especially since the Covid-19 pandemic demanded many rely on more digital means of communication. With the popularity of digital applications, guidance about preventing misuse and ensuring standards for professional conduct is warranted.[34] The digital applications can be a blessing and a curse. As a blessing, they can facilitate communication across time and distance and promote interaction; especially where it may not have been otherwise possible to communicate. As a curse, digital communications can create glitches because expectations differ regarding the appropriate use. Because emailing and texting are two-dimensional communications, the reader only gets part of the message. The nonverbal, energetic elements of tonality, facial expression, gesture, pitch, pacing, and environmental context are all missing. Can you think of a time when you sent an email to someone and their interpretation was totally different from what you had intended? Without the nonverbal cues, email can easily be misinterpreted.

Faculty who are Traditionalists and Baby Boomers may be uncomfortable with the informal tone of emails and texts from students. For example, difficulties may arise when a student sends an email or text in which the salutation uses the faculty member's last name without the title, or begins very informally with "Hey!" or "Yo." Sometimes a distressed student may send an emotionally charged email to a faculty member rather than speaking to the faculty member in person. Finally, legal challenges have arisen because the email or text was inadvertently forwarded to someone who found it offensive. In these situations, it is critical for institutions to develop policies regarding the appropriate use of digital communication and to address unprofessional digital behaviors as soon as they arise.[35] Respect for others is the key moral component in this discussion. One medical school advises students to "think before you post."[34] We advise students not to send an email unless they are sure that they could comfortably say the precise content of the message to the person, face to face, and in a respectful manner. We ask our students to do an Internet and social media search of themselves with their full name and any other familiar or additional names (nicknames) they may have used in the past as it is a typical expectation that clinical sites, clinical faculty, patients/clients, and employers will do the same. Now try a quick search of your own name. What did you find? Did you find anything you were surprised about? How do think your Internet and social media presence will or will not change as you transition and progress in your professional formation as a developing health care professional?

What are your thoughts about policies and procedures regulating email or text conversation between students and faculty? Can you imagine as a student receiving an email or text from a faculty member that offends you and that you wish it had not been sent? What would it contain? Why would it offend you?

Likewise, as a student, can you imagine sending an email or text to a faculty member that might be offensive? What would the circumstances be? How could it be misinterpreted?

Health professional organizations and health care companies are proactively addressing the need for policies related to digital communications and the use of social media. You may also wish to review social media tips and policies within your specific health profession to determine the similarities or differences and how you shall proceed in your day-to-day use of social media and with your patients/clients, peers, and colleagues as we enter a new era with telehealth PPIs. We will examine aspects of communication related to telehealth specifically in Chapter 20.

One final comment: Recent research has indicated that we cannot truly multitask the way that our technology leads us to believe that we can.[33] The mental balancing required to multitask has been shown to shortchange some of the areas of the brain related to memory and learning.[36] Research is revealing that our use of digital technology has begun to alter our attention span. We are beginning to rewire our brains for speed rather than mindfulness. In the health care professions, we must be cognizant of how digital technology impacts us and our patients in positive and negative ways. Then we must make every effort to ensure that we use it for the highest good of all concerned.

# MINDFULNESS IN PRACTICE

Mindfulness-Based Stress Reduction (MBSR) is recognized in the health literature as a helpful tool that is cost effective for individuals coping with clinical and nonclinical problems.[37–49] Study populations have included patients/clients experiencing pain,[38] cancer,[39] heart disease,[40] depression,[41,42] asthma,[43] post-traumatic stress disorder,[44] and anxiety.[48] In addition, MBSR is helpful in stress management with healthy subjects,[49] and HCPs with compassion fatigue and burnout,[45] along with developing HCPs' resilience.[46] MBSR has also helped to decrease ruminative thinking and anxiety in healthy subjects while increasing empathy and self-compassion.[47–49] Mindfulness is the practice of cultivating nonjudgmental awareness of each moment in our day-to-day lives.

Originally developed by Zinn at the University of Massachusetts Stress Reduction Clinic, MBSR includes formal and informal meditation and yoga practices, which are designed to promote moment-to-moment awareness in participants. Research on the usefulness of MBSR and variations continues in a variety of disciplines, including health care, law, psychology, and education.[50,51] Willgens and Sharf[52] described how mindfulness meditation was taught to physical therapy professional students as a means of promoting intrapersonal awareness for those who face challenges in their clinical education experiences. Learning mindfulness meditation appears to be a potentially powerful tool for assisting HCP students who face challenges in integrating effective skills and abilities in the clinical setting.

# POSITIVE PSYCHOLOGY AND E.M.P.A.T.H.Y.

Another helpful tool for HCPs is the utilization of **positive psychology**. Positive psychology evolved out of humanistic psychology and promotes using the scientific method to understand the positive, adaptive, creative, and emotionally fulfilling aspects of human behavior.[53] Positive psychology examines how different cultural groups experience well-being, including positive human traits, such as kindness (e.g., sending a simple, hand-written thank you note), curiosity, and the ability to work in teams, as well as human values, interests, talents, and abilities. All these positive human characteristics in clinicians contribute to one's therapeutic presence as a HCP. HCPs can benefit from applying positive psychology strategies for themselves; you can too, by using this chapter's exercises for promoting your own well-being.

Huta and Hawley[54] found that positive emotions can help to fight psychological disorders such as depression. Think about how a random act of kindness can positively impact your day. Compton and Hoffman[53] discovered that a greater capacity for empathy correlates with higher life satisfaction and more positive relationships. Contemporary research in medical education has focused on teaching HCPs PPIs through nonverbal detection techniques and expressions of empathy, including assessing the nonverbal behaviors that are described in the acronym E.M.P.A.T.H.Y.:[55]

- Eye contact
- Muscles of facial expression
- Posture
- Affect
- Tone of voice
- Hearing the whole patient
- Your response

More attention is now being focused on nonverbal displays to ensure effective PPI in health professions curricula. Empathy is essential for detection of emotions in patients. If there is a mismatch between verbal cues and nonverbal cues, there may be a lack of congruence in the patient's communication about their condition. In order to better understand the patient's perspective, it is vitally important for the clinician to recognize and address any incongruences during PPIs.

In addition to recognizing nonverbal cues in their patients, HCPs need to be aware of their own nonverbal cues and how they are being interpreted by the patient and other staff members. The E.M.P.A.T.H.Y. behaviors can be included in assessment tools for evaluating students' interpersonal and communication skills in patient care and team building.[55] Prior to clinical experiences, developing HCPs may not have received enough specific feedback on their nonverbal behavior and its impact on patients and colleagues. By bringing nonverbal behaviors to the student's conscious attention, the developing HCP has an opportunity to change the behavior to promote better and more effective communication. Developing HCPs sometimes feel that "this is just the way I have always been." As you develop in your professional formation as a HCP, your behaviors must change to reflect professionalism in all your interactions.[56,57] Seek this feedback proactively on your nonverbal communication and work on improvements with your clinical faculty and patients.

Another important aspect of positive psychology is resilience. Resilience is defined as the ability to adapt positively to a challenge, risk, adversity, or negative event. The American Psychological Association has identified factors that promote the development of resilience, as follows:[58]

- Making connections with family, friends, or community
- Avoiding seeing crises as insurmountable problems
- Accepting that change is part of living
- Moving toward one's goals
- Taking decisive action
- Looking for opportunities for self-discovery
- Nurturing a positive view of oneself
- Keeping events in perspective
- Maintaining a hopeful outlook
- Taking care of oneself by attending to one's own needs and feelings

Through combining NLP skills, positive psychological attitudes and behaviors, E.M.P.A.T.H.Y. behaviors, and mindfulness strategies in communication, the HCP enhances the ability to be a therapeutic presence in the health care environment. By integrating the skills for one's own well-being, the clinician is better equipped to be a therapeutic presence for clients, families, and coworkers. By cultivating these skills and developing resilience, you shall enhance the development of your own professionalism and optimal communication skills. Now that the Millennials surpass Gen Xers as the largest labor force in the United States and we have multiple generations represented in health care teams and patients, communicating to establish rapport and reduce negativity has become even more relevant today.[59]

# THE MAP VERSUS THE TERRITORY DESCRIBED BY THE MAP

A final critical concept in NLP is that the map is not the territory it describes. The map is a symbol for the territory but it is not the territory itself. Each individual has a perception of the world from their own point of view, such as the generational differences described. The perceptual filter is our bias with which we experience the world around us. As HCPs, we must be mindful of our bias, lest it become prejudice. Conflicts may occur between us because we have different maps of reality, as described in the digital miscommunications. Each of us has personal models of the world (explanatory models, as will be described in Chapter 13) with our own sets of filters that may include visual, auditory, or kinesthetic PRSs, as well as ways of sorting or categorizing stimuli in the environment. For example, one individual may observe a glass as half full and another individual may observe the same glass as half empty. The glass is exactly the same, but each individual perceives it according to their own sorting style. Different sorting styles also function as filters for how the individual perceives a situation in the environment. Another example might be a patient who perceives exercise as an unpleasant requirement in the recovery process, whereas another patient might perceive it as a blessing in their recovery process.[18]

If we choose to be successful in our communications with our patients, families, colleagues, and support staff, we must recognize that each person has a different map (or explanatory model) and different filters for the territory in which we all find ourselves. Using NLP, we can learn to respect and appreciate the different maps and filters. Laborde[17] suggested using the acronym "MYOUR" as a way to remember and summarize the communication skills in NLP. "MY" is what I want, "YOUR" is what you want, and "OUR" is making sure everyone gets it. Once we appreciate the different maps and filters that we all have, we are in a better position to work together toward common goals.

# CONCLUSION

It is important to remember that NLP, positive psychology, E.M.P.A.T.H.Y., and mindfulness provide us with tools to help us to connect with our patients/clients, their families, and our colleagues. As HCPs, we must be willing to be sensitive and flexible to *match, pace,* and *lead* for the benefit of others. Utilizing summarization techniques such as *collecting, linking,* and *transitioning* assists in developing communication rapport. Whether our patient prefers visual, auditory, or kinesthetic cues, there is no one approach. The HCP who is able to understand and adapt to the patient's/client's way of thinking and receiving will have much better results with PPI. The HCP's task is to make the therapeutic relationships as smooth, helpful, and free from conflict as possible. By practicing the basic NLP principles and techniques, positive psychology strategies, E.M.P.A.T.H.Y, and mindfulness, you will be greatly equipped for building your PPI rapport, calming negative PPIs, and promoting well-being in yourself and in your patients/clients. The exercises that follow will give you a start in the process.

# REFERENCES

1. Bloom B S. *Taxonomy of Educational Objectives: The Classification of Educational Goals.* New York, NY: Longman, Green and Company; 1956.
2. Ferrari C, Ciricugno A, Cattaneo Z. Cerebellar contribution to emotional body language perception. *Adv Exp Med Biol.* 2022;1378:141–153. doi: 10.1007/978-3-030-99550-8_10. PMID: 35902470.
3. May W, Morgan B, Lemke JC, et al. Model for ability-based assessment in physical therapy education. *J Phys Ther Ed.* 1995;9:3–6.
4. Kontney L, May W, Iglarsh A. *Professional behaviors for the 21st century,* 2009–2010. https://www.marquette.edu/physical-therapy/documents/professional-behaviors.pdf. Accessed October 13, 2024.
5. Schmoll B. Physical therapy today and in the twenty-first century. In: Scully RM, Barnes MR, eds. *Physical Therapy.* Philadelphia, PA: Lippincott Raven; 1989.
6. Ketter P. Understanding driving forces behind managed care is crucial for survival. *Phys Ther Bull.* 1997;12(29):6–7.
7. Musolino GM, ed. *Davis' Patient Practitioner Interaction: Instructor's Manual.* 7th ed. Milton Park, Abingdon, Oxfordshire: Routledge, Taylor & Francis Group; 2024.
8. Wheatley MJ. *Leadership and the New Science: Discovering Order in a Chaotic World.* 3rd ed. San Francisco, CA: Berrett-Koehler Publishers; 2006.
9. Jantsch E. *The Self-Organizing Universe: Scientific and Human Implications of the Emerging Paradigm of Evolution.* Philadelphia, PA: Elsevier Science & Technology Books; 1980.
10. Davis C. *Integrative Therapies in Rehabilitation: Evidence for Efficacy in Therapy, Prevention & Wellness,* 4th ed. Thorofare, NJ: SLACK; 2017.
11. Zohar D. *The Quantum Self: Human Nature and Consciousness Defined by the New Physics.* New York, NY: Harper Collins Publishers; 1991.
12. Stein E. *On the Problem of Empathy.* 3rd ed. The Hague, The Netherlands: Martinus Nijhoff; ICS Publications; 1989.
13. Davis CM. *A Phenomenological Description of Empathy as It Occurs Within Physical Therapists for Their Patients.* Dissertation. Boston University; 1982.
14. Rosenzweig S. Emergency rapport. *J Emerg Med.* 1993;11(6):775–776.
15. Jepson CH. Neurolinguistic programming in dentistry. *J Calif Dent Assoc.* 1992;20(3):28–32.
16. Konefal J. *Chronic Disease and Stress Management.* Denver, CO: NLP Comprehensive International Conference; 1992.
17. Laborde G. *Fine Tune Your Brain.* Palo Alto, CA: Syntony; 1989.
18. O'Connor J, Seymour J. *Introducing NLP: Psychological Skills for Understanding and Influencing People.* San Francisco, CA: Conari Press; 2011.
19. Bandler R, Grinder J. *The Structure of Magic.* Palo Alto, CA: Science and Behavior Books; 2005.
20. Perls FS, Miller MV, Wyson J. *Gestalt Therapy Verbatim.* Gouldsboro, ME: Gestalt Journal Press; 2007.
21. Satir V. *The New Peoplemaking.* Palo Alto, CA: Science and Behavior Books; 1988.
22. Gordon D, Meyers-Anderson M. *Phoenix: Therapeutic Patterns of Milton H. Erickson.* Cupertino, CA: Meta Publications; 1981.
23. Bateson G. *Steps to an Ecology of Mind.* Chicago, IL: University of Chicago Press; 1999.
24. Mehrabian A, Ferris S. Decoding of inconsistent communications. *J Pers Soc Psychol.* 1967;6:109–114.
25. Ellison DL, Meyer CK. Presence and Therapeutic Listening. *Nurs Clin North Am.* 2020 Dec;55(4):457–465. doi: 10.1016/j.cnur.2020.06.012.
26. Egbert LD, Battit GE, Welch CE, Bartlett MK. Reduction of postoperative pain by encouragement and instruction of patients: a study of doctor-patient rapport. *N Engl J Med.* 1964;270:825–827.
27. Inui TS, Yourtee EL, Williamson JW. Improved outcomes in hypertension after physician tutorials: a controlled trial. *Ann Intern Med.* 1976;84(6):646–651.
28. Korsch BM, Gozzi EK, Francis V. Gaps in doctor-patient communication: 1. Doctor-patient interaction and patient satisfaction. *Pediatrics.* 1968;42(5):855–871.
29. Kleinman A. Concepts and a model for the comparison of medical systems as cultural systems. *Soc Sci Med.* 1976;12:85–93.
30. Lattanzi JB, Masin HL, Phillips A. Translation and interpretation services for the physical therapist. *HPA Resour.* 2006;6(4).
31. Passmore J, Rowson T. Neuro-linguistic programming: A critical review of NLP research and the application of NLP in coaching. *Int Coaching Psychol Rev.* 2019;14:57–69.

32. Lancaster LC, Stillman D. *When Generations Collide: Who They Are. Why They Clash. How to Solve the Generational Puzzle at Work*. New York, NY: Harper Business; 2003.

33. Frontline. *Life on the virtual frontier: distracted by everything*. Frontline, Digital Nation. https://www.pbs.org/wgbh/pages/frontline/digitalnation/. Accessed October 12, 2022.

34. Farnan JM, Paro JA, Higa JT, Reddy ST, Humphrey HJ, Arora VM. Commentary: the relationship status of digital media and professionalism: it's complicated. *Acad Med*. 2009;84(11):1479–1481.

35. Hickson GB, Pichert JW, Webb LE, Gabbe SG. A complementary approach to promoting professionalism: identifying, measuring, and addressing unprofessional behaviors. *Acad Med*. 2007;82(11):1040–1048.

36. Freeman J. *The Tyranny of Email*. New York, NY: Scribner; 2009.

37. Zhang L, Lopes S, Lavelle T, Jones KO, Chen L, Jindal M, Zinzow H, Shi L. Economic evaluations of mindfulness-based interventions: a systematic review. *Mindfulness (NY)*. 2022 Aug 30:1–20. doi: 10.1007/s12671-022-01960-1.

38. Chen JA, Anderson ML, Cherkin DC, Balderson BH, Cook AJ, Sherman KJ, Turner JA. Moderators and nonspecific predictors of treatment benefits in a randomized trial of Mindfulness-Based Stress Reduction vs. Cognitive-Behavioral Therapy vs. Usual Care for Chronic Low Back Pain. *J Pain*. 2022 Sep 27:S1526–5900(22)00413-8.

39. McCloy K, Hughes C, Dunwoody DL, Marley DJ, Gracey DJ. Effects of mindfulness-based interventions on fatigue and psychological wellbeing in women with cancer: a systematic review and meta-analysis of randomised control trials. *Psychooncology*. 2022 Oct 11.

40. Geiger C, Cramer H, Dobos G, Kohl-Heckl WK. A systematic review and meta-analysis of mindfulness-based stress reduction for arterial hypertension. *J Hum Hypertens*. 2022 Oct 10.

41. Hutchison M, Russell BS, Starkweather AR, Gans KM. Outcomes from an online pilot Mindfulness Based Intervention with adolescents: a comparison by categories of risk. *J Child Fam Stud*. 2022 Sep 29:1–13.

42. Zhang B, Fu W, Guo Y, Chen Y, Jiang C, Li X, He K. Effectiveness of mindfulness-based cognitive therapy against suicidal ideation in patients with depression: A systematic review and meta-analysis. *J Affect Disord*. 2022 Sep 25;319:655–662.

43. Higgins ET, Davidson RJ, Busse WW, Klaus DR, Bednarek GT, Goldman RI, Sachs J, Rosenkranz MA. Clinically relevant effects of Mindfulness-Based Stress Reduction in individuals with asthma. *Brain Behav Immun Health*. 2022 Sep 14;25:100509.

44. Somohano VC, Kaplan J, Newman AG, O'Neil M, Lovejoy T. Formal mindfulness practice predicts reductions in PTSD symptom severity following a mindfulness-based intervention for women with co-occurring PTSD and substance use disorder. *Addict Sci Clin Pract*. 2022 Sep 16;17(1):51.

45. Pérez V, Menéndez-Crispín EJ, Sarabia-Cobo C, de Lorena P, Fernández-Rodríguez A, González-Vaca J. Mindfulness-Based Intervention for the reduction of compassion fatigue and burnout in nurse caregivers of institutionalized older persons with dementia: a randomized controlled trial. *Int J Environ Res Public Health*. 2022 Sep 11;19(18):11441.

46. Taylor H, Cavanagh K, Field AP, Strauss C. Health care workers' need for headspace: findings from a multisite definitive randomized controlled trial of an unguided digital mindfulness-based self-help app to reduce healthcare worker stress. *JMIR Mhealth Uhealth*. 2022 Aug 25;10(8):e31744.

47. Truhlar LM, Durand C, Cooper MR, Goldsmith CW. Exploring the effects of a smartphone-based meditation app on stress, mindfulness, well-being, and resilience in pharmacy students. *Am J Health Syst Pharm*. 2022 Sep 7:zxac240.

48. Witarto BS, Visuddho V, Witarto AP, Bestari D, Sawitri B, Melapi TAS, Wungu CDK. Effectiveness of online mindfulness-based interventions in improving mental health during the COVID-19 pandemic: a systematic review and meta-analysis of randomized controlled trials. *PLoS One*. 2022 Sep 21;17(9):e0274177.

49. Chiesa A, Serretti A. Mindfulness-based stress reduction for stress management in healthy people: a review and meta-analysis. *J Altern Complement Med*. 2009;15(5):593–600.

50. Rogers SL, Jacobowitz JL. *Mindfulness and Professional Responsibility*. Miami, FL: Mindful Living Press; 2012.

51. Scholeberlein D. *Mindful Teaching and Teaching Mindfulness*. Boston, MA: Wisdom Publications; 2009.

52. Willgens AM, Sharf R. Failure in clinical education: using mindfulness as a conceptual framework to explore the lived experiences of 8 physical therapists. *J Phys Ther Educ*. 2015;29(1)70–80.

53. Compton WC, Hoffman E. *Positive Psychology: The Science of Happiness and Flourishing*, 3rd ed. Belmont, CA: Sage Publications; 2019.

54. Huta V, Hawley L. Psychological strengths and cognitive vulnerabilities: are they two ends of the same continuum or do they have independent relationship with well-being and ill being? *J Happiness Stud*. 2010;11(1):71–93.

55. Riess H, Kraft-Todd G. E.M.P.A.T.H.Y.: a tool to enhance nonverbal communications between clinicians and their patients. *Acad Med*. 2014;89(8):1108–1112.

56. Masin HL. Education in the affective domain: a method/model for teaching professional behaviors in the classroom and during advisory sessions. *J Phys Ther Educ*. 2002;16(1):37–45.

57. Masin HL. Integrating the use of the generic abilities, clinical performance instrument, and neurolinguistic psychology processes for clinical education intervention. *Phys Ther Case Rep*. 2000;3(6):258–266.

58. American Psychological Association. The road to resilience. https://www.apa.org/topics/resilience. Accessed October 12, 2023.

59. Fry R. Millennials overtake Baby Boomers as America's largest generation. Pew Research Center. https://www.pewresearch.org/short-reads/2020/04/28/millennials-overtake-baby-boomers-as-americas-largest-generation/ Accessed October 12, 2024.

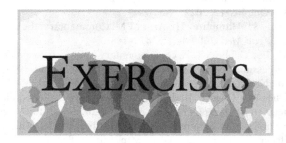

# EXERCISE 1: CLINICAL ENCOUNTERS

1.  Sit across from someone in your class. One person will role-play the therapist and one person the client. Role-play a situation that you remember from a patient–therapist interaction that you have observed. Talk to the patient as you normally would without paying any special attention to matching or mirroring.

    a.  What do you experience as the therapist?

    b.  What do you experience as the patient?

    c.  Do you experience rapport with each other? Why or why not?

2.  Sit across from another person in your class. Again, one person is the therapist and one person is the client. Role-play the same situation that you recall from a patient–therapist interaction that you have observed. This time, the therapist will subtly match the body posture, gesture, hand movements, and breathing of the patient.

    a.  What do you experience as the therapist?

    b.  What do you experience as the patient?

    c.  Do you experience rapport with each other? Why or why not?

# EXERCISE 2: UNDERSTANDING PREFERRED REPRESENTATIONAL SYSTEMS—PREDICATES

1. Sit across from another person in your class. One person tells a story about their favorite vacation. The other person listens to the story and responds as they normally would.

   a. What do you experience as the storyteller?

   b. What do you experience as the listener?

   c. Did you experience rapport? Why or why not?

2. Sit across from another person in your class. One person tells a story about a favorite vacation. The other person listens to the story and pays close attention to predicates—the use of visual, auditory, or kinesthetic words and phrases. The listener responds by matching the PRS of the storyteller.

   a. What is the PRS of the storyteller? How do you know?

   b. What is the PRS of the listener? How do you know?

   c. Did you experience rapport? Why or why not?

   d. Describe a clinical situation where use of predicates may be helpful to establish.

# EXERCISE 3: EYE ACCESSING ACTIVITY

Prior to initiating this activity, review and refer to Figure 12.1 Eye Accessing.

1. Get together with someone in your class. Ask that person the following questions and record their eye movements below. The person responding to the questions can have the eye motion chart on their lap facing the person asking the questions so that the person asking the questions can more readily identify what each eye accessing movement indicates. The thought process and the eye accessing are what you want to understand in this exercise. The verbal responses are not important.

   a. What color is the couch in your living room?

   b. What did you see on your way to class?

   c. What would your ideal house look like?

   d. What would you look like with pink hair?

   e. What is the sound of a busy signal on the telephone?

   f. How would your voice sound underwater?

   g. Recite a nursery rhyme in your head.

   h. How does silk feel next to your skin?

2. What did you discover about eye accessing with your partner?

3. How might you use eye accessing in a clinical situation to enhance rapport?

# EXERCISE 4: ENHANCING ONE'S OWN WELL-BEING

Imagine several evidence-based strategies, described below, that have been shown to be effective in promoting one's own well-being. Choose one different activity to practice each week during this class. Journal about your experience implementing that strategy; continue as you enter the real world as a HCP during your internship, clinical, or field work experiences.

1. Savoring—Practice savoring something good that has happened to you by sharing your positive experience with others while it is happening or afterwards. Create a symbol of the event to remind you of the positive experience such as a photo or souvenir of the experience.

2. Gratitude—Write a letter of gratitude to someone who has impacted your life in a positive way and explain why you are grateful to that person. If possible, deliver it in person. If not, email, mail or fax the letter and follow-up with a phone call.

3. Three good things—Reflect on the positive events you experience each day by writing them in a journal each day followed by your explanation for why this good thing happened.

4. Ways to increase positive emotions:

   a. Become kinder—practice random acts of kindness.

   b. Find healthy distractions to keep your mind off your troubles (e.g., the joy of a simple walk).

   c. Enjoy natural settings nearby—notice the details in nature.

   d. Be sociable with strangers and acquaintances.

   e. Apply your strengths and virtues in your daily habits.

   f. Practice mindfulness by reaching your highest potential—strive for the best, not the mediocre.

   g. Meditation—take a quick but relevant 5 minutes or a deeper 30 minutes.

   h. Help others—anticipate others' needs, open doors, pick up dropped items, let someone in your lane.

   i. Practice gratitude—express your thankfulness to others daily.

   j. Savor positive feelings—write them down, place them in a positive jar, and pull them out when you are feeling bad; reflect on the positive when experiencing the negative.

   k. Share your favorite positivity, meditation, and/or well-being app with a friend.

   l. Visualize your future—tomorrow, next week, next month, 6 months, 1 year, 2 years, 5 years—who are you becoming and how are you developing as a professional? Where are you going? What shall you plan to accomplish? Envision your successful and preferred futures.

# EXERCISE 5: MINDFUL EATING

1. Turn off all distractions, including your phone, social media, Internet, etc.

2. Put a raisin in your hand.

3. Focus on the raisin as if you have never seen one before. Imagine that you have just arrived from another planet and you have been given some raisins. Notice how the raisins look and feel in your hand. Notice the textures and colors of the raisins.

4. Bring a raisin to your nose and smell it. Notice if you have thoughts like, "What is the purpose of this strange exercise?" or "I hate raisins." When you have these thoughts, just acknowledge them, and bring your awareness back to the raisin.

5. Bring the raisin to your ear and squeeze it and roll it around. Notice if you hear anything.

6. Bring the raisin slowly to your mouth and notice if your mouth begins to water.

7. Slowly put the raisin in your mouth and move it gently around with your tongue.

8. When you are ready, intentionally bite down on the raisin and notice where it goes in your mouth. Notice how it tastes.

9. Slowly chew the raisin and notice how its consistency changes as you chew.

10. When you are ready to swallow, notice your intention to swallow and then track the sensations of the raisin as it moves from your mouth to your esophagus and into your stomach.

11. Take a moment to congratulate yourself for taking this time to experience mindful eating.

12. How might the present moment awareness that you have experienced in this mindful eating experience be useful to you in your patient interactions?

# 13

# MINDFUL MATTERS

## COMMUNICATING WITH CULTURAL SENSITIVITY

*Gina Maria Musolino and Helen L. Masin*

## OBJECTIVES

*The learner should be able to*:

- Examine the impact of culture and population trends on the delivery of health care.

- Explore and appreciate one's own and others' cultural heritage.

- Appreciate the National Standards for Culturally and Linguistically Appropriate Services (CLAS) in health and health care.

- Value the utilization of professional interpreters and cultural assessment tools.

- Distinguish the impact of spiritual beliefs, as cultural constructs, affecting health outcomes.

- Examine intercultural communication and cultural competence continuum research.

- Describe the benefits of a mindset of cultural humility, striving for cultural competence and working toward cultural safety in practice to progress health equity.

- Acquire a problem-solving approach that assists health care professionals (HCPs) in enhancing intercultural communication skills utilizing the 5-C Model.

- Compare and contrast the influence of the health care delivery system environments with respect to communication and culture.

- Examine resources that describe the lives and culture shifts of individuals living with disabilities and/or the lives of their families and friends and within health care environments.

Have you ever experienced culture shock? How did you know? With the ever-increasing options for global travel and information exchange via the Internet and other technologies, people who come from different cultures are meeting through work, play, travel, and shared interests or due to relocation from adverse situations. With the expanded

DOI: 10.4324/9781003525554-13     *257*

exposure to different cultures, it has become extremely important to develop both appreciation of and respect for people whose culture differs from one's own. To be effective, developing professionals and HCPs must learn to communicate with cultural sensitivity and to work effectively with patients, families, significant others, colleagues, staff, and support personnel.

# CULTURE SHOCK—WHAT IS IT?

**Culture shock** has been defined as the stress experienced when individuals cannot meet their everyday needs as they would in their own culture. They may have difficulty communicating, making themselves understood, or figuring out why the locals are behaving in a certain way. In response to the stress of culture shock, one may feel a sense of loss and a sense of shock that others behave so differently and seem to have such a different world view.[1]

When culture shock occurs, familiar ways of behaving that you learn through socialization in your own culture do not work in the new culture. Culture shock may occur when you visit another country; when you move from one type of climate to another; when you talk with people who are members of a different generation from yours; when you meet people who have a different sexual orientation from yours; when you meet people who have a disability; or when you meet people who have a different race, religion, or political view from your own. Culture has the broadest connotation when viewed in this way. If these differences pose challenges to communication among people in daily life, you can imagine the impact of these differences in patient care. Do patients truly understand our communication? While cultural and literacy challenges exist, we must make every effort to provide patients with information and education that they can understand, in all forms of patient–practitioner interactions (PPIs).

As HCPs, we are entrusted to putting the needs of our patients first. To do this effectively, the HCP must be aware of and appreciate the cultural mores and expectations of the individual from the world view of that person. Once the other person's world view is understood, it may be easier to establish a therapeutic relationship. One also cannot assume that just because a person is from a certain culture that they ascribe to all the values, beliefs, traditions, habits, patterns, and expectations of that specific culture; there may indeed be variations or even subcultures. The goal of this chapter is to introduce you to intercultural communication in health care to assist you in developing awareness and skills to work effectively in our increasingly diverse communities.

## *A Novel Experience*

As an early career therapist, working in an early intervention program for infants and toddlers with disabilities in Miami, Florida, an opportunity presented to develop a feeding and eating program. Having developed a similar, successful program in the public school system in Maryland, I was delighted to share my experiences with my colleagues in my new setting. I suggested that the classroom teachers begin the feeding program with a food-play activity. The therapeutic objective was to encourage the children to play with the food on their tray. Through play, it has been shown that children will eventually want to bring the food to their mouths to explore it, laying the foundation for the essential hand-to-mouth, self-feeding behavior.

Based on my previous success with this approach in Maryland, I enthusiastically asked the nutritionist at the program to give me several jars of baby food to use for the food-play activity. Many of the children in the program were former premature infants who were generally extremely tactile defensive around their mouths and often resistant to eating food other than in a bottle. I poured out the jar on the tray of the corner chair of one of the toddlers. The child enthusiastically placed both hands into the food and smeared it all over the tray and all over himself and eventually brought his hands to his mouth to taste the food. Of course, I felt extremely pleased that he had been so engaged in the activity and that he had indeed brought his hands to his mouth and tasted the food. Because this child had a history of tactile defensiveness, this was an excellent response—a real success. The next day I hoped to use the food-play activity with several of the other children in the program.

The next day, I suggested that the preschool teachers might want to join me to help introduce the activity with several of the other children with tactile defensiveness. As the teachers politely declined, one by one, I wondered why they were not enthusiastic about my suggestion. I proceeded to work with another child and was again delighted to see that the food play also helped him develop the hand-to-mouth skill. After several more successful days with the food-play activity, I was hopeful that the preschool teachers would finally join in the activity. Because they still politely declined, I decided to ask them whether they had any concerns about the activity. They all said that it made them feel extremely uncomfortable. When I asked them what caused them to feel uncomfortable with the activity, they responded that you are viewed as a bad mother in their culture (Cuban) if you have a messy child. The food-play activity was simply too threatening to them because it challenged their cultural norms about what was acceptable behavior for good mothers with their children.

Once I understood the cultural origins related to the intervention, I had a much better understanding of the teachers' and parents' concerns. I politely explained to the teachers that my intention had not been to offend them or the mothers, and I asked whether there might be an alternative way that we could address the problem. After talking with them, we decided to implement a solution that addressed my concerns, as well as the mothers' concerns. We decided that we would have the children in diapers for the food-play activity. That way, we could bathe them after the activity and then put their clean clothes back on them. Thus, the children had the benefit of the food play without the messiness. The teachers, parents, children, and I were all pleased. If we had not taken the time to understand the cultural norms involved in this situation, the teachers and families might have been labeled as noncompliant and the children would not have had the benefit of the food-play learning experience that was so valuable for the development of their independent feeding skills.

I quickly realized that I wanted to learn as much as I could about the cultures of the children and families with whom I was working. Through my reading and research, considering matters of diversity, population trends,[2] and the Miami-Cuban culture and values specifically, I learned a great deal, enabling me to provide more culturally competent care to my patients and families.

*Can you think of other cultural concerns that might occur in therapeutic settings with interventions? Have you experienced culture concerns first-hand yourself or witnessed others?*

# THE 5-C MODEL OF COMMUNICATION[3]

Using the 5-C Model of communication (conversation, collaboration, cooperation, compromise, and consensus) when working with parents, families, caregivers, and educators with children with disabilities will help to foster a partnership for successful rehabilitation. Having these open and honest discussions takes both courage and risk-taking by all. Yet the benefits outweigh the risks. The model simply entails working through differences using key communication strategies over time for a resulting collaborative plan, together. While the 5-C Model is also effective for any negotiation–conflict–resolution opportunity, it is particularly effective for families and caregivers supporting those with disabilities, because without full engagement of all parties, the opportunities and successful outcomes may be limited. Consider how the 5-C Model of Communication was utilized in the personal experience scenario above and how you will implement it for your effective cultural communications as a HCP:

**Conversation:** Ask/Tell/Ask Exchanges with open-ended queries, "Asking why?" "Tell me more" "Asking for more information"; then answering with "yes, and …" rather than "yes, but …"

**Collaboration:** Open and Honest dialogue, meetings with all vested stakeholders, in a round table format where all are equal partners and able to speak freely and express themselves, away from any interventions, to set the stage for success.

**Cooperation:** Sharing the goals and planned priorities working together as a team.

**Compromise:** Listening to each other through deeper conversations to realize when alterations and compromise may be beneficial in the shared efforts and strategies to achieve therapeutic goals.

**Consensus:** Requires repeat communications in multi-modal formats, over time.

# CULTURAL DIVERSITY IN THE UNITED STATES

HCPs' ability to work effectively with culturally diverse families requires HCPs to acknowledge their own cultural backgrounds and to develop a general understanding of specific cultures.[4] Cultural background is often a powerful force in the relationship between HCPs and the families they serve.[4] As we have learned through the PPI chapters, therapeutic use of oneself in health care is critical for relationships to facilitate therapeutic presence.

To understand the need for culturally competent health care, one must first recognize the increasing diversity in the United States (U.S.). According to the 2022 U.S. Census Bureau data, the percentage of the estimated total population distribution was as follows:[2]

- 75% White alone, non-Hispanic

- 18.9% Hispanic (any race)

- 13.6% Black or African American alone

- 6.1% Asian alone

- 1.3% American Indian and Alaska Native alone

- 0.3% Native Hawaiian and Other Pacific Islanders alone

- 2.9% Two or More Races

Some Census respondents identified with more than one classification due to being multiracial. The U.S. is projected to become a majority-minority nation for the first time in 2043.[2] Based upon the 2043 projection, the White (non-Hispanic) population will remain the largest single group; however, no group will make up a majority. The population of people who are "Two or More Races" is projected to be the fastest growing racial or ethnic group over the next several decades, followed by Asian and Hispanic populations. Further projections from the U.S. Census Bureau predict for the year 2060 that the population distribution in the U.S. shall increase from 326 million to 404 million, reaching 400 million by 2058.[2] By 2030, the turning point year for *all* Baby Boomers (see Chapter 2) with 73.1 million (21%) projected to be 65 years of age or older, referred to as "a graying nation" for 1 in 5 Americans.[2] By 2060, the older U.S. population is projected to consist of 95 million (25%), or 1 in 4 persons.[2] Beginning in 2030, net international migration is expected to overtake natural increase as the driver of population growth in the U.S. because of population aging.[2] The racial and ethnic composition of younger cohorts is expected to change more quickly than for older cohorts.[2] In 2060, over one-third of children are expected to be non-Hispanic White compared with over one-half of older adults.[2] These shifts in U.S. population distribution and diversity[2] are notable for the impacts for HCPs, especially in regions of non-pluralistic representation of HCPs, as compared with those served.[4] Additionally, the aging societies may have fewer working-age HCPs available to serve, and the number of HCPs is not yet meeting today's societal needs, especially in rural regions. This was further compounded by the Covid-19 pandemic, pandemic fatigue, and career shifting due to pandemic demands.

# CULTURE AND RELATIONSHIPS

The quantum physics of our universe is revealing the primacy of relationships.[5] In other words, each aspect of the universe is affected by its relationship with every other aspect of the universe. In quantum physics, nothing exists independent of its relationship with something else, which challenges our traditional Cartesian models of a linear, quantifiable universe. What is critical is the relationship created between two or more elements. Systems influence individuals, and individuals call forth systems.[5] It is the relationship that evokes the present reality. Which potential becomes real depends on the people, the events, and the moment.[5]

For example, in organizations, we may ask which is most important—the system or the individual? The quantum physicist will answer, "It depends." It is not an either/or question. It is important to recognize the relationship that exists between the person and the setting. Relationships will always be different and will generate different responses depending on the person at that moment in time. People, like quantum particles, are "fuzzy." They may go from being predictable to being surprising, just as wave packets of matter include potentialities for both forms—particles and waves. If we can appreciate both the fluctuating "waves" and the interacting entropy of "particles" in ourselves as well as others, we have a better chance of developing the potential in all of us—we must be tolerant of ambiguity and embrace life's randomness—which will aid in being fluid and flexible and not rigid, in both thought and action.

The potential for being a wave or a particle depends on the environment, culture, and context. If we can understand our own environment/culture/context and that of our clients, we have a better chance of developing a strong therapeutic relationship. Given this quantum physics paradigm of the primacy of relationships and the fuzziness of people, we have more appreciation for our own culture and the cultures of our patients and clients. With this paradigm perspective, we have better chances of developing effective therapeutic presence and interprofessional relationships.

The importance of understanding one's cultural world view was emphasized when the U.S. government mandated that care for children be delivered in a culturally competent manner. The federal legislation that began with Public Law (PL) No. 94–142 in 1975 required that public school education be provided for all children from 6 to 21 years of age, regardless of handicapping conditions. This law was modified as PL No. 94–457 (Education of the Handicapped Act of 1986) to include public school education for all children aged 3 to 21 years. The law specified that health services, including physical and occupational therapy, should be provided for all children in a "culturally competent" manner. The two laws were subsequently reauthorized as PL No. 101–119 Individuals with Disabilities Education Act (IDEA). Over time, Congress has amended IDEA for school-aged children and for babies and toddlers, resulting in the 2004 Individuals with Disabilities Education Improvement Act (IDEIA), PL No. 108–446[6] and in 2015 amended the IDEA through PL 114–95, Every Student Succeeds Act.[6] Infants and toddlers, birth through age 2, with disabilities and their families receive early intervention services under IDEA Part C. Children and youth ages 3 through 21 receive special education and related services under IDEA Part B. The law ensures that all children with disabilities receive services and governs how states and public agencies provide for early intervention, special education, and related services, such as evaluations, re-evaluations, and individualized education programs (IEP). We are now going to focus on the aspects related to cultural competence; however, you may be interested to know that additional training, legal and policy updates, grant and related supportive resource information on IDEA is available through the U.S. Department of Education website (https://sites.ed.gov/idea/).

## CULTURAL COMPETENCE

What constitutes cultural competence? Cultural competence has been defined as "the set of congruent behaviors, attitudes, and policies that come together in a system, agency, or among professionals to work effectively in cross-cultural situations."[7] HCPs must recognize the importance of culture in PPI and incorporate culture, assessment of cross-cultural relations, cognizance of the dynamics of cultural differences, expanses of cultural knowledge, and readily modify services to meet culturally unique needs. The concept of cultural competence is also referred to as **cultural sensitivity or intercultural communication**. The term **cross-cultural** refers to comparative studies in multiple cultures. The study of people from different cultures interacting together is termed **intercultural communication**. This chapter highlights results of cultural competence continuum research related to enhancing one's therapeutic effectiveness.

## IMPACT OF CULTURE ON THERAPEUTIC EFFECTIVENESS

Given the continuing increase in diversity of the U.S. population, the ability to successfully communicate in culturally diverse settings is essential for all HCPs. Training in cross-cultural communication enhances the effectiveness of therapists working with clients whose cultures differ from their own.[8] In order to appreciate the importance of developing skill in intercultural encounters, one must first understand the nature of culture itself.

Culture has been referred to as "acquired knowledge people use to interpret experience and generate behavior,"[9] which may consist of a specific framework of meanings within which a population, individually and as a group, shares its ways of life. Margaret Mead (1901–1978) was an American cultural anthropologist, and curator of ethnology at the American Museum of Natural History, who conducted expeditions to Samoa and New Guinea, with 24 field trips to six South Pacific peoples. She defined culture as follows:

> *Abstractions from the body of learned behavior which a group of people who share the same traditions transmit to their children and, in part, to adult immigrants who become members of the society. It covers not only the arts and sciences, religion and philosophies to which the word culture has historically applied, but also the system of technology, the political practices, the small intimate habits of daily life, such as the way of preparing or eating food, or of hushing a child to sleep, as well as the method of electing a prime minister or changing the constitution.*[10]

Given these definitions, one can begin to grasp how, and in what ways, culture is more of a continuum, and that culture is a critical element in understanding how someone responds to illness or disability. Cross-cultural research of culture is, therefore, notably variable and certain cultural concepts do not have the same meaning in all cultures.[11] For example, good health to someone in the U.S. may mean an absence of bacteria or viruses or illness. To someone in China, good health may mean harmony between yin and yang. Therefore, HCPs must understand general and specific components of culture-related health concepts.

**Culture-general** concepts are applicable across all cultures. **Culture-specific** concepts are unique to a particular group. People learn to express symptoms of distress in ways that are acceptable to others in the same culture. For example, in India, stress-related disorders are often suspected when the patient is suffering from an upset stomach. In the U.S., stress-related disorders are often associated with painful headaches. Compared with other countries, there is a notable difference in the widespread promotion of pain-relieving prescriptions and over-the-counter relief options in the U.S.[11] Internationally, Pain Science research[12] provides alternative approaches to pain, especially for those with impacts due to chronic pain, to self-empower patients/clients to manage symptoms and focus on the individual's pain experience in daily life. Functional imaging of the brain has clearly illuminated the veracity of pain concerns.

Understanding the context of pain in the patients'/clients' culture assists the HCP in how to approach therapeutic communication and education. HCPs must explain to patients/clients why they experience pain and utilize their precise narrative and embed for the educational opportunity, by asking the patients/clients about their pain specifically. HCPs must be therapeutically present with their patients/clients utilizing the empathic communication skills you have learned through PPI (Chapters 6 and 8) and provide the patients/clients with techniques to manage their pain and empower self-care. HCPs need to validate the pain that patients/clients are experiencing as real, then proceed to explain the pathway from the most distal impacting structures, and then make the relationship to the brain and how neuropathways and receptors influence the mind–body connections. HCPs must respect the patients'/clients' concept of pain, acknowledging the pain through their unique lived experiences, recognize that pain has psychological, biological, physiological, and social aspects, and that pain is expressed in both verbal and nonverbal ways. Culture may or may not influence how, when, or why pain is expressed or repressed. Pain almost always results in adverse effects on the function, and the social and psychological well-being, of those who are impacted, including family members, caregivers, and significant others; however, those coping with chronic pain, first-hand, may have deeply entrenched adaptive behaviors or compensation as a result. These coping mechanisms may have cultural components and should be respected, while some coping strategies may be maladaptive and/or present as negatively influencing compensatory movements; this is where being fluid comes into play. HCPs must gradually dissect pain behaviors and adaptations through effective communication, remaining open to cultural influences and possibilities. Often warranted, HCPs work collaboratively with a comprehensive pain management team approach to care. Pain is usually a motivating factor for seeking health care. Pain should not only be acknowledged by HCPs but addressed by considering the many potential impacting factors. This is only accomplished through open, therapeutic presence and a listening ear, with astute visual appraisal (scanning for nonverbal pain manifestations, e.g., bracing, guarding, a grimace, frown, wrinkled nose, squeezed/clasped eyes, withdrawal, rapid blinking, distorted facial expressions, etc.) for fully understanding the context of the patient's/client's lived experiences.

As part of the socialization in one's own culture, one learns that certain complaints about distress are acceptable and elicit understanding, whereas other complaints are unacceptable. Hence, culture-specific attitudes, values, and beliefs may also influence how pain is manifested or not. Some cultures encourage effervescent, verbal expressions of pain (moaning, yelling, catastrophizing) while others promote hiding the perceptions of pain displays both verbally and nonverbally, encouraging stoicism. Hence, understanding the cultural basis for a patient's/client's symptoms and signs (or not) becomes more critical for accurate evaluation of the presenting problem, which should be documented, and leads to more accurate clinical diagnosis/es, prognosis/es, plan/s of care and therapeutic alliance/s. The International Association for the Study of Pain (IASP)[12] provides a cultural-global definition of pain as an "unpleasant sensory and emotional experience associated with, or resembling that associated with, actual or potential tissue damage," and is expanded upon with six key notations and the etymology of the word "pain" for further valuable context:[12]

- Pain is always a personal experience that is influenced to varying degrees by biological, psychological, and social factors.
- Pain and nociception are different phenomena. Pain cannot be inferred solely from activity in sensory neurons.
- Through their life experiences, individuals learn the concept of pain.
- A person's report of an experience as pain should be respected.
- Although pain usually serves an adaptive role, it may have adverse effects on function and social and psychological well-being.
- Verbal description is only one of several behaviors to express pain; inability to communicate does not negate the possibility that a human or a nonhuman animal experiences pain.[12]

# CULTURE AND BELIEF SYSTEMS

To understand the ramifications of culture in health care, one must also understand the relationship with beliefs, attitudes, and behavior. **Beliefs** are what people think is true, **attitudes** are how people feel about something (affective domain), and **behaviors** are what people do.[13] Because culture impacts all three of these areas, HCPs must be sensitive to clients' beliefs, attitudes, and behaviors regarding their illness, injury, or disability as important components of evidence-based practice. When the HCP understands what the patient/client is experiencing, the patient/client is more likely to feel that they can be helped. Belief in the possibility of positive outcomes is central to the delivery of and acceptance of health services.[14] To understand the belief systems of their clients, HCPs must first understand the explanatory model of the client.

Kleinman[15] first described the explanatory model as the explanations that are offered for the etiology, onset of symptoms, pathophysiology, course of sickness, and treatment for the particular problem being addressed. On the cultural level, there may be differences between the explanatory model of the family and the explanatory model of the HCP. These differences can hamper effective delivery of health care. However, by respecting the explanatory model of the patient/client, the HCP PPI may be enhanced. For optimal healing to occur, there must be a fit between the expectations, beliefs, behaviors, and evaluation of the outcome between the client and the HCP.

# RESEARCH IN INTERCULTURAL COMMUNICATION

Understanding cultural and transcultural variables is critical to working effectively with different ethnic groups.[16–18] For example, the amount of time spent with the patients influenced patient satisfaction with medical care for respondents identifying as Black within the U.S. population, receiving treatment for hypertension.[17] Additionally, when clients' belief systems were explored and respected by HCPs, an increased compliance with nursing interventions transpired with mothers identifying as Hispanic and Haitian.[16] Coard et al.[18] emphasized that "parent–child conversations about race-related issues serve a protective function for minoritized families and are necessary to help children of color thrive in the US." HCPs need to be aware and facilitate, where appropriate. Ethnic differences appear to be vital determinants of observed differences in health behavior; ethnicity is particularly relevant to what an individual believes and how one behaves regarding various health practices.[17]

# CULTURE AND HEALTH CARE

Cultural differences in relation to health care are reflected in many facets of daily life. Some of the critical cultural issues that may assist HCPs in better understanding their clients include: (1) understanding the characteristics of collectivistic (high-context) cultures and individualistic (low-context) cultures; (2) understanding Eastern and Western perceptions of locus of control and how they differ; (3) the concept of face, heard so often in discussions of Asian cultures; (4) nonverbal intercultural communication patterns; (5) *personalismo*, a concept critical to understanding expectations of Hispanic culture; and (6) somatization.

In addition to exploring these differences, HCPs must understand differences related to disability, racism, ageism, sexism, sexual orientation, and intergenerational expectations (see Chapters 2 and 7). Provided at the end of this chapter are numerous resources for your consideration, chronicling the life experiences of individuals and their families living with disabilities, medical conditions, and diseases and/or those affected by race, class status, or aspects of culture and ethnicity. The shared lived experiences provide insight into the challenges faced by persons with disabilities, their altered status in society or culture, and the effects on the lives of their families, caregivers, and friends. Environmental conditions, such as those living in poverty, those experiencing homelessness, and those lacking a minimal formal education, are variables that transcend all cultures.

# HIGH-CONTEXT AND LOW-CONTEXT CULTURES

First, let's examine the difference between high- and low-context cultures. Cultures that are usually associated with individualism (low-context) include North America (the U.S. is considered the most individualistic), Western Europe, Australia, and New Zealand. Cultures that are usually more associated with collectivism (high-context) include Asia, Africa, Central and South America, and Pacific Island societies.[11]

For HCPs to understand more fully the meaning of these cultural distinctions, they must first be cognizant of their own culture. Saunders's[19] classic works identified numerous characteristics of the Anglo-European culture and/ or Western medical culture that may impact the patient–practitioner relationship. Because the majority of HCPs currently are from Anglo-European roots, it is helpful to understand those values that impact health care, which include the need for personal control over the environment, the need for change, time dominance, human equality, individualism, privacy, self-help, competition, future orientation, action/goal/work, openness/honesty, practicality/ efficiency, and materialism.[20] These values may conflict with other cultures that may espouse collectivistic beliefs, attitudes, and behaviors.

Collectivistic cultures differ from individualistic cultures in critical ways. Collectivism refers to the tendencies of a system that emphasizes the importance of the "we" identity over the "I" identity, group rights over individual rights, and ingroup-oriented needs over individual wants and desires. Individualism refers to the tendencies of a system in emphasizing the importance of individual needs over group needs. The Western Cartesian (individualistic) tradition tends to perceive the self in opposing dualistic terms, whereas the Eastern (collectivistic) tradition tends to perceive the self in a complementary, relational, whole perspective.[21] Differences in world views create very different perceptions for the people who are members of these cultures.

In cross-cultural interactions, low- and high-context cultures reveal marked differences. Low-context cultures, such as most North American and Northern European societies, place emphasis on individualism and individual goals, facts, the management of time, nonverbal communication, privacy, and compartmentalization.[22] Essentially task oriented, they focus on data to provide the answers to living well. Progress is measured in acquiring tangibles or material goods, and goals are action oriented and geared to produce short-term material profits. The driving force of low-context cultures is work. The usual place in which a person is honored is at work. Low-context societies honor individuals who are financially successful. Emotions may be considered inappropriate in most social and work settings.[22]

Low-context individuals, such as U.S. chief executive officers (CEOs) of major corporations are often highly individualistic, directive, and dominating. CEOs tend to be results oriented, independent, strong willed, and quick to make decisions. CEOs may also be impatient, time conscious, solution oriented, and self-contained. They may have a high need to be recognized for performance. When working in groups, low-context individuals need less time to develop relationships in the group, so new and progressive programs can be changed easily and quickly. However, these individuals may create less cohesion and stability in the group and are less committed to group agreements or planned actions. Individualists find that clearing their plans with others may interfere too much with their desire to do their own thing.[22]

In contrast, collectivistic, or high-context cultures and peoples, place emphasis on relationships, group goals, the process, and surrounding circumstances, with time as a natural progression, verbal communication, communal space, and interrelationships.[23] The high-context norms are primarily group oriented. High-context cultures place the relationships of the cultural group before that of an outgroup, such as a university, company, or country. The ties to family and community are strong. In general, feelings and emotions are valued, and expression of feelings is encouraged. Religious and spiritual beliefs are highly valued. Behavior is perceived in a complex way. Nuances of meaning are important in nonverbal communication cues, and the status of others is viewed in context.

To reiterate, Asian cultural norms are considered high context. The personal characteristics that are valued are being indirect, highly affiliative and team oriented, systematic, steady, and quiet. The person is expected to be patient, loyal, dependable, sharing, and respectful; generally slow in making decisions; and a good listener. A longer amount of time is needed for individuals to become acquainted with, and trusting of, each other, but once the trust is established the communication is fast. In general, the culture has strong links to the past and is slow to change. The society is highly stable and works as a unified group. The group members feel comfortable with the constant psychological presence of a group. The members are loyal to the group. They demonstrate cooperation and contribution to the group without the expectation of immediate reciprocity and show public modesty about individual abilities.[23] Individuals are more committed to group agreements and planned actions.

The critical importance of understanding the cultural beliefs and norms of clients became apparent while providing physical therapy at a preschool for a 2-year-old boy with cerebral palsy and a history of grand mal seizures. His family had recently immigrated to Miami from Haiti. All the professional staff were extremely concerned about him because he was having grand mal seizures at the preschool. The staff contacted the mother to determine whether she was giving him the phenobarbital that had been prescribed by the neurologist. She assured the staff that she was giving her son the medication. When the seizures continued, the staff called the mother again and had a Creole translator speak with her about the phenobarbital. However, the boy continued to have seizures at school. Extremely concerned about him, his mother was invited to school and asked to demonstrate how she was administering the phenobarbital. This turned out to be the critical question that had not been asked. His mother demonstrated that she administered the phenobarbital to him by bathing him in the medication. No one had even considered that the medicine would be given in any way other than by mouth. An assumption was made based on the Western medical model of oral administration of the medication. Fortunately, after explaining that the medicine had to be administered orally to be effective, once the mother understood this, she followed through with the oral administration. She explained that in the part of Haiti where she had lived, medicine was administered by bathing in it. Whenever people have experiences during which they must make adjustments, they learn that culture is much more than an abstraction.[11]

Another example is when some mothers refuse to place their infants on the floor, as in their culture it would be dishonorable for their children to be where soiled shoes tread—while others believe babies should not be on the floor until over 100+ days. *How could you reconcile these cultural beliefs to assure a child has needed "tummy time" for normal developmental milestones to emerge—yet still honor the cultural values and expectations?*

Whenever a patient/client is not responding in the way one would have anticipated, it is important to ask whether cultural differences might be causing the difficulty. HCPs may ask, "Which of these symptoms is familiar to me, given my own cultural background, and which seem strange?" The symptoms will seem strange if the HCP has not encountered them in their own socialization. According to Turner,[24] there are three questions that a HCP should ask when working with clients to avoid potential biases:

1. How is this client like all human beings?

2. How is this client like some human beings?

3. How is this client like no other human being?

By asking these three questions, the HCP can avoid stereotypes and generalizations and move toward the person's unique problems, needs, and resources.

# THE CONCEPT OF FACE

The concept of face, regarded as a universal construct, refers to the sense of self-respect or self-esteem that people demonstrate in communicating with each other. The management of face differs from one culture to the next. Managing face involves maintaining a claimed sense of self-dignity or regulating a claimed sense of self-humility in interaction.[21] Three possible issues related to face communication include dignity–humility, respect–deference, and imposition–nonimposition. As anyone who has ever done business in the East will tell you, if one wishes to be successful in keeping face, one must understand the cultural background of face work issues, as well as the norms and boundaries inherent in face work negotiation.[21]

In a study by Hagland et al., the issue of face dialectics proved to be critical to one hospital's retention of Asian nurses.[25] In reviewing the employment records of the Asian nurses, the administration learned that the Asian nurses were leaving after only 90 days of employment. The hospital policy required that all employees receive performance evaluations after 90 days of employment. The Asian nurses were not accustomed to receiving negative feedback face to face, which is a Western norm. As a result, the nurses would immediately quit their jobs after the performance evaluation rather than lose face. Misunderstandings are likely to occur more frequently, with increasing diversity in the health care workforce, unless education in intercultural communication becomes a part of pre-employment and ongoing in-service education training for all HCPs and support staff.

*What ideas can you think of that might solve this problem to avoid the loss of face yet still provide adequate feedback to the Asian nurses?* In general, one can predict that in individualistic cultures, individual pride is more likely to be overtly expressed, whereas individual shame is more likely to be demonstrated through other ego-based emotional reactions, such as anger, frustration, or guilt. In contrast, in collectivistic cultures, relational shame or face loss, such as face embarrassment or face humiliation, is more likely to be experienced, and individual-based pride is more likely to be suppressed. Overall, the individualistic cultures stress ego-based emotional expressions and individual self-esteem, whereas collectivistic cultures value other focused emotions management and protection of collective self-esteem.

Belenky et al.,[26] through gender-based research, indicated that Euro-American males tended to engage in the "morality of justice," whereas Euro-American females tended to engage in the "morality of caring." The ego-based emotions are associated with morality of justice, whereas the other focused emotions are associated with the morality of caring. In other words, in a moral dilemma between doing the right thing vs. doing the caring thing, people from individualistic cultures will choose the right action over the caring action. Doing the caring action is more reflective of the high-context or collectivistic world view. *How does this relate to your professional Code of Ethics? What principles are pertinent and why? Take a moment to journal.*

Numerous scholars have noted that individualists in Western cultures tend to perceive emotion, cognition, and motivation as located in the mind, whereas collectivists in Eastern cultures tend to perceive these three constructs as stemming primarily from the heart.[27] Western vocabularies tend to emphasize the relationship between self-conception and cognition, whereas Eastern vocabularies and metaphors tend to emphasize self-conception and emotional harmony.[27]

# CULTURAL ISSUES OF TIME, SPACE, AND ENVIRONMENTS

Hall and Hall[28] identified time and space as factors of "context" that are universal in all cultures. They distinguished between **monochronic time** and **polychronic time**. In low-context cultures, monochronic time is used. The individual pays attention to time and does only one thing at a time. Time is used to compartmentalize events, functions, people, communication, and information flow.

In high-context cultures, polychronic time is used. In this paradigm, many things may happen or get attention at the same time (multitasking). There is more involvement with people and events. People take precedence over time and schedules. Emphasis is placed on completing human interactions. In low-context perception of monochronic time, information flow and communication are restricted. Meetings and communication in low-context cultures are used to pass on information and/or determine information from which to evaluate and make decisions. In the high-context perception of polychronic time, information flows freely among all participants. Because the information is available to everyone, it is expected that people will use intuition and understand automatically. In high-context cultures, meetings are held to reach a consensus about what is already known. Each person has invisible boundaries of personal space or territory, which often implies ownership or power when linked to physical location. Spatial changes influence and give meaning to human interaction, even more so than the spoken word. Spatial cues, such as distance between the speaker and listener, are perceived by all the senses. Cultures may vary as to which senses are most attuned to spatial cues. For example, appropriate distance between speaker and listener in Anglo cultures is about 2.5 to 3 feet. In Middle Eastern cultures, it is about 2 to 2.5 feet. A popular example of this norm in North American culture is shown when the speaker expresses annoyance that someone is "in my face." However, the Middle Eastern speaker may be confused as to why the North American listener keeps moving away from them during conversations. Social distancing due to the Covid-19 pandemic challenged all norms.

In some cultures, spatial cues may be primarily perceived by vision, hearing, touch, or kinesthetic prompts. Vision, hearing, and kinesthetic cues are important components of HCP communication, as described in Chapter 12.

For low-context, monochronic societies and individuals, personal space is perceived as private, controlled, and often large. For high-context polychronic societies or individuals, space is frequently shared with subordinates and centralized or shared in an information network. Time and space are closely linked because access to individuals is often determined by location and timing.[22] Correspondingly, one finds in athletic events on the international scale, such as with the World Cup Soccer games, crowds and teams always maintain highly close contact, whereas North American soccer events generally present with greater personal space maintained by all participants. You may also have some experience within time and space cultural differences with "Southern hospitality" and "Cuban time." With Southern charmers, you may always be welcome to come over anytime and stay indefinitely, front porch sitting is more formal and open to all, while back porch sittings is for deeper, more intimate conversations and purposes. In Cuban time, if you arrive too early, it may be considered rude, and it is better to arrive an hour or more late. In contrast, most U.S. health care facilities maintain strict time schedules with precise adherence to time and specific planned utilization of space and equipment. Hence, these approaches to time and space may be problematic and lead to cultural clashes with HCPs and their patients or coworkers.

However, some regions experience therapy as a shared cultural experience vs. a singular experience. While participating in outpatient services in Hawaii, a clinical experience student was surprised to experience "island time" in which participants attend therapy during the day (scheduled at any time), make an event of the therapy sessions, and everyone brings nourishment to the clinic for all to partake in throughout the day. It is a shared cultural experience vs. a singular experience. Certain patient units are also geared toward more inclusive participation by the families, such as joint camps for pre- and postoperative joint replacement rehabilitation. At joint camp units, patients are allowed and encouraged to designate and bring a family member to participate directly in their care on a regular basis, and the patients participate in group rehab sessions, along with the individual care. Group therapy fosters support and a culture of shared experiences in a formal networking process, with the opportunity for informal interactions during meal breaks and planned recreational therapy. Many support groups for specific conditions and diseases benefit from group approaches to coping, management, and recreational and conditioning activities. Families and patients benefit from the collective experiences of all participants sharing and exchanging thoughts, ideas, and strategies. Many groups develop their own unique culture or ways of interacting, so if one group does not work, one might try another.

In addition, variations in the types of setting in which one works may have an impact on your concentration and that of your patients' abilities and stressors. For example, the Neonatal Intensive Care Unit (NICU) and the Intensive Care Unit (ICU) are very fast-paced and involve caring for critically ill patients with life-sustaining measures, with multiple lines, tubes, and patient-monitoring devices. NICU/ICUs, while hectic, also strive to reduce the negative environmental impacts on the patients. Patients who desire to move on from the intensive setting quickly, nevertheless are unable to do so until they are stable (Table 13.1).

The acute care setting is somewhat fast-paced and moves patients toward discharge quickly due to the high cost of services in the more acute settings, and the patients are less medically ill in acute care than the patients in the ICUs. The goal in acute care is discharge to the next level of care or return to home. The rehabilitation and long-term care settings are more moderately paced and involve longer stays for the patients, with less focus on life-sustaining measures and more focus on function and daily living skills. As you look back on the reflections in Chapter 11 of how developing HCPs are transforming society, you will note variations in the lived experiences of the developing professionals within the various types of health care settings.

TABLE 13.1

## OVERVIEW COMPARISON OF TREATMENT SETTINGS

| SETTING CRITERIA | GENERAL ACUTE AND/OR INTENSIVE | REHAB HOSPITAL | SNF/ SUBACUTE REHAB | HHA/ALF | LT ACUTE CARE | OUT-PATIENT | SCHOOL BASED | HOSPICE | PUBLIC HEALTH IHS/GOV VISN | INDUSTRY |
|---|---|---|---|---|---|---|---|---|---|---|
| **Patient audience** | Captive | Captive | Captive | Earned/ captive | Captive | Earned | Captive | Captive | Earned/ captive | Earned/ captive |
| **Patient expecta-tions** | o Save my life<br>o Get me well | o Get me well<br>o Help me function at maximum capacity | o Get me well<br>o Take care of me with dignity<br>o Help me reach my goals | o Get me well<br>o Teach me to manage myself in my home environment | o Save my life<br>o Get me better<br>o Help me reach greater function while addressing my serious condition(s) with longer time, patience | o Get me well<br>o Get me ready to get back to work/sports<br>o Help me function at maximum capacity<br>o Don't keep me waiting | o Help me reduce my physical limitation in order to maximize my ability to learn<br>o Help me play | o Control my pain<br>o Take care of me with dignity until it is my time to die<br>o Caring attitude any environment | o Get me well but keep me in harmony with my values and beliefs | o Get me well<br>o Get me ready to go back to work safely |
| **Primary services provided** | o Life-sustaining services<br>o Medical stabilization<br>o Diagnostic Services | Intensive team-oriented rehab ≥6 hours/day | o Primarily geriatrics<br>o Maybe life-sustaining subacute unit/beds | Primarily geriatrics rehab | o Acute care, LT, avg >25 days transferred from ICU/ CCU; longer inpatient stay<br>o Movement and function | o Acute to subacute<br>o Diagnostic and minor surgical<br>o Movement and function for chronic diseases | Develop-mental peds rehab | Palliative care | Same as with acute, OP, and home health, et al | o Primarily orthopedics, some neuro, cardio<br>o Burns/falls/ traumas |
| **Role of PT** | o Early mobilization<br>o Pain control<br>o Wound care<br>o Consult/ screening | o Functional mobility: return to life/ community<br>o Work with rehab team | o Functional mobility<br>o Establish patient movement programs for nursing/ care providers | o Functional mobility in home environ-ment<br>o Patient movement program family/ caregiver involve-ment | o Improvements of function and mobility<br>o Work with rehab team and very closely with nursing | o Manager of PT department<br>o Direct/ primary hands-on<br>o OP may be offered in homes | Direct hands-on, then consult/ advise teachers/ aides and parents/ caregivers | o Some direct hands-on<br>o Some consulting | o Direct/ hands-on<br>o Medical mission-aries<br>o Often primary | o Direct/ hands-on<br>o Consultation/ screenings |

*(continued)*

TABLE 13.1 (CONTINUED)

## OVERVIEW COMPARISON OF TREATMENT SETTINGS

| SETTING CRITERIA | GENERAL ACUTE AND/OR INTENSIVE | REHAB HOSPITAL | SNF/ SUBACUTE REHAB | HHA/ALF | LT ACUTE CARE | OUT-PATIENT | SCHOOL BASED | HOSPICE | PUBLIC HEALTH IHS/GOV VISN | INDUSTRY |
|---|---|---|---|---|---|---|---|---|---|---|
| **Availability of support staff** | Excellent, especially for life-sustaining activities | Excellent for broad spectrum of team members | Fair/adequate | You may be sole provider | ○ Excellent to good<br>○ Similar to inpatient hospital with longer stays, 3 to 6 concurrent diagnoses, comorbidities | Could be sole practitioner or broad spectrum of disciplines | Sole practitioners with nonprofessional staff within earshot or aides | ○ Nursing support<br>○ Support staff varies<br>○ Home services: sole | As with acute, OP and home health, etc. | ○ Usually sole practitioner/employer<br>○ Consults |
| **Discharge criteria** | When medically stable | Depends on payer source, usually 20 to 60 days max | ○ Medicare<br>○ Managed care when can be handled at home | ○ When no longer homebound<br>○ When reached max potentials<br>○ When functional goals met or fluctuating | ○ Ready to return to home or stable to LT care if still requiring custodial care with feeding and dressing or assisted living<br>○ Pain managed | ○ Payer source often determines<br>○ Medicare: when reached max potential<br>○ RTW<br>○ Managed care: contract<br>○ Commercial: highly variable | ○ Usually continues through public school education<br>○ Public Law 94–142 requires | ○ When pain is controlled<br>○ Comatose/ deceased | When goals are met or patient refuses | ○ With successful RTW FT, part-time<br>○ Disability determination<br>○ Functional Capacity Evaluation<br>○ Alternate duty determined |

ALF = assisted living facility; CCU = critical care unit; FT = full-time; GOV = government; HHA = home health agency; ICU = intensive care unit; IHS = Indian Health Service; LT = long-term; OP = outpatient; PT = physical therapy; RTW = return to work; SNF = skilled nursing facility; VISN = Veteran's Integrated Health Service.

Rehabilitation units strive to provide more intensive rehabilitation therapies, typically for several hours each day, with at least two or more services, to improve the patient's ability for daily function and sustained quality movement. Subacute rehabilitation may be in a specialty hospital that may provide acute and long-term rehabilitation services. Extended care or skilled nursing facilities provide for therapies, predominantly for elderly patients who require longer-term nursing care, rehabilitation, and other services. The pace of inpatient facilities is often census driven and based upon the fragility of the patients receiving services. The pace may fluctuate from fast to moderate to slow, depending upon admissions, support staff, and diagnoses being treated. The outpatient setting is fast paced to very fast paced; however, the patients can self-mobilize, in general, and commute to attend therapy. Generally, outpatient services address predominantly musculoskeletal and neuromuscular injuries and impairments that may be limiting a person's life function or role in society. Those receiving outpatient rehabilitation services generally attend formal therapy sessions in less frequent bouts (two to three times a week or several times a month) depending upon the conditions and impairments and functional limitations being addressed, with all receiving home and education programs to address movement improvements. Some patients/clients also receive outpatient services for ongoing alterations in movement abilities and function due to chronic disease processes and the impact on the movement systems.

Rehabilitation services, as mentioned previously in the chapter when discussing IDEIA,[6] are provided in the school and preschool settings. The educational environment is the setting for preschool, elementary, and secondary education facilities and is coordinated with families and teachers.[6] In traditional home health settings, rehab services are provided in the patient's residence. Traditional home health may serve the elderly and children who are unable to otherwise attend therapy in outpatient or school-based services.[6] Home health may also occur in the patient's room within a care facility, group home, or elsewhere in the community. In today's society of accessibility, home care is also provided in the home at the convenience, preference, or request for the patient, for actual outpatient therapy services provided within the home, as a service option. Home care involves the added stressor of travel between locations for the HCP (rather than the patient), with one-to-one therapy within the home that may involve the family unit. In-home, outpatient therapy services are particularly popular with aging populations, who are less safe to drive, and rural populations where travel is not possible or resourced. Hospice care provides therapy services in the chronic phases of disease for functional abilities and pain management. Respite care is also a viable option for shorter-term caregiving. The pace is highly variable within in-home care environments and the context variable with real-world applications.

Rehabilitation services may also be provided for within industries or occupational work environments; through local, state, and federal government agencies, such as Veterans Health and Indian Health Services (IHS); and in research centers with private or government funding. Each setting has its own culture and expectations for care by the professional staff members. Veterans often present with complex and multi-systems concerns and with multiple conditions, and they may be impacted heavily by psychological concerns such as posttraumatic stress disorder (PTSD) and/or concussive syndromes. Rehabilitation centers with IHS may not be fully resourced with needed HCPs, and patients may receive infrequent care; therefore, one may encounter more chronic conditions that have not been addressed in early phases or may serve as the primary provider. HCPs may also need to consider greater efforts toward primary prevention to assist in the potential gaps in care. Physical and occupational therapy rehabilitation services have been provided in the IHS only since the late 1950s and early 1960s. Today, all rehab services continue to expand in tribal programs, and cultural appreciation is key as an IHS HCP. Patients/clients want to get well, but in harmony with their values and beliefs (see Table 13.1). IHS offers services addressing patients with diabetes; pediatric, cardiopulmonary, mental health, and orthopedic conditions; specialty hand and foot care; wound care; health promotion; neurological rehabilitation; prosthetics/orthotics clinics; gender-health programs, and others. A strong generalist with the ability to provide community outreach and preventative education is needed in IHS. Sometimes, student loan repayment opportunities for a dedicated service and time commitment are available for service in remote and rural areas for HCPs to address the underserved needs (visit the www.va.gov and www.ihs.gov websites to learn more about these unique cultural settings and practice opportunities). Additionally, telehealth and tele-rehabilitation further emerged as a necessity of the Covid-19 pandemic and continue today where and whenever deemed appropriate by the HCPs with changing legislative actions and reimbursement as a result. This two-way, real-time, visually augmented, two-dimensional communication poses unique challenges, yet assists in communication for care, where health care may not have otherwise been delivered. As haptic technologies develop, HCPs may be able to reach out with enhanced virtual connections in both 3D and 4D realities.

As you can see, a wide variety of practice environments exist for HCPs in rehabilitation services. While during your training you shall focus on the skills to enter (entry-level generalist) practice in a variety of settings initially, as a generalist, your preferences for the setting type, cultural exchanges, context, time, and environmental influences may further guide your decision making in your preferred practice setting and pursuit of a future specialization. In any event, as a HCP one must acculturate to the people we serve to effect a change within the HCPs' PPI.

In the exercises at the end of the chapter, you will further explore a patient's journey through the health care system. For now, so that you may begin to understand the patient's perspectives, in the context and cultures of the health care environment, select a few videos from the Johns Hopkins website that explore what it is like to experience being a patient in an ICU setting (www.hopkinsmedicine.org/pulmonary/research/outcomes-after-critical-illness/oacis-videos-news). After reviewing, share and discuss with your classmates what you learned, how it will change your communication approach, and how you felt after viewing. *Take a moment to journal your thoughts and reflections.*

# HIDDEN DIMENSIONS OR IMPLICIT MEANINGS IN CULTURE

To understand the complete or true meanings in intercultural communication, one must appreciate the multiple hidden dimensions of unconscious culture. Context will largely determine the message that the person receives.[28] In collectivistic, high-context communication, much of the information is already understood, either internalized in the individual or in the physical context of the situation.[28] Only a small amount of the meaning is in the explicit transmission or coding of the message. For example, in high-context cultures, the mere presence of an official representative at a meeting, regardless of whether something is said by the official, indicates that the meeting is understood to be important by all those present. In contrast, in low-context, individualistic communication, most information is in the explicit coding of the message, rather than within the individual or the situational (context).[28]

It is up to each person to perform the critical function of correcting for distortions or omissions, in the messages received.[28] To be truly effective in intercultural communication, one must know the degree of information or context that must be supplied to correctly interpret another individual's verbal and nonverbal behavior. The context or the information surrounding the event that gives it meaning varies from culture to culture, and it is often the critical factor in determining whether individuals from different cultures communicate effectively.

For the Anglo-American HCP working with Native American clients, understanding the context of the situation is critical to effective intercultural communication; for example, the very different cultural interpretations of silence in Native American communication compared with Anglo-American communication.[11] For the Native American, silence is a culturally acceptable response to ambiguity.[11] For the Anglo-American, small talk is a culturally acceptable response to ambiguity.[11] For the Anglo-American HCP who does not understand the Native American context of silence, silence may inappropriately be perceived as disinterest or noncompliance.

# NONVERBAL COMMUNICATION

Nonverbal communication refers to information exchange (or difficulties in such an exchange) that does not require oral or written forms of language. These include gestures, positioning of the body, and tenseness of the facial expressions (see the section "Neurolinguistic Psychology and Rapport" in Chapter 12). Unfortunately, there are few cultural universals, except the recognition that all cultures use both verbal and nonverbal means, and that people should avoid drawing any conclusions regarding nonverbal behaviors without a great deal of knowledge. Such knowledge involves developing an understanding of specific gestures, expressions, and uses of the body, as well as a full grasp of the context of communication; and asking questions to confirm meaning.

For example, the distance that people keep from each other is a potent means of nonverbal communication. In the U.S., when people first meet each other, they usually stand about 2.5 to 3 feet apart. If they stand closer, it may be interpreted as a sign of more than casual interest in each other. However, in Latin America, the typical distance people stand from each other while conversing is about 2 feet. Reduced distance does not convey a special message of "desire for more interaction in the future."[28] For HCPs working with clients from Latin America, this information is critical to understanding the context of the intercultural communication.

# *PERSONALISMO*

As a new therapist working in Miami, it was initially surprising to receive invitations to attend celebrations at the homes of the children in treatment. It was confusing too, when the parents of the children asked questions regarding my parents, marital status, and siblings. Fortunately, consulting with my colleagues at the preschool, who served as my cultural informants, it became clear as to why the families were so interested in my personal life. They politely informed me that the families wanted to get to know me as a person, as well as a professional—also known as the concept of *personalismo* in the Hispanic culture—and that it is very important in establishing rapport with the families. Understanding the cultural context of the communication was essential!

# SOMATIZATION

Somatization, a behavior more common among Asians, Africans, and Latin Americans than North Americans, refers to the tendency to report physical symptoms when a person is experiencing psychological distress. The patient does not present any identifiable organic causes for the problem but experiences symptoms that are real and troublesome. Somatization is more frequently seen in cultures where complaints about anxiety, worries, and depression are perceived as signs of weakness. In many cultures, people have much less tolerance for mental illness than for physical illness. Therefore, the context of the communication must be understood by the HCP to have effective intercultural communication. The concepts of *nervios* and *ataques de nervios* may present with symptoms of heart palpitations, sleep disorders, and generalized body pains. These somatic symptoms may reflect chronic feelings of stress that are related to various life challenges.

# SIX UNIVERSAL ASPECTS OF HEALTH CARE IN ALL CULTURES

Scholars have examined interactions between HCPs and people seeking help in different parts of the world.[8,11,14] HCPs include people with advanced degrees in highly industrialized nations and native healers, shamans, and herbalists in less industrialized nations. Six universal concepts in the delivery of health care were identified:

1.  The health care specialist applies a name to a problem.

2.  The qualities of the HCP are important.[14] The HCPs must be perceived by clients to be **caring**, **competent**, **approachable**, and **concerned** with identifying and finding solutions to the problem. (With minority groups in the U.S., HCPs must communicate a sense of **credibility**, that they can be of help. In addition, they should be able to offer health-related benefits of some kind as soon as possible. If the HCP does not establish credibility, the client is not likely to return for an appointment.)

3.  The HCP must establish credibility using symbols and trappings of status that are familiar in the culture.

4.  The HCP places the client's problems in a familiar framework (this implies recognition of the client's explanatory model[15] by the practitioner).

5.  The HCP applies a set of techniques meant to bring relief (this implies recognition of the client's explanatory model[15]).

6.  Interactions between the clients and the practitioners occur at a special time and place (this implies recognition of the client's explanatory model[15]).

To achieve these six universal requirements in the intercultural environment, HCPs must be educated about their own culture, as well as the cultures of the clients, families, colleagues, and support staff with whom they work. Many researchers recommend training in cultural sensitivity to provide optimal care through application of knowledge of culture and cultural differences. In fact, counselors trained in cultural sensitivity were rated higher in the dimensions of expertise, trustworthiness, ability to show positive regard, and empathy compared with counselors not trained in cultural sensitivity.[11] There is a difference between the pseudo-tolerance that results from "putting the lid on" one's intolerance and the genuine tolerance that stems from developing an open, courageous, and loving heart. Intolerance comes from fear. Knowledge and sensitivity training go a long way to quell the fear of what is different and to yield true tolerance for and enjoyment of the differences among us. The HCP must demonstrate a willingness to bring knowledge to interactions with different clients and be able to take culture into account when discussing important topics related to alleviating pain and stress.

# CULTURALLY AND LINGUISTICALLY APPROPRIATE SERVICES (CLAS) STANDARDS

Culturally and linguistically appropriate services (CLAS) standards have been mandated by the Office of Minority Health (OMH) of the U.S. Department of Health and Human Services (HHS).[29] CLAS standards are designed to advance health equity, improve quality, and help eliminate health care disparities by establishing a blueprint for health care organizations to provide services that are respectful, understandable, effective, and equitable. The National CLAS[29] standards include 15 mandates that are organized by theme. The Principal Standard calls on organizations to "provide effective, equitable, understandable and respectful quality care and services that are responsive to diverse cultural health beliefs and practices, preferred languages, health literacy, and other communication needs."[29] Remaining standards are divided into three themes: (1) Governance, Leadership, and Workforce; (2) Communication and Language Assistance; and (3) Engagement, Continuous Improvement, and Accountability; with an implementation checklist for organizations to self-assess capacities.

One standard specifically mandates that health care organizations must provide language assistance services in the patient's preferred language in writing and verbally, offering language assistance services to each patient with limited English proficiency.[29] Modern technology has enhanced translation capabilities through the use of language applications, such as Babbel, MediBabble©, Duolingo, Google Translate, Foreign Services Institute, and BBC languages (free online lessons in languages of the world); smart phone apps have dramatically reduced the need to rely too heavily on human interpreters. However, the responsibilities and accountabilities for translation for HCPs and cultural nuances may not be obvious with all technological applications. You might wish to check out a few of the language apps to begin your exploration for those patients you will serve with limited English proficiencies. If you commonly work with non-English-speaking persons, or those with limited English proficiency, as many of us do in certain parts of the country that are more multilingual and multicultural, you will likely need to become more proficient in languages such as Spanish, Chinese, Tagalog, Creole, Vietnamese, Arabic, French, Farsi, German, Korean, Russian, and Italian because these are some of the non-English languages most frequently spoken in the U.S.[30] There are several counties in the U.S. where more than 100 languages are spoken (in California, Washington, Arizona, Illinois, and New York). Take advantage of Spanish courses for medical professionals. Becoming proficient in American Sign Language is also a helpful skill. Two-way communication is needed with patient care, and this can only happen if we are communicating with our patients' preferred language, or one that they understand, and doing so in an equitable manner, regardless of individual differences. HCPs must take reasonable steps to provide meaningful access for those who have limited English proficiency. Excellent guidance has been provided by Juckett and Unger[31(p 476)] on the use of medical interpreters:

> *More than 25 million Americans speak English "less than very well," according to the US Census Bureau. This population is less able to access health care and is at higher risk of adverse outcomes such as drug complications and decreased patient satisfaction. Title VI of the Civil Rights Act mandates that interpreter services be provided for patients with limited English proficiency who need this service, despite the lack of reimbursement in most states. Professional interpreters are superior to the usual practice of using ad hoc interpreters (i.e., family, friends, or untrained staff). Untrained interpreters are more likely to make errors, violate confidentiality, and increase the risk of poor outcomes. Children should never be used as interpreters except in emergencies. When using an interpreter, the clinician should address the patient directly and seat the interpreter next to or slightly behind the patient. Statements should be short, and the discussion should be limited to three major points. In addition to acting as a conduit for the discussion, the interpreter may serve as a cultural liaison between the provider and patient. When a bilingual clinician or a professional interpreter is not available, phone interpretation services or trained bilingual staff members are reasonable alternatives. The use of professional interpreters (in person or via telephone) increases patient satisfaction, improves adherence and outcomes, and reduces adverse events, thus limiting malpractice risk.*

Unfortunately, despite the awareness of the vital need for the utilization of interpreters, these services are underused, resulting in less access to health care, suboptimal care, with increased hospital-based admissions, leading to increased serious medical events and deficient health literacy.[31-33] Effective and appropriate use of professional interpreter services decreases clinically significant errors and increases the quality of care.[32-33]

## SPIRITUALITY AS CULTURE AND HEALTH CARE

As you will read in Chapter 15, current descriptive literature suggests that spirituality and/or religion are linked with health outcomes. Koenig et al.[34] reviewed 1,600 studies and found that better health outcomes over time were associated with individuals who had a religious or spiritual practice compared with controls. HCPs can conduct cultural/spiritual screenings with their patients to ascertain whether they have a religious/spiritual practice. Four questions to ask are:

1. What are your sources of health, strength, comfort, and peace?
2. Are you part of a religious or spiritual community?

3.   What spiritual practices do you find most helpful to you personally?

4.   Are there any specific practices or restrictions I should know about in providing your care?

Well-being and spirituality are vital for basic human experiences. Spirituality exists in our connection to other humans, our environment, and the unfolding universe and the transcendent. HCPs can have an impact on the patient's health and healing if they acknowledge and address the patient's spirituality as part of their assessment.[35,36] Using assessment tools, the HCP can learn how the belief system of the patient may impact how the patient deals with their illness or disorder.[35] Numerous assessment tools are available, including the Well-being Health Assessment (takingcharge.csh.umn.edu/wellbeing-assessment) and the Berg Cultural/Spiritual Assessment Tool (cshmodules. umn.edu/Integrativehealingpractices/culture/tool/cf0049.pdf).

## PROMOTING AND VALUING THE CULTURAL COMPETENCE CONTINUUM FOR HEALTHCARE: TOOLS, GUIDES, RESOURCES, AND RESEARCH

Contemporary tools have been developed to assess and promote cultural competence in educational programs for HCPs and through the OMH.[29] OMH provides information, continuing education, and resources to learn about and implement health care promoting a culture of safety along the cultural competence continuum. Access to OMH Think Cultural Health website is via the U.S. Department of Health and Human Services (HSS). Pause now, to explore the OMH site (thinkculturalhealth.hhs.gov/education), select a HCP cultural competency course or refresher, as applicable, to complete. Then review the resources in the library (https://thinkculturalhealth.hhs.gov/resources/ library), paying particular attention to the how-to guides, especially Providing CLAS, Culturally Capable materials, and Communication Styles; self-assess your abilities utilizing the checklists, including Effective Cross-Cultural Communication and Working Effectively with an Interpreter; along with the tools, RESPECT model and ADDRESSING framework, spend some time considering Kleinman's eight questions (Explanatory Model).[15] *Reflect and journal about how you will utilize these newly acquired tools and resources for your culturally aware approach to health care for your patients and clients.*

## KLEINMAN'S[15] QUESTIONS

- What do you call your problem? What name do you give it?

- What do you think has caused it?

- Why did it start when it did?

- What does your sickness do to your body? How does it work inside you?

- How severe is it? Will it get better soon or take longer?

- What do you fear most about your sickness?

- What are the chief problems your sickness has caused for you (personally, family, work, etc.)?

- What kind of treatment do you think you should receive? What are the most important results you hope to receive from the treatment?

Next take some time to review the video units (thinkculturalhealth.hhs.gov/resources/videos) and explore the remainder of the site. *Journal about your impressions and how your beliefs and values have been changed because of your learning and review.* Be prepared to discuss further with your peers key takeaways and impacting perspectives. You may be asked to discuss and share some of the activities you have completed and learning gleaned during your in-class discussion sessions. You will find many of the resources helpful to refer to once again, as you transition from classroom to clinical realms.

Several of the Special Interest and Catalyst Groups within the APTA Academy of Leadership & Innovation provide educational programming at national conferences and offer other resources and networking opportunities related to a wide variety of topics, including global health initiatives, health disparities, social responsibility, cultural competence, disability issues, service-learning, justice, equity and inclusion, pro bono clinics, and ethical practice in resource-limited settings domestically and internationally.[37]

Musolino et al.[38,39] demonstrated that the utilization of interprofessional educational modules for cultural competence and mutual respect produced measurable gains in cultural competence for interprofessional health professions students enrolled in the modules at the University of Utah. The participating students were from physical therapy, medicine, pharmacy, and nursing disciplines. The students enrolled in the modules demonstrated significant progression on comparative postscores in the cultural constructs of attitudes, knowledge, and skills, but not in encounters and desires. Researchers recommend that efforts be made to introduce more culturally competent interactive practice opportunities in health care settings and the cultural competence and mutual respect interprofessional education modules to reduce health care disparities and medical errors for clinicians working in diverse communities.

Another study, by Musolino and Feehan,[40] demonstrated that service-learning opportunities also promoted the development of cultural competence in students who worked in community-based facilities for school-aged children from 7 to 13 years old from Hispanic migrant farm worker families and low-income Black communities in Southwest Florida. In addition, 31% of the participating children were deaf or hard of hearing or had physical and/or mental disabilities. The physical therapy students were involved in teams whose goals were to increase awareness of the physical therapy profession in diverse communities. HCP students developed and implemented interactive learning opportunities to educate the school children about the various aspects of the profession of physical therapy. The physical therapy student projects enhanced their personal development as self-reflective and more culturally aware physical therapy professionals. In addition, the physical therapy students were recognized with the National Student Assembly award, Student Outreach for Cultural Diversity Awareness. There are also many books, research articles, and media resources describing the personal experiences of individuals living with disabilities,[2–43] with a representative sample provided at the end of this chapter to explore.

Cultural humility incorporates a lifelong commitment to self-evaluation and self-critique, to redressing the power imbalances in the patient–HCP dynamic, and to developing mutually beneficial and nonpaternalistic clinical and advocacy partnerships with communities on behalf of individuals and defined populations.[44] Cultural humility addresses matters of social injustice and entails the desire to learn from others about their culture and cultural experiences, in a mutually respectful manner.[44–47] Bangs et al.[48] share that cultural competence and cultural humility require specificity for the HCP for each individual patient/client, and require ongoing and lifelong processes that emphasize HCP-PPI focused on collaborative decision-making in a reciprocally respectful manner. Cultural safety refers to acknowledging the barriers to clinical effectiveness arising from the inherent power imbalance between provider and patient.[49] Campinha-Bacote[45] provides clarity for HCPs for the various constructs along the cultural competence continuum and describes the "Process of Cultural Competemility" in the delivery of health care. Campina-Bacote[46,47] shares that cultural competence and culture humility are harmonious terms and conjoined them, coining the term "cultural competemility." The term is defined as "as the synergistic process between cultural humility and cultural competence in which cultural humility permeates each of the five components of cultural competence: cultural awareness, cultural knowledge, cultural skill, cultural desire, and cultural encounters."[46(p 5)] The amalgamation has high likelihood in accelerating the need for practical application either alongside or within patient-centered care models for HCPs treating patients across the many complexities of cultural identity.[45–47] More practically, Campinha-Bacote[45] implores HCPs to address health inequities by asking themselves "Have I ASKED myself the right questions?" in their journey toward Cultural Competemility. Reflect on the ASKED[45] pneumonic queries as you continue your HCP professional development:

# ASKED[45]

- **Awareness:** Am I aware of my prejudices and biases, as well as the presence of racism and other "isms?"
- **Skill:** Do I know how to conduct a culturally specific history, physical, mental health, medication and spiritual assessment in a culturally sensitive manner?
- **Knowledge:** Do I have knowledge regarding different cultures' worldview, the field of biocultural ecology, and the importance of addressing social determinants of health?
- **Encounters:** Do I have sacred and unremitting encounters with people from cultures different from mine and am I committed to resolving cross-cultural conflicts?
- **Desire:** Do I really "want to" engage in the process of competemility?

# CONCLUSION

According to the World Health Organization (WHO), more than 16% of the world population has a disability, and children with disabilities face even higher levels of discrimination than their peers without disabilities.[50] Persons with disabilities are further challenged to have a sense of belonging that includes four interactive components: "interacting with similar persons, navigating norms and expectations, negotiating meaningful roles, and engaging in social relationships."[50] We will further discuss matters of disabilities upcoming in Chapters 17 and 18 specifically.

Clinical practice today offers HCPs many challenges and opportunities. **Ethnocentrism**, the belief that one's own culture is the best, will be challenged, and HCPs need to continue to expand their thinking to become tolerant of differences and ambiguity while civilly addressing matters of social injustice. Researchers are challenged to develop the best culturally appropriate intervention programs in the areas of health, education, and worker productivity while addressing ways to reduce stressors related to HCP intercultural interactions. Yet combining experience with current best practices offers many guidelines, tools, and queries to continue your professional development on your journey along the cultural competence continuum. This chapter has made you more aware, and enhanced your knowledge and skills, yet you need to have more clinical encounters to increase your competence along with the desire to know more to further address your, and society's, need for greater *cultural competemility*.

Basic information regarding the benefits and pitfalls of intercultural interactions will continue to be widely discussed, just as preventive health behaviors are discussed today.[11] Opportunities will abound as discussions regarding tolerance, understanding, and mutual enrichment evolve and are disseminated. Women, persons of color, and those who identify differently will continue to have increasing choices in their lives, and people will analyze the role that culture and cultural differences play in their lives and in the policies of their societies, especially with health care policy. If HCPs put time and effort into understanding cultural influences on their own behavior and the behavior of others, they will no doubt enjoy the challenges, enrichment, and the stimulation that intercultural interactions can bring.[11]

If we adopt the quantum physics paradigm regarding the primacy of relationships and their fuzziness, we have a new model to assist us in appreciating and valuing our diversity. With our new awareness of, and appreciation for, our relationships with one another, we can introduce unconditional compassion, or love, into our organizations. According to Wheatley,[5] Chopra,[51] and many very wise people from the beginning of time, love in the broadest sense is the most potent source of power that we have available to us. Love, including respect and caring, is most thwarted when we emphasize how different we are from one another. Knowledge and sensitivity to cultural differences will facilitate our therapeutic presence and our sense of oneness with those fellow human beings who are our patients, clients, their families and caregivers, and our health care colleagues. Finally, a few guided exercises follow to help you on your way to greater self-awareness and cultural sensitivity and cultural humility today! Before embarking on the meaningful chapter exercises to enhance your cultural capacities, please take a moment to reflect on the poignancy of the words imparted by MLK and consider how you, as a HCP, are able to address this matter of justice for society:

*Of all the forms of inequality, injustice in health care is the most shocking and inhumane.*

—Dr. Martin Luther King Jr.

# REFERENCES

1.  Mitha K, Sayeed SA, Lopez M. Resiliency, stress, and culture shock: findings from a global health service partnership educator cohort. *Ann Glob Health*. 2021;87(1):120.
2.  Current Population Reports Estimates. Washington, DC: *US Census Bureau*;2022. Available: https://www.census.gov/quickfacts/fact/table/US/RHI125221 Accessed March 5, 2023.
3.  Bud PS, Jacobson TL. *Navigating Special Education: The Power of Building Positive Parent-Educator Partnerships*. Thorofare, NY: Slack; 2023.
4.  Zhang C, Bennett T. Facilitating the meaningful participation of culturally and linguistically diverse families in the IFSP and IEP Process. *Focus on Autism and Other Developmental Disabilities*. 2003;18(1):51–59.
5.  Wheatley MJ. *Leadership and the New Science: Discovering Order in a Chaotic World*, 3rd ed. San Francisco, CA: Berrett-Koehler Publishers; 2011.
6.  *Individuals With Disabilities Education Improvement Act* Amendments of 2004 (Pub Law No. 108–446, Federal Register Vol 71, No 156).
7.  Butler M, McCreedy E, Schwer N, Burgess D, Call K, Przedworski J, Rosser S, Larson S, Allen M, Fu S, Kane RL. *Improving Cultural Competence to Reduce Health Disparities*. Rockville, MD): Agency for Healthcare Research and Quality (US); 2016 Mar. Report No.: 16-EHC006-EF. PMID: 27148614.

8. Majda A, Bodys-Cupak IE, Zalewska-Puchała J, Barzykowski K. Cultural competence and cultural intelligence of healthcare professionals providing emergency medical services. *Int J Environ Res Public Health.* 2021;18(21):11547.

9. Spradley J, McDurdy D, Shandy D. *Conformity and Conflict: Readings in Cultural Anthropology,* 15th ed. New York, NY: Pearson Education; 2015.

10. Mead M. Cultural problems and technical change in United Nations Educations Scientific and Cultural Organization, Paris. In: Saunders L, ed. *Cultural Differences and Medical Care.* New York, NY: Russell Sage Foundation; 1954:247–248.

11. Brislin RW. *Understanding Culture's Influence on Behavior,* 2nd ed. Independence, KY: Cengage Learning; 2000.

12. Raja SN, Carr DB, Cohen M, Finnerup NB, Flor H, Gibson S, Keefe FJ, Mogil JS, Ringkamp M, Sluka KA, Song XJ, Stevens B, Sullivan MD, Tutelman PR, Ushida T, Vader K. The revised International Association for the Study of Pain definition of pain: concepts, challenges, and compromises. *Pain.* 2020;161(9):1976–1982.

13. McMaster HS, LeardMann CA, Speigle S, Dillman DA; Millennium Cohort Family Study Team. An experimental comparison of web-push vs. paper-only survey procedures for conducting an in-depth health survey of military spouses. *BMC Med Res Methodol.* 2017; 17(1):73.

14. Sue S, Zane N, Nagayama Hall GC, Berger LK. The case for cultural competency in psychotherapeutic interventions. *Annu Rev Psychol.* 2009;60:525–548.

15. Kleinman A. Concepts and a model for the comparison of medical systems as cultural systems. *Soc Sci Med.* 1978;12(2B):85–93.

16. DeSantis L. Health care orientations of Cuban and Haitian immigrant mothers: implications for health care professionals. *Med Anthropol.* 1989;12(1):69–89.

17. Harwood A. *Ethnicity and Medical Care.* Cambridge, MA: Harvard University Press; 1982.

18. Coard SI, Kiang L, Martin Romero MY, Gonzalez LM, Stein GL. Talking through the tough: identifying facilitating factors to preparation for bias and racial–ethnic discrimination conversations among families from minoritized ethnic–racial groups. *Family Process.* 2023; 00:1–16.

19. Saunders L. *Cultural Differences and Medical Care.* New York, NY: Russell Sage Foundation; 1954.

20. Shilling B, Branan E. *Cross-Cultural Counseling: A Guide for Nutrition and Health Counselors.* Washington, DC: US Department of Agriculture and United States Department of Health and Human Services; 1989.

21. Ting-Toomey S. Intercultural conflicts: a face-negotiation theory. In: Kim Y, Gudykunst W, eds. *Theories in Intercultural Communication.* Newbury Park, CA: Sage; 1988:213–238.

22. Graham M, Miller D. *The 1995 Annual: Volume 1, Training.* San Diego, CA: Pfeiffer and Co; 1995.

23. Tirandis HC. In: Graham M, Miller D, Eds. *The 1995 Annual: Volume 1, Training.* San Diego, CA: Pfeiffer and Co; 1995.

24. Turner H. Interacting successfully with people from other cultures. In: Brislin RW, ed. *Understanding Culture's Influence on Behavior.* Fort Worth, TX: Harcourt Brace Jovanovich; 1993:325.

25. Hagland MM, Sabatino F, Sherer JL. New waves. Hospitals struggle to meet the challenge of multiculturalism now—and in the next generation. *Hospital.* 1993;67(10):22–25, 28–31.

26. Belenky M, Clinchy B, Goldberg N, Tarul J. *Women's Ways of Knowing: The Development of Self, Voice, and Mind.* New York, NY: Basic Books; 1997.

27. Wiesman R, Koester J, eds. *Intercultural Communication Competence.* Newbury Park, CA: Sage; 1993.

28. Hall ET, Hall MR. *The Dance of Life: The Other Dimension of Time.* Sioux City, IA: Anchor Publications; 1984.

29. US Department of Health & Human Services, Office of Minority Health, *National Standards for Culturally and Linguistically Appropriate Services in Health and Health Care (National CLAS Standards),* Think cultural health. Available: https://think-culturalhealth.hhs.gov/clas/standards Accessed April 5, 2023.

30. United States Census Bureau. *What Languages Do We Speak in the United States.* Available: https://www.census.gov/library/stories/2022/12/languages-we-speak-in-united-states.html Accessed March 5, 2023.

31. Juckett G, Unger K. Appropriate use of medical interpreters. *Am Fam Physician.* 2014 Oct 1;90(7):476–480. PMID: 25369625.

32. Boylen S, Cherian S, Gill FJ, Leslie GD, Wilson S. Impact of professional interpreters on outcomes for hospitalized children from migrant and refugee families with limited English proficiency: a systematic review. *JBI Evid Synth.* 2020 Jul;18(7):1360–1388.

33. Brown CM, Bland S, Saif N. Effective communication with refugees and immigrants. *Prim Care.* 2021;48(1):23–34.

34. Koenig HG, McCullough ME, Larson DB. *Handbook of Religion and Health.* 2nd ed. New York, NY: Oxford University Press; 2012.

35. Saguil A, Phelps K. The spiritual assessment. *Am Fam Physician.* 2012;86(6):546–550.

36. Snapp M, Hare L. The role of spiritual care and healing in health management. *Adv Mind Body Med.* 2021;35(1):4–8.

37. American Physical Therapy Association. Academy of Leadership & Innovation (Health Policy & Administration—The Catalyst), *Special Interest & Catalyst Groups.* www.aptahpa.org. Accessed April 5, 2023.

38. Musolino GM, Torres Burkhalter S, Crookston B, Harris RM, Chase-Cantarini S, Babitz M. Understanding and eliminating disparities in health care: development and assessment of cultural competence for interdisciplinary health professional at the University of Utah: a 3-year investigation. *J Phys Ther Educ.* 2010:24(1):25–36.

39. Musolino GM, Babitz M, Burkhalter ST, et al. Mutual respect in healthcare: assessing cultural competence for the University of Utah Interdisciplinary Health Sciences. *J Allied Health.* 2009;38(2):e54–e62.

40. Musolino GM, Feehan P. Enhancing diversity through mentorship: the nurturing potential of service learning. *J Phys Ther Educ.* 2004;18(1):29–42.

41. Galanti GA. *Caring for Patients From Different Cultures,* 5th ed. Philadelphia, PA: University of Pennsylvania Press; 2015.

42. Campinha-Bacote J. Cultural desire: the key to unlocking cultural competence. *J Nurs Educ.* 2003;42(6):239–240.

43. Campinha-Bacote J. The process of cultural competence in the delivery of healthcare services. In Douglas M, Pacquiao D, eds. Core Curriculum in Transcultural Nursing and Health Care. *J of Transcultural Nursing.* 2010;21 Suppl 1:119S–127S.

44. Tervalon M, Murray-Garcia J. Cultural humility versus cultural competence: a critical distinction in defining physician training outcomes in multicultural education. *J Health Care Poor & Underserved.* 1998;9(2):17–25.

45. Campinha-Bacote J. A path to antiracism through the lens of cultural humility. *J Transcult Nurs.* 2021;32(2):191.

46. Campinha-Bacote J. Cultural competemility: a paradigm shift in the cultural competence versus cultural humility debate—part I. *OJIN: The Online Journal of Issues in Nursing.* 2018;24(1).

47. Ballard T, Campinha-Bacote J. Cultural Competemility Training and Use of a Standardized Assessment Tool in Reducing Misdiagnosis of Black Patients with Schizophrenia Spectrum Disorders and Psychotic Disorders. *J Am Psychiatr Nurses Assoc.* 2024 Nov 26:10783903241269046. doi: 10.1177/10783903241269046. Epub ahead of print. PMID: 39600043

48. Bangs D, Hayward LM, Donlan P. Cultural competence and cultural humility: a dialogue on adopting a multimodal approach in physical therapist education. *J Phys Ther Educ.* 2022; 36(2):128–132.

49. Laverty M, McDermott DR, Calma T. Embedding cultural safety in Australia's main health care standards. *Med J Aust.* 2017;207(1):15–16.

50. Long T. Inclusion, participation, belonging = surviving, thriving, flourishing. *Ped Phys Ther.* 2024;36(3): 298–306.

51. Chopra D. *The Path to Love.* New York, NY: Random House; 1998.

52. Trees DW, Smith JM, Hockert S. Innovative mobility strategies for the patient with ICU-acquired weakness: a case report. *Phys Ther.* 2013;93(2):237–247.

# SUGGESTED READINGS

Albom M. *Tuesdays With Morrie.* New York, NY: Doubleday; 1997. A journalist interviews an older man who had been his college professor; shares his experiences living with and dying from amyotropic lateral sclerosis (ALS).

Ambrose SE. *Band of Brothers: E Company, 506th Regiment, 101st Airborne from Normandy to Hitler's Eagle's Nest,* 2nd ed. New York, NY: Simon & Schuster; 2001. Follows Easy Company of the US Army 101st Airborne Division's mission in World War II Europe, from Operation Overload through VJ Day, exploring the trials of service and resulting PTSD and disabilities.

Beck M. *Expecting Adam: A True Story of Birth, Rebirth, and Everyday Magic.* New York, NY: Times Books; 1999. A PhD candidate shares her pregnancy and life as mother of a child with Down syndrome.

Campbell O. *Women in White Coats: How the First Women Doctors Changed the World of Medicine.* Toronto, Ontario, Canada: Park Row Books; 2021.

Cahalan S. *Brain on Fire: My Month of Madness.* New York, NY; Simon and Schuster; 2012. The author describes her truly terrifying bout with and eventual recovery from encephalitis.

Cohen RM. *Blindsided: Lifting a Life Above Illness.* New York, NY; HarperCollins; 2005. Richard is a television writer who develops multiple sclerosis, affecting his vision and balance, followed by a diagnosis of cancer.

Crimmins CE. *Where Is the Mango Princess? A Journey Back From Brain Injury.* New York, NY; Vintage Books; 2001. Written by a woman whose husband sustains a severe traumatic brain injury (TBI) in a boating accident; follows his acute rehabilitation and living with the residual deficits.

Coughlin R. *Grieving: A Love Story.* New York, NY; Random House; 1993. A widow tells the story of her husband's death from cancer.

Fox, Michael J. *No Time Like the Future: An Optimist Considers Mortality.* New York, NY: Flatiron Books; 2021. Advocate and actor shares personal stories and observations about illness and health, aging, the strength of family and friends, and how our perceptions about time affect the way we approach mortality; while considering the drama of medical madness associated with confronting early onset Parkinson's Disease.

Galli R. *Rescuing Jeffrey.* Chapel Hill, NC: Algonquin Books; 2000. A father's story of his high school son's spinal cord injury (SCI) due to a diving accident.

Gerlach H. *Happily Ever After: My Journey with Guillain-Barré Syndrome and How I Got My Life Back.* Bloomington, IN: Trafford Publishing; 2012. Just 3 weeks after giving birth, young Holly notices her fingertips are numb and her legs weak. She was paralyzed, admitted to the ICU, and placed on a ventilator; she could not speak, move, or hold her daughter. Was her life over? Explores her intensive physiotherapy and recovery.

Graboys T. *Life in the Balance: A Physician's Memoir of Life, Love, and Loss with Parkinson's Disease and Dementia.* New York, NY: Union Square Press; 2008. Dr. Graboys, a successful cardiologist, musician, athlete, husband, and father affected by Parkinson's disease and Lewy body disorder, describes his descent into immobility and dementia.

Grealey L. *Autobiography of a Face.* Boston, MA: Houghton Mifflin; 1994. After undergoing 5 years of treatment for cancer, a woman is left with facial disfigurement and subsequent reconstructive surgeries.

Halpin B. *It Takes a Worried Man: A Memoir.* Manhattan Beach, CA: Open Road Distribution; 2015. One father's raw account of his experiences after his young wife is diagnosed with breast cancer.

Hartsell EB. *Abled in a Disabled World.* Haymarket, VA: Curry Brothers Marketing and Publishing Group; 2020.

Heffernan DD. *An Arrow Through the Heart: One Woman's Story of Life, Love, and Surviving a Near-Fatal Heart Attack.* New York, NY: Free Press; 2002.

Hornbacher M. *Wasted: A Memoir of Anorexia and Bulimia*. New York, NY: Harper Perennial; 1998. A young woman with both anorexia and bulimia, further complicated by substance abuse.

Housden M. *Hannah's Gift: Lessons From a Life Fully Lived*. New York, NY: Bantam Books; 2002. A mother tells the story of her three-year old daughter's struggle and death from cancer.

Knapp C. *Drinking: A Love Story*. New York, Bantam Dell Doubleday Publishing, 1996. The author describes her 20-year struggle with alcoholism, rehabilitation, and recovery.

Kyle C, McEwen S, DeFelice J. *American Sniper: The Autobiography of the Most Lethal Sniper in U.S. Military History*. New York, NY; Morrow: Harper Collins Publishers; 2014. Explores the intense life of a US Navy Seal sniper serving in battle and its PTSD effects.

Levine A. *Run Don't Walk: The Curious and Courageous Life Inside Walter Reed Medical Center*. New York, NY: Penguin Publishing Group; 2014. *M\*A\*S\*H* meets *Scrubs* in a sharply observant, darkly funny, and totally unique debut memoir from a physical therapist.

Long T. Inclusion, participation, belonging = surviving, thriving, flourishing. *Ped Phys Ther*. 2024;36(3): 298–306.

Lydon J. *Daughter of the Queen of Sheba: A Memoir*. Boston, MA: Houghton Mifflin; 1997. NPR reporter writes a memoir of growing up with a mentally ill mother and providing her care.

Papadopoulos I, Koulouglioti C, Papadopoulos C, Sgorbissa A. *Transcultural Artificial Intelligence (AI) and Robotics in Health and Social Care*. New York, NY: Elsevier; 2022. Provides HCPs a deeper understanding of the incredible opportunities brought by the emerging field of AI robotics.

Parker S. *Tumbling After: Pedaling Like Crazy After Life Goes Downhill*. New York, NY: Crown Publishers; 2002. A wife copes after her husband sustains a C4 SCI after a bicycle accident.

Purnell LD, Frenkl EA, eds. *Textbook for Transcultural Health Care: A Population Approach: Cultural Competence Concepts in Nursing Care*, 5th ed. New York, NY: Springer; 2020. Discusses individual competences and evidence-based practices as well as international standards, organizational cultural competence, and perspectives on health care in a global context. The individual chapters present selected populations, offering a balance of collectivistic and individualistic cultures.

Redfield Jamison K. *Night Falls Fast: Understanding Suicide*. New York, NY: Knopf Publishing Group; 2000. An internationally acknowledged authority on depression—Dr. Jamison has also known suicide firsthand: after years of struggling with manic-depression, she tried at age 28 to kill herself. A powerful and life-altering book providing critical reading for those wanting to understand the tragic epidemic of suicide.

Redfield Jamison K. *An Unquiet Mind: A Memoir of Moods and Madness*. New York, NY; Alfred A. Knopf, Doubleday Publishing Group; 1997. A renowned psychologist describes mercurial living with bipolar disorder and her support system; explores from both the healer and healed perspectives and related struggles.

Rothenberg L. *Breathing for a Living: A Memoir*. New York, NY; Hyperion Books; 2003. A 19-year-old college student with cystic fibrosis shares her memoir, a moving account that follows through her double lung transplant and rehabilitation.

Schlosser E. *Fast Food Nation: The Dark Side of the All-American Meal*. New York, NY: Mifflin Harcourt Publishing; 2001. Explores the fast-food industry, related cultural perspectives, and the dark side of the industry related to immigration and the modern tale of Upton Sinclair's *The Jungle* (1906), which exposed the poor conditions in the meat-packing industry.

Sheff D. *Beautiful Boy: A Father's Journey Through His Son's Addiction*. Boston, MA; Houghton Mifflin Company; 2008. A father tells the story of his journey through his son's methamphetamine addiction.

Skloot R. *The Immortal Life of Henrietta Lacks*. New York, NY; Crown Publishing, Random House; 2010. Engaging reading about the immortal cellular line of Henrietta Lacks from her cervical cancer cells in 1951, and the many ethical, racial, and class issues that emerged; considers matters of informed consent.

Simon C. *Mad House: Growing Up in the Shadow of Mentally Ill Siblings*. New York, NY: Penguin; 1998. Part memoir, part practical guide, a reporter describes growing up with two schizophrenic siblings.

Suskind R. *A Hope in the Unseen: An American Odyssey From the Inner City to the Ivy League*. New York, NY: Broadway Books, Random House; 1999. Follows Cedric Jennings, a young black teen from the disadvantaged Southside DC district with a single mother, as he traverses high school to the Ivy League and emerges a man.

Suskind R. *Life, Animated: A Story of Sidekicks, Heroes, and Autism*. Glendale, CA: Kingswell; 2014. Follows the life of the author's son, Owen Suskind, afflicted with autism, and how Ron and his wife, Cornelia, communicated with Disney characters as a vehicle for enhanced understandings.

Wilde Hawking J. *Traveling to Infinity: My Life with Stephen*. Surrey, UK: Alma Books; 2010. Shared by Hawking's wife, Stephen Hawking's (renowned astrophysicist) courage and determination in the face of a crippling motor neuron disease; relevance of assistive and rehabilitation technologies.

# SUGGESTED VIEWING

*12 Years a Slave*. 20th Century Studios. 2013. A biographical period drama film, adaptation of the 1853 slave memoirs written by Solomon Northup. Born a free New York state African American man, Northup was kidnapped by two conmen in 1841 and sold into slavery and forced to work on plantations for 12 years, before being finally released. This story sheds a heart-wrenching but much needed light on the horrifying condition that African American people sold into slavery faced.

*American Sniper.* Warner Bros. 2014. Story of Navy S.E.A.L. sniper saving countless lives on four tours of duty, yet cannot leave the war behind when returning home.

*Band of Brothers.* HBO. 2001. The story of Easy Company in the U.S. Army 101st Airborne Division and their mission in World War II Europe from Operation Overlord to V-J Day.

*Body and Soul: Dianna & Kathy.* New Day Digital. 2007. Two women with significant disabilities live together and take care of each other so they can live independently; demonstrates the use of assistive technology and a symbiotic culture.

*Darius Goes West: The Roll of His Life.* Indie Film. 2006. A teenager with Duchenne muscular dystrophy goes on a cross-country trip, leaving home for the first time, with his 11 best friends; MTV hosts to find someone to "pimp" his chair.

*Emmanuel's Gift.* First Look Home Entertainment. 2005. Young African man with a congenital deformity advocates for disability rights biking in Africa.

*Fast Food Nation: The Dark Side of the All-American Meal.* 20th Century Fox, 2007. Shedding light on how the fast food industry wields power over our nation, fuels obesity and exploitation of minorities and teenagers.

*Hale.* Fondly known as the Godfather of the Disability movement in Berkeley, California, Hale Zurich is a living legend. Diagnosed with Cerebral Palsy as a child, Zurich went on to study Russian and Math at UC Berkeley in the 1970s. He also helped found Berkeley's groundbreaking Center for Independent Living, which has become a nationwide model. Hale's work has ever since affected everything from ramps to curb cuts, to even the way buildings are built today.

*Hidden Figures.* Twentieth Century Studios. 2016. Addresses issues of racism, sexism, and workplace discrimination about three brilliant African American female scientists and their extraordinary contributions during the space race.

*Including Samuel.* Institute on Disability, University of New Hampshire. 2009. School inclusion issues for a child with cerebral palsy.

*McFarland, USA.* Walt Disney Pictures. 2015. Inspired by a 1987 true story, follows novice runners from a socioeconomically deprived, predominantly Latino high school; considers matters of ethnicity, class, and culture.

*MILK.* Universal Pictures. 2008. The challenges and victories faced by Harvey Mail. Milk became the first openly gay person to be elected as a member of a public office in California. A human rights activist, Milk spent his entire life fighting against the prevalent homophobia in California.

*My Angel My Hero: Dancing with Parkinson's.* 3-Dimensions Films. 2013. Filmed over 6 days, shares the beat of a teenager's life in his fight against Parkinson's disease.

*So Much, So Fast.* Indie Films. 2006. Chronicles a young husband and father's struggles with ALS and his devoted family support.

*Superman: The Christopher Reeve Story.* 2024. Follows Reeves rise to star power as Superman, then tragedy hit with a fatal horse-riding accident (1995) that left him paralyzed from the neck down. He then became an activist for spinal cord injury research, treatments, and disability rights.

*The Collector of Bedford Street.* New Day Digital. 2005. Adult with developmental disabilities lives on his own and struggles with independence.

*The Divide: Confronting Racism in American Healthcare. The Pipeline to Compassionate Care.* The Commonwealth Fund. www.commonwealthfund.org

*The Imitation Game.* StudioCanal. 2014. Follows Turing, genius British mathematician who helped decode German messages during World War II. A beautiful depiction of the science behind Germany's perceived upper hand, it also brings to light the psychological horrors faced by the members of LGBTQIA+ community, especially during those early years.

*The Soldier's Heart.* PBS Frontline. 2005. Explores the psychological impact of combat; Iraq/Afghanistan veterans and PTSD.

*The Theory of Everything.* Working Title Films. 2014. Examines the relationship between Stephen Hawking, famous physicist, and his wife.

*Through Deaf Eyes.* PBS. 2007. Explores the 200-year history of the deaf community in America.

*You're Not You.* Entertainment One. 2015. A classical pianist's journey coping with ALS with the support of her home care assistant.

*Wonder.* Lionsgate. 2017. Follows a boy with Treachers Collins Syndrome trying to fit in.

*Worlds Apart: A Four-Part Series on Cross-Cultural Health Care.* Fanlight Productions. 2003. www.fanlight.com or via YouTube.

# SUGGESTED WEB RESOURCES

## *U.S. Department of Health & Human Resources: Office of Minority Health—Think Cultural Health*

https://thinkculturalhealth.hhs.gov/education/physicians A practical guide to culturally competent care.

https://cccm.thinkculturalhealth.hhs.gov/ Video resources and case guides for e-learning for culturally competent care geared toward medicine and nursing specifically.

https://thinkculturalhealth.hhs.gov/resources/library A resource library of helpful tools, guides, checklists for cultural health care.

https://thinkculturalhealth.hhs.gov/resources/videos Video case studies (pediatrics, surgery, obstetrics and gynecology) about culturally and linguistically appropriate clinical encounters to learn more about applying the National CLAS Standards in daily health care.

https://thinkculturalhealth.hhs.gov/resources/presentations Collection of presentations on various cultural and linguistically appropriate services and the National CLAS Standards.

## Quality Interactions

www.qualityinteractions.com Website filled with resources and accredited training activities to improve health equity. Quality Interactions' mission is to improve health equity and reduce costly inequities in health care systems through accredited cultural competency, quality care for those with limited English proficiency, cross-cultural communication, implicit bias training, etc. Health professionals' education courses to address cross-cultural skills to reduce health disparities and improve health care for all patients (cost-associated continuing education modules).

## Georgetown University National Center for Cultural Competence (NCCC)

https://nccc.georgetown.edu/ Website designed to increase the capacity of health care and mental health care programs to design, implement, and evaluate culturally and linguistically competent service delivery systems to address growing diversity, persistent disparities, and to promote health and mental health equity. Includes a plethora of self-assessment instruments and resources.

## The Cross-Cultural Health Care Program

www.xculture.org Serves to bridge communities and health care institutions to advance access to quality health care that is culturally and linguistically appropriate. Provides resources (cost-associated) and training for individuals and institutions with the goal of systems change.

## EthnoMed

http://ethnomed.org EthnoMed is Harborview Medical Center's ethnic medicine website containing medical and cultural information about immigrant and refugee groups. Information is specific to groups in the Seattle area, but much of the cultural and health information is of interest and applicable in other geographic areas. EthnoMed is a joint program of the University of Washington Health Sciences Libraries and Harborview Medical Center. The objective of the website is to make information about culture, language, health, illness, and community resources directly accessible to health care providers who see patients from different ethnic groups. EthnoMed was designed to be used in clinics by care providers in the few minutes before seeing a patient in clinic. For instance, before seeing a Cambodian patient with asthma, a provider might access the website to learn how the concept of asthma is translated and about common cultural and interpretive issues in the Cambodian community that might complicate asthma management. A practitioner could also download a patient education pamphlet in Khmer (Cambodian language) to give to the patient.

## Health Begins—Upstream Movement

https://healthbegins.org/ Designed to address the relationship between health and health care today, addressing social determinants of health through a variety of platforms and services.

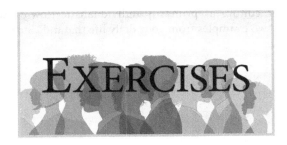

# EXERCISE 1: CULTURE SHOCK ACTIVITY

1.  Have you personally experienced culture shock? Write a brief description of what you experienced. What did you see, hear, and feel? What was the context of the situation that shocked you?

2.  Ask someone you know and admire whether they have ever experienced culture shock. Write a brief description of what they experienced.

3.  List similarities and differences in what you and your colleague or friend described.

4.  What are the implications of culture shock for individuals of non-North American cultures when they immigrate to your state? What provisions does your state make for immigrants requiring government support?

# EXERCISE 2: WHAT IS YOUR CULTURE/ETHNICITY?

1. Would you describe your culture as primarily individualistic (low-context) or primarily collectivistic (high-context)? Write out two examples from your daily life that indicate which context best describes your perception of your culture.

   a.

   b.

2. Describe the culture of someone you know whose culture is different from yours. Write out two examples from your observations of that person that validate your perception of that individual's culture as high or low context.

   a.

   b.

3. What did you learn from this activity? What did you take for granted before that has become more apparent through this activity?

4. What implications does this have for your clinical practice? What do you expect will be the nature of your patients' cultural backgrounds?

# EXERCISE 3: CLINICAL DILEMMA

1. You are a therapist from an Anglo-European background working in an outpatient clinic that serves a primarily Hispanic patient population. You notice that your clients are frequently late for their appointments. Based on your knowledge of high- and low-context cultural differences, what might be the possible reasons for the lateness?

2. What strategies can you use to address these differences?

   a. What is the worst thing you can do? Why?

   b. What is the wisest thing you can do? Why?

3. What challenges and opportunities are presented to you personally in this clinical dilemma?

# EXERCISE 4: PHYLLIS TRAVELS TO THE LONG-TERM ACUTE CARE CENTER (LTAC)[52]

The patient you are about to view is Phyllis, a 73-year-old woman with necrotizing, multilobar pneumonia; septic shock; and atrial fibrillation, with resulting profound muscle weakness due to the prolonged bed rest. She required 5 days of vasopressors, a tracheostomy (respiratory failure), and percutaneous endoscopic gastrostomy. She was ventilator dependent initially. Phyllis was in the ICU for a total of 6 weeks and then was able to move on to acute, long-term rehabilitation care. Following weeks of long-term acute care rehabilitation center therapies, she went home. Phyllis was in the long-term acute care hospital for a total of 10 weeks from her date of admission to final discharge.

View the video[52] showing Phyllis as she travels through the health care system from the ICU to acute, long-term care and outpatient rehabilitation services (https://academic.oup.com/ptj/article/93/2/237/2735537?login=true) or via YouTube (www.youtube.com/watch?v=rAEjjcjob-Y). The video is also available on the Hopkins website reviewed earlier in the chapter, along with other ICU and Covid-related patient videos (www.hopkinsmedicine.org/pulmonary/research/outcomes-after-critical-illness/oacis-videos-news). The video of Phyllis is provided with permission for educational instruction purposes by Darin Trees, PT, DPT, CWS with Solara Rehabilitation Hospital, LTAC, Conroe, TX.[52]

Reflect on your impressions:

1. How was the HCP communication adjusted in the varying settings Phyllis went through in her recovery?

2. How were her family members supportive in the process?

3. What surprised you?

4. What did you consider about cultural context and pace in each setting?

5. What did you find perplexing, confounding, or impressive?

Here is another YouTube link to a short video that you might also find informative:

*Holly Gerlach's Journey: From Guillain-Barré Syndrome to Happily Ever After* www.youtube.com/watch?v=VwQzjj9aQnQ (extended version www.youtube.com/watch?v=huN8iIWXNCs).

# EXERCISE 5: REFLECTIONS AND RUMINATIONS FOLLOWING MULTIMEDIA READING/VIEWING

Choose one book and/or multimedia resource to review from the additional resources provided at the end of the chapter.

1.  What did you learn about the situation described?

2.  What did you learn that you were not previously aware of regarding the condition?

3.  How did you feel after reading/viewing the book/media resource? Remember that feelings are expressed in one word.

4.  What would you like to share with your classmates as a result of reading/viewing this book/media resource?

5.  How will what you learned from this book/media resource impact your interactions with individuals and their families in your future practice as a HCP?

6.  What is one thing you will change in your approach to patient care as a result of the learning in this resource?

# 14

# HEALING ATTITUDES

## THE HELPING INTERVIEW

*Gina Maria Musolino and Carol M. Davis*

## OBJECTIVES

*The learner should be able to*:

- Value the importance of effective communication in the initial stages of the therapeutic relationship with the patient/client.
- Differentiate the vital characteristics to conduct a helping interview.
- Effectively demonstrate the essential skills of the helping interview for healing.
- Explain key points necessary for a successful interview for people of all ages.
- Portray the qualities of a helpful interviewer through adaptive communication abilities by demonstrating empathy, compassion, mindfulness, and emotional intelligence.
- Develop and practice one's interviewing skills.
- Adapt verbal and nonverbal communication with patient–practitioner interactions (PPIs).
- Apply the skills of peer and self-assessment for professional formation of helping interviews, working toward reflective, mindful practice.
- Seek to appreciate the impact of inclusive communication skills, social determinants of health, and diverse influences during the helping interview process.
- Recognize the need to integrate the social determinants of health in the interview process along with the impact on health.

## ARTFUL PATIENT—PRACTITIONER INTERACTIONS

This chapter focuses on another specific application of communication skills: the art of establishing a relationship with our patients and gleaning from them the information we need to be of most help. First impressions often count, and the importance of obtaining the patient's trust from the outset of our interaction together is invaluable to the healing process. Interviewing is much more than obtaining a patient history. The interview serves as the cornerstone

DOI: 10.4324/9781003525554-14

for the structure of care we give. Patients come to us worried and often in pain. They feel vulnerable and in need of our help and understanding. They want, often desperately, to put this problem behind them and to get on with their lives, and they know they cannot do it themselves. They come to us hoping that we will listen carefully, that we will know something about their problem, and that we will be able to help alleviate their worries. Patients sincerely want to trust that they have made a wise decision in coming to us. Not only do they want physical and psychological comfort, but they also want another human being to resonate with their distress.[1] All of this emotion, in varying degrees of intensity, depending on the patient and the problem, is presented to us upon our initial contact with the patient. However, most people will utilize maximum coping skills, and few will fully reveal the extent of their feelings about their problem.

Most adults will convey varying degrees of ability to remain in control in an environment that appears at best strange and at worst hostile. As heath care professionals (HCPs), the burden is on us to recognize that the patient feels at a distinct disadvantage and is in an unfamiliar environment and an altered situation. HCPs must reassure and support even those who convey a remarkable sense of confidence and comfort. During the interview process, if one utilizes an insensitive approach, this often will lead to the patient's/client's increased distress, possibly wielding a lasting impact on their ability to adjust and adapt. The insensitive encounter with the HCP may potentially lead to resentment and an increased litigation risk, as initially discussed in Chapter 4. HCPs may find these interactions stressful, and in the absence of effective training and sufficient practice, one may adopt inappropriate ways of patient–practitioner interaction (PPI) and coping with the likely emotional downfall.[2] At the initial patient/client encounter (which may also include support network persons, significant others, and/or family members), interest, genuineness, acceptance, and unconditional positive regard are critical to establishing a healing relationship with the HCP for the most effective PPI. As we have said many times before, the nature of the relationship we have with our patients is critical to the helping and healing process. Encapsulating the emphasis of the healing attitude with a HCP's helping interview is the wisdom imparted by one considered to be the Father of Modern Medicine:

> *It is much more important to know what sort of patient has a disease than what sort of disease a patient has.* —William Osler

# EMPATHY, COMPASSION, EMOTIONAL INTELLIGENCE, AND MINDFUL COMMUNICATION

Empathy remains a core element of any PPI. Empathy is an understanding of what another person is going through; that is, feeling for someone. Being empathic ensures that a HCP is attentive to the emotions of another—their patients/clients. Utilizing empathic interpersonal communication enhances patient satisfaction and therapeutic alliances with your patients. With specific practice, empathy skills, which establish true rapport and trust, can be improved upon and empathic behaviors successfully trained.[3]

The word *compassion* derives from Latin and means "to suffer together." In a therapeutic relationship, compassion requires a HCP to be responsive to the suffering of another, specifically your patients/clients, to help prevent and relieve their suffering. Compassion can only arise from self-reflection and knowing oneself, as we have discussed in Chapter 1 and Chapter 10. Compassion encompasses expressing concern for the physical and emotional or mental pain that results from disease or injury and the associated discomforts a person experiences. Compassion is not only an emotional connection but also a motivator in shared humanity. Compassion motivates us to relieve the pain and suffering of others. Compassion occurs when empathy is accompanied by the desire to be helpful.

For example, in day-to-day life a compassionate act might be to give up a more accessible seat to someone with a disability or someone who is elderly. As we discussed in Chapter 11, servant leaders practice compassion daily. Compassion leads to enhanced psychological well-being for all. Compassionate HCPs speak with kindness, listen carefully without judgments, encourage, and are happy for another's success. Compassionate HCPs apologize when they have made mistakes, accept others for who they are, and forgive others for making mistakes.

Compassionate HCPs must self-monitor for signs and symptoms of compassion fatigue, in themselves and colleagues, as discussed in Chapter 5, and seek self-care and/or referrals if needed. Compassionate HCPs are respectful, altruistic, express gratitude and appreciation, and show respect for others. When you are compassionate you are mindful of people's thoughts, emotions, and experiences, which leads to enhanced emotional intelligence (EI).

Furthermore, one must employ a degree of emotional intelligence to effectively conduct a helping interview. EI is described simply as the "ability to first recognize and understand emotions in yourself and others, along with your ability to use this awareness to effectively manage your behavior and relationships."[4] EI is not just about identifying or acting on a single emotion, but also understanding the range of emotions in yourself and others and then using that information to navigate relationships. EI is even more important today in a world that continues to evolve in recognition of justice and in becoming ever more cognizant of diversity, equity, and inclusion, as discussed in Chapter 7. You will personally reap rewards by enhancing your performance and supporting your well-being, through EI development. EI assists you in the ability to enhance your networks and foster meaningful relationships with others, and most importantly your patients and clients.

EI entails the acute awareness of your own emotions and triggers to manage your emotional responses in positive ways. Additionally, EI includes a social element, which pertains to building your social awareness to understand what's going on around you and how others may react, and then using that insight to build relationships. EI can change over time, so you must constantly be aware, and practicing this skill, to achieve your patient and career goals. EI consists of four quadrants: intelligence, self-awareness, self-management, and social awareness.

Emotions are complex and consist of a broad array of potential reactions. While you don't need to change who you are, or your emotions themselves, you do need to be aware of how you can satisfactorily manage your emotions to have more joy in your life and career. Getting your emotions in "flow" is a positive psychology method to practice in an activity you do well so that you can capitalize on your performance to support your well-being. Finding your flow helps to recharge your energy and build resilience, while disrupting negative thoughts allows you to stay in flow. You must also recognize triggers and find ways to defuse yourself so that emotions do not explode, implode, or get in the way of healthy, productive relationships.

- What are your flow activities?
- What activities challenge and stretch you in a positive way?
- What makes you feel so engaged that time can pass without you even noticing?
- What activating events serve as negative triggers?
- What emotions tend to hijack your ability to respond?
- What are the consequences of your reaction and/or responses?
- How can you disrupt the negative triggers and replace them with more useful beliefs to help you achieve a better result/outcome?
- What, then, will be the effective outcome or improved result?

Learning to shift your perspective will allow you to regain your flow, and you will not only be surprised at how easily you can employ these methods, but you will also be stronger and more capable in your abilities. You will have a sense of accomplishment and realize that it feels much better to overcome negative triggers than the ridiculous, useless energy it took to have a negative reaction. Continue to practice saying "Yes, and..." rather than "Yes, but..." Consider the "What ifs?" not the "What nots." These efforts provide opportunities for communicating differences of ideas and thoughts, while moving toward more productive, creative options rather than stifling the potentials.

With our patients we can also deploy efforts to connect with more perspective by asking:

- Tell me more about where you are coming from.
- I really want to understand your perspective on this; what am I missing?

These queries benefit the HCP by homing in on the potential solutions and building stronger relationships as the other person feels heard and understood. Certainly, everyone wants to be heard, acknowledged, and understood. Listen intently and strive to become more authentically adaptable with your PPI.

Mindfulness is that state of being actively present in the moment, without rushing to judgment or interpretation. Mindfulness, compassion, empathy, and emotional intelligence are critical elements for interactions with others, and in terms of navigating our own range of emotions, and all need to be deployed for effective, helpful interviewing.[4]

Empathy leads to feelings of awareness and understanding toward others' emotions that are being experienced. Compassion is that emotional response with the desire to help. Mindfulness, empathy, compassion, and emotional intelligence are needed to effectively communicate with your patients and colleagues in health care. According to Barrett-Lennard, broadly speaking, empathic communication includes the following: "(i) an inner process of listening, reasoning, and understanding, (ii) the communication of this awareness by the empathizing person, and (iii) the perception of being understood by the counterpart."[5] Effective communication with patients and interprofessional colleagues remains critical to effective clinical care. Further solidifying the skills and behaviors needed for PPI, in a systematic review of 52 studies in medical education, researchers identified the following key behaviors as effective in initial interviews to facilitate empathy and compassion:

1. Eye level is parallel with the patients' (e.g., sitting versus standing, elevating the bed, ect.) during the interview

2. Detecting patients' nonverbal cues of emotion

3. Recognizing and responding to opportunities for compassion

4. Nonverbal communication of caring (e.g., eye contact, congruent facial expressions)

5. Verbal statements of acknowledgement, validation, and support

These behaviors were found to improve patient perception of the health care providers' empathy and/or compassion.[6]

While communication is indeed an essential, foundational element for clinical practice, it remains complex. Yes, with practice, HCPs can enhance their PPI communication skills and abilities, but challenges are evident to achieve effective communication with patients; being cognizant of these hurdles will assist in your training progressions. In a qualitative study of patient communication with medical students and experienced clinicians, eight predominant challenges were unequivocally identified: "time constraints and chaotic environments, rapport building, patient characteristics, reluctance, omissions, assumptions, decision-making, and keeping conversations focused."[7] It is very likely that these same challenges will present to you as a developing HCP. However, with dedicated and mindful practice, along with true fidelity for honest peer and self-assessment, your skills and abilities as a compassionate communicator will be enhanced over time.

You might find it interesting that research has demonstrated through functional magnetic resonance imaging[8,9] that when people experience empathy, brain pain centers are activated, and when compassion is experienced, reward pathways are activated. Hence, PPI should emphasize empathic and compassionate communication to address pain and motivate recovery. Unfortunately, despite a plethora of support that better communication results in health care cost savings (ordering unnecessary diagnostics and referrals) and HCPs' well-being, evidence illustrates compassion crises and fatigue in health care today.[10] Let's ensure you do not fall into these mindless traps by staying healthy, addressing and managing HCP stress (see Chapter 5), and becoming efficient and effective in your PPI communications through practice.

Let's carefully examine the overarching dimensions of empathic communications in Table 14.1 to begin to get a sense of the specifics we are striving for in effective PPIs.[3] Do any of these dimensions surprise you? Which dimensions do you anticipate might be challenging for you? Why? Which might come more naturally for you? Why? These dimensions lay the foundation for effective PPI. Now let's further consider HCPs' attitudes and questioning strategies for PPI.

| TABLE 14.1 |
|---|
| **EMPATHY-RELATED COMMUNICATION SKILLS** |
| **Instructions:** For each empathic dimension, complete peer and self-assessment feedback on each dimension and provide the gift of substantive, constructive suggestions for continued improvement for professional formation development. |
| **Empathic Dimensions** |
| **1. Active listening** (reflective, responsive, open) |
| **2. Understanding the situation** (describe, restate, relate) |

TABLE 14.1 (CONTINUED)

## EMPATHY-RELATED COMMUNICATION SKILLS

3. **Understanding the problems** (asks appropriate questions, clarifications, restate, reiterate, revisit)

4. **Understanding feelings** (reflect, clarifications, supportive gestures, nods, leaning in, sensing, attending and responsive to emotions)

5. **Empathic expressions** (responsive understanding patient experiences, reflect concerns, and perspectives, combined with a capacity to communicate this understanding)

6. **Explanations** (of the diagnosis, medications, rehab potential, treatments, etc.)

7. **Shared decision-making** (purposeful collaboration, goal setting, incorporates life)

8. **Communicating hope** (clear expression of capacities without overpromise)

9. **Being competent** (professional, listens with whole self, efficient, capable, instills confidence, knowledgeable)

10. **Verbal expression** (inner conviction, articulate with sensitivity, utilizes appropriate pacing; avoids the use of meaningless words/phrases, e.g., 'um', 'like', appropriate tone, inflection, volume, culturally aware)

11. **Nonverbal expression** (fully present; focused; utilizes matching; not distracted; appropriate eye accessing, not staring; open body posture, e.g., not crossing arms or legs controls own emotions, etc.)

12. **Degree of coherence in the interview** (lack of medical jargon or explanations when utilized; understandable language with use of summarizations, e.g., connection, linking, transitioning; integration of interview elements, systematic approach with logical order and integration with consistent connections; realistic)

**Comments/Suggestions for Improvements:**

_____

_____

Adapted from: Wündrich M, Schwartz C, Feige B, Lemper D, Nissen C, Voderholzer U. Empathy training in medical students - a randomized controlled trial. *Med Teach.* 2017; Oct;39(10):1096-1098.

# HELPFUL ATTITUDE AND SKILLFUL QUESTIONING

Not only is it important to convey a healing attitude for our patients at the outset in the interview, but it is also imperative that the patient feel listened to and understood so that all of the information can surface that will lead to the most adequate and complete description of the problem/s and/or concern/s. Your patient/client will tell you everything you need to know—yet you often must be the one to notice the need, initiate, and make the ask—and this helps to ensure best practice efforts and safer PPI, and opens up the communication for the most effective therapeutic relationship. Thus, pragmatically, effective clinical reasoning and clinical decision-making depend on skillful interviewing, which begins with a healing attitude and proceeds with artful questioning. Let's take a closer look at both.

# THE HEALING ATTITUDE OF THE INTERVIEW

A good interview depends on appropriate attitude, good timing, and artful phrasing.[11] The nature of the questions and the process of the interview session will flow out of the beliefs that the questioner holds about such things as one's self-esteem, the appropriate nature of one's role in healing, and what patients are like as people. Let's take a look at some ideas, beliefs, and attitudes that facilitate a healing interview.

Positive self-esteem helps one assume a stance of "I'm okay and so are you. Neither of us is perfect, but each of us, I choose to believe, is doing the best we can to move forward in this world, and I want to help you get back to the business of life as soon as possible." This attitude fosters a healthy, collegial relationship with the patient and keeps the locus of control within the patient. Likewise, it hinders any tendency on the HCP's part to lay blame on the patient for behavior that might have contributed to the problem that they are coming to us for within the rehabilitation process.

A helpful belief of the nature of one's role in healing is to assist the person needing help to identify and cope with their problems quickly and return to a feeling of being in control of their life as soon as possible. Patients are simply people who have problems/concerns that they would solve by themselves if they could, but they need our professional help to identify the problems/concerns, clarify the nature and causes of the problems/concerns, and solve their problems/concerns so they can get on with living.

# OBSTACLES TO CONVEYING A HEALING ATTITUDE

People who have an attitude that facilitates healing are able to accept their patients just as they are without judging them. These HCPs will often have identified and dealt with biases and prejudices about certain behaviors, such as alcohol and drug abuse, laziness, smoking, use of profanity, and obesity. They will have reconciled their abhorrence of some behaviors, such as rape and murder, and are willing to be therapeutically present to people accused of such behaviors. As much as possible, they will be aware of and willing to underplay and/or eliminate deeply held prejudices about race, socio economic status, religion, culture, gender, age, and/or sexual orientation, and self-monitor implicit biases, as discussed in Chapters 7 and 8.

How does all this happen? Obviously not overnight. The previous paragraph describes a mature person whose ego is not bound by the fear that emanates from immature judgmental and dualistic thinking. Behavior that is accepting is nonjudgmental or non-blaming in nature. As much as we might abhor a person's behavior, it is helpful to believe that the person would have acted differently if they had had more information, felt less helpless, and been less impulsive.

Remember from Chapter 2 that many of the immature judgments and prejudices we continue to carry as adults stem from fear that we developed as children from the messages we heard from adults around us. As adults, we must confront the inappropriateness and negativity of these judgments and work to establish more whole, accepting, self-affirming beliefs.

The gains of good interviewing skills justify the need for continued practice and professional development in this skill throughout your career; positive outcomes include:

> *increased time efficiencies, improvements in accuracy and completeness of data, improved clinical diagnoses, fewer needs for more test and measures, increased patient compliance and satisfaction, increased mutual understanding and learning in each PPI encounter with the resultant of patients taking a more active role in their care.[12]*

One of the purposes of this text is to assist you in this maturation process by helping you to identify harmful attitudes and behaviors that would interfere with the healing nature of the interview. Practicing our active listening skills and assertiveness skills helps in an interview. True active listening and speaking out of an awareness of your own rights helps one to diminish a tendency to project one's own weaknesses and to minimize a judgmental attitude.

# INTERVIEWING ADOLESCENTS

More than 3 million teenagers in the United States have chronic illnesses, mental health concerns, and disabilities. They are a diverse group, but at this developmental stage, adolescents share some behavioral similarities that are important to understand and be sensitive to during the interview and during treatment.[12] Teenagers are preoccupied with their bodies and peer acceptance and may be embarrassed by certain questions or feel that some questions are trivial or none of the business of the HCP.

> *The willingness of a teenager to share personal or intimate information depends on the perceived receptiveness of the provider. ... It is usually not difficult for patients and providers to discuss routine chronic medical conditions such as diabetes and asthma. Control of these conditions in some teenagers, however, may be related more to dietary indiscretions and marijuana or cigarette consumption, respectively, than to insulin or inhaler use. Such health-compromising behaviors must be identified before they can be dealt with; comments, facial expressions, or body language indicating disapproval can undermine the patient's willingness to disclose confidential behavior.[12]*

Remember from Chapter 12 that practicing the principles of neurolinguistic psychology will assist you in matching, leading, and pacing the patient to help solidify trust. A nonjudgmental and supportive attitude toward lesbian, gay, bisexual, transgender, and questioning youth (and adults) can help cushion the stigma they may perceive from family and peers. Likewise, teenagers who are depressed usually suffer from fear of exposure, and the stigma of having a mental illness, and need the support of the HCP.

Sleep disturbance, decreased appetite, hopelessness, lethargy, continual thoughts about suicide, illogical thoughts, and/or hallucinations are signs that the patient may have an undiagnosed depression and should be referred for medical follow-up immediately, with the support of the parents or guardians. However, with questioning in the interview, these symptoms may be determined to be contextual—that is, the teen may have no energy to do homework, exercise, or house chores but have unlimited energy to attend concerts, participate in flash mobs, go to the mall with friends, play video games, use social media, and/or party. Likewise, these symptoms may also be secondary to an undiagnosed substance abuse problem, and further follow-up is required. Reassure adolescents that the information they provide will be kept confidential, unless the threat of harm to the patient or others is revealed. Discussions about sex, their bodies, or use of substances should always take place in a private area. If an adult accompanies the patient, first solicit appropriate information from the adult, but then request that the adult leave the room for the remainder of the interview.

With regard to compliance with a treatment plan, recognition of a parental problem is important. Teenagers need the support of parents to meet goals set in therapy. Adolescence is a time of testing boundaries. Chronically ill teenagers are often nonadherent with their therapy secondary to a need to feel in control and test limits or for other reasons due to altered beliefs and values. The struggle for independence clashes with the need to follow a routine to improve or maintain health.[12] Local peer support groups can help, as can an open and trusting communication with the HCP. Emphasize the positive outcomes of adherence to quality of life and have patients actively participate in developing a realistic treatment program.[12]

# INTERVIEWING OLDER PATIENTS

Patients in their eighties, nineties, and older (the "old-old"—in contrast to the "young-old" in their sixties and seventies) are products of a traditional upbringing (Traditionalists and Boomers) and respond most positively to certain respectful behaviors that may seem trivial to younger clinicians (see Chapters 2 and 12). They often respond best if the HCP addresses them by their last names, shakes hands warmly, establishes good eye contact, walks with them to the treatment area, and makes small talk about family and the weather before starting the interview. Many old-old patients are concerned that any new thing wrong with them may spell the initiation of a downward slope toward death, so they will be looking for reassurance and information about the nature of the illness or disability that is limiting them and will want a realistic perspective about a return to their previous level of function.

Once, as a new HCP, I had established a great rapport with Mr. Moe, who was progressing along quite nicely in his outpatient rehabilitation. The Catholic Health Services, hospital-based rehab department, and outpatient services were informal, and everyone went by first names. One day, Mr. Moe, a conservative Catholic, was sharing his World War II stories; he had not previously talked at all about any of these experiences. He related these stories as we were working on his exercises for his low back pain from a rotated innominate with muscle imbalances. As he was lying supine looking at the ceiling and I was monitoring the quality of his movement performance, it must have struck a memory for him. He shared some unfortunate and moving details related to his time as a Naval air pilot in the bombardment squadron in the South Pacific. I would not be surprised if this may even have been one of the few and only times he talked about his Veteran experiences. Unfortunately, I, being clueless and a novice HCP, made the mistake of interpreting this disclosure as meaning I could now be more informal with him in terms of his namesake. I called him Archie, his first name, as he was departing therapy. Mind you, this gentleman came dressed in his seersucker suit and jacket to therapy daily; the only thing informal was that he did not always wear a tie, making him seem a bit more approachable. He took immense pride in his appearance, health, and philanthropic service to society. He also would walk the 2 miles to the hospital and back to his home each session, no matter the weather. As I called him Archie as he was putting on his hat, luckily I noticed him raise his eyebrows at me and wrinkle his forehead slightly, in the triangle of concern, in utter dismay, and appear quite startled as his eyes enlarged (almost as if I had assaulted him!). If I had not been watching his nonverbal communication through his facial expressions, I may have completely missed that I had offended him greatly. I immediately restated and said, "I'm very sorry, I mean Mr. Moe," which quickly brought a gleam back to his eye, and he tipped his hat back to me and said, "Thank you and see you on Friday." He seemed quite relieved the next visit that I continued to refer to him as Mr. Moe! We were back in sync in our HCP PPI. I also discovered, after his death many years later, that he was one of the sustainers of the hospital and quietly served on the Board of Directors and in many realms of community service as a silent partner. He had made a fortune as a founder of a thermoplastics company that made foam air packaging, was very well off, and never let anyone really know his wealth status—a true Traditionalist of the more silent Greatest Generation. I was very relieved that I was able to reestablish the appropriate therapeutic relationship in this HCP PPI and continue his care. And, if you were wondering, he fully recovered from his low back pain. This raises the point to also clarify preferred pronouns with your patients/clients if it is not clear up-front.

Older people often suffer from hearing loss (or other diminished senses, such as depth perception or vision changes) but do not appreciate being shouted at or patronized as if they are stupid. Do not speak louder than is appropriate; speaking more slowly, clearly, and in a moderate tone is more helpful. Ask how you can best communicate if the patient is having difficulty hearing you; you may need to be in a quiet area when doing your intake or ongoing work with the elderly. Taking the time to get a thorough and true interview at the outset will pay off in the long run. Careful questioning about previous illnesses, medications, and comorbid conditions is critical to making an accurate diagnosis and planning an effective treatment. Likewise, a good understanding about support at home and the home environment is critical to planning an effective treatment.

In sum, interviewing old-old and oldest old, patients takes longer, but a thorough interview that establishes trust and rapport is absolutely necessary for successful treatment and recovery. Older patients may need a break, and ensure that they are hydrating during the interview process to help sustain them (unless they are on fluid restrictions for some reason). Some older patients will be very difficult to communicate with, especially if they have held the identity of victim all their lives and want you to fix all their problems for them. They can be quite demanding, and it is important to set clear limits of what is possible in treatment. Explain your role in the HCP PPI relationship and not only what you are willing to do, but also what the patient must do for a successful recovery. Rehabilitation is a therapeutic partnership and requires trust, unconditional positive regard, and a commitment by patient and provider, hopefully with supportive networks, including family members, significant others, and/or caregivers. Perhaps you will find a certain deep pleasure in getting to know older patients, because many enjoy sharing their wisdom and humor, which can be the high point of your day. We learn much from our patients who have traveled the journey of life before us, and the geriatric population has many lessons and insights to share. Older people will amaze you with their resilience and can often be a pure joy! Most love to share their life stories and teach you, too.

# THE INTERVIEW

## Good Timing

With regard to timing, an effective interviewer avoids interruption (which often reveals an underlying harmful attitude of "this person is not very important to me") and listens carefully, effectively using silence. Those who are uncomfortable with silence will miss much of what a person will say when given a chance to pause and reflect. Time is positively manipulated to indicate a seriousness of attention and level of involvement. A specific uninterrupted amount of time is set to be spent listening to the patient carefully as they tell you the story of the problem.

## *Artful Phrasing*

Artful phrasing, a skill that is learned over time, involves using the right kind of question (open vs. closed, direct vs. indirect) at the right time; avoiding jargon, slang, and dialect; and tuning one's words and gestures to reassure the patient that they are being attended to at a serious and thoughtful level.[11] The patient will tell you everything you need to know if only you ask! Be careful not to end before you begin … lots of practice is needed to perfect this important skill for best HCP PPI.

# STAGES OF THE INTERVIEW

There are three stages in the interview: initiation, or statement of the purpose of the interview; development or exploration; and closure.

1.  The initiation of the interview takes place as you, the interviewer, explain who you are, why you are here, and the purpose of the interview.

2.  The body of the interview is the development or exploration stage. In it, the interviewer leads an exploration on the part of the patient, perhaps beginning with the open-ended question, "What brought you here today?" A good interviewer will guide the patient down a meaningful path, assisting the patient to explore their problem but not allowing the patient to go too far afield from the problem. Active listening helps the patient to clarify and zero in on the unique aspects of their situation. The interviewer listens carefully and sorts the information, jotting down significant revelations as they prepare for the clinical examination. The body of the interview unfolds in a unique story that the patient is invited and encouraged to tell. The helpful interviewer confirms to the patient that they are being carefully and humanely listened to by a skilled and caring HCP. When moving from one topic to another, it is helpful to use a transition statement. An example would be, "I think I understand the nature of your headaches; is it okay with you to shift now to the pain in your lower back?"

3.  The closing of the interview takes place at a time that has been predetermined by the interviewer. If it becomes obvious that the interview is not complete, the interviewer does not just let the session drop but says, for example, "We're beginning to run out of time for this session and I realize you haven't yet finished. What still needs to be covered?" Then a second session is scheduled, or the interviewer may begin the physical examination and continue discussing the problem with the patient during the exam. I offer a note of caution here, however. To begin the physical examination before allowing the patient to tell as complete a personal story as time allows is a mistake. As an interviewer, you cannot expect to establish a relationship and obtain meaningful information while engaging in palpation and physical evaluation methods. Your brain will address what you see and feel before it will attend to what it hears.

# BODY OF THE INTERVIEW—INFORMATION GATHERED

Table 14.2 provides sample opening queries for the PPI to initiate the interview and consider, in an open-ended manner, aspects of the social determinants of health (SDoH). SDoH were adopted by the Centers for Disease Control from the World Health Organization and incorporated within Health People 2030 as leading health indicators (https://health.gov/healthypeople). Examples of the SDoH (see Chapter 1, Figure 1.1), well-being, and quality of life, which may have negative or positive influences, include:

- Income and social protection and support
- Education
- Unemployment and job insecurity/opportunities
- Working life conditions
- Food insecurity, access to nutritious foods, and physical activity opportunities
- Polluted air and water
- Language and literacy skills

| TABLE 14.2 |
| :--- |
| ## PPI: OPENING QUERIES—ADDRESSING SOCIAL DETERMINANTS OF HEALTH (SDoH) |
| ○ What brings you here? |
| ○ What do you call your problem/concern? |
| ○ What causes your problem/concern (or henceforth, insert the terminology utilized by the patient/client, that is what the patient/client "calls their problem/concern")? |
| ○ What kind of treatment do you think would be best for your problem? |
| ○ How has this problem affected your life? |
| ○ What frightens you or concerns you most about your problem? |
| Adapted from: Johnson TM, Hardt E, Kleinman A. Cultural factors in the medical interview. In Lipkin M, Putnam SM, Lazare A, eds. *The Medical Interview*. New York, NY: Springer-Verlag; 1995. |

- Safe and affordable housing, basic amenities, and the environment
- Transportation and neighborhoods, including safe streets and green spaces
- Early childhood development
- Social inclusion and nondiscrimination, social norms, and attitudes
- Structural conflict
- Access to affordable health services of decent quality
- Historical trauma and microaggressions, exposure to violence or conflict

Consider how each of these SDoHs may impact your patients'/clients' care and accessibility needs for care. You may need to delve more deeply into the SDoH as you build your therapeutic relationship and the patient becomes more comfortable and trusting of you. However, these open-ended, preliminary queries provide an appropriate place to begin to learn more about your patients'/clients' lived experiences and social determinants that influence and impact their health. Additional SDoH resources and links to informatics data are provided at the end of this chapter for your exploration and utilization.

Couple the queries in Table 14.2 that begin to address SDoH with the following key questions. This will build upon the opening queries to form the structure of the body of the interview. It will also set the boundaries for a meaningful story from the patient:

- What is the patient's reason for seeking health care? Why did they come today?
- What is the patient's perception of the problem? What is it? Why did it begin? What are the consequences of the problem?
- What impact, if any, does the problem have on the patient's life? How does the patient feel about it? Does it affect work, relationships, and quality of everyday life?
- What are the characteristics of the problem? When did it begin? Precipitating factors? Where is it located? What is its quality and severity? What alleviates the problem? What makes it worse? What factors are associated with it?
- What does the patient expect from this visit? What does the patient hope that you will do?

# NONVERBAL COMMUNICATION

The nonverbal communication of the interviewer can facilitate or hinder the quality of the interview. Revisiting Chapter 12 on neurolinguistic psychology and Chapter 13 on cultural sensitivity, and reviewing nonverbal communication in more depth, will help you develop your use of this important communication skill.

Key nonverbal elements of a helping interview include wise use of space and the environment (posture toward each other and at the same eye level, eliminating physical and perceived barriers); time (uninterrupted level of involvement; sufficient and adequate overall time, allowing for needed breaks); appropriate posture (leaning in, avoiding rigid posture or slouching or defiant gestures, keeping both feet on the ground, open arms); voice inflection (appropriate speed and volume, warmth, and genuine curiosity conveyed vs. flatness or excessive use of "you know" or "like"); elimination of distracting body movements (twitching, shaking foot, tapping pencil); avoiding closed postures (no crossed legs, ankles, arms) and maintaining good eye contact (not constantly looking down at your paper or clipboard) so that you can utilize good pacing and timing, along with monitoring the patient's nonverbal communication and being fully present with the patient in the moment (so you can readily and responsively match, pace, and lead); and eliminating any and all distractions (social media, audible sounds from your devices, documentation barriers [i.e., looking at a computer screen instead of the patient, interruptions by support staff, etc.]).

## THE INTERVIEW—A UNIQUE COMMUNICATION FORM

The interview represents a different form of communicating from what we have learned growing up in our families and with our friends. The interview is the very first opportunity to convey a professional healing attitude, and it must be learned and practiced in order to develop skill. Behind every word needs to be an attitude of willingness and awareness that will result in congruence.

The words and the inner attitude must be in harmony in order for the interview to be therapeutic. The interviewer must feel confident, peaceful, at one with self, and genuinely willing to establish a healing relationship. You will need to practice many times before you feel fully comfortable, even with the process. Each time, you shall gain in skill level and become more comfortable in establishing the healing relationship, which is essential to the work of the HCP in effective PPI.

## MORE ON THE INTERVIEW ATTITUDE—WHAT WE ARE

Alfred Benjamin[13] said:

> When interviewing, we are left with what we are. We have no books then, no classroom lessons, and no supporting person at our elbow. We are alone with the individual who has come to seek our help. How can we assist them? The same basic issues will confront us afresh whenever we face an interviewee for the first time. In summary they are:
>
> 1. Shall we allow ourselves to emerge as genuine human beings, or shall we hide behind our role, position, and authority?
> 2. Shall we really try to listen with all our senses to the interviewee?
> 3. Shall we try to understand with the person empathetically and acceptingly?
> 4. Shall we interpret their behavior in terms of their frame of reference, our own, or society's?
> 5. Shall we evaluate their thoughts, feelings, and actions and if so, in terms of whose values: theirs, society's, or ours?
> 6. Shall we support, encourage, urge them on, so that by leaning on us, hopefully they may be able to rely on their own strength one day?
> 7. Shall we question and probe, push and prod, causing them to feel that we are in command and that once all our queries have been answered, we shall provide the solutions they are seeking?
> 8. Shall we guide them in the direction we feel certain is the best for them?
> 9. Shall we reject their... thoughts and feelings, and insist that they become like us, or at least conform to our perception of what they should become?

These are the central attitudinal questions that underlie every helping interview, and the response to each reveals the values that form our attitudes. When you read the above questions carefully, you will see that Benjamin[13] phrased a few to encourage a negative response, as if to have us examine our attitudes very carefully in order to be clear about our helping intentions. The humanistic values (and their subsequent actions) we discussed in previous chapters lead to developing a healing attitude. Once that attitude is established, and with continued practice and refinement, skillful and artful questions will become second nature. The helping interview will become one of the most important tools in the HCP's repertoire of healing behaviors.

Automatically, you will assume an active listening stance and convey a warm and genuine interest in your patient. Once this practiced routine becomes second nature, less stress will be attached to it, and you will experience magnificent pleasure listening to most of your patients tell their stories.

# THE NONHELPFUL INTERVIEW

What would a nonhelpful interview look and sound like? Sometimes it is useful for us to explore a concept by describing its opposite. One interpretation of the opposite of a healing interview might go like this:

> The clinician enters the treatment area where the patient has been waiting for quite a while. Without looking up from the patient record or acknowledging the patient in any way, the clinician begins to read the chart and mumbles, "Mr. Zuck?"
>
> The patient replies, "Yes," and the clinician continues to read.
>
> Clinician:  "So, what's wrong with you?"
>
> Patient:  "I'm not sure. I hurt my back. I can't work."
>
> Clinician:  (No response but thinks to herself, *Oh no, another back. This is the third malingerer I have seen today.*)
>
> Clinician:  "Well, take off your shirt and climb up on the table."
>
> She leaves the area, returns 10 minutes later, and, without speaking, begins the physical examination.

This, as you can see, is not really an interview at all. No rapport has been established, no active listening was done, and no meaningful information was gathered. The HCP valued only the information she would get from her physical examination. The patient was reduced to a thing—another low back in a parade of low backs.

How would you feel if you were the patient? Would you, as many patients do, make excuses for the poor, overworked therapist whom you are grateful has made the time to see you? Or have you decided already that here is a person without manners who will treat you only as a thing, another event in a long and uninteresting day? Would you throw up your hands in frustration and bury your disappointment one more time, further convinced that no one really cares about your pain and that you must endure this alone without the understanding help of another person?

Whatever treatment gets accomplished in the previous example, it will be of far less quality than it could be had the clinician used helping interview skills.

# RUMINATIONS AND CONCLUSION

If you have ever been fortunate enough to have observed an expert clinician at work, you have seen a person who truly values the interview and devotes the kind of attention to it described in this chapter. The greatest obstacles to consistent use of the helping interview are overwork, burnout, and/or compassion fatigue (see Chapter 5). The more we feel overextended in our day, and the more we feel that we are repeatedly facing irresolvable problems, the more difficult it will be to come outside of ourselves with a therapeutic presence for the interview. Therefore, the very foundation of the helping interview is a commitment to the discipline required to keep a balance in our lives so that we are rested and have good energy to give to our work. Also, we are required to keep a rein on the extent to which we commit ourselves to the work that must be done, avoiding giving up the right to keep a reasonable pace.

People who feel consistently overworked are avoiding the responsibility they have to keep control of the workload and to fight for that right. Each patient we see ideally deserves 100% of our professional ability. It is our responsibility to make sure that we have as much of ourselves to give as we can. Chapter 5 expanded significantly on burnout and compassion fatigue and helped you learn to balance your life and manage HCP stress so that this ideal is attainable.

The exercises for this chapter are critical to effective learning. Conducting a useful interview requires maturation, experience, and practice. Practice in peer and self-assessment shall assist you in developing as a mature HCP. As discussed in Chapter 10, Musolino[14] described self-assessment skills as not only essential for HCPs, but also crucial to becoming a reflective practitioner[15,16] and moving along the professional development continuum from novice to expert practice.[17] Musolino's[14] study findings paralleled Schön's[15,16] concept of reflective practice and supported Bandura's[18–21] social learning theory in the resulting developed, conceptual model of self-assessment. Recall that feedback is necessary to convert reflective practice didactic skills into actual clinical abilities and may require a transformative process for novice clinicians.[14,21] Musolino[14] emphasized the influence of critical thought and reflective action through the process of self-assessment and the need for guided feedback to effect a change toward mindful practice.[22] Constructive feedback is not only a gift, but an art of sharing crucial insights to assist another to be an excellent HCP in PPI. Doing peer and self-assessment and truly critically reflecting and being mindful will enhance not only your interview skills, but also your communication skills as a developing reflective practitioner and HCP. It is challenging and uncomfortable at first, but thriving on feedback shall ensure that you reach your full potential, along with your abilities to truly help your patients and clients. Do not forget that your patients are also great resources for feedback too.

One of the most efficient ways to correct mistakes and improve style is to review videos of yourself interviewing in a role-play and, if possible, with a patient, then to receive specific feedback in all learning domains (affective, cognitive, and psychomotor, see Chapter 3, Appendix) as you watch the video. In this chapter's exercises, you shall find that the reviewer assessment forms are exceptional guidance documents for your practice sessions with peer and self-assessment to facilitate your progress toward reflective practice. Maturation and experience lead to quiet self-confidence and relaxation wherein the "third ear" (see Chapter 6) is automatically engaged. Practicing interviewing will help you value and develop the artful balance of scientific discovery with compassionate intuition—the true amalgamation of the art and science of reflective practice in health care is to help others reach the full potential of their movement system.

Remember to be honest, objective, and constructively critical in your peer and self-assessment feedback. Feedback is a true gift, and your future patients are counting on your abilities to be a true partner in the care of their health. The only way to achieve an effective patient–HCP partnership is through the initial establishment of good rapport. Seif and Brown[23] described a similar learning activity using videorecording. They described physical therapy students who participated in two video-recorded sessions of simulated interviewing and examinations and completed peer and self-assessment during a three-part, musculoskeletal series, prior to their first clinical education experience. The peer and self-assessment debriefing sessions provided feedback on areas for improvement and continued growth in areas of strength, with detailed specific information for continued progression in interviewing skills. The students in this study described the learning activity of peer and self-assessment, utilizing video recordings for assisting in the development of clinical and communication skills for patient care. Additional helpful HCP resources for screening,[24] measurements,[25] and interviewing skills for self-assessment[26,27] and review[28] are available at the end of the chapter.

Don't forget to write a journal about this experience. What new perspectives did you gain from reviewing the Singh et al.[28] article? How will these insights impact your PPI? What did you learn about yourself as an interviewer? What feelings did you have as you received feedback and/or watched yourself on video? Does videorecording help you identify with patients even more than simply role-playing? What new knowledge did you gain from exploring the additional resources for screening and measurements? Will these screening tools impact your practice?

Again, have fun as you learn and grow and mature into the role of a healing HCP. Be patient with yourself, it takes practice! Keep paying it forward with positive actions and constructive feedback for improved professional formation with your peers. Again, you might find it interesting to know that researchers have found that with compassion training, one actually elicits on the neural level networks, including the

> *medial orbitofrontal cortex, putamen, pallidum and ventral tegmental area—brain regions associated with positive affect and affiliation. Hence, deliberate cultivation of compassion is in itself a coping strategy that fosters a positive affect (affective domain), and strengthens resilience, even when confronted with the distress of others.*[8,29]

Ah, the golden rule prevails: "do unto others as you would have done unto yourself," and it remains true that "people don't care how much you know until you care about them as a person first." Exercising compassion enhances neuroplasticity in the brain, enabling adaptive coping and self-soothing physiological benefits,[30] i.e., being compassionate with others yields upregulating positive affects and is beneficial for HCPs. This ability to better cope with emotional adversity is supported by the "neurophysiological alterations in cardiovascular, endocrine and neural systems supporting positive emotions and emotion regulation."[30(p 107)] Let's end this chapter with a pause for the cause, reflecting on the words of the ancient Greek philosopher, Plato: "Be kind, for everyone you meet is fighting a harder battle."

# REFERENCES

1. Perlman HH. *Relationship: The Heart of Helping People*. Chicago, IL: University of Chicago Press; 1983.
2. Fallowfield L, Jenkins V. Communicating sad, bad, and difficult news in medicine. *Lancet*. 2004;363(9405):312–319.

3. Wündrich M, Schwartz C, Feige B, Lemper D, Nissen C, Voderholzer U. Empathy training in medical students—a randomized controlled trial. *Med Teach.* 2017 Oct;39(10):1096–1098.

4. Pionke JJ, Graham RA. Multidisciplinary scoping review of literature focused on compassion, empathy, emotional intelligence, or mindfulness behaviors and working with the public. *J Library Admin.* 2021;61:2, 147–184.

5. Barrett-Lennard GT. The phases and focus of empathy. *Br J Med Psychol.* 1993;66:3–14.

6. Patel S, Pelletier-Bui A, Smith S, Roberts MB, Kilgannon H, Trzeciak S, et al. Curricula for empathy and compassion training in medical education: A systematic review. *PLoS ONE.* 2019;14(8): e0221412. doi: 10.1371/journal. pone.0221412.

7. Gilligan C, Brubacher SP, Powell MB. "We're All Time Poor": Experienced clinicians' and students' perceptions of challenges related to patient communication, *Teach & Learn Med.* 2022;34:1, 1–12.

8. Lamm C, Decety J, Singer T. Meta-analytic evidence for common and distinct neural networks associated with directly experienced pain and empathy for pain. *Neuroimage.* 2011; 54(3):2492–2502.

9. Klimecki OM, Leiberg S, Ricard M, Singer T. Differential pattern of functional brain plasticity after compassion and empathy training. *Soc Cogn Affect Neurosci.* 2014;9(6):873–879.

10. Epstein RM, Franks P, Shields CG, Meldrum SC, Miller KN, Campbell TL, et al. Patient-centered communication and diagnostic testing. *Ann Fam Med.* 2005;3(5):415–421.

11. Enelow AJ, Forde DL, Brummel-Smith K. *Interviewing and Patient Care.* 4th ed. New York, NY: Oxford University Press; 1996.

12. Feldman MD, Christensen JF, eds. *Behavioral Medicine: A Guide for Clinical Practice.* 5th ed. New York, NY: McGraw Hill; 2019.

13. Benjamin A. *The Helping Interview.* 3rd ed. Boston, MA: Houghton Mifflin; 1981.

14. Musolino GM. Fostering reflective practice: self-assessment abilities of physical therapy students and entry-level graduates. *J Allied Health.* 2006;35(1):30–42.

15. Schön DA. *Educating the Reflective Practitioner: Toward a New Design for Teaching and Learning in the Professions.* San Francisco, CA: Jossey-Bass; 1990.

16. Schön DA. The theory of inquiry: Dewey's legacy to education. *Curriculum Inquiry.* 1992;22:119–140.

17. Jensen G, Denton B. Teaching physical therapy students to reflect: a suggestion for clinical education. *J Phys Ther Educ.* 1991;5:33–38.

18. Bandura A. *Self-Efficacy: The Exercise of Control.* New York, NY: W.H. Freeman; 1997.

19. Bandura A. Self-efficacy: toward a unifying theory of behavioral change. *Psychol Rev.* 1997;84(2):191–215.

20. Bandura A. *Social Learning Theory.* Englewood Cliffs, NJ: Prentice-Hall; 1977.

21. Bandura A. The self-system in reciprocal determinism. *Am Psychologist.* 1978;33:344–358.

22. Epstein RM. Mindful practice. *JAMA.* 1999;282(9):833–839.

23. Seif GA, Brown D. Video-recorded simulated patient interactions: can they help develop clinical and communication skills in today's learning environment? *J Allied Health.* 2013;42(2):e37–e44.

24. The Psych Congress Network. http://www.psychcongress.com. Accessed January 3, 2023.

25. Carlson JF, Geisinger KF, Johnson JL. *The Twenty-first Mental Measurements Yearbook.* Lincoln, NE: Buros Center for Testing, Department of Educational Psychology, University of Nebraska-Lincoln; 2021.

26. Seif GA, Kraft SV, Bowden MG, Boissonnault JS. Intra-rater Reliability of the ECHOWS Tool for Real-time Assessment of Physical Therapy Student Interviewing Skills: A Pilot Study. *Health Professions Educ.* 2019;5(2):146–151.

27. Boissonnault JS, Evans K, Tuttle N, Hetzel S, Boissonnault WG. Reliability of the ECHOWS Tool for Assessment of Patient Interviewing Skills. *Phys Ther.* 2016; 96(4):443–445.

28. Singh S, Orlando JM, Alghamdi ZS, Franklin KA, Lobo MA. Reframing clinical paradigms: strategies for improving patient care relationships. *Phys Ther.* 2021;101(7):1–13. doi: 10.1093/ptj/pzab095.

29. Klimecki OM, Leiberg S, Lamm C, Singer T. Functional neural plasticity and associated changes in positive affect after compassion training. *Cereb Cortex.* 2013 Jul;23(7):1552–1561. doi: 10.1093/cercor/bhs142. Epub 2012 Jun 1. PMID: 22661409.

30. Förster K, Kanske P. Upregulating positive affect through compassion: psychological and physiological evidence. *Int J Psychophysiol.* 2022 Jun;176:100–107. doi: 10.1016/j.ijpsycho.2022.03.009. Epub 2022 Mar 28. PMID: 35358613.

# SUGGESTED READINGS AND RESOURCES FOR SCREENING AND MEASUREMENTS

## Tools to Assess and Measure Social Determinants of Health—Rural Health Information Hub Toolkit

www.ruralhealthinfo.org/toolkits/sdoh

Provides numerous community and individual standardized measurement tools for SDoH for health care screening. Community-based measures and mapping tools are detailed, along with health impact assessment, decision-support tools. International Classification of Disease (ICD) Codes are provided to provide identification for potential health hazards related to SDoH, along with a plethora of resources linked from national affiliated organizations to help better address and understand SDoH. While no one tool is sufficient for everyone, additional SDoH-specific screening tools are available (e.g., Protocol for Responding to and Assessing Patients' Assets, Risks and Experiences, PRAPARE, Health Related Social Needs Screening Tool, Hunger Vital Sign, Abuse Assessment Screens, and EveryONE Project) via the American Academy of Family Practice (www.aafp.org/fpm).

## Academy of Communication in Healthcare

https://achonline.org/
Organization and website for all HCPs dedicated to anyone looking to improve patient care, teamwork, patient satisfaction, and developing their individual communication skills.

## Psych Congress Network

www.hmpglobalevents.com/psychcongressportfolio
As you may have discovered already in your helping interview practice sessions, even the apparently healthy may present with the need for screening for other issues and concerns. There are many standardized screening tools to help you screen for psychological concerns if your HCP PPI and helping interview lead you to believe that further work-up and referral may be appropriate for your patients and clients (e.g., Patient Health Questionnaire-9; Bech, Hung, and Hamilton Scale for Mood Disorders, Primary Screen for Mental Disorders and the Beck Depression Inventory-II, which is a 21-item self-report, multiple-choice inventory with a resulting scaled score of severity, with 81% sensitivity and 92% specificity).[24] The Psych Congress Network houses much information about many of the HCP practice tools for scales and screeners for diagnoses, such as attention deficit hyperactive disorder, alcohol abuse, anxiety disorders, Asperger's, bipolar disorder, cognitive impairment, depression, psychosis, post-traumatic stress disorder, sexual dysfunction, and suicide, as well as Structured Diagnostic Interview Instruments for neuropsychiatric function, Drug Use Questionnaire, and Well-Being Index. The Psych Congress Network serves as a resource to get you started and also includes trending topical information. Topics vary, and include exploration of subjects such as caregiver burden, blogs for HCP support, and HCP expert interviews. The site covers additional psychological aspects of diverse trending areas, such as the effects of pharmacotherapeutics, current efforts related to medical marijuana, and related approaches for HCPs PPI for motivational interviewing. The Psych Congress Network Psychiatry & Behavioral Health site also includes mental health and wellness apps related to meditation, nutrition, exercise, mental health, cognitive behavioral therapy, and sleep applications. As a HCP in training, you may also find it helpful to explore and try the applications as you go through the stressful times and the best of times.

## The Mental Measurements Yearbook

https://buros.org/       https://buros.org/mental-measurements-yearbook
Founded in 1938, and published by the Buros Center for Testing, named for late author Oscar Krisen Buros, *The Mental Measurements Yearbook*[25] is the classic biannual text that includes timely, consumer-oriented test reviews; provides evaluation information; and aids HCPs in selecting, promoting, and encouraging informed test selections. *The Mental Measurements Yearbook* includes descriptive information and professional reviews and is updated every two years. The tests cover psychology and education mental measurements. It is the classic go-to text to determine the best tests for target populations, scoring, publication resources, access, and webinar information.

## ECHOWS Tool

The ECHOWS Tool[26,27] (E: Establishing rapport; C: Chief complaint; H: Health history; O: Obtain psychosocial perspective; W: Wrap-up; and S: Summary of performance) is an instrument for assessment of physical therapist students' patient interviewing skills with standardized patients. The ECHOWS instrument maintains excellent intrarater reliability and good interrater reliability. A training guide for users is provided with the ECHOWS instrument. The ECHOWS is a helpful assessment to use for additional practice and allows for student, peer, and faculty/clinical instructor feedback for interviewing skills, with either standardized or real patients. The ECHOWS may also be used as an assessment tool for debriefing purposes, with videorecorded interviews and role-play practice with standardized or real patients, as in Exercise 2 at the end of this chapter.

## *Perspective Article*[28]

https://doi.org/10.1093/ptj/pzab095
Singh S, Orlando JM, Alghamdi ZS, Franklin KA, Lobo MA. Reframing clinical paradigms: Strategies for improving patient care relationships. *Phys Ther.* 2021;101(7):1–13.

A meaningful perspective article providing information and additional resources to support therapeutic relationships with patients and members of their support networks from the viewpoint of a parent and disability researcher. Specific examples, tools, and techniques are provided and discussed that may be immediately implemented. Helpful tables are available that provide positive and negative examples for respectful communication techniques as well as a simple *plan-do-check-act* framework for patient-centered interactions. An insightful article to review before practicing Exercise 2.

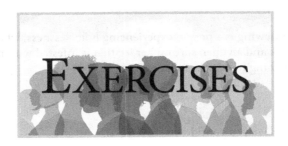

# EXERCISE 1: RESPONDING TO SITUATIONS

The following are situations in which you might likely find yourself as you interact with patients in the clinical setting. These situations are posed to help you explore in advance what you might feel in the situation, what underlying concerns may be in the situation, and some specific things you might say or do in a situation such as this.

1. You are scheduled to interview Dr. Reynolds and report your findings to your clinical supervisor. Dr. Reynolds has been waiting for you for more than an hour, pacing up and down in the waiting area. When you go out to introduce yourself to her, she turns to you angrily and says, "You clinicians don't give a damn about other people's time. Do you realize how long I've been waiting out here?"

   ○ How might you feel at this moment?

   ○ What might the patient's underlying concerns include?

   ○ What are some specific things you might say or do at this point to try to salvage the interview?

2. You walk into the patient's room, and they are watching a Netflix movie on their phone and texting with their friends. You introduce yourself, and the patient never even takes their eyes off the phone. They act as if you are not present in the room.

   ○ How might you feel?

   ○ What might the patient's situation be? Have you considered the SDoH?

    ○  What are some specific things you might say or do in this situation?

3.  The person you are interviewing is a person experiencing homelessness, who has not bathed in a long time. She has a severe body odor and an open sore on her leg that is infested with maggots. As she begins to speak to you, she asks for something to spit her tobacco into.

    ○  What might you feel? Have you considered the SDoH?

    ○  What might be underlying the patient's behavior?

    ○  What might you say and do to ensure a helping interview?

4.  You begin an interview with Mr. Selker, who is 89 years old, with a good, open-ended question, but soon after you begin he starts talking about his favorite football team. As you try to keep him on track about his problem, he consistently digresses to the topic of football. He is hard of hearing and seems to not understand what you are saying to him.

    ○  How might you feel?

    ○  What may be underlying this patient's behavior? Have you considered the SDoH?

    ○  What might you do to salvage the interview in the given amount of time allotted?

5.  You are trying to conduct an interview with a patient, but each time you ask her a question, she looks to her husband and he answers it for her.

    ○  What might you feel?

    ○  What might be underlying this situation?

    o  What are some things you might say or do to get more information from the patient herself? Have you considered the SDoH?

6. You are interviewing a teenager who has a sports injury. She has had type 1 diabetes mellitus since childhood and indicates that she is very tired of having to have insulin injections each day. She feels like an outsider with her friends. She loves playing sports, but it interferes with her insulin regimen, and she is feeling hopeless that she will never be accepted as a normal person. She tells you she wants to die.

    o  What might you feel?

    o  What might be underlying this situation? Have you considered the SDoH?

    o  What might you say or do at this point to maintain a helping quality to the interview? (Practice your active listening skills of reflection and clarification. How serious is this wish to die, and has it been followed up by others?)

7. You are interviewing a patient, and the patient suddenly leans forward, grabs your arm, and says, "You are so attractive. I'd like to see you, you know, have a date with you. How about it?"

    o  How might you feel?

    o  What might be underlying the patient's behavior? Have you considered the SDoH?

    o  What might you say or do to get the interview back on track?

8. You are interviewing an elderly patient who is sitting in a wheelchair. You believe that he is able to understand you, but his responses are quite slow and labored. Suddenly you notice a stream of urine running down his leg and onto the floor. He seems not to pay attention to this.

    o  What might you feel?

    o  What decision must you make at this point of the interview?

     ○  What might you say or do to ensure that the interview remains helpful in nature? (Practice self-transposal. What would you want someone to say to you? To do?)

9.  You are asked to interview a patient who only speaks Spanish. You cannot elicit meaningful information using rudimentary sign language. No one is close by who could translate for you.

     ○  What might you feel?

     ○  What decision must you make at this point?

     ○  How can you solicit accurate information and informed consent? Be creative. (Sign language alone is not legally adequate.) Have you considered the SDoH?

     ○  Can you ethically or legally proceed without informed consent?

# EXERCISE 2: VIDEORECORDING AN INTERVIEW

This exercise is offered to help you develop skills in conducting the helping interview and in critiquing your skills and the skills of your classmates. It consists of a role-play of an interview that, ideally, should be videorecorded. Divide the class into several small groups, with each small group serving as an observation and feedback unit.

The exercise begins with each class member receiving a description of the patient they are to portray. This description should include all pertinent personal and illness (symptom) information so that the acting can be carried out for the respective role completely. Completion of the Patient Information Form is important to this process. Students are to be invited to submit patient descriptions from their experiences or simply make up a description of a patient's situation. Each student should complete a Patient Information Form.

Class members number off, but first divide the class in half. If there are 50 students, number off 1 through 25, then start over and number 1 through 25 again. The two number 1s will interview each other. Each will role-play their own patient described on the Patient Information Form.

When videorecording is done in small groups, an instructor should be with each group. The group should meet for as many sessions as it takes for each person to interview for 5 to 8 minutes. At that time, the interview may not be over, but the instructor will call for an end.

During the interview, many thoughts and feelings are taking place. During the video playback, the interviewer has control of the pause button and should stop the recording at any point they wish to discuss the action and to review the distinct options that are available at that moment.

The patient is invited to ask for the recording to be stopped as well, but the interviewer is in charge of the playback. Once the recording is stopped, the interviewer and the patient are invited to discuss thoughts and feelings, and classmates may feel free to question, emphasizing a noncritical, curious attitude.

During the interview, observers are asked to complete the Reviewer Assessment Form. After the interview, the patient is asked to complete the Patient Assessment Form.

During the discussion of the interview, reviewers may add comments on their assessment form. At the end of the entire process, the interviewer completes the Interviewer's Self-Critique Form.

The total time for each interview session should be 20 to 30 minutes.

## An Alternative Plan

Time and resource constraints may require that the patient and clinician meet outside class, arrange to have their interview videorecorded, and then bring the recording to class for discussion and feedback. Classmates (reviewers) should have a summary description of the patient before viewing the video, but again, the class completes the Reviewer Assessment Form as they are watching the video for the first time.

The most important learning for this exercise grows out of the class discussion, not out of the video itself. Feedback is best received when it is specific and given with kindness. Insights that contribute to learning are most effective when they are stimulated in a supportive and nonpunitive atmosphere.

You are reminded to journal about the experience. What was it like to play the role of an interviewer in front of a camera and your classmates? What did you learn about yourself? What behaviors do you intend to develop?

## *Patient Information Form*

Please answer the following questions about the situation you will be representing in your role as a patient. This exercise will be most useful if you answer each item as accurately, completely, and authentically as would a patient who actually has the problem.

1. What is your reason for seeking care?

2. Why are you coming in to see the clinician now?

3. What other complaints or concerns have you had, consider also specifically the SDoH?

4. What do you think or fear the problem might be?

5. What do you think the consequences of the problem might be?

6. What are your past experiences with this problem?

7. How have your activities of daily living been modified as a result of this problem?

8. What other impact has this problem had on your life?

9. What has been the chronology of events in the development of this problem?

10. What is (are) the location(s) of the symptom(s)?

11. What is (are) quality(ies) of the symptom(s)?

12. What is (are) the quantity(ies) of the symptom(s) (e.g., frequency, duration)?

13. What factors have you noted aggravate or alleviate the problem?

14. In what setting does the problem seem to occur (i.e., what have you noted seems to precipitate the problem)?

15. What other manifestations or symptoms have you noted that seem to be associated with the problem?

16. What are your expectations of this visit to the therapist?

17. Describe your personal situation and characteristics.

18. What is the state of your underlying health?

19. What has been your past personal and medical history?

(Adapted from Course in Health and Human Values, University of Miami School of Medicine, 1982–1985.)

# Reviewer Assessment Form

Circle the appropriate letters. Y = yes, N = no, NA = not applicable.
(Note: Where indicated, use space under items to describe and give specific examples of what the interviewer did.)

Your Name: _____

Interviewer's Name: _____

## BEGINNING OF THE INTERVIEW

*Did they:*

1. Greet the patient in a friendly, attentive, respectful manner? . . . . . . . . . . . . . . . . . . . . . . . . Y  N  NA

2. Address introductions of themself and the patient, using the patient's name and
   their own name? . . . . . . . . . . . . . . . . . . . . . . . . . . . . . . . . . . . . . . . . . . . . . . . . Y  N  NA

3. Define the purpose of the interview? . . . . . . . . . . . . . . . . . . . . . . . . . . . . . . . . . . Y  N  NA

4. Help the patient get physically comfortable? . . . . . . . . . . . . . . . . . . . . . . . . . . . . Y  N  NA

## EXPLORING THE PATIENT'S CONCERNS: GATHERING INFORMATION

*Did they:*

5. Use questions appropriately?

   a. Use a general open-ended approach to help establish the reason(s) for the patient's visit? . . . . Y  N  NA

   b. Use a topic-oriented approach to explore new topics, including the SDoH, using specific
      questions only as needed? . . . . . . . . . . . . . . . . . . . . . . . . . . . . . . . . . . . . . . . Y  N  NA
      *Give example:*

   c. Avoid premature closed questions that can be answered "yes" or "no"? . . . . . . . . . . . . . . Y  N  NA

   d. Ask one question at a time? . . . . . . . . . . . . . . . . . . . . . . . . . . . . . . . . . . . . . . . . Y  N  NA

   e. Refrain from using leading questions? . . . . . . . . . . . . . . . . . . . . . . . . . . . . . . . . . . Y  N  NA
      *If used, give example:*

6. Nonverbally communicate attentiveness and openness?

   a. With a relaxed, open posture? . . . . . . . . . . . . . . . . . . . . . . . . . . . . . . . . . . . . . . Y  N  NA

   b. With facilitating gestures, like head nodding? . . . . . . . . . . . . . . . . . . . . . . . . . . . . Y  N  NA

   c. With natural, varied eye contact? . . . . . . . . . . . . . . . . . . . . . . . . . . . . . . . . . . . . Y  N  NA
      *Describe:*

7. Verbally communicate attentiveness and openness?

   a. Using encouraging phrases, like "Please, go on"? . . . . . . . . . . . . . . . . . . . . . . . . . Y  N  NA

   b. Repeating key words or feelings? . . . . . . . . . . . . . . . . . . . . . . . . . . . . . . . . . . . . Y  N  NA

   c. Paraphrasing, reflecting back the essence of what the patient is saying and/or feeling? . . . . . Y  N  NA
      *Describe:*

8. Remain silent where appropriate?

   a. Give the patients an adequate opportunity to ask questions? . . . . . . . . . . . . . . . . . . Y  N  NA

   b. Not interrupt patient? . . . . . . . . . . . . . . . . . . . . . . . . . . . . . . . . . . Y  N  NA
     *Describe:*

9. Respond to patient in a warm and sympathetic manner? . . . . . . . . . . . . . . . . . . . Y  N  NA
   *Describe:*

10. Organize the interview in an orderly fashion?

   a. Proceed from the general to the specific? . . . . . . . . . . . . . . . . . . . . . . . Y  N  NA

   b. Proceed from the less personal to the more personal? . . . . . . . . . . . . . . . . . . Y  N  NA

   c. In history taking, proceed from present to past history? . . . . . . . . . . . . . . . . Y  N  NA

   d. When changing topics, make transitional statements? . . . . . . . . . . . . . . . . . Y  N  NA
     *Describe:*

11. Speak clearly, using appropriate language without jargon? . . . . . . . . . . . . . . . . . . Y  N  NA

## Closing the Interview (Complete Only if Interviewer Got This Far)
*Did they:*

12. Summarize what was said? . . . . . . . . . . . . . . . . . . . . . . . . . . . . . . . Y  N  NA

13. Check whether there were any further concerns or questions? . . . . . . . . . . . . . . . . Y  N  NA

14. Let the patient know what will happen next? . . . . . . . . . . . . . . . . . . . . . . . Y  N  NA

15. Other strategies interviewer used that facilitated the interview:

16. Other strategies interviewer used that blocked the interview:

(Adapted from Course in Health and Human Values, University of Miami School of Medicine, 1982–1985.)

# Patient Assessment Form

Name of Patient: _____

Name of Interviewer: _____

In response to the following, please be as specific as possible.

1. Behavior that facilitated my ability to communicate (e.g., your use of silence, which gave me a chance to collect my thoughts).

2. Behaviors that blocked my ability to communicate (e.g., your use of leading questions, like "You don't have a sore throat, do you?").

3. Information and feelings, if any, that I was unable to share with you.

4. What I wished you had done or asked me.

(Adapted from Course in Health and Human Values, University of Miami School of Medicine, 1982–1985.)

# Interviewer's Self-Critique Form

Circle the appropriate letters. Y = yes, N = no, NA = not applicable.
Note: Where indicated, use space under items to describe and give specific examples of what you did.

Name: _____    Date: _____

## BEGINNING OF THE INTERVIEW

*Did I:*

1. Greet the patient in a friendly, attentive, respectful manner? . . . . . . . . . . . . . . . . Y  N  NA

2. Address introductions of myself and the patient, using the patient's name and my own name? . . Y  N  NA

3. Define the purpose of the interview? . . . . . . . . . . . . . . . . . . . . . . . . . . . . . Y  N  NA

4. Identify and reflect on my initial impressions of the patient? . . . . . . . . . . . . . . . . Y  N  NA

## EXPLORING THE PATIENT'S CONCERNS: GATHERING INFORMATION

*Did I:*

5. Use questions appropriately?

   a. Use a general open-ended approach to help establish the reason(s) for the patient's visit? . . . . Y  N  NA

   b. Use a topic-oriented approach to explore new topics, including the SDoH, using specific
   questions only as needed? . . . . . . . . . . . . . . . . . . . . . . . . . . . . . . Y  N  NA

   c. Avoid premature closed questions that can be answered "yes" or "no"? . . . . . . . . . . . . Y  N  NA

   d. Ask one question at a time? . . . . . . . . . . . . . . . . . . . . . . . . . . . . . . Y  N  NA

   e. Refrain from using leading questions? . . . . . . . . . . . . . . . . . . . . . . . . . . Y  N  NA
   *If used, give example of leading questions to avoid in future:*




6. Nonverbally communicate attentiveness and openness?

   a. With a relaxed, open posture? . . . . . . . . . . . . . . . . . . . . . . . . . . . . . . Y  N  NA

   b. With facilitating gestures, like nodding my head? . . . . . . . . . . . . . . . . . . . . Y  N  NA

   c. With natural, varied eye contact? . . . . . . . . . . . . . . . . . . . . . . . . . . . . Y  N  NA
   *Describe how use of nonverbals felt during interview:*




7. Verbally communicate attentiveness and openness? . . . . . . . . . . . . . . . . . . . . . . Y  N  NA

   a. Using encouraging phrases, like "Please, go on"? . . . . . . . . . . . . . . . . . . . . . Y  N  NA

   b. Repeating key words or feelings? . . . . . . . . . . . . . . . . . . . . . . . . . . . . . Y  N  NA

   c. Paraphrasing, reflecting back the essence of what the patient is saying and/or feeling? . . . . . Y  N  NA
   *Describe:*




8. Remain silent where appropriate?

   a. Give the patient an adequate opportunity to respond to questions? . . . . . . . . . . . . . Y  N  NA

   b. Not interrupt patient? . . . . . . . . . . . . . . . . . . . . . . . . . . . . . . . . . . Y  N  NA
   *Describe positives and negatives of verbal communication:*

9. Reflect on my own feelings and attitudes toward the patient?. . . . . . . . . . . . . . . . . . . . . . . Y  N  NA
   *Describe:*

10. Organize the interview in an orderly fashion?
    a. Proceed from the general to the specific?. . . . . . . . . . . . . . . . . . . . . . . . . . . . . Y  N  NA
    b. Proceed from the less personal to the more personal? . . . . . . . . . . . . . . . . . . . . Y  N  NA
    c. In history taking, proceed from present to past history?. . . . . . . . . . . . . . . . . . . Y  N  NA
    d. When changing topics, make transitional statements? . . . . . . . . . . . . . . . . . . . . Y  N  NA
    *Describe:*

11. Speak clearly, using appropriate language without jargon? . . . . . . . . . . . . . . . . . . . . . Y  N  NA

## CLOSING THE INTERVIEW (COMPLETE ONLY IF YOU GOT THIS FAR)

*Did I:*

12. Summarize what was said?. . . . . . . . . . . . . . . . . . . . . . . . . . . . . . . . . . . . . . . . Y  N  NA
13. Check whether there were any further concerns or questions? . . . . . . . . . . . . . . . . . . Y  N  NA
14. Let the patient know what will happen next? . . . . . . . . . . . . . . . . . . . . . . . . . . . . Y  N  NA
15. Other strategies I used that facilitated the interview:

16. Other strategies that blocked the interview:

(Adapted from Course in Health and Human Values, University of Miami School of Medicine, 1982–1985.)

These exercises are also available online at www.routledge.com/9781638220039.

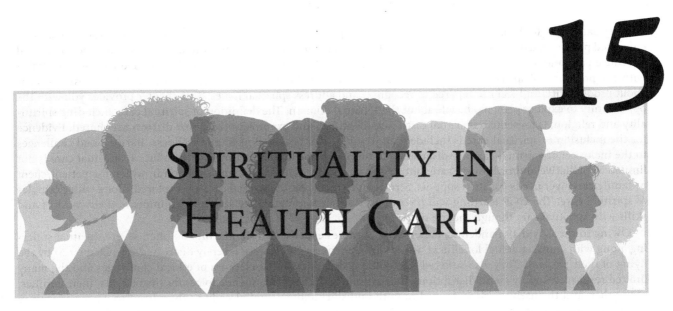

# 15

# SPIRITUALITY IN HEALTH CARE

*Gina Maria Musolino and Darina Sargeant*

## OBJECTIVES

*The learner should be able to:*

- Explore the role of the spiritual domain in providing spiritual health care for patients/clients.
- Discover the components of the biomedical and biopsychosocial models of health care and contrast their implications to holistic care and the relationship to the human movement system.
- Contrast constructs associated with the spiritual domain: spirituality, spirit, religion, religiousness, and religiosity.
- Value the interaction between the spiritual domain and health and wellness.
- Foster understanding, appreciation, and respect for the diversity and individuality of patients' values, beliefs, culture, and spirituality regarding health.
- Compare various levels of spiritual distress in patients.
- Describe challenges, barriers, and opportunities addressing spiritual care for health.
- Administer spiritual assessment and screening tools.
- Appreciate the role of hospital chaplains and clergy as health care team partners for patients'/clients' optimal health.
- Explore personal levels of comfort and value with the spiritual domain.
- Encourage spiritual self-care through attention to the purpose and meaning of one's own life and work, mindfully examining how this influences patient–practitioner interaction (PPI).

Let's begin by considering the first-hand impressions on spirituality from a cancer survivor, thriver, psychologist, and author:

> *Spiritual healing is often experienced as a state of harmony, balance, greater well-being and joyfulness.*
> —Susan Barbara Apollon

Upon reflection, describe how these words make you feel and how they might impact you as a developing health care professional (HCP). Take a moment to write a journal entry.

DOI: 10.4324/9781003525554-15

Spirituality is a tool that can assist the health care professional in providing holistic patient-centered care and enhanced patient outcomes. Literature supports the inclusion of spirituality and/or religion as a coping tool, a method to reduce pain and anxiety, a means to improve quality of life, and a source of hope. HCPs are often uncomfortable with the provision of spiritual care because they perceive it to be beyond their scope of practice, express concerns about productivity, and feel unprepared to recognize and address spiritual issues. This chapter provides you with the opportunity to explore personal beliefs about the spiritual domain. The definition of spiritual care, including spirituality and religion, is presented. Spiritual distress is identified, and examples of spiritual distress are shared. Evidence for the inclusion of spiritual care is included, as are models of health, illness, and wellness. Barriers and challenges to the inclusion of spiritual care are discussed, and tools for spiritual screening are introduced. Spiritual care is not limited to palliative and/or hospice care, but also has a role in wellness and any situation in which the patient/client or family/caregiver needs spiritual support. Strategies to incorporate spiritual care are explored, along with examples of spiritual care. The HCP learning will have opportunities to practice the strategies to improve their comfort and skills with spiritual care though the use of the exercises at the end of the chapter.

Owing to the Covid-19 pandemic, patients and families experienced significant and often severe spiritual suffering along with transcendental loneliness, while simultaneously HCPs were severely distressed (see Chapter 5) by the dying of their patients. They also suffered existential distress due to the plethora of ethical challenges and the many limited resources, supply chain disruptions, and extremely difficult treatment choices for the patients, their families, each other, and themselves. Many turned to faith and spirituality, if not already in their lives, to cope and endure while continuing to provide care and support. HCPs with appropriate training are able to readily offer spiritual support to patients, families, and support networks. HCPs accomplish spiritual support through taking a basic spiritual history to assess for spiritual distress, providing empathic listening and compassionate caring (see Chapters 6, 7, and 12), acknowledging grief and sadness and offering support, while often sharing a sacred and inclusive moment incorporating spirituality in health care. The pandemic led to the eruption of the need for health care to address patients and HCPs as **bio-psycho-social-spiritual beings**.

HCPs collaborate with patients/clients from diverse cultures who have spiritual needs ranging from maintaining health and wellness to facing life-altering circumstances. As culturally competent practitioners and moral agents, HCPs are expected to interact with patients/clients using ethically caring responses. Because spirituality and religion are part of an individual's cultural identity, knowledge of the spiritual domain can be used by HCPs to enhance culturally competent and ethically caring responses.[1,2] The spiritual needs of the patient are not always obvious, so the practitioner must be mindful and listen for them, as in the following example:

Ray is a 45-year-old over-the-road truck driver who recently had a repair of a right rotator cuff tear. Ray's surgeon believes the surgery was successful and anticipates that Ray will be able to return to driving his truck without residual problems. Ray has expressed to his physical therapist, Amy, that he still has a lot of pain and expected to be moving better by now. He tells Amy, "As a young man, I led a pretty wild life, so maybe God is punishing me—maybe that's why I am not getting better." Amy thinks she should talk with Ray about his statement, but she is afraid that her employer or coworkers may think she is overstepping her boundaries as a physical therapist. She decides not to talk to Ray and to just drop it, even though she can see he is terribly upset and his focus on this issue seems to be primarily on his mind. She actually believes that this preoccupation is interfering with motivation to do his home exercises, almost as if he feels that he deserves to be punished.

# SPIRITUAL VERSUS RELIGIOUS

In this chapter, the term **spiritual domain** is used to refer to any concepts associated with the patient's religious and spiritual needs. The spiritual domain influences the patient's/client's perception of the impact of illness and assists the individual in coping with the illness and promoting psychological well-being.[2-4] Knowledge of illness and health models, the spiritual domain, spiritual distress, coping strategies, and aspects of health and wellness will assist the HCP in assessing the patient's/client's spiritual needs. The spiritual domain cannot be limited to illness alone because it is a component of wellness and is a growing focus area for HCP interested in the overall health of the general population and themselves.

Jensen and Mostrom[5] indicated that the level of comfort a physical therapist has in addressing the patient's spiritual/religious needs is related to the HCP's personal comfort with the spiritual domain. The purpose of this chapter is to introduce developing HCPs to key concepts of the spiritual domain, allowing them to explore personal beliefs about the spiritual domain and apply that knowledge to ensure a caring response with all patients/clients and their families.

# MODELS OF ILLNESS AND HEALTH

Historically, HCPs have practiced in an environment guided by the biomedical model of illness in which the focus of treatment is primarily on illness as a biological process. This model is reductionist or single factor in nature and focuses on a biochemical explanation of illness, such as a disease process, presence of microorganisms, or accidents and their resulting biochemical and physiological changes. This is not a holistic model of care. Little attention is given to psychological or social factors present in the individual's life. According to Wade and Halligan,[6] the patient is viewed as victim and, as such, has limited to no responsibility in the cause or outcomes. The biomedical model of illness reflects the separation of mind and body, with a focus on illness, rather than health.

Most HCPs have moved away from this unifactorial view of illness and disease. For example, the American Physical Therapy Association (APTA) adopted the World Health Organization's (WHO) International Classification of Functioning, Disability, and Health (ICF) that is grounded in the biopsychosocial model of health,[7] which considers physical, emotional, and environmental factors present in the individual's life. In the profession of physical therapy, Sahrmann[8,9] focuses on the movement system in physical therapy and not only considers the physiological system that produces movement in the body at all levels (subcellular, cellular, and system), but also the interaction with the environment; modifiers in the nervous system, including psychosocial factors; and personal characteristics, thus building on the ICF model. The individual's accessibility to preventative care, routine health practices, social support, and exposure to various toxins and environmental pollutants can all impact the individual's health and wellness. Thus, the individual has the responsibility to make choices that lead to improved health. The patient/client becomes an active participant in the health care process. The biopsychosocial model of health is rooted in the unity of the mind, body, and spirit and, hence, is multifactorial in nature.

The biopsychosocial model recognizes that there are micro- and macro-level processes that influence health. The micro-level processes include cellular disorders and chemical imbalances. Macro-level processes consider social support, including cultural, family, religious, and spiritual support systems; psychological well-being, including the presence of depression; and environmental factors, such as pollution, accessibility of health care, and education. In sum, the WHO model includes all the factors in the ICF and recognizes that health is dependent on attention to the biological, social, and psychological needs of each person, including the spiritual.

In addition, Puchalsiki[10] suggested that the patient-centered care model, along with the biopsychosocial model, supports the inclusion of spiritual care because these models consider not only the physical aspect of an illness, but also the emotional, social, and spiritual aspects of care. Patient values and preferences, including quality of life and religious/spiritual beliefs, are considered and inform the decision-making process in the patient-centered model of care.

Patient's/client's/families' beliefs about their health locus of control can also be a determinant in clinical outcomes (SDoH). Patients/clients and their families may or may not believe that they are responsible for their health or that they can return to a healthy state even in the presence of a disability or illness. Contemporary HCPs must be aware of each of these factors in screening patients/clients and in developing a plan of care that is individualized and achievable and addresses health and wellness, healing, pain mediation, coping strategies, quality of life, and end-of-life care.[11,12]

The assumptions associated with the models of health and illness can lead to vastly different patient–practitioner interactions. In the most simplistic terms, the biomedical model is hierarchical in nature, with the HCP supplying answers to the health problems and providing a "cure." The patient is the passive recipient of care. Although the patient is not an equal partner in the decision-making process, the HCP expects cooperation from the patient. The cooperative or fully engaged patient will follow the directions given by a HCP without fail, whereas the uncooperative or less engaged patient will not (see Chapter 16) follow the HCP's instructions.

In contrast, the biopsychosocial and patient-centered care models encourage the HCP and the patient to work together to find solutions to problems to enhance the healing process. Understanding the complexity of pain and its impact on the movement system[8] necessitates attention to the contextual factors present in the patient's/client's life. Deep listening and attention to the patient's values and beliefs are critical in understanding how these contextual factors affect healing and the return to a functional and meaningful life. PPI needs to be an exchange of ideas, with all participants valuing the shared information.[13] The relationship between the patient/client and the HCP may serve as a motivator and source of support to the patient and is more egalitarian in nature. The HCP's attitude toward the patient can become a barrier to health and healing if the relationship between the patient and therapist is not based on mutual trust and acceptance. Knowledge of and comfort with the spiritual domain can help prepare the HCP as a positive influence in the healing process, with a *bio-psycho-social-spiritual* approach for health care.[10]

# RELIGION, RELIGIOUSNESS, RELIGIOSITY, SPIRIT, AND SPIRITUALITY

The literature pertaining to the spiritual domain is complex and multidimensional and focuses on the impact of religion, religiousness, religiosity, and spirituality related to patient outcomes with varying levels of consensus.[2,14–21] Definitions of religion and spirituality are different, depending on the approach of the researcher or authors. In general, many authors consider **spirituality** an internal search for the transcendent or sacred based on a personal belief system, and religion is considered external to that process. One view of religion defines it as the rules, rites, and rituals that are an external or exoteric manifestation of beliefs and, as such, separate from spirituality.[22] Spirituality is described as the search for the sacred and forms the substantive approach to religion.[23] "The sacred is the common denominator of religious and spiritual life. It represents the most vital destination sought by the religious/ spiritual person, and it is interwoven into the pathways many people take in life."[24] According to Anandarajah and Hight:[25]

> *Spirituality is a complex and multidimensional part of the human experience. It has cognitive, experiential and behavior aspects. The cognitive or philosophic aspects include the search for meaning, purpose and truth in life and the beliefs and values by which an individual lives. The experiential and emotional aspects involve feelings of hope, love, connection, inner peace, comfort, and support. These are reflected in the quality of an individual's inner resources, the ability to give and receive spiritual love and the types of relationships and connections that exist with self, the community, the environment, and nature, and the transcendent (e.g., power greater than self, a value system, God, cosmic consciousness). The behavior aspects of spirituality involve the way a person externally manifests individual spiritual beliefs and inner spiritual state.*

While Puchalski[10] defines a bit more pragmatically:

> *Spirituality is a dynamic and intrinsic aspect of humanity through which persons seek ultimate meaning, purpose, and transcendence, and experience relationships to self, family, others, community, society, nature and the significant or sacred. Spirituality is expressed through beliefs, values, traditions, and practices.*

It remains clear that definitions of spirituality are multifactorial, including religious heritage, culture, generation, and nationality; a visual construct assists when considering the complexities of spirituality in health care. Investigators de Brito Sena, Damiano, Lucchetti, and Peres[26] conducted a systematic review of the literature pertaining to spirituality and discovered that spirituality consisted of 24 different dimensions, which, not surprisingly, most often related to connectedness and the meaning of life. According to the researchers, spirituality presents as a human and individual aspect which led to their construction of a representative, quantifiable framework for the construct (Figure 15.1) to assist in integration and understanding for health care.[25]

**Figure 15.1** Spirituality Framework (From de Brito Sena MA, Damiano RF, Lucchetti G, Peres MFP. Defining spirituality in healthcare: a systematic review and conceptual framework. *Front Psychol.* 2021 Nov 18;12:756080. doi: 10.3389/fpsyg.2021.756080.)

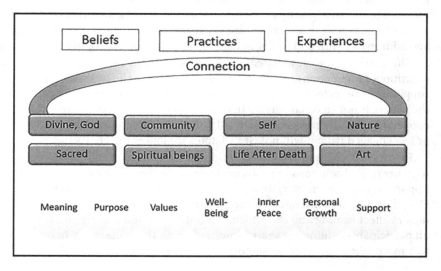

The framework consists of three axes, is not hierarchical, and is considered to be fluid depending upon one's individual context and experiences. The starting point, first axis (upper section) is composed of beliefs, practices, and experiences, promoting connection. These aspects are assessed via validated instruments; e.g., Spiritual Involvement and Beliefs Scale (SIBS) and Spiritual Well-Being Scale (SWBS).[27] The second axis (middle section) consists of potential aspects which may be connected through spiritual beliefs, practices, or experiences. Finally, the third axis (lower section) refers to the development of values, personal growth, and sensations of meaning, purpose in life, well-being, support, and inner peace through connection with something that can affect the behavior of the individual.

Other views of religion consider spiritual or internal beliefs as essential and inseparable components of religion. Psychologists who center their work in the spiritual domain speak of religion as having a substantive and functional purpose in an individual's life. This description of religion is characterized by the search for meaning "related to the sacred" or religiousness.[23] **Religiosity** is a term used in the literature to describe the degree to which a person's life is influenced by religious beliefs and practices.

When spirituality is solely viewed as an extension of religion, it is labeled **religious spirituality**. When spirituality is perceived as independent of religion, it is labeled **secular spirituality**. Hill and Pargament[24] contended that the division of religion and spirituality implies that spirituality is good, whereas religion *can be* bad. Although some patients/clients may have a poor or negative experience with traditional religion, that experience tends to be the exception for most people.[24] Individuals display varying levels of conviction in their religious beliefs, so it is important for HCPs to listen for clues about the level of importance of religion, faith, and spirituality in the patient's/client's life. Notably, scoping review results indicated lesbian gay bisexual (LGB) persons consider spirituality "as a more resonating construct"[28 (p 649)] than religion; yet not all LGB communities were represented the reviewed eligible studies.[(pp 650–51)] For some, forms of spiritual expression were anchored to religious practice, while others were belief and faith expressions outside formal religious confines. Spiritual expressions were associated with LGB satisfaction and life direction.[28]

Being a religious and/or spiritual person does not equate to being immune from illness, however religious persons cope more readily with illness and going through the healing process; spirituality has also been associated with a longer lifespan due to mental health coping strategies.[29] For many patients/clients, religion is always a guiding force, whereas for others it becomes more important during times of illness or injury.

# RELIGION, SPIRITUALITY, AND HEALTH CARE

Strict religious beliefs can sometimes be at odds with medical practice, such as when a religion forbids the use of blood or blood products or the use of vaccines for prevention of illness. For many people, however, religion, faith, and/or spirituality offer tremendous help in coping with pain, uncertainty, spiritual suffering, and/or any change they may be experiencing.[30–34]

Some individuals may also use religion in a maladaptive manner; just as in the case of Ray, they may believe that the pain or illness they are experiencing is a punishment for a past transgression and decide against treatment that could restore their health.[35] It is important to gather information about a patient's spiritual needs during initial assessment in order to provide holistic care. But all HCPs must exercise caution not to proselytize or force their own religious beliefs on others, judge individuals with different belief systems as inferior or unworthy of assistance, or in any way discriminate based upon the patient's or their own religious beliefs.[2,15,36] Also, one must not assume that, because a person ascribes to a certain religion, they practice every tenet of that faith or belief in daily life. HCPs should explore how faith and religion, beliefs, and practices are part of those individuals' spiritual practices or not. HCPs should become familiar with these practices but make no assumptions for individual patients and consider each patient's/client's individual spiritual history.

For individuals who harbor negative feelings toward traditional religions, spirituality viewed separately from religion can be a reasonable alternative coping strategy. They can ignore the negative thoughts associated with religion and focus instead on hope and finding meaning in the situation. Leaders in patient-centered spiritual care include physicians Koenig[16] and Puchalski,[10] who believe that HCPs cannot ignore a patient's/client's spiritual or religious beliefs because both assist the patient/client to cope and find meaning in all experiences, including health care.

# SPIRITUALITY

Although spirituality has numerous definitions in the literature, the consistent components include the search for meaning and purpose in life; connection with others, nature, or a higher being; and transcendence or movement beyond oneself.[2,24,37] Spirituality is a characteristic of all cultures.[2] In Western culture, spiritual development is grounded in the theories of Jung, Erickson, Frankl, Kohler, and Fowler and is influenced by Eastern cultural beliefs and practices.[38] Scandurra's[39] definition—"[s]pirituality is a fundamental, everyday-life process involving and connecting to self, others, nature, and to a larger meaning or purpose"—is useful for persons who may not have a belief in a supreme being. For the purposes of this chapter, we will refer to spirituality as an internal set of beliefs and needs that function to help discover the sacred and meaning in life, and religion will refer to one external way that people act on their need for spirituality in their lives.

As altruistic HCPs, we want to do everything possible to help our patients get back into functional life again, to heal and thrive. That is our primary purpose, no matter what discipline we practice. Illness and injury interrupt our lives, and once the original insult has been assimilated or chronic disease becomes a reality of their lives, patients often start asking the larger questions about meaning and purpose of these events in their own lived experiences.

In addition, spirituality is considered a component of wellness that can contribute to health and well-being. Hettler[40] defined wellness as "an active process through which people become aware of, and make choices toward a more successful existence." Hettler developed a hexagon model of wellness in which he identified six dimensions of wellness: social, occupational, spiritual, physical, intellectual, and emotional. Spirituality as a component of wellness is associated with balance in life, as well as quality of life. Other wellness models offer similar categorizations, e.g., Ardell's Model in Three Domains, Robins' Seven Dimensions of Wellness, and either implicitly or explicitly include spirituality as a dimension.[41] Ardell's model explores wellness in three domains: physical, mental, and meaning and purpose.[41]

As individuals, HCPs give so much of themselves to others, and in the care of others, we need a place to replenish ourselves. Assuming that spirituality is a connection with others or with a greater being and nature and/or transcendence beyond self, HCPs can utilize spirituality to help their patients find meaning in their lives and to find balance in their own personal and professional lives. In addition, HCPs have a professional responsibility to address the health and wellness of society and of individuals in special populations.[42] The APTA House of Delegates[43] has encouraged knowledge of all components of wellness as essential for physical therapy practice because, as HCPs we must play a positive role in the promotion of healthy lifestyles for persons with and without existing disabilities and we must advocate and create programs for wellness, injury prevention, and improved quality of life.[44] The APTA Vision,[45] discussed in Chapter 11, embraces the profession's impact on society: "Transforming society by optimizing movement to improve the human experience." What is the vision of your chosen profession and the tenets or guiding principles to uphold or achieve the vision? Explore how you have seen HCPs impact society or how you plan to within your chosen profession. Consider the impact on the human spirit in your explorations.

# RESEARCH EVIDENCE SUPPORTING SPIRITUAL CARE—POSITIVE HEALTH IMPACTS

The incorporation of spirituality into holistic patient care is reported to contribute to health, wellness, pain control, delayed morbidity, reduction of depressive symptoms, and healing. Koenig[2,16] cited numerous studies that support the role of spirituality and religion in the promotion and maintenance of health. Udermann's[46] literature review, exploring the role of spirituality on health and healing, discovered a positive association between spirituality and health. The field of psychoneuroimmunology considers the complex interconnection of the mind, body, and spirit through the study of the limbic system and its influence on the autonomic nervous system. Chronic stress is linked to the development of autoimmune diseases, chronic illness, and pain.[47] Seybold's[48] literature review relating health to religiosity and spirituality, reported many health benefits associated with spirituality and religious practices:

- Increased longevity and decreased morbidity as a result of healthy habits (no smoking, moderate diet and alcohol intake)
- Social support
- Increased self-esteem
- Increased self-efficacy
- Increased levels of serotonin during meditation
- Decreased pain
- Decreased cortisol levels

- Increased blood flow to the frontal lobes with decreased blood flow to the parietal lobes during prayer and meditation

- Reduced sympathetic nervous system activity and increased parasympathetic nervous system activation

Increased activation of the parasympathetic nervous system through religious or spiritual engagement promotes relaxation, improved sleep, decreased heart and respiratory rates, and decreased blood pressure, and can result in improved autoimmune function, less depression, and an improved sense of well-being and general health.[49-51] The literature supports the use of the spiritual in assisting patients/clients and families in coping with life-altering events and pain.[10,14,16,52] Mactavish and Iwasaki[53] reported that individuals with disabilities utilize the spiritual domain for stress coping in different ways—through organized religion, culturally defined activities, prayer, meditation, exercise, or time away from others spent in connecting with the transcendent. Idler and Kasl[54] found that elderly persons who attended church services regularly demonstrated less functional decline or disability over time and lower ratings on pain scales. A study of 132 men and women with stage B heart failure (asymptomatic, but at elevated risk for the development of symptomatic heart failure due to structural changes in the heart) examined a potential association between depression and spiritual well-being in patients with asymptomatic heart failure as a means of slowing disease progression, improving quality of life, and reducing death. Researchers determined that higher levels of spiritual well-being and a greater sense of life meaning and peace were positively associated with fewer depressive symptoms,[55] suggesting that spiritual care interventions could be a potential treatment consideration for patients with asymptomatic heart failure. These spiritual interventions can include such activities as journaling, having a connection to nature, meditation, prayer, yoga, utilizing a spiritual coach, art, music, and guided imagery.

Some research does exist supporting the value of the spiritual domain in rehabilitation care for screening, building trust, coping with pain and improved outcomes, discovering a sense of purpose, interacting with compassion, coping in matters of life and death, and promoting relaxation during physical therapy procedures.[56-61] Pressman et al.[59] used an index of religiousness and ambulatory status at discharge to demonstrate a correlation between distances walked and level of religiousness. Elderly women with higher levels of religious practice exhibited better ambulation status and a lower level of depression following hip fractures.[59] The researchers concluded that the lower level of depression present in elderly women with strong religious practices contributed to improved physical therapy outcomes. Mackey and Sparling[62] reported in their qualitative study that older women with terminal cancer found strength, acceptance, and improved quality of life through their spiritual beliefs. They identified that this acceptance and improved quality of life were accomplished by the physical therapist listening carefully to reminiscences and stories about the important meanings in their lives. Similar skills are utilized in nursing. Johnston-Taylor[63] addressed dimensions of listening for HCPs, including the following:

- *Intellectual—The HCP can reiterate the intellectual or factual content of what the patient has said in a way that the patient recognizes.*

- *Emotional—The HCP can identify and reflect to the patient the deepest feelings or significance of what they have said.*

- *Physical—The HCP maintains an awareness of the nonverbal and postural messages sent from the patient's body (e.g., voice quality, posture, facial expressions, the look in their eyes) as well as the HCP's own body's physical responses to the incoming messages (e.g., neck tension, flushed face, knot in the stomach). These messages then inform the HCP's responses. For example, a nurse feels exhausted and slumps her shoulders while listening to a patient talk about several losses. Such information can inform the nurse that the losses are tiring for the patient, as well as for herself.*

- *Spiritual—The listener has an awareness of the Holy in the relationship, a sense of divine presence, and consequently an openness to whatever transpires in the conversation.*

Quality of life is individually determined and has different meanings for different persons. Stuifbergen et al.[44] indicated that quality of life is a complex construct dependent on three sets of factors: context, antecedent variables, and health-promoting behaviors. It is highly subjective and depends on context, such as the perceived severity of the condition. Antecedent variables include barriers, resources, self-efficacy, and acceptance. Barriers may include those imposed by society or those perceived by the person. Resources may include financial, emotional, and cultural resources, to name a few. Religious and spiritual support has been shown to be a positive influence on an individual's quality of life. Belief in self and the ability to overcome a circumstance can influence an individual's health and quality of life.[64] Acceptance of what has occurred or will occur allows the individual to focus on the possibilities rather than the limitations. As noted earlier, the presence of health-promoting behaviors demonstrates the individual's belief in the ability to influence outcomes.

The spiritual dimension should be considered a fundamental component of the quality of life and well-being of patients with neurological diseases, significantly influencing coping abilities with disease.[65] In a systematic mapping review of the literature,[65] researchers charted the knowledge of the spirituality experienced by people with neurological and neurodegenerative disorders and its influence on outcomes and the ability to cope with the disease. Most studies noted positive correlations with improved health, higher quality of life and well-being with the adoption of religious beliefs and/or spirituality.[66] Evidence suggests that spiritual practices help decrease the stress-producing hormones and increase the numbers of neurotransmitters for pain relief.[67]

Despite so many positive outcomes reported in the literature, several researchers believe that many of the study methodologies are flawed.[68] Therefore, HCPs must approach the literature critically while considering the expressed needs of the patient/client/family when making decisions about the inclusion of spiritual care. One cannot ignore the potential ramifications of the growing body of literature, and HCPs are encouraged to be ever mindful of the spiritual influence in their patients'/clients' lived experiences within the health care arenas.

The spiritual domain can be an excellent source of strength for coping with loss, potential loss, pain, and the dying process. It can also contribute to an improved quality of life and improved ability to cope with depressive symptoms, such as loss of hope and withdrawal from social interaction.[2,16,59,69–72] In a study reported by Murphy et al.,[73] patients with amyotrophic lateral sclerosis "who were more religious or spiritual had more hope" and used prayer and attendance at church to help them cope with the changes they experienced. In a study by Anderson et al.,[74] 74% of individuals who sustained spinal cord injuries as children or adolescents reported that their spiritual beliefs helped them to cope with the injury. Kaufman et al.[75] reported a slower progression of Alzheimer's disease in people with higher levels of spirituality and private religious activities. In a study conducted with 293 Indonesian individuals with congestive heart disease, the researchers concluded that higher levels of spirituality were associated with fewer depressive symptoms, less anxiety, and less anger.[76]

Now, let's reflect on the action of a caregiver by considering the following example of spirituality and religious faith in action:

Louise is a professional woman, age 58 and married with three children, who was diagnosed with pancreatic cancer. Louise receives chemotherapy on a weekly basis depending on her blood count. One evening, Louise experienced extreme nausea and vomiting that was accompanied by severe pain. She was unable to take oral pain medications due to nausea. As she lay on the bathroom floor, she said aloud, "God, you promised me that you would not give me more pain than I could manage. I cannot handle this. You have to take it away." Louise considered going to the emergency department for a pain shot but believed that she would not be a priority there and was afraid that she may be even more uncomfortable lying on a stretcher. Her husband lifted her from the floor and took her to her bed. As she lay down, she continued to pray to God to uphold His promise. Louise reported that she fell asleep and was pain free when she awoke. She remained pain free throughout the night. Louise reported that her pain returned in the morning but not to the level she had experienced the preceding evening. Louise believed that God kept His promise. She said that she knew that pain was a reality in her life, but she said she could cope with it knowing that God had not deserted her.

In this example, Louise used her spiritual and religious beliefs to provide hope that she would not be abandoned and that her pain could be controlled. Her belief in a power beyond herself provided her with hope, which allowed her to relax and sleep. Recent science has confirmed that negative symptoms can be mitigated by a change in belief emphasizing hope and optimism.[77]

What would be your level of comfort if Louise shared her story with you the next day? As a HCP working with special populations, in this case a person who has cancer, you must not only be aware of the specific physical and cognitive needs of the patient, but you must also be aware of the patient's spiritual needs. As a future health care professional, you must ask yourself, "Would I be able to listen and respond to what Louise has shared?" Or would you quickly move past it by changing the focus of the conversation?

Discomfort with a patient's/client's/family's spiritual needs may be a reality, but ignoring a patient's religious or spiritual needs is not acceptable. By ignoring their statements, you may cause the patient/client embarrassment and undermine the trust relationship you established. Baetz and Bowen[31] shared important perspectives:

*Asking patients about their religious or spiritual beliefs may allow for exploration of potential positive or negative forms of coping or beliefs that would otherwise go unnoticed. Sensitive inquiry and referral to appropriate sources to deal with spiritual struggles are encouraged as part of patient-centered care.*

Redirection of the conversation away from personal disclosures, such as religious, faith, or spiritual beliefs, undermines the patient–therapist relationship and ultimately diminishes the likelihood that the HCP's interventions will be successful. The patient will likely feel embarrassed and be less likely to share other personal information that could inform the HCP's clinical decisions. Mackey and Sparling[62] believed that physical therapists can help patients who are receiving hospice care to improve the quality of life by listening to the patient's thoughts about the meaning of life through reminiscence. This is an excellent illustration of using spiritual care and listening to help a patient cope with impending death (see Chapter 19). On occasion, differences in religious beliefs between patients and caregivers can lead to misunderstanding. Consider the following example:

Kathy Winslow is a nurse in a skilled nursing facility who is working with Mrs. Randall, a 78-year-old patient with a diagnoses of congestive heart failure and Parkinson's disease. Mrs. Randall asked Kathy if she would have a priest come to see her for anointing of the sick. Kathy is concerned that Mrs. Randall is depressed and is giving up rather than fighting to get better. Kathy tells Mrs. Randall that she will contact the priest for her. Kathy feels very troubled and considers calling the doctor to report Mrs. Randall's depression.

In this situation, the nurse is not comfortable with a religious ritual requested by the patient. Kathy does not realize that Mrs. Randall finds solace in receiving grace afforded through the anointing of the sick sacrament. On the surface, she is being supportive of Mrs. Randall's wishes by agreeing to contact the priest. However, her concern about the patient being depressed may be unfounded and may lead to unnecessary medical and pharmaceutical interventions and result in Kathy being less emotionally available to Mrs. Randall. If Kathy speaks with the chaplain/priest and shares her concerns, the chaplain/priest can explain the purpose of this sacramental ritual as not preparing the patient for death, but rather as providing spiritual strength. Open dialogue about spirituality and religion is paramount for true patient-centered care.

# OVERCOMING DISCOMFORT

How can you address the person's spiritual needs if you are not comfortable with the spiritual domain? Becoming familiar with signs of spiritual distress can be helpful in identifying an individual who is at risk and could benefit from spiritual care. At the very least, you must acknowledge the sacredness of the person's statement by reflecting to the person the importance of the statement (see Chapter 8). In the example of Louise, you might say, "Your faith in God seemed to help you relax enough to get the rest you needed last night" or "I have worked with other people who had similar experiences." The patient then knows that you have heard what was said and recognizes that you did not negatively judge their admission. Depending on your level of comfort, you might disclose more in your response with a statement such as, "Focusing on God has helped me deal with pain in my life, also." Then you must assess the patient's reactions to determine whether there is any level of discomfort present for the patient, and you would need to modify your actions accordingly. Once again, it is never appropriate to detail your own religious beliefs in the hopes of convincing patients to believe as you believe (proselytizing). Your role as a clinician is to support and assist through active listening and empathy. Even if patients ask you to go into detail about your beliefs, the patients are most often seeking support of their own beliefs. Simply redirecting the conversation to them and the patient's concerns will be most helpful. For example, say, "I'm more interested in what you believe and how that is helping you cope, or not, at this time."

# SPIRITUAL DISTRESS

Patients in religious- and non-religious-based institutions experience varying levels of spiritual distress: spiritual pain, spiritual alienation, spiritual anxiety, spiritual guilt, spiritual anger, spiritual loss, and spiritual despair.[78] Likewise, the concept of spiritual care has implications for HCPs in any setting—inpatient, outpatient, home care, telehealth, and school systems. HCPs who collaborate closely with patients are often the first to notice the signs of spiritual distress. The most basic level involves spiritual pain, in which patients may experience a loss of support from their normal spiritual or religious sources. The patient may be physically unable to attend services if they are homebound or lacking transportation resources; may be unable to watch religious programs; may be hesitant to read the Bible late into the night out of concern for disturbing a roommate, if hospitalized; or may feel unable to pray or find a sense of peace because of feeling overwhelmed with the situation. Spiritual alienation is precipitated by material concerns, such as financial resources, pain, and an inability to take care of family obligations or fear of the unknown that takes the person's attention.

Patients often express their concerns to HCPs by indicating that they need to return home to take care of a loved one or that they do not know how they will pay for all the care they are receiving. Spiritual anxiety is the fear that the persons or group who normally provide spiritual support will judge the person as no longer worthy of such support. Spiritual guilt is associated with feelings of sinfulness, such as the person who believes that somehow having more faith would have protected them from this situation or the belief that they are being punished for leading a bad life. Patients sometimes say this in jest, but further probing by the HCP may reveal that these are very real concerns for the person. Spiritual anger may be manifested by blaming others or God for what has happened. Spiritual loss is the feeling that the patient no longer has the support of others or God, and there is a loss of meaning in life. The most severe manifestation of spiritual distress is spiritual despair. Once hope is lost, the person believes that they have no future and often gives up. Any level of spiritual distress could affect the health care outcomes because the patient's/client's ability/desire to focus on tasks will likely diminish. The HCP is responsible for noticing spiritual distress and communicating that observation to the appropriate persons. This may involve a referral to pastoral care; contact with nursing, physicians, psychology, or social service; contact with family members with the patient's permission; or a gentle encouragement to the patient to contact their own clergy/rabbi, pastor/priest, shaman, or other spiritual leader.

# SPIRITUAL DOMAIN IN PATIENT CARE

Not all HCPs engage in end-of-life care or in care of patients with permanently life-altering events. However, every HCP has or will have patients who are afraid of the potential outcome of their injuries or illnesses, who have short-term, life-altering events with which they must cope, or who have acute or chronic pain. It is irrelevant whether the injury/illness is transient or permanent because the normal routine of the patient is altered and coping strategies will need to be adapted to meet their changing emotional, physical, and spiritual needs.

HCPs must recognize when to incorporate spirituality into patient care as well as when a patient's spiritual needs are beyond their scope of practice. Clinicians should pay attention to cues that patients may give, such as religious symbols in their room, statements about God, search for meaning or purpose in what they are experiencing, feelings of despair or loss of support, and the methods they use to cope with the situation.[79] As stated previously, at the very least, HCPs have a responsibility to provide holistic, patient-centered care, including responding to the patient's physical, intellectual, emotional, and spiritual needs. Hospitalized or homebound persons often lose their spiritual and social support systems because they cannot physically attend religious services or have more limited contact with persons who normally provide them with spiritual support.[47] At a time when individuals require additional emotional and spiritual support, there is generally less support available. The Joint Commission recognized this need and created a regulation requiring HCPs to consider the spiritual and religious needs of patients.[80,81] The regulation may be technically addressed by asking patients about their religious affiliation, but that question alone does not truly assess the spiritual and religious needs of the patients/clients. The Joint Commission provided guiding queries for supporting patient spiritual and/or religious needs:[81]

- Who or what provides the patient with strength and hope?
- Does the patient use prayer in their life?
- How does the patient express their spirituality?
- How would the patient describe their philosophy of life?
- What type of spiritual/religious support does the patient desire?
- What is the name of the patient's clergy, ministers, chaplains, pastor, rabbi, or other spiritual leader?
- What does suffering mean to the patient?
- What does dying mean to the patient?
- What are the patient's spiritual goals?
- Is there a role of church/synagogue in the patient's life?
- How does your faith help the patient cope with illness?
- How does the patient keep going day after day?

- What helps the patient get through this health care experience?
- How has illness affected the patient and their family?

It cannot be stated often enough that HCPs must be vigilant to avoid judgment about a person's beliefs or non-beliefs. HCPs should not make patients feel uncomfortable with explicit and/or unsolicited conversation about personal religious or spiritual beliefs. Although the HCP may feel comfortable offering to pray for the patient, this should only be done after the HCP has clearly established that the patient values prayer. For some patients, the offer for prayer would be viewed as proselytization, and the patient–practitioner relationship could be negatively impacted.

What should the practitioner do if the patient discloses that they feel that they deserve this illness? When a patient discloses this level of spiritual distress, it is imperative that the HCP recognizes that the level of spiritual care needed by the patient is beyond their skills/scope. Referral to persons trained in spiritual care is required. The HCP can remain aware and supportive of the patient's spiritual care but cannot be the sole source of spiritual care when the individual's needs are more complex.

# HELPFUL TOOLS TO ASSIST

How can the HCP address the patient's spiritual needs given limited time with patients and limited knowledge of world religions? Knowledge of all the religions that exist is not an expectation HCPs should have for themselves because that would be unrealistic. The nuances are too complex and too subject to personal interpretation to allow accurate understanding across multiple religions. Instead, it is appropriate to ask the patient questions about how the clinician can support their spiritual or religious beliefs and needs. The patient should be able to identify rules and rituals that may alter how you interact with the individual and the family. A spiritual history, which is a screen for spiritual needs, can be quickly conducted by the health care professional. Short questionnaires exist that allow the clinician to quickly determine how to support the patient and can be readily incorporated into the initial subjective examination or later as needed. Tools such as © FICA,[19] SPIRITual History,[22] B-E-L-I-E-F,[82] and HOPE[25,83] provide the HCP with the information in 5 minutes or less. Each of these questionnaires has common elements related to inquiry about the beliefs or faith life of the patient, how the beliefs support the patient in daily life and during times of stress, and how the HCP can support their beliefs during care.

HCPs should familiarize themselves with these tools to determine which tool works best for a given patient or situation. Although the HCP may be the person who initially identifies spiritual distress, referral to the chaplain or spiritual advisor is necessary because the spiritual staff have the training to perform a more formal spiritual assessment and formulate a spiritual plan of care.[2,25,84] The most basic method a HCP can use to determine whether a patient would like spiritual assistance is by asking the person for permission to contact pastoral care personnel or a chaplain and requesting a visit if the patient displays signs of spiritual distress. A team approach to spiritual care is essential and demands ongoing communication with the patient/client, family members, spiritual leaders, and HCP.

Developed by a team at Brown University School of Medicine, many HCPs elect to employ the spiritual assessment, HOPE tool within the initial patient interview.

**HOPE Questions:**[25]

**H**: Sources of hope, meaning, comfort, strength, peace, love, and connection

**O**: Organized religion

**P**: Personal spirituality and practices

**E**: Effects on health care and end-of-life issues

One can approach these queries by introducing the fact that many patients/clients have religious or spiritual beliefs affecting their health care choices; so, I would like to inquire:

*(H) Where do you find hope and/or comfort with of health matters, illness, or pain? When things get tough, what keeps you going?*

*(O) Tell me if organized religion has a place in your life, or in your family's or support networks'?*

*(P) Are there spiritual beliefs and/or practices essential or vital to you personally?*

*(E) Are there ways that your personal beliefs affect your health care choices or might provide guidance as we discuss decisions about your care or care near the end of your life?*

Mr. Cunningham experienced a myocardial infarction 3 days ago, which has left him reeling with confusion and fear. He is currently awaiting discharge from a stepdown unit following the insertion of a stent, and his physician has ordered physical therapy for weakness and fatigue. He is scheduled to begin cardiac rehab in two weeks. When his physical therapist, Erin, came to his bedside to evaluate and examine him, she recognized immediately that his anxiety and fear seemed to dominate his responses to her questions. More than once, he mentioned that he did not understand how God could allow this to happen after all he had done to take care of himself, and he felt afraid to get back into life again for fear of what God would do next. He asked Erin, "Why do you think this happened to me?"

Erin decided to do a quick FICA[19,25,73–85] spiritual history and screening in order to plan how to arrange for Mr. Cunningham's support. She told him she recognized that he seemed to be struggling with spiritual questions, and although this was not her area of professional expertise, she asked his permission to gather a little more specific information to better know how to help him. Here is how she proceeded with the FICA:[19,84]

- **F (Faith)**: "Mr. Cunningham, do you consider yourself a religious or spiritual person?" He responded, "Yes, I've gone to the Lutheran church regularly since I was a child."

- **I (Importance and influence)**: "How important is your religion to you?" He responded, "It really serves as a cornerstone of my life. My faith in God and my ability to worship regularly keeps me going."

- **C (Community)**: "Besides attending church regularly, do you feel like you are a member of a spiritual community?" He said, "Yes, I look forward to meeting my pastor and my friends after church for coffee hour, and I am a Deacon in the church, so I help serve the congregation."

- **A (Address or application)**: "It seems as if these questions are foremost on your mind, and your rehab will benefit greatly once you get a chance to talk about this with your pastor or spiritual community members. What can I do to help you get your religious and spiritual questions answered?" Mr. Cunningham hesitated and then said, "Well, I have been fussing about calling my pastor. He is so busy. And I just can't shake this feeling that somehow I am at fault for all of this and I feel so guilty."

Erin then offered to have a chaplain talk with him. She also offered him the option to have his social worker help contact his pastor. Both solutions reinforce the idea that once these issues around faith and meaning were talked out, he very likely would feel more at ease and freer to engage fully in his rehab program.

Any of these assessment tools are helpful to ascertain the spiritual domain. Sometimes a full spiritual screening evaluation is not even necessary. If the HCP practices in a hospital, assisted living, skilled nursing facility, or other inpatient facility, spiritual care can be accomplished in several ways: by listening attentively to the patient, using reflective communication skills (i.e., reflection of content, feeling, and meaning), offering a warm blanket when the patient is cold, remarking on pictures of family and friends at the patient's bedside or in the home, or offering to keep the person in their prayers if the patient has made it clear that prayer is important to them. If the HCP is seeing the patient in an outpatient setting or home care, the clinician could ask the patient whether they have someone with whom to discuss spiritual or religious questions or who can provide spiritual support. The HCP should feel comfortable enough to ask probing questions if the patient discloses spiritual concerns during the subjective interview or normal conversations. In addition, clinicians can be respectful of the spiritual care of the patient if they happen upon a shared spiritual interaction by stepping outside or silently standing by during a spiritual interaction between the patient and pastoral care. The presence of the HCP is comforting to the patient and indicates that the therapist recognizes the value of prayer for the patient.

Sometimes a patient may ask the HCP to pray with them during care. This can be an uncomfortable situation for many HCPs. It may be more comfortable to ask the patient to lead the prayer because the patient knows what petitions to include in the prayer. For the HCP who is comfortable leading prayer, it is generally less likely to offend the patient if the clinician invokes guidance throughout the treatment session, as well as patient relaxation, as part of the prayer.

# CHALLENGES SUPPORTING PATIENTS' SPIRITUAL NEEDS

What should the HCP do if the patient is offended by questions within the spiritual domain? Just as many HCPs are not comfortable with the spiritual domain, there will be patients/clients who prefer not to talk about personal beliefs. In approaching a delicate subject such as spirituality or religion, it is helpful to preface the interaction with a statement such as "Sometimes patients want their HCP to be aware of religious or spiritual beliefs, so I need to ask you some questions about that. Is that okay with you?" If the patient says no, then naturally you would not proceed further. If the patient says yes, you can ask them to tell you what is important for you to know. Another approach would be to say, "I need to ask you some questions about how I might support your religious or spiritual beliefs while you are my patient." You would then proceed with one of the tools noted earlier and/or guiding queries[81] for religious/spiritual assessment (© FICA,[19,72–85] SPIRITual History,[22] B-E-L-I-E-F,[82] and HOPE[25,83]).

What should the HCP do if the patient loses focus on therapy and focuses instead on converting the HCP to their religious beliefs? There is a danger in asking about religious and spiritual beliefs because the individual may view the question as an opportunity to convert you to their religious beliefs. The HCP can manage this situation by thanking the patient for sharing information about their religious beliefs and then redirecting the conversation to the task at hand.

In summary, HCPs must stand with patients/clients in their spiritual pain. How can HCPs accomplish this when they do not have training as spiritual leaders? When the HCP remains in touch with their humanity and acknowledges personal mortality, it is easier to be present with the patient. Quite simply, a gentle touch, a nod, or some other affirmation that the patient is not alone can be shared by the health care professional, thereby establishing the human connection during a time of potential alienation and fear.

There are times when the patient's spiritual needs are more intense and require more advanced skills than reminiscencing, listening, or standing silently as prayer occurs. During the patient's/client's times of escalated spiritual needs, the HCP should make a referral to professionals trained in spiritual care, such as chaplains and/or pastoral care.

# BARRIERS TO INCORPORATING SPIRITUAL CARE

As noted earlier, barriers to incorporating spiritual care are ever present. Barriers may include concerns regarding scope of practice, preference for the biomedical model, productivity requirements, and personal discomfort with the spiritual domain. For many HCPs, one barrier to providing spiritual care to the patient is the concern that spiritual care is beyond one's scope of practice and should not be part of the HCP's plan of care. As noted earlier, to provide holistic care, the patient's spiritual domain must be considered as physical symptoms and signs are affected by the mind and spirit.

A second possible barrier to incorporating spiritual care for some HCPs is that they may be more comfortable with the reductionistic point of view afforded by the biomedical model, preferring not to delve into the societal, spiritual, and personal factors that influence health and return to a meaningful life. Because many professional associations have adopted the WHO model/ICF and the patient-centered care model, it is less likely today that HCPs will consider the biomedical model superior to the biopsychosocial model.

A third possible barrier is productivity, which is a very real concern for HCPs. Listening to patients and addressing their spiritual needs appear to use more time, but when a patient believes that the clinician has their best interests in mind, the level of trust increases, and the patient is more likely to respond in a positive manner to the interventions suggested by the HCP, therefore resulting in less time needed overall. Ultimately, this often results in fewer refused treatments, better control of pain, and increased functional ability when the patient–practitioner relationship is based on mutual trust and an ethically caring response that is attentive to the patient's values, beliefs, and practices.

Finally, the HCP's level of comfort with the spiritual domain can indeed be a barrier to implementing spiritual care for patients, their families, support networks, and caregivers.[10,82,84–88] Many studies have reported maladaptive coping strategies of HCPs and caregivers.[87] In a study conducted with 108 pediatricians, the researchers[86] noted that physicians who were less comfortable in addressing spirituality/religion were less likely to value referral to pastoral care personnel/chaplains than those physicians who recognized the value of the chaplain in the pediatric and oncology settings. Both spiritual needs and spiritual coping strategies are warranted in integrating spirituality in health care; along with a spiritually sensitive approach for spiritual health care with patients, families, caregivers, as well as peer colleagues.[85–88] Increasing your knowledge about the spiritual domain and pastoral care professionals/chaplains will be helpful, and exploration of your level of comfort with the spiritual domain is necessary. At the end of this chapter, you will find exercises to assist you in reviewing and/or developing your comfort zone with the spiritual domain.

# CONCLUSION

HCPs may enhance the quality of PPIs by increasing their level of comfort with the spiritual domain. Knowledge of the evidence that supports and refutes the inclusion of spiritual care as part of holistic patient care remains essential for the HCPs to determine the value of including spiritual care as part of the plan of care. Exploration of the spiritual domain informs HCPs of the most effective and efficient methods to include the provision of spiritual support to patients as an important aspect of holistic, patient-centered care. Let's end the chapter considering the Blessing of the Hands for HCPs offered for DPT HCP learners about to transition from classroom to clinical education practice settings, embarking on patient-centered health care.

# BLESSING OF THE HANDS

*In the name of God, compassionate and merciful,*
*Almighty and Righteous,*
*We bless you;*
*May this anointing of your hands yield refined strength and sure skill,*
*to optimize the human movement system.*
*May your hands be proficient to facilitate movement for all lives*
*as you touch others with God's Grace.*
*May your hands provide adept joint mobilization*
*while also mobilizing the spirit in the lives of those you serve.*
*In the skillful palpation of tissues,*
*may your fingers carefully discern and sense the wonder*
*of a body fearfully and brilliantly created by God.*
*Through your sense of touch,*
*may you be mindfully competent in clinical reasoning,*
*By your touch,*
*may others come to understand and discover more fully*
*God's healing relief.*
*As the spirit works to restore health to the soul,*
*may your empathic caring do the same,*
*as you optimize purposeful, fluid movement to restore*
*functional abilities and mobilities for your patients and clients.*
*As the Divine is a very present help in time of trouble,*
*may you inhibit and modulate pain, offering relief,*
*working through Jesus' hands.*
*God of healing, wholeness, and holiness,*
*these Doctor of Physical Therapy learners reflect your Glory*
*in ability, knowledge, and clinical reasoning;*
*in passion and compassion,*
*with power and tenderness, through the art and science of healing.*
*We praise you for them and we honor them as healers.*
*We ask you to watch over them to give them your spirit*
*to keep them and their patients safe,*
*to strengthen them in the practice of their profession*
*and to be for them a source of hope and joy.*
*We pledge our prayerful and practical support to these Healers*
*and to their work.*
*We pray that they shall collaborate to cure,*
*gently speak to instruct, and soothe,*
*boldly and bravely educate to facilitate movement,*
*and with their touch foster health, with your love and power*
*that they shall be renewed, blessed, and fulfilled.*
*Let your strong and gentle hand bestow blessings upon them,*
*and with their patients now and always.*
*Amen.*

From prayer written and offered by Rev. Kelli W. Taylor, MDiv. University Chaplain, shared with permission and adapted by Dr. Gina Maria Musolino, PT, DPT, EdD, MSEd, 2022.

# REFERENCES

1. Elkins M, Cavendish R. Developing a plan for pediatric spiritual care. *Holist Nurs Pract.* 2004;18(4):179–186.
2. Koenig H. *Medicine, Religion, and Health: Where Science and Spirituality Meet.* West Conshohocken, PA: Templeton Foundation Press; 2008:54–112.
3. Krok D. The role of meaning in life within the relations of religious coping and psychological well-being. *J Relig Health.* 2015;54(6):2292–2308.
4. Drutchas A, Anandarajah G. Spirituality and coping with chronic disease in pediatrics. *R I Med J (2013).* 2014;97(3):26–30.
5. Jensen GM, Mostrom E. *The Handbook of Teaching and Learning for Physical Therapists.* 3rd ed. St. Louis, MO: Elsevier, Butterworth-Heinemann; 2013.
6. Wade DT, Halligan PW. Do biomedical models of illness make for good healthcare systems? *BMJ.* 2004;329(7479):1398–1401.
7. Borrell-Carrió F, Suchman AL, Epstein RM. The biopsychosocial model 25 years later: principles, practice, and scientific. *Ann Fam Med.* 2004;2(6):576–582.
8. Sahrmann SA. The human movement system: our professional identity. *Phys Ther.* 2014;94(7):1034–1042.
9. Sahrmann S, Bloom N. Update of concepts underlying movement system syndromes. In: Sahrmann S. *Movement System Impairment Syndromes of the Extremities, Cervical and Thoracic Spines.* St. Louis, MO: Elsevier; 2011:1–34.
10. Puchalski C. Restorative medicine. In: Cobb M, Puchalski C, Rumbold B, eds. *Oxford Textbook of Spirituality in Healthcare.* New York, NY: Oxford University Press; 2014:197–210.
11. Hematti S, Baradaran-Ghahforokhi M, Khajooei-Fard R, Mohammadi-Bertiani Z. Spiritual well-being for increasing life expectancy in palliative radiotherapy patients: a questionnaire-based study. *J Relig Health.* 2014;54(5):1563–1572.
12. Siddall PJ, Lovell M, MacLeod R. Spirituality: what is its role in pain medicine? *Pain Med.* 2015;16(1):51–60.
13. May S. Patient satisfaction with management of back pain: part 2: qualitative study into patients' satisfaction with physiotherapy. *Physiotherapy.* 2000;87:10–20.
14. Astrow AB, Puchalski CM, Sulmasy DP. Religion, spirituality, and health care: social, ethical, and practical considerations. *Am J Med.* 2001;110(4):283–87.
15. Highfield MF, Cason C. Spiritual needs of patients: are they recognized? *Cancer Nurs.* 1983;6(3):187–192.
16. Koenig HG. *Spirituality in Patient Care: Why, How, When, and What,* 3rd ed. West Conshohocken, PA: Templeton Foundation Press; 2013.
17. Koenig HG, Larson DB, Larson SS. Religion and coping with serious medical illness. *Ann Pharmacother.* 2001;35(3):352–359.
18. Peterman AH, Fitchett G, Brady MJ, Hernandez L, Cella D. Measuring spiritual well-being in people with cancer: the functional assessment of chronic illness therapy—Spiritual Well-Being Scale (FACIT-Sp). *Ann Behav Med.* 2002;24(1):49–58.
19. Post SS, Puchalski CM, Larson DB. Physician and patient spirituality: professional boundaries, competency, and ethics. *Ann Intern Med.* 2000;132(7):578–583.
20. Zinnbauer B, Pargament K. Capturing the meanings of religiousness and spirituality: one way down from a definitional Tower of Babel. *Res Soc Sci Stud Relig.* 2002;13:22–54.
21. Zinnbauer B, Pargament K, Scott A. The emerging meanings of religiousness and spirituality: problems and prospects. *J Pers.* 1999;67:889–919.
22. Maugans T. The SPIRITual history. *Arch Fam Med.* 1996;5:11–16.
23. Zinnbauer B, Pargament K. Religiousness and spirituality. In: Paloutzian RF, Park CL, eds. *Handbook of the Psychology of Religion and Spirituality,* 2nd ed. New York, NY: Guilford Press; 2014:21–42.
24. Hill PC, Pargament KI. Advances in the conceptualization and measurement of religion and spirituality. Implications for physical and mental health research. *Am Psychol.* 2003;58(1):64–74.
25. Anandarajah A, Hight E. Spirituality and medical practice: using the HOPE questions as a practical tool for spiritual assessment. *Am Fam Physician.* 2001;63(1):81–89.
26. de Brito Sena MA, Damiano RF, Lucchetti G, Peres MFP. Defining spirituality in healthcare: a systematic review and conceptual framework. *Front Psychol.* 2021;18(12):756080.
27. Hyman C, Handal, PJ. Definitions and evaluation of religion and spirituality items by religious professionals: a pilot study. *J Relig Health.* 2006;45:264–282.
28. Ledesma GCM, Reyes MES, Delariarte CF. Meaning in life, death, anxiety, and spirituality in the lesbian, gay, and bisexual community: a scoping review. *Sex Cult.* 2022 Nov 9:1–23.
29. Skoko I, Topić Stipić D, Tustonja M, Stanić D. Mental health and spirituality. *Psychiatr Danub.* 2021 Spring–Summer;33(Suppl 4):822–826.
30. Delgado-Guay MO. Spirituality and religiosity in supportive and palliative care. *Curr Opin Support Palliat Care.* 2014;8(3):308–313.
31. Baetz M, Bowen R. Chronic pain and fatigue: associations with religion and spirituality. *Pain Res Manage.* 2008;13(5):383–388.
32. Wachholtz AB, Pargament KI. Migraine and meditation: does spirituality matter? *J Behav Med.* 2008;31(4):351–366.
33. Wachholtz AB, Pearce MJ. Does spirituality as a coping mechanism help or hinder coping with chronic pain? *Curr Pain Headache Rep.* 2009;13(2):127–132.

34. Wachholtz AB, Pearce MJ, Koenig H. Exploring the relationship between spirituality, coping, and pain. *J Behav Med.* 2007;30(4):311–318.

35. Groopman J. *The Anatomy of Hope: How People Prevail in the Face of Illness.* New York, NY: Random House; 2005.

36. Miller WR, Thoresen CE. Spirituality, religion, and health. An emerging research field. *Am Psychol.* 2003;58(1):24–35.

37. Narayanasamy A. Learning spiritual dimension of care from a historical perspective. *Nurse Educ Today.* 1999;19(5):386–395.

38. Sargeant D. Teaching spirituality in the physical therapy classroom and clinic. *J Phys Ther Educ.* 2009;23(1):29–35.

39. Scandurra A. Everyday spirituality: a core unit in health education and lifetime wellness. *J Health Educ.* 1999;30:104–109.

40. Hettler B. Wellness: encouraging a lifetime pursuit of excellence. *Health Values.* 1984;8:13–17.

41. Rush Thompson C. *Prevention Practice and Health Promotion: A Physical Therapist's Guide to Health, Fitness, and Wellness,* 2nd ed. Thorofare, NJ: SLACK; 2015.

42. Emmons R, Paluotzian R. The psychology of religion. *Ann Rev Psychol.* 2003;54:377–402.

43. American Physical Therapy Association. *Physical fitness for specialized populations. Health Priorities for Populations and Individuals.* Available: https://www.apta.org/apta-and-you/leadership-and-governance/policies/health-priorities-populations-individuals Accessed January 15, 2024.

44. Stuifbergen AK, Seraphine A, Roberts G. An explanatory model of health promotion and quality of life in chronic disabling conditions. *Nurs Res.* 2000;49(3):122–129.

45. American Physical Therapy Association. *Vision, mission, and strategic plan.* https://www.apta.org/apta-and-you/leadership-and-governance/vision-mission-and-strategic-plan Accessed January 15, 2024.

46. Udermann BE. The effect of spirituality on health and healing: a critical review for athletic trainers. *J Athl Train.* 2000;35(2):194–197.

47. Drench ME, Noonan A, Sharby N, Ventura S. *Psychosocial Aspects of Healthcare,* 3rd ed. Upper Saddle River, NJ: Pearson Prentice Hall; 2012.

48. Seybold KS. Physiological mechanisms involved in religiosity/spirituality and health. *J Behav Med.* 2007;30(4):303–309.

49. Daaleman TP, Kaufman JS. Spirituality and depressive symptoms in primary care outpatients. *South Med J.* 2006;99(12):-1340–1344.

50. Daaleman TP, Perera S, Studenski SA. Religion, spirituality, and health status in geriatric outpatients. *Ann Fam Med.* 2004;2(1):49–53.

51. Yohannes AM, Koenig HG, Baldwin RC, Connolly MJ. Health behavior, depression and religiosity in older patients admitted to intermediate care. *Int J Geriatr Psychiatry.* 2008;23(7):735–740.

52. Banks JW. The importance of incorporating faith and spirituality issues in the care of patients with chronic daily headache. *Curr Pain Headache Rep.* 2006;10(1):41–46.

53. Mactavish J, Iwasaki Y. Exploring perspectives of individuals with disabilities on stress-coping. *J Rehabil.* 2005;71:20–31.

54. Idler EL, Kasl SV. Religion among disabled and nondisabled persons II: attendance at religious services as a predictor of the course of disability. *J Gerontol B Psychol Sci Soc Sci.* 1997;52(6):S306–S316.

55. Mills PJ, Wilson K, Iqbal N, et al. Depressive symptoms and spiritual wellbeing in asymptomatic heart failure patients. *J Behav Med.* 2015;38(3):407–415.

56. Reynolds F. *Communication and Clinical Effectiveness in Rehabilitation.* Edinburgh, Scotland: Elsevier; 2005.

57. Kim J, Heinemann A, Bode R, Sliwa J, King R. Spirituality, quality of life, and functional recovery after medical rehabilitation. *Rehabil Psychol.* 2000;45:365–385.

58. McColl M, Bickenbach J, Johnston J, et al. Changes in spiritual beliefs after traumatic injury. *Arch Phys Med Rehabil.* 2000;81:817–823.

59. Pressman P, Lyons JS, Larson DB, Strain JJ. Religious belief, depression, and ambulation status in elderly women with broken hips. *Am J Psychiatry.* 1990;147(6):758–760.

60. Fisher MF, Cohn JC, Harrington SE, Lee JQ, Malone D. Screening and assessment of cancer-related fatigue: a clinical practice guideline for health care providers. *Phys Ther.* 2022;102(9):pzac120.

61. van Oorsouw R, Oerlemans A, Klooster E, van den Berg M, Kalf, J, Vermeulen H., et al. A sense of being needed: a phenomenological analysis of hospital-based rehabilitation professionals' experiences during the COVID-19 pandemic. *Phys Ther.* 2022;102(6):pzac052.

62. Mackey KM, Sparling JW. Experiences of older women with cancer receiving hospice care: significance for physical therapy. *Phys Ther.* 2000;80(5):459–468.

63. Johnston-Taylor E. *What Do I Say? Talking With Patients About Spirituality.* Philadelphia, PA: Templeton Foundation Press; 2007.

64. Womble MN, Labbé EE, Cochran CR. Spirituality and personality: understanding their relationship to health resilience. *Psychological Rep.* 2013;112(3):706–715.

65. de Diego-Cordero R, Martos-Lorite I, Vega-Escaño J. Spiritual dimension in neurological and neurodegenerative diseases: a systematic mapping review. *J Relig Health.* 2022; Oct 15:1–19.

66. Sarrazin JP. The relationship between religion, spirituality and health: a critical review from the social sciences. *Findings* 2021;18(36):409–442.

67. Gomes MV, da Xavier ADSG, de Carvalho ESDS, Cordeiro RC, Ferreira SL, Morbeck AD. Waiting for a miracle: Spirituality/Religiosity in coping with sickle cell disease. *Revista Brasileira De Enfermagem.* 2019;72(6):1554–1561. doi: 10.1590/0034-7167-2018-0635.

68. Powell L, Shahabi L, Thoresen CE. Religion and spirituality. Linkages to physical health. *Am Psychol*. 2003;58(1):36–52.

69. Ecklund EH, Cadge W, Gage EA, Catlin EA. The religious and spiritual beliefs and practices of academic pediatric oncologists in the United States. *J Pediatr Hematol Oncol*. 2007;29(11):736–742.

70. Fanos JH, Gelinas DF, Foster RS, Postone N, Miller RG. Hope in palliative care: from narcissism to self-transcendence in amyotrophic lateral sclerosis. *J Palliat Med*. 2008;11(3):470–475.

71. Lin HR, Bauer-Wu SM. Psycho-spiritual well-being in patients with advanced cancer: an integrative review of the literature. *J Adv Nurs*. 2003;44(1):69–80.

72. Robinson MR, Thiel MM, Backus MM, Meyer EC. Matters of spirituality at the end of life in the pediatric intensive care unit. *Pediatrics*. 2006;118(3):e719–e729.

73. Murphy PL, Albert SM, Weber CM, Del Bene ML, Rowland LP. Impact of spirituality and religiousness on outcomes in patients with ALS. *Neurology*. 2000;55(10):1581–1584.

74. Anderson CJ, Vogel LC, Chlan KM, Betz RR. Coping with spinal cord injury: strategies used by adults who sustained their injuries as children or adolescents. *J Spinal Cord Med*. 2008;31(3):290–296.

75. Kaufman Y, Anaki D, Binns M, Freedman M. Cognitive decline in Alzheimer disease: impact of spirituality, religiosity and QOL. *Neurology*. 2007;68(18):1509–1514.

76. Ginting H, Näring G, Kwakkenbos L, Becker ES. Spirituality and negative emotions in individuals with coronary heart disease. *J Cardiovas Nurs*. 2015;30(6):537–545.

77. Lipton B. *Biology of Belief*. Carlsbad, CA: Hay House; 2011.

78. O'Brien M. The need for spiritual integrity. In: Yura H, Walsh MB, eds. *Human Needs and the Nursing Process*. Norwalk, CT: Appleton-Century-Crofts; 1982:85–115.

79. Stanworth R. Spirituality, language and depth of reality. *Int J Palliat Nurs*. 1997;3:19–22.

80. *The Joint Commission: Advancing Effective Communication, Cultural Competence, and Patient- and Family-Centered Care: A Roadmap for Hospitals*. Oakbrook Terrace, IL: The Joint Commission, 2010.

81. The Joint Commission. *A Trusted Partner in Patient Care*. Available: https://www.jointcommission.org/ Accessed January 15, 2024.

82. Clark P, Drain M, Malone M. Addressing patients' emotional and spiritual needs. *J Comm J Qual Saf*. 2003;29:659–670.

83. McEvoy M. An added dimension to the pediatric health maintenance visit: the spiritual history. *J Pediatr Health Care*. 2000;14:216–220.

84. Puchalski C, Ferrell B. *Making Health Care Whole: Integrating Spirituality into Patient Care*. West Conshohocken, PA: Templeton Foundation Press; 2010.

85. George Washington Institute for Spirituality and Health. *FICA Spiritual Assessment Tool*. https://smhs.gwu.edu/gwish/clinical/fica. Accessed January 15, 2024.

86. King SD, Dimmers MA, Langer S, Murphy PE. Doctors' attentiveness to the spirituality/religion of their patients in the pediatric and oncology settings in the Northwest USA. *J Health Care Chaplain*. 2013;19(4):140–164.

87. Leidl BF, Fox-Davis D, Walker FO, Gabbard J, Marterre B. Layers of loss: a scoping review and taxonomy of HD caregivers' spiritual suffering, grief/loss and coping strategies. *J Pain Symptom Manage*. 2023 Jan;65(1):e29–e50.

88. Casaleiro T, Caldeira S, Cardoso D, Apóstolo J. Spiritual aspects of the family caregivers' experiences when caring for a community-dwelling adult with severe mental illness: a systematic review of qualitative evidence. *J Psychiatr Ment Health Nurs*. 2022;29(2):240–273.

# SUGGESTED READINGS AND RESOURCES

Allen JT, Koenig HG. *A Theology of God Talk: The Language of the Heart*. London: Taylor & Francis; 2021.

Cobb M, Puchalski C, Rumbold B, eds. *Oxford Textbook of Spirituality in Healthcare*. New York, NY: Oxford University Press; 2014.

Wish G. GW School of Medicine and Health Sciences (gwu.edu). https://gwish.smhs.gwu.edu/ Institute for Spirituality & Healthcare: Conducting research, educating practitioners, and impacting health care policy worldwide; offers online interprofessional spiritual health care training, © FICA tool, and spiritual health care resources and references.

Henahan MP, Koenig HG. *Integrating Spirit and Psyche: Using Women's Narrative in Psychotherapy*. London: Taylor & Francis; 2018.

Koenig HG, McCall JB. *A Practical Guide to Hospital Ministry: Healing Ways*. New York, NY: Haworth Press; 2018.

Leidl BF, Fox-Davis D, Walker FO, Gabbard J, Marterre B. Layers of loss: A scoping review and taxonomy of HD caregivers' spiritual suffering, grief/loss and coping strategies. *J Pain Symptom Manage*. 2023 Jan;65(1):e29–e50.

Peteet JR, Koenig HG, VanderWeele T. *Handbook of Religion and Health*. New York, NY: Oxford University Press; 2023.

Puchalski C, Jafari N, Buller H, Haythorn T, Jacobs C, Ferrell B. Interprofessional spiritual care education curriculum: a milestone toward the provision of spiritual care. *J Palliat Med*. 2020 Jun;23(6):777–784.

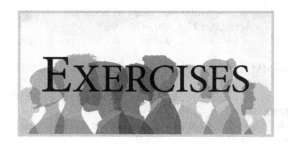

# EXERCISE 1: ASSESSING PERSONAL LEVELS OF COMFORT WITH SPIRITUALITY

1.   What does the word *religion* mean to you?

2.   What does the word *spirituality* mean to you?

3.   Create a timeline of meaningful spiritual or religious events in your life.

4.   How comfortable do feel you are with the idea of giving spiritual care as a health care professional? Please explain.

5.   If there are aspects of giving spiritual care that make you uncomfortable, what are your plans to increase your level of comfort?

# EXERCISE 2: INTERVIEW A FAMILY MEMBER OR FRIEND

1.  If you have a spiritual or religious belief system, how do you use it to support you during times of illness?

2.  How would you feel if your doctor or other HCP asked about your religious or spiritual needs?

3.  When do you think is the best time for the doctor or other HCP to ask about your spiritual or religious needs?

4.  How should your doctor or other HCP support religious or spiritual beliefs?

5.  Show the Spirituality Framework (Figure 15.1) to your family members or friends to visually cue them in characterizing their spirituality. Ask if they can describe each dimension (where applicable) of the construct to you in terms of their beliefs. Did you find that the framework brought about more information and insights?

# EXERCISE 3: PRACTICE YOUR SKILLS

## *Case Study 1*

Selma Brown is a 50-year-old female with a 20-year history of multiple sclerosis. During the interview, she shared with you, the HCP, that after her initial diagnosis she remained as active as possible. She exercised and walked regularly and was careful not to over fatigue herself. Prior to her diagnosis of multiple sclerosis, Mrs. Brown was an avid bicyclist and hiker and worked as a flight attendant. She was able to work for almost 15 years after her diagnosis. As Mrs. Brown shares the details of her life with you, she begins to cry. About six years ago, Mrs. Brown had a major exacerbation of her symptoms. While in the hospital, she tried to help herself as much as possible during bed baths and activities of daily living. One day a nurse asked her, "Why bother helping me so much? You're going to end up wheelchair dependent anyway." Mrs. Brown says, "That was the day I gave up." Her husband divorced her five years ago because he could not "deal with her problem."

Mrs. Brown lives alone in a one-story home. She shares with you that her house is totally accessible because, prior to her divorce, she had good insurance and had the house adapted for her use. She uses a motorized wheelchair and can transfer independently. She no longer has insurance and is seeing you as an outpatient at a county hospital.

When the physical therapist requested Mrs. Brown's input on what she hopes to achieve by coming to physical therapy, Mrs. Brown says she really wants to be able to stand again. She tells the therapist that she wants to be more independent and realizes that walking is out of the question. "I know I will never get back to where I was, but I really want to be as independent as possible. The people from my church offer me a lot of help, but I want to be able to reach plates in my cabinet without falling when the ladies are not around. I prefer to talk with them rather than having them doing everything for me. I just want to be me again. I can't go on this way!"

1.  What information has Mrs. Brown given you about her quality of life?

2.  How will you address the despair Mrs. Brown has shared with you?

3.  What do you know about Mrs. Brown's support system?

## *Case Study 2*

Alma Bender is an elderly female presenting with cachexia, who is experiencing an overall decline in independent function. Her medical history includes spinal stenosis, breast cancer, severe scoliosis, and an aortic aneurysm that needs to be repaired. Her 60-year-old daughter, who is bipolar, lives with her. Mrs. Bender was admitted to the hospital 4 days ago secondary to a diagnosis of pneumonia. You received an order to evaluate and treat Mrs. Bender.

During your initial interview, Mrs. Bender indicates to you that she is very worried about her daughter because her daughter can't live alone. Mrs. Bender feels that she doesn't have much time left on this earth. She wakes up each morning with pain in her back and a feeling of impending doom about her health. She feels like she is failing her daughter. She is worried about what will happen to her daughter if she doesn't stay as independent as possible. She wants to be able to get home as soon as possible so that her daughter can come home from the nursing home in which she is currently living.

As her health care professional, you have listened carefully to Mrs. Bender and have reflected her content and feelings back to her. Mrs. Bender has expressed gratitude to you for being such a nice person and says, "Your mother must be very proud of you." Mrs. Bender then begins to cry. You feel awkward but ask her what is wrong. She shares with you, "I am afraid to die because my daughter needs me." As you work with Mrs. Bender on transfers, you hear her say under her breath, "Oh God, please help me. I need your help."

1.  How can you communicate your awareness of Mrs. Bender's spiritual needs to her?

2.  What is your level of comfort in discussing her spiritual health with Mrs. Bender?

3.  What are the pros and cons of addressing Mrs. Bender's spiritual needs?

4.  How has your ability to make a connection with Mrs. Bender assisted you in establishing a plan of care that is most likely to have a positive outcome?

# *Case Study 3*

You are a HCP working in a moderately large hospital with a rehab floor. Several of the patients you see participate in the endurance program developed for persons with cancer. Mr. Ryder was recently diagnosed with lung cancer. Surgery was performed, and Mr. Ryder has been referred to the endurance program. You will treat Mr. Ryder for the first time today. As part of your initial evaluation, you have decided to use the © FICA.[19,25,73–85] Spiritual History Tool. Go to the George Washington Institute for Spirituality and Health[85] website (https://smhs.gwu.edu/gwish/clinical/fica) to learn more about the FICA Spiritual Assessment Tool. Develop your FICA approach to gather Mr. Ryder's spiritual history. You may wish to refer to the example earlier in the chapter utilizing the FICA questionnaire.

- F (Faith, Belief, Meaning):

- I (Importance and Influence):

- C (Community):

- A (Address/Action in Care):

1.  Develop a transitional statement you will use to put Mr. Ryder at ease when asking about a sensitive issue such as spirituality/religion.

2. Mr. Ryder appears depressed with his diagnosis and unsure of the future. What are some tactics you could incorporate into your plan of care to address his needs?

3. Mr. Ryder is genuinely concerned about his fatigue and his inability to get down on the floor because he wants to play with his grandchildren on the floor again. How would working on floor transfers support this man's spiritual needs?

# EXERCISE 4: SPIRITUAL AUTOBIOGRAPHY

1.  Clearly state your personal beliefs about spirituality, faith, and/or religion. Or state that, after you have reflected on your beliefs, you are not comfortable sharing this information.

2.  Include examples of defining moments in personal spiritual, faith, or religious development. Indicate that key moments have not been part of your experience, or indicate in #1 that you not comfortable sharing beliefs or examples.

3.  Utilize the Spirituality Framework (Figure 15.1) to fully describe your spirituality, considering each dimension, as applicable; then contrast yours with a peer. Remember to consider utilizing this framework as a helpful visual aid for your patients'/clients' spirituality. Practice with a peer through one of the patient cases described in the chapter or based upon your own lived experiences.

# EXERCISE 5: ANNOTATED BIBLIOGRAPHY

1.  Provide a one-paragraph summary of the key points of an article (not the abstract) about spirituality or religion as related to the provision of spiritual care by HCPs.

2.  Craft a discussion question based on the article content that will stimulate discussion with your classmates. Be prepared to share the query for round table discussions.

# 16

# PRINCIPLES AND PRACTICES FOR EFFECTIVE PATIENT/ CLIENT EDUCATION

## PROMOTING HEALTH BEHAVIORS THROUGH HEALTH LITERACY, TRANSFORMATIVE HEALTH MODELS AND THEORIES

*Gina Maria Musolino and Kathleen A. Curtis*

## OBJECTIVES

*The learner should be able to*:

- Describe health behavior and health literacy.
- Explore concepts of providers' perceptions and patient responsibility examining Brickman's Models[1] of helping and coping for health behaviors.
- Compare and contrast health behavior theories to better understand why patients sometimes act in ways that go against promoting their health.
- Appraise evidence supporting the use of technology and interactive approaches to promote health behavior change.
- Demonstrate principles of effective patient education.
- Develop effective instructional planning guidelines for patient and family education goals with appropriate supporting instructional materials.
- Examine the influence of language and culture on health-related communications.
- Construct and evaluate patient/client education materials considering health literacy and readability levels.
- Design health behavior change plans with measurable learning domain goals.

DOI: 10.4324/9781003525554-16

- Provide peer-teaching facilitation for a peer's behavior change efforts considering the Transtheoretical Model of Change.
- Teach instructional tips when working with groups and/or peer teams to promote healthy choices.
- Conduct a mini-needs assessment for a health behavior with a targeted group.
- Evaluate health behavior needs assessments, considering educational interventions and available health resources.

The health care professional (HCP) entered a note in the patient's medical record. An excerpt:

> The patient returns for follow-up today with essentially no change in his condition ... Questionable compliance with the prescribed treatment program. Plan: review importance of continuing daily medication.

What happened? The patient forgot, didn't have time, didn't have the money, didn't want to? It was too much trouble, too complicated, didn't meet his needs, couldn't fit it in with his lifestyle? He didn't understand, doesn't speak English, has too many children, lost the instructions, or felt it was just not that important?

Most HCPs would find one of these reasons to explain the patient's noncompliance with the treatment program. The reasons may be valid, but the patient's inability or choice not to follow through with the provider's instructions may result in serious illness, disability, or death.

On the other hand, it may be a person's active choice not to proceed with care; not noncompliance per se, just their desires, beliefs, or values that may be incongruent with care plans.

If HCPs really want to influence patient behavior, they must understand health behavior and health literacy.

## WHAT IS HEALTH BEHAVIOR?

*Health behavior* is a series of actions we take to maintain, promote, or improve our well-being. Health behaviors might include getting immunizations and vaccinations, making regular dental visits, having a mammogram, Pap smear, colon cancer screening, using condoms with sexual activity, doing activities designed to reduce anxiety or stress, being mindful of what you are eating and drinking, or starting a regular stretching and cardiovascular exercise program. What health behaviors do you practice regularly in these three categories? Take a moment to journal on these behaviors:

1. Screening examinations
2. Health promotion activities
3. Treatment of chronic illnesses or conditions

## WHAT IS HEALTH LITERACY?

Millions of adults have difficulty following self-care instructions due to limited health vocabulary and poor understanding of information and concepts. *Health literacy* (HL) is simply the patient's ability to read and understand all types of health-related materials. One of the first HL studies documented that 1 in 3 English-speaking patients, and 1 in 2 Spanish-speaking patients at public hospitals had marginal health literacy.[2] It is estimated that if all counties in the United States (U.S.) had high health literacy, then there would be 1 million fewer Medicare hospital visits with 25.4 billion dollars in savings each year.[3] Individuals with low HL lack sufficient health background knowledge and often have difficulty reading and understanding labels, appointment information, and medication instructions.

As a social determinant of health (SDoH), the degree of HL makes a significant difference in health outcomes and is often overlooked. Individuals with lower levels of HL report worse overall health. When asked to self-report overall health, adults with higher degrees of health had higher average HL scores than did adults who self-reported worse overall health levels. It takes additional time and costs more to provide quality care to patients with low HL.[3,4] Low HL is associated with poor health outcomes, including increased hospitalization rates, fewer preventive screenings, and higher rates of disease and mortality. For older adults there are positive associations between HL and medication adherence.[4]

The Institute of Medicine defines HL as "the degree to which individuals can obtain, process, and understand the basic health information and services they need to make appropriate health decisions."[5] At least 88% of U.S. adults have HL that is inadequate to navigate the health care system or promote their well-being.[6] It is estimated that only 12% of the populations are truly health literate and HL remains a leading cause of world-wide mortality.[6,7] Without

HL patients/clients may not be able to conduct needed self-care and are at a higher risk for mortality. Lower HL has a notable increased risk of death.[8] Inadequate HL is linked to poor disease management, perceived noncompliance with treatment recommendations, and medication errors by patients or caregivers.[9]

Hence, not surprisingly, lower levels of HL have been associated with persons' chronic disease and with lower vaccination rates.[10,11] Canadian[12] investigators, utilizing the Test of Functional Health Literacy in Adults (TOFHLA)[13] completed a prospective, multi-center cohort investigation. General medicine patients admitted in two urban, tertiary care hospitals presented with the following HL levels: 50% adequate, 32% inadequate, and 18% marginal.[12] Study patients with inadequate HL were more likely to revisit emergency services than those with adequate HL.[12] Whether for patients or HCPs, HL plays an irreplaceable role in disease prevention and management.[9,10–14]

Healthy People 2030[14] extended the HL definition to include *organizational* health literacy, emphasizing the responsibility of providers and health-related organizations to disseminate understandable information and eliminate health inequities. In line with Healthy People 2030:[14]

> ***Personal*** *health literacy is the degree to which individuals have the ability to find, understand, and use information and services to inform health-related decisions and actions for themselves and others.*
>
> ***Organizational*** *health literacy is the degree to which organizations equitably enable individuals to find, understand, and use information and services to inform health-related decisions and actions for themselves and others.*

In an era where cost containment has reduced the availability of follow-up services, low HL presents an ever-present danger to population health and raises the question of who is responsible for one's well-being: the patient or the provider?

# WHO IS RESPONSIBLE ⋯ IN SICKNESS AND IN HEALTH?

If you are like most people, you are highly likely to seek medical assistance when you have a painful problem. Imagine yourself visiting your physician for diagnosis and treatment of a minor but very irritating and painful skin infection. Your skin is cultured, and you are given a prescription medication to put on your skin every day and an oral medication to take by mouth for 10 days. After 4 or 5 days, the lesion clears up and you discontinue your oral medication. A resistant strain of the same organism then shows up in the same location 2 weeks later. Your physician tells you that you will now have to undergo a complicated, prolonged course of treatment that is riskier to you and those around you. In addition, you will not be allowed to work at your job in the hospital due to the possibility of spreading this infection to immune-compromised patients.

## *Who Is Responsible Now?*

If the patient doesn't do what they are told to do, is it the provider's fault? Most providers would say no! Do you believe the patient is responsible for the previous situation? How would you feel as the patient in this case?

Our beliefs about the patient's responsibility influence how willing we are to help our patients. Brickman et al.'s[1] four models of helping and coping provide a framework for understanding how the concept of responsibility ties into the messages we give to patients in many patient education situations. The four models vary in provider perceptions of the patient's responsibility for causing the problem and for taking action to solve the problem. Here are the rules:[1]

1. If providers believe that patients are not responsible for causing their problems, they are more willing to help (*Medical and Compensatory Models*).

2. If providers believe that the patients are responsible for causing their problems, they are less willing to help (*Enlightenment and Moral Models*). If patients see themselves as not responsible for their problem and providers see them as responsible for the problems, conflict may result. Patients may be angry and resentful of the providers' assigning blame to them.

3. If providers see patients as not responsible for the solutions to their problems (such as the treatment), they are likely to take most of the responsibility for patients and therefore do less patient education (*Medical and Enlightenment Models*).

4. If providers see patients as responsible for the solutions to their problems, they are likely to involve the patient in solving the problem and then hold the patient responsible (*Compensatory and Moral Models*).

Put yourself in the provider's shoes. What are your feelings about your patient's problems in this case? Who is responsible? If your provider holds you responsible for the solution, they may consider you unreliable and feel that their efforts have been wasted and are likely unappreciated, even though they may feel some sense of obligation to provide further treatment. Brickman's Models[1] (Table 16.1) helps to explain the relationship of HCPs' perceptions of

| TABLE 16.1 |
| --- |

| BRICKMAN'S[1] MODELS OF HELPING AND COPING APPLIED TO PATIENT EDUCATION: PROVIDER PERCEPTIONS OF PATIENT RESPONSIBILITY | | |
| --- | --- | --- |
| | **PATIENT RESPONSIBLE FOR CAUSING PROBLEM** | **PATIENT NOT RESPONSIBLE FOR CAUSING PROBLEM** |
| **PATIENT RESPONSIBLE FOR SOLUTION** | *Moral Model*<br>Patient admonished for causing problem. Patient education of high value but probably less likely to happen. | *Compensatory Model*<br>The provider has sympathy for the patient's problems. Patient education is highly valued. Provider highly motivated to provide it. |
| **PATIENT NOT RESPONSIBLE FOR SOLUTION** | *Enlightenment Model*<br>Patient education of less value. Patient likely to be admonished for causing problem. Provider will be responsible for solution, which minimizes need for patient education. | *Medical Model*<br>Patient education of less value. Provider has sympathy for patient. Provider will be responsible for patient. Provider will be responsible for solution, which minimizes need for patient education. |

Adapted from Brickman P, Rabinowitz VC, Karuza J Jr, Coates D, Cohn E, Kidder L. Models of helping and coping. *Am Psychol.* 1982;37(4):368–384.

responsibility to their willingness to help. As you can see, only one set of conditions (Compensatory Model) exists in which the provider is highly motivated to help, and the patient is seen as responsible for participating in the solution to the problem.

As you are reading, some of you have already begun worrying about your health. Consider your perceptions about your own illnesses or problems or commitment to your personal health. Then consider, would most patients see themselves as causing their obesity, their hypertension, their HIV or Covid-19 infection? Do you think your HCPs hold the same perceptions of your responsibility for these health problems? It would be interesting to find out, because the answer to this question has everything to do with the way patients are treated and cared for by their HCPs. The behavior change exercise at the end of this chapter may help you gain insight into the challenges of changing your own personal health behaviors and what we are often imposing with our patients/clients, as we facilitate their own health behavior changes. In designing effective patient education approaches, it is essential that we understand what influences health behavior. Researchers have published widely on this area for the past 60 years, and there are still many questions. However, there are several key schools of thought that can help HCPs to feel more informed about how to proceed with their patients.

# HEALTH BEHAVIOR THEORIES

## *Health Belief Model*

Perhaps the most influential theory of health behavior is the *Health Belief Model.*[15] This model helps to frame why people fail to participate in programs or behaviors that prevent or detect disease.[15] For example, when the evidence is clear that smoking is harmful to one's health, why would a young person begin to smoke? Why would a HCP, fully aware of the risks and diseases associated with smoking, continue to smoke?

The Health Belief Model[15] consists of six components: *perceived severity, perceived susceptibility, perceived benefits, perceived barriers, cues to action, and self-efficacy.* The Health Belief Model[15] proposes that the likelihood of an individual doing something to protect against a health threat is related to their perceptions, willingness to take action, and self-efficacy:

1. Perceived Susceptibility to the health threat? (e.g., *How likely is it that I will have this problem?*)

2. Perceived Severity of the health threat? (e.g., *How serious is this problem?*)

3. Perceived Benefits of the recommended behavior? (e.g., *What will I gain by doing this?*)

4. Perceived Barriers or costs of the recommended behavior? (e.g., *What are the obstacles that stand in my way or the costs to me of taking this action?*)

5. Cues to action: Factors that activate "readiness to change" (e.g., *I am ready to change? What will it take for me to change?*)

6. Self-efficacy: Confidence in one's ability to take action (e.g., *Am I capable of changing? Can I do this? Might I fail?*)

Essentially, discordant perceptions may be evidenced with messages received or the validity of the information communicated and received. Thus, a person could simultaneously hold the belief that smoking is a potentially harmful behavior and, because of conflicting beliefs such as "My grandfather smoked for 55 years and died when he was 87" or "I will gain weight if I attempt to quit," this person will not take the essential action to reduce the health threat even though they may cognitively recognize it. However, this person may later see a cross-section of a blackened, physical lung on display at a community health fair that clearly compares a healthy lung with one damaged by smoking; the first-hand witnessing of this visual cue may then cause the person to act. However, they may then question their ability (self-efficacy) to be successful as they are so used to the habit of smoking. The utility of the model is that it aids in identifying a person's perceptions and where their willingness to take action resides. This likely assists the HCP in best courses of action (or in-action) in collaboration with patients for patient-centered health care. HCPs must meet their patients/clients along the care continuum.

## *Locus of Control*

Another widely accepted theoretical approach uses the concept of *locus of control*, which refers to our perceptions that the outcomes and rewards we experience are either under our control or out of our control.[16] Remember that we first discussed this theory in Chapter 9 on assertiveness.

Individuals with an internal locus of control generally believe that their personal actions and choices have a direct bearing on the outcomes they experience. In contrast, individuals with an external locus of control feel that events are caused by fate, powerful others, or other factors out of their control. This orientation has significance in information-seeking behavior because individuals with an internal locus of control are more likely to seek information about their health problems and choices. Some studies have reported that individuals with an internal locus of control experience more favorable health outcomes than matched subjects with an external locus of control.[17] However, an external locus of control may work very well for some individuals who prefer to follow the directions of an expert.

HCPs who are offering educational interventions for their patients or clients need to keep in mind that individuals may not only vary in beliefs regarding the problem and ease of solving the problem (health belief model), but they may also vary in the degree to which they believe that their choices and actions will influence the outcomes they experience. In a study at the Royal Free Hospital in London, physical therapists sent a message designed to increase perceived control to 39 first-time patients with a variety of disabilities who were scheduled for outpatient physical therapy services.[18] The patients who received the letter reported significantly higher levels of perceived control and were more satisfied with information than the control group, who only received a letter about their appointment time.[18] The sample message in Figure 16.1 illustrates an effective means to influence patient perceptions of locus of control.

## *Self-Efficacy*

Another perspective in understanding health behavior comes from social learning theory (as discussed in Chapter 10).[19] Self-efficacy is an individual's sense that they can successfully carry out a particular health behavior needed to result in a desired outcome. Self-efficacy is influenced by one's own past experiences, observations of the experiences of influential others, and valued verbal and emotional support of others.[20] Self-efficacy and social learning theory have tremendous implications for patient education in that we can promote the use of peer educators who model the desired behavior, providing emotional support.

Bandura[19-20] also discussed how the environment influences our choices. Providing and suggesting to patients a variety of environments in which to be successful may assist in compliance efforts. For example, a patient with a forward head position may benefit from simple chin tuck exercises; cue the patient to complete a few at every red stop light, rather than asking them to do multiple bouts all at once. By breaking down the exercise activity into simple cues and short periods of time, the patient may not be as overwhelmed. Incorporating the exercise into the patient's daily routine will assist in reminding them without being additive to their day. You may also cue the patient that every time

Royal Free Hospital
222 Hospital Rd
Anytown, England 12345

This is to let you know that you are now being offered physiotherapy at the Royal Free Hospital to help you to overcome your particular health problem. By concentrating on your difficulties, you will be shown how you can control your symptoms and problems as quickly and as effectively as possible.

You may be offered advice and instructions about your symptoms or problems and given a home program. It will be up to you to follow these if you want to recover quickly.

Experience has shown that the more effort you can put in, the more quickly results will be achieved. The therapists are there to help you to resolve your problems.

You may find it helpful to enlist friends and relatives to help you to follow any home program you are given. May we wish you a speedy recovery.

Sincerely,
Royal Free Hospital

**Figure 16.1** Message to patients at the Royal Free Hospital. (Adapted from Johnston M, Gilbert P, Partridge C, Coolins J. Changing perceived control in patients with physical disabilities: an intervention study with patients receiving rehabilitation. *Br J Clin Psychol*. 1992;31[pt 1]:89–94.)

they think about the time of day or answer a phone call or text, they should think about their posture and self-correct. Utilizing the environment and everyday occurrences that fit the patient's lifestyle may lead to greater degrees of compliance. A busy mother and wife with three young children, who works full-time is not going to be able to dedicate a solid, lengthy time frame to a home program, but intervals of exercise might work. Utilize the patients' changing environments to assist you in achieving their rehabilitation goals.

## Theory of Planned Behavior

Ajzen's[21] theory of planned behavior incorporates the concept of social influence and intention in addition to self-efficacy. This theory uses three elements to explain individual behavior: (1) behavioral intentions, which reflect an individual's attitude (consequences and desirability) about the behavior; (2) the individual's perceptions of the subjective norms (attitudes of important others, such as family, friends, and society) about the performance of the behavior; and (3) the individual's perceptions of control (difficulty) over performance of the behavior. Ajzen's[21] theory can be used to understand diverse and complex health behaviors, such as refraining from alcohol use and adherence to a recommended exercise program. The planned behavior approach takes into account that our behavior is influenced by our intentions and our beliefs about the attitudes of others, in addition to our perceptions of self-efficacy.

## Health Promotion Model

Pender[22] built upon some of these ideas and identified modifying factors (demographic, biologic characteristics, interpersonal influences, situational and behavioral factors) that may influence perceptions of self-efficacy, health status, perceived benefits, and barriers. Pender's model[22] also incorporates internal and external cues to action, further increasing the likelihood of engaging in health-promoting behaviors.

Educational messages may serve as external cues to influence an individual to continue a behavior. For example, the use of internal cues, such as "I feel much better when I exercise," or external cues, such as "heart-healthy" symbols on a restaurant menu or health information in the news or social messaging increases the likelihood of continuing beneficial behaviors.

## Transtheoretical Model of Change

The transtheoretical model[23,24] describes stages that individuals progress through as they change health behaviors. The model includes five stages of change[23-25]—*precontemplation, contemplation, preparation, action, and maintenance*—which allow for a nonlinear, or even cyclical, progression through them before sustained behavior change can occur (Table 16.2). This integrative transformation model is particularly helpful in understanding change, such as starting an exercise routine or stopping smoking. With this orientation to patient education, a HCP is aware of the activities that would support the patient in various stages of the change process and able to identify the stage(s) in which the patient/client presents in real time.[24,25] Let's look at a few instances in which this applies.

In a gender-specific, community-based health promotion program with livestock farmers in Ireland, researchers[26] implemented the Transtheoretical Model of Change[23,24] in a pragmatic manner in real-time environments. The farmers experience inequities in access to care due to the rural nature of their work and lives. Hence this "hard to reach" group of higher risk men were recruited to participate in a cardiovascular prevention program. Through this large-scale, primary prevention public health effort, investigators reached out to a cohort of 1,400 farmers with a resultant 868 participating in The Farmers Have Hearts—Cardiovascular Health Program. The study implemented a health behavior change intervention using three modes of delivery based upon farmers' preferences for health: coaching by phone, mobile-health text messages, or a combination of both; a control group was also utilized. Utilizing the Transtheoretical Model of Change, the farmers were coached based upon where they were in the stages of change. The researchers provided the health change intervention over 52 weeks, with their preferred same-gender providers, were nonjudgmental in delivery, meeting the farmers on "their turf," while accounting for farming season demands. The focus was on personalized and achievable changes with choices related to the progressive plans. The resultant outcomes were farmers' sense of empowerment, increased health awareness, and participant satisfaction. Physical health checks and cardiovascular tests and measures were completed pre/during/post the interventions. The health checks occurred at regularly scheduled agricultural events (e.g., sale barns, farmers markets) with farmers selecting when and where they wanted to have the checks completed. Participants were also provided with related patient education materials and self-monitoring tools, which were noted as extremely helpful for this self-sufficient population.[26]

| TABLE 16.2 | | |
|---|---|---|
| **TRANSTHEORETICAL MODEL OF CHANGE[23–25] PATIENT EDUCATION IMPLICATIONS** | | |
| **STAGE** | **PATIENT-CHANGE READINESS** | **IMPLICATIONS FOR PATIENT EDUCATION** |
| **Precontemplation** | Not intending to change | Help clients identify personal priorities and lifestyle goals. Establish trust and rapport to eventually provide insight into negative risk behaviors. |
| **Contemplation** | Intend to change within **6 months** | Provide motivational messages of pros and cons of risk behavior. Tie into goals. Support decision making and help clients evaluate pros/cons of the behavioral change. |
| **Preparation** | Actively planning to change in **next 30 days** | Seek commitment to risk behavior change and starting date. Support decision to take action with discussion of resources and coping skills. |
| **Action** | Has initiated change within the **past 6 months** | Support behavioral change and adaptive replacement of risk behaviors with new lifestyle practices. Provide information about social and medical resources that facilitate change. Teach self-management strategies to prevent relapse. |
| **Maintenance** | Has successfully modified behavior **for greater than 6 months** | Prevent relapse and encourage long-term change. Review skills for managing situations triggering relapse to prior behaviors. Reinforce new lifestyle habits and achievement of goals. |

Adapted from Basler HD. Patient education with reference to the process of behavioral change. *Patient Educ Couns.* 1995;26:93–98; and Nolan RP. How can we help patients to initiate change? *Can J Cardio.* 1995;11(suppl):16A–19A.

Let's now consider a single subject example:

> Jeanette, a health care professions student, feels that she should begin an exercise program after a class on cardiovascular risk factors. She visits her physician to have her cholesterol checked. She looks through American Heart Association literature, reviews the American College of Sports Medicine guidelines, and scores more than 90% on her class test on the material 2 weeks later. Her friends talk about stopping at the gym almost daily; however, she has yet to go with them and join in the gym exercise activities.

One of the main messages that the Transtheoretical Model of Change[23,24] proposes is that if education is introduced when someone is in a precontemplative phase, it does not result in a behavior change. The transtheoretical model[23,24] is especially important when considering the implementation of programs for major changes in life habits, smoking cessation, weight loss, and exercise programs. HCPs must emphasize readiness and give the patient responsibility and control. Also important to keep in mind when using this orientation is that the health behavior may be cyclical; therefore, we could often expect to see progress, setbacks, and periods of high and low compliance. Tolerance of those ups and downs with a general commitment to get back on track seems to be the key to incorporating the health behavior in one's life on a regular basis (see Table 16.2).

## *Motivational Interviewing*

Motivational interviewing (MI)[27,28] is a cognitive-behavioral approach that uses the Transtheoretical Model of Change,[23,24] mentioned previously, as a framework. The key premise is that people may best be persuaded by self-discovered reasons, rather than those in others' minds. HCPs use MI to help an individual to identify and change behavior related to health issues. The approach includes techniques to promote understanding of one's thought processes and emotional reactions to a health problem and how those thoughts and feelings result in common behavior patterns. MI is a collaborative conversation that is focused on engaging (*connecting*) for change, focusing on the reasons for change, evoking (*why and how*) and discovering a person's motivation for change, along with ensuring a planned commitment (*action*) to change. In what are often referred to as "mini-counseling sessions," HCPs utilize many of the communication skills first discussed in Chapters 6 and 8. MI incorporates open-ended queries with affirmations, reflective listening, and re-cap summaries for collaborative change.

Once the stage of change is determined, the key to behavior change using MI is to challenge habitual thought patterns and encourage and support alternative behaviors. This approach has been used effectively to institute interventions to traditionally overcome addictive behaviors, practice safer sex, and more recently to promote healthier behaviors with chronic disease, pain management, nutrition, osteoporosis prevention, telerehabilitation for post-op total joint arthroplasty and therapeutic activities post stroke, telehealth to promote community dwelling ambulation, functional mobility, and preventative home exercise programs.[29–36]

# WHICH APPROACH TO TAKE?

Given the variety of approaches that health behavior theorists[5,16–25,27] have taken to explain why patients choose or do not choose to take recommended action, HCPs have quite a few things to consider. How can we incorporate this information into good patient education? What educational activities are needed?

# PRINCIPLES OF EFFECTIVE PATIENT EDUCATION

*Education is the kindling of a flame, not the filling of a vessel.*
—Socrates

Patient education skills are just as critical to our success as the discipline-specific skills and activities that we learn as part of our professional training. HCP–patient education, instructional skills, and strategies take practice and development. Just as not all patient care skills are applicable to all patients, not all patient education skills are applicable either. However, in general, the following assist to positively influence patient behavior:

- Build rapport with the patient, an essential ingredient for all other aspects of the process.
- Set the agenda for change with the patient. The patient's priorities, the difficulties they perceive, and the realities of resource limitations are critical to this process.

- Communicate clearly and effectively. Focus on the message you want to send.
- Evaluate the patient's readiness to learn or intention for behavior change.
- Assess the patient's language skills, beliefs, cultural background, SDoH, environment, coping skills, and abilities that will help or hinder the change process.
- Customize your approach to the patient, their readiness, and associated needs.
- Assess barriers (cognitive, emotional, physical, social, or support systems) to carrying out recommendations.
- Problem solve with patients to generate solutions to apparent problems and concerns.
- Use appropriate teaching resources (videos, web-based, smart phone or other technological resources, written materials, peer support, family/caregivers, active learning approaches, and other HCPs) to facilitate the learning process.

Notice that this list does not include giving the patient a poorly visible photocopy of something you found in the files or even a computer-generated, custom-made list of exercises. Foremost is understanding the process of individualized behavior change as the key to effective patient education. Once you have assessed that the patient is ready, willing, and able to make the recommended change, there is sufficient time to introduce the appropriate instructional materials as reinforcements of the change process. Assess where the patient is in the change process and proceed with appropriate interventions. Now, how can you deliver your message in the most effective manner?

# ACTIVE AND PASSIVE APPROACHES TO LEARNING

Consider how to engage the patient as a partner in their education and best use of active, instead of passive, learning strategies. Passive learning approaches require the learner to acquire the information through listening, reading, or watching others. In contrast, active learning strategies require learners to process information, solve problems and respond or take action.[37] Evidence confirms that high-frequency contact through team-based interactive approaches encouraging patient participation and including feedback were associated with a higher effectiveness of lifestyle change in metabolic syndrome.[38] Examples of differences between passive and active learning are provided in Table 16.3.

| TABLE 16.3 | | |
|---|---|---|
| COMPARISON OF PASSIVE AND ACTIVE LEARNING APPROACHES | | |
| | PASSIVE | ACTIVE |
| Examples | Lectures, reading assignments, demonstrations, watching videos | Problem solving, feedback, peer support, discussion, experiments, role-play, journaling, writing, interactive participation, debate |
| Advantages | ○ Can present a large volume of information in a short time period<br>○ Easier for teacher and learner<br>○ Teacher and learner expectations are simpler and easier to meet<br>○ Aligned with traditional testing and assessment techniques | ○ Relevant and action oriented<br>○ Incorporates learner feedback and increases relevancy to culture and environment<br>○ Encourages learner to problem solve and apply to individual circumstances<br>○ Encourages innovation and transfer of knowledge or the experiences of others to new situations |
| Disadvantages | ○ Does not prepare learner for application or provide instructor with feedback of learner understanding and ability to use information<br>○ Lower-level rote processing of information is unlikely to lead to innovation, new discoveries, or adherence to treatment recommendations | ○ Learners may be uncomfortable using active learning strategies, especially if they are accustomed to passive strategies<br>○ May be more time consuming<br>○ May require flexibility and more interaction by instructor or provider |

# INSTRUCTIONAL PLANNING GUIDELINES

Let's look at some ideas used by leading instructional designers. The key elements of any instructional sequence answer the following questions:

- What is the problem and what are the patient's (learner's) goals?

- What is the learner's state of readiness for the recommended action?

- What do you want the learner to know, feel, or do? When? How often? Where? With whom?

- What is the key content that must be presented to accomplish these outcomes?

- What learning experiences will help to transmit this content and teach these skills?

- What key steps, decisions, and activities must the learner do to follow the recommendations?

- What materials can reinforce, supplement, or draw attention to the content or process?

- How will you know that you have been successful in teaching?

- How can you evaluate that the learner has learned what you were trying to teach?

Refer to these instructional planning guidelines and respond to the questions with respect to the following case revisited:

> Our patient has returned seeking treatment for a recurrent skin infection. The patient has already failed to take medication consistently on one occasion. The patient must now undergo a complicated, prolonged course of antibiotic treatment using medications with high potential for toxicity and will not be allowed to work in the hospital due to the possibility of spreading this antibiotic-resistant infection.

# PRESENTATION TIPS AND EDUCATIONAL ACTIVITIES

Whether you are teaching one-on-one or in a group situation, you may find it useful to incorporate the following ideas in your presentation:

- Present the most important content first. *("First, we are going to practice rising from the bed by side lying first.")*

- Be brief and emphasize the main point. *("Bend forward as you begin to stand up.")*

- Organize the information into topics, clusters, or categories. *("There are three steps to this process.")*

- Give specific one- to two-step instructions. *("Test your blood sugar 1 hour prior to meals.")*

- Repeat vital information in a variety of ways. *("You can see it again here—you have to bend your knees, not your back.")*

- Use a variety of instructional cues by considering visual, auditory, and kinesthetic prompts to address all varieties and types of ways in which learners prefer to receive information. Reinforce key principles by repeating in a way that addresses all potential learning styles through a variety of instructional modalities of dissemination. *(E.g., Verbally explain good body mechanics and provide auditory cues; physically demonstrate proper body mechanics, implementing visual cues; guide the learner in physically performing an activity of daily living, such as lifting a box or vacuuming, using good body mechanics; implementing one activity with learning reinforcements.)*

- Present at the comprehension level of the learner. *("We'll review some anatomy terms first before we get into the specifics of the technique." "Let's break down the movement activity into three parts first, then we will put them all together after we go through each.")*

Now consider the Sluijs **Checklist for Educational Activities**[39] in Table 16.4. The checklist was developed and validated by physical therapists, but the elements could be adapted and applied across multiple professions.[39] The checklist is helpful when you are providing home programming activities for patients/clients, caregivers, and their families. Examining the checklist, are there elements that you found surprising or unexpected? How would you choose to prioritize these elements for the aforementioned case? How might your approach be different if you were instructing a caregiver? Would you include all elements in every situation? Why are the various elements relevant?

| TABLE 16.4 |
|---|
| ### CHECKLIST[39] FOR EDUCATIONAL ACTIVITIES |

| **TEACHING AND PROVIDING INFORMATION ABOUT DIAGNOSIS** | |
|---|---|
| ○ About diagnosis and complaints<br>○ About the cause of diagnosis/illness/pathology<br>○ About the prognosis, health-related quality of life, and psychosocial implications | ○ Illustrative materials to clarify<br>○ Miscellaneous or additional related/relevant topics<br>○ Assessment of patient's/client's understanding |
| **INSTRUCTIONS FOR HOME EXERCISES/ACTIVITIES** | |
| ○ Explaining home exercises/activities<br>○ Frequency of each exercise/activity<br>○ Number of sessions per day<br>○ Exercise/activity specific instructions<br>○ The build-up of the exercise/activity program<br>○ The build-up of each exercise/activity<br>○ Exercise/activity information—precautions/contraindications/indications/risk | ○ Instructions written by the HCP and documented properly<br>○ Integrating exercises and daily activities<br>○ Motivating the patient to comply<br>○ Monitoring the patient's compliance<br>○ Resolving compliance problems<br>○ Miscellaneous or remaining topics |
| **ADVICE AND INFORMATION** | |
| ○ Rest intervals and expectations/outcomes<br>○ Self-care activities<br>○ Safety precautions/concerns<br>○ Correct posture and movement<br>○ General health education<br>○ Stress management<br>○ Caregiver/family member education | ○ Explanation of treatment, benefits<br>○ Relating goals and outcomes<br>○ Incorporating patient's/client's values and beliefs<br>○ Support from current evidence<br>○ Any referral needs and/or follow-up<br>○ Contact information |
| Adapted from Sluijs EM. A checklist to assess patient education in physical therapy practice: development and reliability. *Phys Ther.* 1991;71(8):561–569. | |

# CULTURE, LANGUAGE, AND LITERACY IN PATIENT EDUCATION

In *Unequal Treatment: Confronting Racial and Ethnic Disparities in Health Care*, Smedley et al.[40] reported that regardless of a patient's insurance status or income, individuals from racial and ethnic minority groups tend to receive a lower quality of health care than do members of nonminority groups. The study documented that stereotyping, biases, and uncertainty on the part of HCPs all contribute to unequal treatment. As discussed in previous chapters, particularly Chapters 7 and 13, a failure to recognize the influence of language or culture can easily lead to undesirable health outcomes. The seminal publication by Smedley et al. served as a wake-up call for both health policy makers and HCPs by documenting numerous examples of poor outcomes related to language barriers and cultural misunderstandings (SDoH). For example, findings indicated that patients with limited English proficiency were less likely to visit physicians and receive preventive services, regardless of economic status, source of care, literacy, health status, or insurance status. Patients with limited English proficiency also reported lower rates of satisfaction with their care. Researchers have found that patients who did not speak the same language as their HCP were more likely to miss appointments or drop out of treatment. Findings indicated that using interpreters seemed to eliminate the likelihood of missed appointments.[40] The National Standards for Culturally and Linguistically Appropriate Services (CLAS) in Health Care[41] mandate that health care organizations:

> *Provide effective, equitable, understandable, and respectful quality care and services that are responsive to diverse cultural health beliefs and practices, preferred languages, health literacy, and other communication needs. Offer language assistance to individuals who have limited English proficiency and/or other*

*communication needs, at no cost to them, to facilitate timely access to all health care and services. Ensure the competence of individuals providing language assistance, recognizing that the use of untrained individuals and/or minors as interpreters should be avoided.*

In the 20 years since the original CLAS report and recommendations were made, some progress has been accomplished through changes in policies, cross-cultural education, and implicit bias training, but the Covid-19 pandemic has shed additional light on the persistence of health care disparities; there is no one solution for these, yet there is a personal responsibility on behalf of each HCP. Work remains, with the need for more sustainable actions to progress health care equality.

# COMMUNICATING WITH THE NON-ENGLISH-SPEAKING PATIENT

Developing sensitivity to verbal and nonverbal language, speech patterns, and communication styles is an important skill for HCPs. Incorporating sensitivity to the potential influence of psychological, social, biological, physiological, cultural, political, spiritual, and environmental aspects of the patient's or client's experience is the obligation of HCPs for appropriate PPIs.

Services for non-English-speaking patients should include informing them that they have the right to receive no-cost interpreter services. Signs and commonly used written patient education materials should be translated for the predominant language groups in a service area.[41]

Try to use the patient's/client's preferred language whenever possible. Use interpreters as needed when bilingual clinicians are not available. Interpreters and bilingual staff should have bilingual proficiency and be trained in interpreting. They should have knowledge in both languages of the terms and concepts needed in the clinical encounter. Family members are not considered suitable substitutes for trained interpreters because they usually lack these skills and knowledge. Avoid using patients' children or grandchildren as interpreters. Numerous online apps are available for accurate language translation. Additional information and video units demonstrating working effectively with interpreters are provided in the Suggested Resources section at the end of this chapter.

# BRIDGING THE HEALTH LITERACY GAP

Poor HL can lead to life-threatening accidents and errors from misunderstandings about dosages or methods of administering medication. It may keep a patient from accessing key services for screening or seeking effective intervention for treatable illnesses. HL has especially serious implications for our older adult populations because older age has been shown to be strongly associated with limited HL, including reading, comprehension, reasoning, and numeracy skills.[42]

Approaches to patient education in conditions when individuals may face HL issues should incorporate interactive techniques and a careful selection of written and online materials. For example, a return demonstration, in which the patient teaches the content back to the educator, may maximize recall. Written materials for low-literacy users serve to illustrate key concepts and aid memory. Follow-up telephone calls, random reminders, email and/or texts, virtual assistants, and return visits also serve as a check for understanding. Random reminders for all patients are helpful, and even more so with limited English proficiency. Additional techniques, such as verbal quizzing, repetition, interactive games, individual coaching with concept mapping, theatrical productions, films, music, and radio have all been used to reach low-literacy populations. A coalition of national organizations with the Institute for Healthcare Improvement worked together to promote awareness and solutions around the issue of low HL and its effect on safe care and health outcomes. It developed a simple educational program called *Ask Me 3*®[43] (www.ihi.org/resources/tools/ask-me-3-good-questions-your-good-health).

This approach encourages individuals to ask their HCPs three simple questions:

1. What is my main problem?
2. What do I need to do?
3. Why is it important for me to do this?

We invite you to view the video on the *Ask Me 3*[43] website and/or YouTube and reflect on the information to reinforce your learning of the method to improve communications as a HCP.

# USE OF TECHNOLOGY IN PATIENT EDUCATION

With the explosion of personal computer use, voice assistants, and web-based information resources, many consumers turn to the Internet for health information. Technological interventions may be effective as a health information delivery system, especially for those with chronic conditions that can be self-managed and for those who lack health care access, in response to the Covid-19 pandemic, or those that just prefer technology-based care for efficiency and quality of life.[26,32–36,44] Evidence-based best practices for effective computer-based health education include use of engaging multimedia approaches, with voiceover and script messaging, opportunities for repetition, creation of a learning environment that allows privacy, designing questions and answers to reinforce key concepts, user control over sequence and information content, and careful integration with existing educational and preintervention procedures.[45]

Evidence supports the use of technology-specific interactive health communication applications to influence knowledge, social support, and clinical outcomes in chronic disease. Interactive health communication applications and web-based systems typically include a combination of health information, behavioral change support, social support, and decision-making support.[46] In addition, research supports positive effects of the use of monitored social networking sites to share data and provide health and fitness messages, links, and videos to address health behavior–related outcomes.[47]

Be wary of relying solely on search engines for information because it is only as credible as the posting source(s). Table 16.5 lists some online resources that may enhance your patient education efforts.

| TABLE 16.5 | |
|---|---|
| **HEALTH CARE RESOURCES: NATIONAL ASSOCIATIONS, GOVERNMENT AGENCIES, SOCIETIES, FOUNDATIONS, AND CORPORATIONS** | |
| American Academy of Orthopaedic Surgeons \| AAOS | aaos.org |
| American Cancer Society \| ACA | cancer.org |
| American Diabetes Association \| ADA | diabetes.org |
| American Heart Association \| AHA | heart.org |
| American Lung Association \| ALA | lung.org |
| American Physical Therapy Association \| APTA | apta.org |
| American Physical Therapy Association \| Choose PT | choosept.com |
| American Occupational Therapy Association \| AOTA | aota.org |
| American Red Cross \| ARC | redcross.org |
| American Speech-Language-Hearing Association \| ASHA | asha.org |
| Arthritis Foundation \| AF | arthritis.org |
| Brain Injury Association of America \| BIAA | biausa.org |
| Brain Trauma Foundation \| BTF | braintrauma.org |
| Centers for Disease Control and Prevention \| CDC | cdc.gov |
| Coalition for the Homeless | coalitionforthehomeless.org |
| Medscape and MedPulse app | medscape.com |
| National Association of Area Agencies on Aging \| NAAAA | healthinaging.org |
| National Coalition to End Homelessness | endhomelessness.org |
| National Homeless Law Center | homelesslaw.org |
| National Institute of Health \| NIH | www.nih.gov |

*(continued)*

| TABLE 16.5 (CONTINUED) | |
| --- | --- |
| **HEALTH CARE RESOURCES: NATIONAL ASSOCIATIONS, GOVERNMENT AGENCIES, SOCIETIES, FOUNDATIONS, AND CORPORATIONS** | |
| National Institute of Arthritis and Musculoskeletal and Skin Diseases \| NIAMSD | niams.nih.gov |
| National Institute of Diabetes and Digestive & Kidney Diseases \| NIDDKD | niddk.nih.gov |
| National Multiple Sclerosis Society \| NMSS | nationalmssociety.org |
| National Parkinson Foundation \| PDF | parkinson.org |
| Michael J. Fox Foundation for Parkinson's Disease \| MJFPD | Michaeljfox.org |
| United Spinal Association \| USA | spinalcord.org |
| National Stroke Association \| NSA | stroke.org |
| National Alliance for the Mentally \| NAMI | nami.org |
| WebMD | webmd.com |

# EVALUATING WRITTEN MATERIAL

Written materials are important adjuncts to the patient education process, whether in print or online. They should be selected or written specifically for the population with whom you are working or the goals of the intervention. Start to collect or bookmark samples of good patient education materials when you see them. Your target audience should be able to read and understand the written materials you choose. Be sensitive to technical terms, long sentences, and complex ideas. Watch the use of jargon and translation of medical language to lay terms. Materials should be written at a sixth- to eighth-grade reading level to reach the most people.

Examine the Flesch Reading Ease Readability Formula and the Gunning Fog Index Readability Formula for evaluating the reading level of written materials (Tables 16.6 to 16.8).

| TABLE 16.6 |
| --- |
| **THE FLESCH READING EASE READABILITY FORMULA** |
| 1. For short pieces, assess the entire selection. For longer pieces, test at least three randomly selected samples of 100 words each. Do not use introductory paragraphs as part of the sample. Start each sample at the beginning of a paragraph. |
| 2. Determine the average sentence length (SL) by counting the number of words in the sample and dividing them by the number of sentences. Count as a sentence each independent unit of thought that is grammatically independent (i.e., if its end is punctuated by a period, question mark, exclamation point, semicolon, or colon). In dialogue, count speech tags (e.g., "he said") as part of the quoted sentence. |
| 3. Determine the word length (WL) by counting all the syllables in the sample as if reading the words aloud. Divide the syllables by the number of words in the sample and multiply by 100. |

*(continued)*

| TABLE 16.6 (CONTINUED) |
|---|

## THE FLESCH READING EASE READABILITY FORMULA

4. These indices are then applied to the formula to compute the reading ease:

$$RE = 206.835 - (1.015 \times SL) - 0.846\ WL$$

where RE is the reading ease score, SL is the average sentence length in words, and WL is the average word length measured as syllables per 100 words.

### Interpretation of the Flesch Reading Ease Score

| Reading Ease | Grade | Description of Style | No. Syllables/ 100 Words | Average Sentence Length |
|---|---|---|---|---|
| 90 to 100 | 5 | Very easy | 123 | 8 |
| 80 to 90 | 6 | Easy | 131 | 11 |
| 70 to 80 | 7 | Fairly easy | 139 | 14 |
| 60 to 70 | 8 to 9 | Standard | 147 | 17 |
| 50 to 60 | 10 to 12 | Fairly difficult | 155 | 21 |
| 30 to 50 | College | Difficult | 167 | 25 |
| 0 to 30 | College graduate | Very difficult | 192 | 29 |

You may also find it useful to use an online generator to evaluate out the readability: www.readabilityformulas.com/free-readability-formula-tests.php

Adapted from Flesch R. *The Art of Readable Writing.* New York, NY: Harper & Row; 1974:184–186, 247–251.

---

| TABLE 16.7 |
|---|

## THE GUNNING FOG INDEX READABILITY FORMULA

1. Select a sample of writing 100 to 125 words long. If the piece is long, take several samples and average the results.
2. Calculate the average number of words per sentence. Treat independent clauses as separate sentences, "In school we studied: we learned: we improved" counts as three sentences.
3. Count the number of words of three syllables or more. In your count, omit capitalized words, combinations of short words such as bookkeeper or workforce, and verbs made into three syllables by adding "-es" or "-ed." Divide the count of long words by the passage length to get the percentage.
4. Add 2 (average sentence length) and 3 (percentage of long words). Multiply the sum by the factor 0.4, and ignore the digits following the decimal point. The result is the years of schooling needed to read the passage with ease. Few readers have more than 17 years of schooling, so any passage over 17 gets a Fog Index of "17-plus."

**(0.4 × [words ÷ sentence]) + (100 × [complex words ÷ words]) = years of schooling needed**

Adapted from Gunning R, Kallan R. *How to Take the Fog Out of Business Writing.* Chicago, IL: Dartnell Books; 1994.
The Fog Index Scale is a service mark licensed exclusively to RK Communication Consultants by D & M Mueller.
For comparison, you may also wish to utilize an online Gunning Fog Index Tool (http://gunning-fog-index.com/)

---

**TABLE 16.8**

## SAMPLE PATIENT EDUCATION MATERIALS WRITTEN AT DIFFERENT GRADE LEVELS

**WRITTEN AT THE 13TH GRADE LEVEL**

The heart usually receives electrical signals from the sinoatrial node, an area in the top right chamber. In ventricular tachycardia, the signals that orchestrate the rhythm originate in the ventricle, located below the atrium. This area of origin results in an erratic beat or rhythm. The erratic beat disables the ventricles from contracting; thus blood is unable to be pumped out adequately. Inadequate blood supply affects all body parts because oxygen and nutrients are located in the blood. When the brain does not receive adequate blood supply, symptoms that include fainting, dizziness, and unconsciousness can occur. Stroke and death are also potential results.

With the knowledge that ventricular tachycardia is an erratic and potentially fatal rhythm that can occur at unpredictable times, physicians usually prescribe medications to control or prevent that rhythm. When medications are unable to keep the erratic beat dormant, the heart may require defibrillation. Defibrillation resets the electrical circuit, allowing the sinoatrial node to once again dominate.

REWRITTEN AT THE 6TH GRADE LEVEL

Electrical signals from the heart's pacemaker keep the heart beating in a normal way. The pacemaker is called the S-A node and is found in the top part of the heart. Signals can also come from the bottom part of the heart. If they come from the bottom part, an irregular or rapid beat result. Several rapid and irregular beats are called V Tach. V Tach means the heart is not able to pump blood. When this happens, the body is not able to get the blood it needs. Blood carries oxygen and food to the body. One of the body parts that needs blood most is the brain. When the brain does not get blood, it can make a person feel faint or dizzy. It can also cause a stroke or death.

Doctors order medicines to try to control or stop this irregular or rapid beat. The medicines usually control this type of beat. Sometimes they do not work. The heart may then need to be shocked. The shock is given by a machine called a defibrillator. The shock usually helps the heart to reset its signals. It then beats in a regular way. All parts of the body can then get the supply of blood they need.

Adapted from Evanoski CAM. Sample patient education materials written at different grade levels. *J Cardiovasc Nurs.* 1990;4(2):1–6.

# PUTTING IT ALL TOGETHER

HCPs who educate patients join in a powerful partnership to achieve goals that each, separately, could not realize. Through understanding factors that influence attention, readiness for change, motivation, principles of instructional design and presentation, and the patient's desire for return to function,[48,49] we are better able to design and carry out effective patient education interventions. Finally, your capabilities in delivering patient education are paramount for effective and efficient health care. Continue your HCP professional formation through utilization of the reliable and validated **Physical Therapy Patient Education (PTPE) Performance Tool**[50] (Table 16.9) to assess your performance.

The combination of assessment of your educational interventions utilizing the **Checklist for Educational Activities**[39] (Table 16.4) along with your capacities as an health care educator through the **PTPE** (Table 16.9) will improve your readiness for direct patient/client education and for coaching for success with health behavior changes.[51-55] You will have the opportunity to do just that in the upcoming exercises at the end of this chapter.

| TABLE 16.9 | | | | | | |
|---|---|---|---|---|---|---|
| **PHYSICAL THERAPY PATIENT EDUCATION (PTPE) PERFORMANCE TOOL**[50] | | | | | | |
| **COMPETENCY** | **CIRCLE ONE NUMBER ONLY** | | | | | |
| 1. Seeks patient perceptions and/or concerns using appropriate questioning | 0 | 1 | 2 | 3 | 4 | Not assessable |
| 2. Uses reflective questioning | 0 | 1 | 2 | 3 | 4 | Not assessable |
| 3. Uses shared decision making | 0 | 1 | 2 | 3 | 4 | Not assessable |
| 4. Selects and uses appropriate learning content tailored to the best interests of the patient | 0 | 1 | 2 | 3 | 4 | Not assessable |
| 5. Uses effective and engaging communication styles, language, anchor materials that are tailored to the patient | 0 | 1 | 2 | 3 | 4 | Not assessable |
| 6. Effectively explains the patient's condition or problem | 0 | 1 | 2 | 3 | 4 | Not assessable |
| 7. Provides self-management education and reinforces patient ability to manage | 0 | 1 | 2 | 3 | 4 | Not assessable |
| 8. Provides family or caregivers with information | 0 | 1 | 2 | 3 | 4 | Not assessable |
| 9. Effectively summarizes information | 0 | 1 | 2 | 3 | 4 | Not assessable |
| 10. Uses the "teach back" (verbal or demonstration) method to evaluate learning | 0 | 1 | 2 | 3 | 4 | Not assessable |
| 11. Identifies when educational needs have been met | 0 | 1 | 2 | 3 | 4 | Not assessable |

\*Not assessable = no opportunity to demonstrate skill/competency.

† 0 = skill/competency not attempted or observed; 1 = a minimal attempt is made to exhibit skill/competency; 2 = skill/competency observed and a minimum skill level is achieved; 3 = skill/competency exhibited to a good standard; 4 = skill/competency exhibited to an excellent standard.

Forbes R, Mandrusiak A. Development and reliability testing of a patient education performance tool for physical therapy students. *J Phys Ther Educ.* 2022;33(1): Table 1. p 66.

# REFERENCES

1. Brickman P, Rabinowitz VC, Karuza J Jr, Coates D, Cohn E, Kidder L. Models of helping and coping. *Am Psychol.* 1982;37(4):368–384.
2. Williams MV, Parker RM, Baker DW, Parikh NS, Pitkin K, Coates WC, Nurss JR. Inadequate functional health literacy among patients at two public hospitals. *JAMA.* 1995 Dec 6;274(21):1677–1682.
3. UnitedHealth Group. *Health Literacy Key to Better Health Outcomes.* Available: https://www.unitedhealthgroup.com/newsroom/research-reports/posts/health-literacy-research-462863.html Accessed January 13, 2024.
4. Schönfeld MS, Pfisterer-Heise S, Bergelt C. Self-reported health literacy and medication adherence in older adults: a systematic review. *BMJ Open.* 2021;11(12):e056307.
5. Nielsen-Bohlman L, Panzer AM, Kindig DA. *Health Literacy: A Prescription to End Confusion.* Washington (DC): National Academies Press (US); 2004.
6. Lopez C, Bumyang K, Sacks K. *Health Literacy in the United States: Enhancing Assessments and Reducing Disparities.* Santa Monica, CA: Milken Institute; 2022.
7. Juvinyà-Canal D, Suñer-Soler R, Boixadós Porquet A, Vernay M, Blanchard H, Bertran-Noguer C. Health literacy among health and social care university students. *Int J Environ Res Public Health.* 2020;17:2273.
8. Fan, Zy, Yang Y, & Zhang F. Association between health literacy and mortality: a systematic review and meta-analysis. *Arch Public Health.* 2021;79:119.
9. Wittenberg E, Ferrell B, Kanter E, Buller H. Health literacy: exploring nursing challenges to providing support and understanding. *Clin J Oncol Nurs.* 2018;22(1):53–61.
10. Rafferty AP, Luo H, Winterbauer NL, Bell RA, Little NRG, Imai S. Health literacy among adults with multiple chronic health conditions. *J Public Health Mgt Pract.* 2021;28(2):E610–14.
11. Feinberg I, Scott JY, Holland DP, Lyn R, Scott LC, Maloney KM, Rothenberg R. The relationship between health literacy and COVID-19 vaccination prevalence during a rapidly evolving pandemic and infodemic. *Vaccines (Basel).* 2022 Nov 23;10(12):1989.
12. Shahid R, Shoker M, Chu LM, Frehlick R, Ward H, Pahwa P. Impact of low health literacy on patients' health outcomes: a multicenter cohort study. *BMC Health Serv Res.* 2022 Sep 12;22(1):1148.

13. Parker RM, Baker DW, Williams MV, Nurss JR. The test of functional health literacy in adults: a new instrument for measuring patients' literacy skills. *J Gen Intern Med*. 1995 Oct;10(10):537–541.
14. U.S. Department of Health and Human Services. *Health Literacy in Healthy People 2030*. Available: https://odphp.health.gov/healthypeople/priority-areas/health-literacy-healthy-people-2030 Accessed January 13, 2024.
15. Rosenstock IM. The Health Belief Model and preventive health behavior. *Health Education Monographs*. 1974;2(4):354–386. doi:10.1177/109019817400200405
16. Rotter JB. Generalized expectancies for internal versus external control of reinforcement. *Psychol Monogr*. 1966;80(1):1–28.
17. Arakelian M. Assessment and nursing applications of the concept of locus of control. *ANS Adv Nurs Sci*. 1980;3(25):25–42.
18. Johnston M, Gilbert P, Partridge C, Collins J. Changing perceived control in patients with physical disabilities: an intervention study with patients receiving rehabilitation. *Br J Clin Psychol*. 1992;31(pt 1):89–94.
19. Bandura A. Self-efficacy: toward a unifying theory of behavioral change. *Psychol Rev*. 1977;84(2):199–215.
20. Bandura A. Human agency in cognitive theory. *Am Psychol*. 1989;44(9):1175–1184.
21. Ajzen I. The theory of planned behavior. *Organ Behav Hum Decis Process*. 1991;50:179–211.
22. Pender NJ, Murdaugh CL, Parsons MA. *Health Promotion in Nursing Practice*, 8th ed. New York, NY: Pearson; 2019.
23. Prochaska JO, DiClemente CC. Transtheoretical therapy: toward a more integrative model of change. *Psychother Theory Res Pract*. 1982;19:276–288.
24. Prochaska JO, Velicer WF. The transtheoretical model of health behavior change. *Am J Health Promot*. 1997 Sep-Oct;12(1):38–48.
25. Basler HD. Patient education with reference to the process of behavioral change. *Patient Educ Couns*. 1995;26:93–98.
26. van Doorn D, Richardson N, Meredith D, Blake C, McNamara J. Study protocol: Evaluation of the "real-world" Farmers Have Hearts—Cardiovascular Health Program. *Prev Med Rep*. 2022 Oct 17;30:102010.
27. Bundy C. Changing behaviour: using motivational interviewing techniques. *J R Soc Med*. 2004;97(suppl 44):43–47.
28. Miller WR, Rollnick S. *Motivational Interviewing: Preparing People for Change*, 2nd ed. New York, NY: Guilford Publications; 2022.
29. Nijs J, Wijma AJ, Willaert W, Huysmans E, Mintken P, Smeets R, Goossens M, van Wilgen CP, Van Bogaert W, Louw A, Cleland J, Donaldson M. Integrating motivational interviewing in pain neuroscience education for people with chronic pain: a practical guide for clinicians. *Phys Ther*. 2020 May 18;100(5):846–859.
30. Van Looveren E, Meeus M, Cagnie B, Ickmans K, Bilterys T, Malfliet A, Goubert D, Nijs J, Danneels L, Moens M, Mairesse O. Combining cognitive behavioral therapy for insomnia and chronic spinal pain within physical therapy: a practical guide for the implementation of an integrated approach. *Phys Ther*. 2022 Aug 4;102(8):pzac075.
31. Berner P, Bezner JR, Morris D, Lein DH. Nutrition in physical therapist practice: tools and strategies to act now. *Phys Ther*. 2021 May 4;101(5):pzab061.
32. Allegue DR, Sweet SN, Higgins J, Archambault PS, Michaud F, Miller WC, Tousignant M, Kairy D. Lessons learned from clinicians and stroke survivors about using telerehabilitation combined with exergames: multiple case study. *JMIR Rehabil Assist Technol*. 2022 Sep 15;9(3):e31305.
33. Giangregorio LM, Thabane L, Adachi JD, Ashe MC, Bleakney RR, Braun EA, Cheung AM, Fraser LA, Gibbs JC, Hill KD, Hodsman AB, Kendler DL, Mittmann N, Prasad S, Scherer SC, Wark JD, Papaioannou A. Build better bones with exercise: protocol for a feasibility study of a multicenter randomized controlled trial of 12 months of home exercise in women with a vertebral fracture. *Phys Ther*. 2014 Sep;94(9):1337–1352.
34. Heij W, Sweerts L, Staal JB, Teerenstra S, Adang E, van der Wees PJ, Nijhuis-van der Sanden MWG, Hoogeboom TJ. Implementing a personalized physical therapy approach (Coach2Move) is effective in increasing physical activity and improving functional mobility in older adults: a cluster-randomized, stepped wedge trial. *Phys Ther*. 2022 Oct 6:pzac138.
35. Kline PW, Melanson EL, Sullivan WJ, Blatchford PJ, Miller MJ, Stevens-Lapsley JE, Christiansen CL. Improving physical activity through adjunct telerehabilitation following total knee arthroplasty: randomized controlled trial protocol. *Phys Ther*. 2019 Jan 1;99(1):37–45.
36. Pellegrini CA, Brown D, DeVivo KE, Lee J, Wilcox S. Promoting physical activity via physical therapist following knee replacement: a pilot randomized controlled trial. *PMR*. 2022 Sep 15.
37. Russell AT, Comello RJ, Wright DL. Teaching strategies promoting active learning in healthcare education. *J Educ Hum Dev*. 2007;1(1):1–12.
38. Bassi N, Karagodin I, Wang S, et al. Lifestyle modification for metabolic syndrome: a systematic review. *Am J Med*. 2014;127(12):1242.e1–1242.e10.
39. Sluijs EM. A checklist to assess patient education in physical therapy practice: development and reliability. *Phys Ther*. 1991;71(8):561–569.
40. Smedley BD, Stith AY, Nelson AR, eds. *Unequal Treatment: Confronting Racial and Ethnic Disparities in Health Care*. Washington, DC: The National Academies Press; 2002.
41. US Department of Health and Human Services. *National Standards for Culturally and Linguistically Appropriate Services in Health Care*. Washington, DC: US Department of Health and Human Services, Office of Minority Health; 2004. Available: https://thinkculturalhealth.hhs.gov/clas/standards Accessed January 22, 2024.
42. Kobayashi LC, Wardle J, Wolf MS, von Wagner C. Aging, and functional health literacy: a systematic review and meta-analysis. *J Gerontol B Psychol Sci Soc Sci*. 2016 May;71(3):445–457.
43. Institute for Healthcare Improvement. *Ask Me 3®: Good Questions for Your Good Health*. https://www.ihi.org/resources/tools/ask-me-3-good-questions-your-good-health Accessed: Nov 10, 2024.

44. Kashikar-Zuck S, Barnett KA, Williams SE, Pfeiffer M, Thomas S, Beasley K, Chamberlin LA, Mundo K, Ittenbach RF, Peugh J, Gibler RC, Lynch-Jordan A, Ting TV, Gadd B, Taylor J, Goldstein-Leever A, Connelly M, Logan DE, Williams A, Wakefield EO, Myer GD; FIT Teens Clinical Trial Study Group and the Childhood Arthritis and Rheumatology Research Alliance (CARRA) Pain Workgroup Investigators. FIT Teens RCT for juvenile fibromyalgia: protocol adaptations in response to the COVID 19 pandemic. *Contemp Clin Trials Commun.* 2022 Nov 29;30:101039

45. Fox MP. Systematic review reporting on studies that examined the impact of interactive, computer-based patient education programs. *Patient Educ Couns.* 2009;77(1):6–13.

46. Lightfoot CJ, Wilkinson TJ, Hadjiconstantinou M, Graham-Brown M, Barratt J, Brough C, Burton JO, Hainsworth J, Johnson V, Martinez M, Nixon AC, Pursey V, Schreder S, Vadaszy N, Wilde L, Willingham F, Young HML, Yates T, Davies MJ, Smith AC. The co-development of "My Kidneys & Me": A digital self-management program for people with chronic kidney disease. *J Med Internet Res.* 2022 Nov 14;24(11):e39657.

47. Petkovic J, Duench S, Trawin J, Dewidar O, Pardo Pardo J, Simeon R, DesMeules M, Gagnon D, Hatcher Roberts J, Hossain A, Pottie K, Rader T, Tugwell P, Yoganathan M, Presseau J, Welch V. Behavioural interventions delivered through interactive social media for health behaviour change, health outcomes, and health equity in the adult population. *Cochrane Database Syst Rev.* 2021 May 31;5(5):CD012932.

48. Randall KE, McEwen IR. Writing patient-centered functional goals. *Phys Ther.* 2000;80(12):1197–1203.

49. O'Neill DL, Harris SR. Developing goals and objectives for handicapped children. *Phys Ther.* 1982;62(3):295–298.

50. Forbes R, Mandrusiak A. Development and reliability testing of a patient education performance tool for physical therapy students. *J Phys Ther Educ.* 2022;33(1):64–69.

51. Michie S, van Stralen MM, West R. The behaviour change wheel: a new method for characterising and designing behaviour change interventions. *Implement Sci.* 2011;6:42.

52. Mather M, Pettigrew LM, Navaratnam S. Barriers, and facilitators to clinical behaviour change by primary care practitioners: a theory-informed systematic review of reviews using the Theoretical Domains Framework and Behaviour Change Wheel. *Syst Rev.* 2022;11(1):180.

53. Bartlett EE. At last, a definition. *Patient Educ Couns.* 1983;7:323–324.

54. McManus DA. The two paradigms of teaching and the peer review of teaching. *J Geoscience Educ.* 2001;49(5):423–434.

55. den Bakker CR, Hendriks RA, Houtlosser M, Dekker FW, Norbart AF. Twelve tips for fostering the next generation of medical teachers. *Med Teach.* 2022;44(7): 725–729.

# Suggested Resources

Australian Heart Foundation, Motivational Interviewing with Dr. Stan Steindl, Clinical Psychologist
www.heartfoundation.org.au
*Dr. Steindl provides Motivational Interviewing techniques, tips with YouTube examples for HCPs. Discusses experiential insights related to MI and the Transtheoretical Model of Change.*

Center for Disease Control (CDC), Health Literacy: Accurate, Accessible and Actionable Health Information for All
www.cdc.gov/health-literacy/php/develop-plan/cdc-plan.html
*Center for Disease Control website with resources for health communicators, public health professionals, and community leaders who seek information and tools on health literacy research, practice, and evaluation. Includes the HL National Action Plan, activities by state and links to HL training modules.*

Deusinger SS, My father's journey: a reading and interview with Susan S. Deusinger, PT, PhD, FAPTA. *Journal of Humanities in Rehabilitation* (jhrehab.org)
www.jhrehab.org/2020/11/17/
*Dr. Deusinger shares her father's 83 year journey in a conversational style describing his journey toward death, a journey touched by loss, illustrating the locus of control with choice, as the highest privilege patients have in health care—a privilege the system struggles to honor. This is the story of her father's beliefs and choices.*

Health Resources and Services Administration (HRSA)
www.hrsa.gov
*Provides toolkits for HL, universal precautions, clear communications, print and web based guides, and video resources.*

Mather M, Pettigrew LM, Navaratnam S. Barriers and facilitators to clinical behaviour change by primary care practitioners: a theory informed systematic review of reviews using the Theoretical Domains Framework and Behaviour Change Wheel. *Syst Rev.* 2022;11(1):180
*Comprehensive systematic review of the Behavior Change Wheel related to capabilities, opportunities, and capacities and the relationship to theoretical domains framework.*

Miller WR, Rollnick S, Butler CC. *Motivational Interviewing in Healthcare: Helping Patients Change Behavior*, 2nd ed. New York, NY: Guilford Publications; 2022
*The decisive guide to MI for HCPs utilizing the engaging, focusing, evoking, and planning approach; incorporates lessons learned from the authors' ongoing clinical practice. Includes a case example addressing vaccine hesitancy.*

U.S. Department of Health & Human Services—Think Cultural Health (hhs.gov)
https://thinkculturalhealth.hhs.gov/resources/videos
*Video units for review on culturally and linguistically diverse care with utilization of an interpreter.*
https://thinkculturalhealth.hhs.gov/assets/pdfs/resource-library/working-effectively-with-interpreter.pdf
*Checklist for effectively working with an interpreter.*

U.S. Department of Health and Human Services, Office of Disease Prevention and Health Promotion—Healthy People 2030 (health.gov)
https://odphp.health.gov/healthypeople
*Provides data driven national objectives to improve health and well being over the next decade; including the Leading Health Indicators for the Nation, and helpful evidence based resources on health behaviors and conditions, populations, settings and systems, and social determinants of health.*

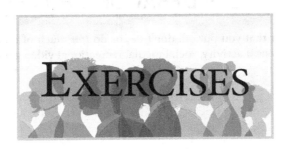

# EXERCISE 1: EXPLORING PROVIDER PERCEPTIONS OF RESPONSIBILITY

For what types of problems do you hold most patients responsible? List a few of these problems below.

# EXERCISE 2: USING THEORY TO UNDERSTAND HEALTH BEHAVIOR CHOICES

1.  Identify a health behavior that you put off, don't do, or do too much of on a daily basis (sleep, dentist, safe sex, healthy nutrition, physical activity, social media, recreational video gaming, etc.). What are your beliefs about these behaviors?

2.  Enter the answers to these in your journal (or here) and be prepared to discuss in class.

    a.  Susceptibility to the health threat? (i.e., How likely is it that I will have this problem?)

    b.  Severity of the health threat? (i.e., How serious is this problem?)

    c.  Benefits of the recommended behavior? (i.e., What will I gain by doing this?)

    d.  Barriers or costs of the recommended behavior? (i.e., What are the obstacles that stand in my way or the costs to me of taking this action?)

    e.  What environmental cues influence you?

    f.  What have you seen and learned from others?

    g.  In what stage (transtheoretical model of change[23-24]) would you place yourself at this moment? Have you moved through various stages recently?

    h.  What can you do to influence your own behavior?

    i.  What beliefs must you change?

    j.  What cues would make it more likely that you'll make the behavior change?

    k.  What forms of social support or decision support would be helpful to you to make this change?

3.  Now, make an **action plan**. Identify the challenge and which domain is most impacting your ability to achieve your goal (affective, cognitive, psychomotor, spiritual); utilize Bloom's taxonomy (see Chapter 3 Appendix—Bloom's Taxonomies) learning domains to select the level and action verbs needed for your short- and long-term goals. Include your personal behavior change goal (in the ABCDE format) and specifically include the following:

    - **Identified Health Behavior Concern to Address (problem):**
    - **Domain most Impacting (Affective, Cognitive, Psychomotor, Spiritual):**
    - **Goal Statement:**
        - A—**Audience** or Who? (You in this case, or "I"):

        - B—**Behavior** or What? (Behavior you wish to change):

        - C—**Condition** or Context? Every behavioral objective should state how or in what context (where) in which the goal occurs:

        - D—**Degree** or How well? (How will you measure how well you are doing or your success and track your progress?):

        - E—**Expected** time frame or by when? (By when will the short- and long-term goals be completed?):

    Put it all together → **Measurable ABCDE—Goal Statement** summarized in one goal statement (Audience/ who, Behavior/what, Condition/context/where, Degree/ how well, Expected time frame/by when?):

    - **Identify Transtheoretical Model Level:**
    - **Stage of Change:**
    - **Specific Action Plan for Change:**

    Develop your plan for action, and include the following: What steps will you take to make the change? What rewards might you build in to reinforce your efforts? How will you employ those who influence you (or not) to assist you in your goal achievement?

    Once you have formulated your goal and specific action plan on how you shall achieve your goal, identify a behavior change partner and work together to monitor, coach, and track each other's progress. Discover how your stage in the transtheoretical model of change[23–24] is impacting your or your partner's progress. Consider how you can facilitate each other based on the stage and progress (or regression) to date.

    As the peer change partner, explore the following key questions when checking in regularly with your partner's progress, which may be supportive through change (modified from Michie et al.[51]):

    - Transtheoretical Model of Change: *What is the current stage of change?*
    - Understanding the behavior: *What problem/s are we trying to solve? What behavior/s need to change, and in what way? What will it take for the desired change/s to happen?*
    - Identifying intervention options: *What intervention/s and/or modified intervention/s are likely to bring about the necessary change?*
    - Identifying implementation options: *What should the specific content of the intervention/s be? How should these be implemented? What adjustment/s are needed along the way?*
    - Relapse prevention: *What are the benefits of changing?*

# EXERCISE 3: EXPLORING THE PERCEPTIONS OF OTHERS

Identify a health behavior topic relevant to your profession (e.g., repetitive stress disorders for computer users, preventing low back pain, preventing sexually transmitted diseases, low-fat diet). Do a mini survey of ten people on campus, in your community, or at your facility about their beliefs on this topic (the cause, the severity of the problem, the effectiveness, and ease of prevention or treatment). You can do this as an in-class activity if the instructor assigns it.

1. List your chosen health behavior.

2. Prepare some questions (open-ended) to gather information.

3. Summarize your results (using data charts and summarizing feedback) and discuss in class.

4. Based on your results, how might your approach differ next time or how will you build upon the exploration? Discuss, as a HCP, how you might address the outcomes in your community of service. Consult the Healthy People 2030 website in the recommended resources for additional information for health behaviors and conditions affecting your chosen population.

# EXERCISE 4: DEVELOPING EFFECTIVE INTERVENTIONS TO PROMOTE HEALTHY CHOICES

Identify a health behavior topic relevant to your profession. You can choose the same topic on which you did a needs assessment in Exercise 2 or 3.

1. How would you organize a patient education approach?

2. What is the problem and your goals?

3. What is the learner's state of readiness for the recommended action?

4. What do you want the learner to know, feel, or do? When? How often? Where? With whom?

5. What is the key content that must be presented to accomplish these outcomes?

6. What learning experiences will help to transmit this content and teach these skills?

7. What key steps, decisions, and activities must the learner do to follow recommendations?

8. What materials can reinforce, supplement, or draw attention to the content or process?

9. How will you know that you've been successful in teaching? How can you evaluate that the learner has learned what you were trying to teach?

# EXERCISE 5: EVALUATING WRITTEN PATIENT EDUCATION MATERIALS

Select a patient education pamphlet, brochure, or consumer education website with at least 30 sentences and analyze its reading level using the Flesch Reading Ease Readability Formula (see Table 16.6) and the Gunning Fog Index (see Table 16.7). Note, additional readability formulas are available online (https://readabilityformulas.com/freetests/six-readability-formulas.php) an alternative to the Fog Index is the SMOG Readability Formula. Be prepared to talk about your pamphlet in a small group.

1.  What messages specifically influence the reader's perceptions of the following:

    a.  The cause of the problem and their susceptibility to the problem?

    b.  The severity of the problem?

    c.  The effectiveness of their actions?

    d.  Ease of taking those actions?

    e.  Barriers to those actions?

2.  How would you improve the brochure?

    The patient returns for follow-up today with essentially no change in their condition … Questionable compliance with the prescribed treatment program. Plan: review importance of continuing daily medication.

# EXERCISE 6: STRETCHING—PRIMING ACTIVITY

## *Putting It All Together: Patient–Family Education Plan*

Please complete this exercise once you have completed Chapters 15 and 16 in this book. The exercise is introduced here to begin to stretch you to think about this patient case as you proceed with your additional learning in the upcoming chapters, and to give you time to develop your educational interventions and practice delivering your patient/family education.

Consider a patient, Kim, within a neurorehabilitation unit who is receiving ongoing therapies twice per day. You are going to instruct her parent and the patient in a home educational program for the long weekends and after hours when therapy is not in session. The patient is a 19-year-old female who was traveling with three friends back to Florida from Mardi Gras. They were drinking and driving; she was not wearing a seatbelt, but everyone else in the vehicle was. They were involved in a motor vehicle accident, and she was thrown from the car through the window and sustained a traumatic brain injury. Kim had graduated from high school, where she had run track, and has been attending the local community college and working at the Gap. Her mom has a high school education and works part-time as a server, and her father completed vocational school and works at the local wheel-manufacturing plant. Kim was living at home at the time of the accident. Her parents are Bible Baptist, raised their child in their religion, and were not aware that she consumed alcohol at all. The mother wants her to get rest so that her brain heals more quickly and does not want to cause her further injury, but the father is very worried about the medical bills and wants her to be discharged as soon as possible. Kim was released from the acute care hospital after 5 days and discharged to the neurorehabilitation unit for a potential 30- to 90-day stay.

Currently, Kim requires the assistance of one to two HCPs, minimally to moderately, for all of her activities of daily living, including bathing and dressing. Kim is able to ambulate with moderate to maximum assistance of one to two HCPs. Her primary problem with upright gait is that she has extreme trunk extension in standing and is therefore unable to maintain her center of gravity within her base of support in upright postures. When ambulating, she tends to lean to the right side, and it becomes more pronounced as she fatigues. However, she is able to sit with the standby assistance of one HCP for short periods of time. She must use a posey vest when seated in the wheelchair, even with the use of the tray table, due to lack of safety recognition and sudden movements.

Kim has a 1- to 2-beat clonus in her right lower extremity and approximately a one-finger-width subluxation at the right glenohumeral joint, with pain with flexion above 90 degrees and beyond 45 degrees of abduction. She tends to hold her arm in a flexed and adducted position across her body, as if it were in a sling. The therapist reported this to the doctor, and a plain x-ray was completed, which ruled out any fracture. The physical and occupational therapists have been doing cotreatments once a day because her endurance for activities is still only about 45 minutes at a time. She is also receiving speech therapy and speaks in a very monotone pattern, without voice inflections. She is having memory problems but is emerging in cognition. She is able to follow 1- to 2-step commands. She is inconsistent in her bowel and bladder control and therefore wears a disposable diaper garment. Kim is able to sign her name, but it is micrographic and excessively slanted, not like she used to write at all.

Kim is experiencing some right-side neglect and has netting over her bed, called a full-enclosure bed or posey bed, that is like a canopy with netting/webbing on all four sides (to avoid needing night restraints so she does not need to be in posey garments during the night) to keep her from wandering at night or injuring herself or others, along with full bed rails. The nursing staff has video monitoring of the room to ensure that suffocation or entrapment is not a concern, and they do rounds every hour. Kim is eating and drinking well and requires minimal to moderate assist of one aide to help with meals due to distractibility and difficulty grasping objects and placing consistently. She has challenges with utensil use and putting on her makeup. She can brush her hair but tends to ignore the right side. We are trying to determine if she might have hemianopia. She is unable to stand and balance on one leg without maximum assistance from one HCP and has trouble maintaining middle line with stationary standing, even in the parallel bars with cueing and the use of a mirror for feedback.

- Glasgow Coma Scale: Eye Opening, 4; Verbal Response, 3; Motor Response, 6
- Rancho Los Amigos Scale: Level V and Level VI (fluctuating)

Develop a **measurable education goal** (in the **ABCDE** format, see Exercise 2) for the patient/family with traumatic brain injury's parent(s) and expand the plan to include the educational elements provided by the Sluijs **Checklist for Educational Activities** (see Table 16.4). Consider in your educational plan the learning style of the family member(s), cultural elements, active teaching strategies, leadership principles, the potential need for conflict resolution, generational differences, effective communication, aspects of interpersonal interactions, the FOG and Flesch formulas, the stage of change determinations, and any need for consultation or referrals. Prepare your educational plan activities based on the educational goal, following the checklist, as applicable related to your selected goal, and be prepared to implement it in a class session designated by your instructor. Don't forget to use peer and self-assessment of your developed patient education plan by assessing your delivery of patient/family education utilizing the **PTPE Performance Tool**[50] (Table 16.9). You may wish to practice videorecording your patient education encounter and then review. Please consider safety aspects related to Kim's emerging coma status. To summarize:

1. Review the case of Kim, above. Note key areas for HCP engagement and status. Note family and social history. Discern what **educational problems** need to be addressed.

2. Develop a **measurable educational learning goal for Kim and her family** (ABCDE format and identify the primary learning domain/s) (refer to Chapter 3, Appendix).

3. Develop an **educational intervention** for Kim and her family based upon the **Checklist for Educational Activities**[39] (Table 16.4) as a guideline, along with the need for any patient/family educational supporting materials.

4. Deliver the patient education intervention and self, peer-assess your delivery utilizing the **PTPE Performance Tool**[50] (Table 16.9). Practice, assess, review, repeat with your peers.

5. Be prepared to demonstrate your patient–family education intervention in class.

As a reminder, patient education is defined as:

**a planned learning experience using a combination of methods such as teaching, counseling and behavior modification techniques which influence patients' knowledge and health behavior.**[53]

These exercises are also available online at www.routledge.com/9781638220039.

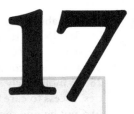

# COMMUNICATING WITH PEOPLE WHO HAVE DISABILITIES

## PERSON-CENTERED PRACTICE

*Gina Maria Musolino and Kathleen A. Curtis*

## OBJECTIVES

*The learner should be able to*:

- Accentuate the power of language and the use of words that reflect our innermost values, feelings, and thoughts.
- Appraise the negative results of labeling people with disabilities.
- Distinguish between descriptors often used inappropriately.
- Explore models of disability and how concepts of disability influence actions.
- Advocate for person-centered/identity-first language as the humane choice that makes a difference in how we view people who have disabilities.
- Be cognizant of the impact of Social Determinants of Health (SDoH) and key legislation related to issues of disability, children with disabilities, and older adults
- Support that individuals with disabilities are human—no more, no less—and that to emphasize what an inspiration they are often serves to dehumanize them as paragons of virtue.
- Appreciate the unique lived experiences of each person with disability.
- Challenge how we might identify and counter our indoctrinated prejudices and/or biases from our culture.

According to the United States (U.S.) national estimates, approximately 1 in 4 Americans (26% of adults), numbering more than 61 million people, report a disability, with over 1 billion people estimated worldwide.[1] This may be a chronic disease process, such as persons with heart disease, sickle cell anemia, epilepsy, or cancer; a sensory disability, such as a hearing or visual impairment; a physical disability, such as persons with an amputation, paralysis, or problem with pain or movement (e.g., walking, climbing stairs); a learning disability, such as persons with dyslexia or attention deficit disorder; a cognitive disability, such as persons with confusion, trouble concentrating, poor memory,

DOI: 10.4324/9781003525554-17

or an inability for decision making; or a disability related to mental health, such as persons with schizophrenia or bipolar disorder; or a combination. The number of people with disabilities today may be underestimated due to the impacts of long Covid still being determined. For those with disabilities, many have additional challenges with health behaviors and conditions with a "more likely" percentage than those without disabilities: 36% more likely being obese, 28.2% more likely smokers, 11.5% more likely heart disease, and 16.3% more likely diabetes.[1] For those with disabilities, access to care and regular care is also problematic with 1 in 3 having unmet health care needs due to cost and 1 in 4 not having regular check-ups.[1]

Some disabilities are not visible to the casual observer; others are obvious. Some disabilities are stable; some are progressive or intermittent in nature.

> *We know that equality of individual ability has never existed and never will, but we do insist that equality of opportunity still must be sought.* —Franklin D. Roosevelt

How many members of your family have a disability? Rates of disability increase with age,[2] with an estimated 61.4% of older adults in the U.S. aged 65 years and older reporting a disability.[3] Disorders of the musculoskeletal, circulatory, and respiratory systems are the three leading causes of disability.[3] Regardless of the type of disability, individuals with disabilities share some common experiences and challenges in their lives. One might assume that all, most, or some people with disabilities have some common characteristics. That assumption is as wrong as assuming that all people of Italian descent like spaghetti or that people who are tall must be good at basketball.

The guidelines in this chapter are intended to enlighten and stimulate you to examine your attitudes, beliefs, and the subtle and not-so-subtle limitations that you may inadvertently place on the value of a person and their own rights, privileges, and potential contribution to the world, based on the diagnosis, conditions, and/or problems they present to you.

## LABELS—THE POWER OF WORDS

Health care professionals (HCPs) spend many years of education and training studying the characteristics of diagnoses, pathologies, and their typical signs and symptoms. In the seemingly endless task to master the extensive classification of diagnostic categories and subcategories, sometimes we lose sight of the fact that real people have these disorders.

Language is a powerful symbol of our understanding of these complex concepts. Our knowledge, attitudes, beliefs, and values determine what we pay attention to and the thoughts we have about what we hear, read, or experience. The language we use reflects, as well as influences, our thoughts and feelings. Our thoughts and feelings determine, to a large extent, how we act. Moreover, language is not just an issue of political correctness; it influences beliefs, attitudes, expectations, and the course of events.

### The Results of Labeling

The experience of persons with disabilities throughout time has been largely negative. Summarily, people with disabilities undergo experiences that stigmatize, dehumanize, disempower, and generally discount their needs. Not only do individuals with disabilities face the discrimination of physical barriers in housing, schools, business, and health care, they often face staggering obstacles in overt and covert discrimination in the job market. Owing to a multitude of factors such as physical or mental restrictions, societal prejudice, or inadequate working conditions and accommodations, persons with a disability have a harder time getting a job than their nondisabled peers. In 2022, the U.S. Department of Labor Statistics reported the employment rate of working-age people (16–64) with disabilities in the U.S. was 38.%, compared with 76.9% of those without disabilities.[4] With fewer employment opportunities, many people with disabilities end up in poverty and/or must depend upon others for daily living. Regrettably, during the novel Covid-19 pandemic, persons with disabilities within the U.S. were disproportionately subject to sources of trauma and stress.[5] Let's look at some beliefs that may underlie these staggering statistics.

## WHAT'S IN A NAME?

Let's consider verbs first. Look at the difference between the active tense and the passive tense. In describing an individual's relationship to an assistive device, one can draw a marked distinction in the meaning of "being confined to a wheelchair" and "using a wheelchair."

There is also an essential distinction between being and having. Can you sense the difference between being a "quadriplegic" and being a "person who has quadriplegia"? Bottom line—describing a person as the attributes of their disability connotes an identity solely as the disability. In addition, the emphasis on the disability draws attention to our perception of difference, which most often increases psychological and social distance. We feel less at one with those we perceive to be most different.

Many terms have been used over the years to refer to people with disabilities. We can also draw a distinction between the terms *disability* and *handicap*. A disability has been defined as a condition of the person. The term *disability* has been debated, in that by pure definition it connotes a problem with ability. Some persons with disabilities prefer to define a disability as meaning *a person may do something a little differently from a person who does not have a disability, but with equal participation and equal results,*[6] hence, *differently abled.* Yet, it is important to ask the person how they would like to be represented and referred to in their lived experiences.[6-7]

Another term, *handicap*, has been used to connote the accrued result of multiple barriers (emotional, physical, social, environmental) imposed by society that prevent an individual who has a disability from assuming a desired role in society. For example, the characteristic that a person cannot walk quickly from place to place is a feature of a disability. The employer who hires a less qualified applicant who walks more quickly, the landlord who rents to another tenant, the university campus and classroom layout that requires a half-mile walk in the 10-minute break between classes—all help to create the handicaps associated with disability.

Today, we speak in terms of the Social Determinants of Health (SDoH), as specifically discussed in Chapters 1 (Figure 1.1), 3, 11, and 14–16.

Various models have been proposed over the years to define the concepts surrounding disability (Table 17.1).[8-10] Notice the distinction between problems at the body organ level, the economic level, the functional activity or performance level, and the level of the cultural or social environment. Health care professionals often focus on factors at the body organ and functional level; the person with a disability experiences most life problems because of factors in the economic, cultural, political, and social environment. Hence, HCPs must shift their mindset to discover the SDoH impacting each person and incorporate in their plans of care the paradigms for that person's lived experience, to truly understand the needs of that person and provide for person-centered care. Can you think of examples of those you have worked with in health care?

The World Health Organization (WHO) International Classification of Functioning, Disability and Health (ICF)[11] is perhaps the most prevalent framework used today, especially in rehabilitation, providing the platform for HCPs paradigm shift. It incorporates health conditions and their effects, as well as environmental factors. The ICF interactive model focuses on the concept of participation (involvement in a life situation), rather than the disorder or disease, impairment, or deviation. Pay attention to whether your focus is on the disease or impairment or the life experience of the individual with a disability. Be sure to acknowledge individual differences. Few people with similar impairments experience the same degree of disability, activity limitation, or participation restriction. Similarly, the cultural, social, political, and physical environment in which a person with a disability lives may vary widely and strongly influences the individual's activities and participation in society.

Both the medical and social model approaches to disability still present with some shortcomings and the "*disability-affirmative, intersectional* approach [Table 17.1] can serve as a strategy for challenging and reforming" what may be perceived as oppressive systems.[9-10]

Derived from Black Feminist literature, the intersectional approach considers that "a disabled individual may hold other marginalized or oppressed identities and these intersecting oppressions may exacerbate health inequities."[9] Brinkman et al.[9] provide a specific example illustrating the intersectional approach:

> *Eugenia, a Black person who uses a wheelchair who is also a lesbian, transgender, and Muslim will have a different lived experience than others. There's every possibility that Eugenia will have to navigate misogyny, racism, Islamophobia, homophobia, and ableism on any given day. Different parts of her identity might be dependent on the others, which means she might experience discrimination for one or many aspects of her identity either simultaneously or in isolation. The oppression can be multi-layered, deeply complex, and no doubt very tiring.*[9]

# INCLUSIVE LANGUAGE

An established standard of good writing, *person-centered/identity-first language*, requires that the writer identifies the person—the woman, transgender, man, child, professor, student, client, physician, receptionist, mother—and then refers to the attribute of having a disability (if it is applicable at all to the discussion; e.g., the man with epilepsy) rather than using the disability as either an adjective (e.g., the epileptic driver) or a noun (e.g., an epileptic). This distinction, although subtle, makes a profound difference in our focus and perceptions. It empowers and provides information rather than stigmatizing and labeling (Table 17.2).[12]

| TABLE 17.1 |
|---|

## MODELS OF DISABILITY[8,9]

| MODEL | CHARACTERISTICS OF MODEL | WHAT HCPS SHOULD KNOW |
|---|---|---|
| **Medical** | Denotes a medical etiology that emphasizes the cause of disability as a medical condition or disorder. Disabilities are treated as diagnostic categories. Individuals with disabilities assume a sick role. | HCPs assume that the cause of a disability is a medical condition. Instead, consider how the individual's social or emotional life affects their physical health. *How do our social expectations or the environment influence the individual's experience of disability?* The medical model minimizes consideration of the social sources of disability, such as stigma, prejudice, and public policy. |
| **Economic** | Relates to the individual's inability or limited ability to work. Medical evaluations of disability are used to predict the likelihood of employment. Links functional physical capacity with employment. | Research indicates that employment of persons with disabilities is influenced greatly by social and economic trends, not by the nature of their disabilities or their functional capacities. |
| **Functional Limitation Paradigm** | Pathology and impairment refer to an individual's medical condition and the related limitations. In contrast, the term disability refers to social function. It is the interaction of an individual's physical or mental limitations with environmental and social factors that determines disability. | Individuals with physical or mental impairments and functional limitations do not necessarily experience disability in the same ways. Individuals may have a disability in one environment and not in another. |
| **Sociopolitical** | At the heart of the disability rights movement is the common understanding that disability is an acceptable form of human variation. In this context, disability is viewed as a policy and civil rights issue, with individuals with disabilities considered an oppressed minority, facing daily prejudice and discrimination. Individuals with disabilities experience architectural, sensory, attitudinal, cognitive, and economic barriers, limiting their full participation in society. | Many HCPs see their role as helping individuals with disabilities adapt to the demands of society. Instead, consider the role of policy to alter the barriers of the social, cultural, economic, and political environments in which persons with disabilities live. Facilitate environmental, societal, and political adjustment to accommodate the needs of individuals with disabilities and ensure full participation. |
| **Disability-Affirmative Intersectional** | Includes all protected characteristics, such as class, ethnicity, sexual orientation, age, religion, disability, and gender. It's the idea that these layers do not exist separately from each other but intersect to form a person's identity, and can magnify the discrimination and marginalization they might experience. | People are complex and multifaceted, with many interwoven attributes making up their identity. Disability is just one part of a person's identity, which may shape but not define them. To fully understand to what extent, it's crucial to look at the whole picture of someone's identity. |

Adapted from Hubbard S. Disability studies and health care curriculum: the great divide. *J Allied Health.* 2004;33(3):184–188; and Brinkman AH, Rea-Sandin G, Lund EM, Fitzpatrick OM, Gusman MS, Boness CL; Scholars for Elevating Equity and Diversity (SEED). Shifting the discourse on disability: Moving to an inclusive, intersectional focus. *Am J Orthopsychiatry.* 2022 Oct 20.

| TABLE 17.2 | |
|---|---|
| **EXAMPLES OF EMPOWERING LANGUAGE[12]** | |
| **USE THIS** | **INSTEAD OF THIS** |
| People who are experiencing disabilities<br>People with mobility disability | Disabled people, person |
| Child without a disability | Normal child (in comparing with a child with a disability) |
| People with obesity | Obese or morbidly obese |
| Patient or persons with Covid-19 | Covid-19 cases |
| People/Person who are/is experiencing homelessness | The homeless |
| People/Person who have/has visual impairments | The blind |
| People/Person who use/uses a wheelchair, crutches, prosthetic, braces, scooter, etc. | Confined to a wheelchair, wheelchair-bound, has to use crutches, unable to walk without braces |
| Individual or person who has (name of the problem) | Language such as:<br>○ Victim of…   ○ Stricken   ○ Poor<br>○ Suffers from…   ○ Crippled   ○ Unfortunate<br>○ Afflicted with…   ○ Diseased   ○ Sick<br>○ Burdened with…   ○ Disabled   ○ Tragic |
| Individual who has (describe what the person has accomplished) | ○ Courageous   ○ Heroic<br>○ Inspirational   ○ Special |
| Use person-centered/identity-first language in verbal and written communication (e.g., a person who has epilepsy, limb difference; person without housing, person living with a mental health condition, person who is incarcerated, etc.) | Referring to the disability or condition as an adjective (the blind man, homeless person, mentally ill, prisoner, etc.), a noun (paraplegics, epileptics), or a passive form (help the handicapped) |
| Ms., Mrs., Mr., Dr., or preferred name—ask | First names or terms of endearment such as "Dear" or "Honey" or "Babe" in nonromantic or professional relationships (see Chapter 9) |
| Adapted from Inclusive Language Guidelines (apa.org)[12] and American Medical Association and Association of American Medical Colleges. (2021) *Advancing Health Equity: Guide on Language, Narrative and Concepts.* Available: ama-assn.org/equity-guide. | |

Unfortunately, research across a variety of disciplines provides evidence that we have a way to go to be compliant as HCPs with person-centered language, and HCPs must work to diminish stigmatizing language, to aid in decreasing psychosocial stressors for persons with disabilities.[6,7,13–16] Language is one conscious choice we can make that makes a substantial difference. We discussed attributes of how to address others in Chapter 7, how we may differ better together. Turn your attention now to beliefs about people with disabilities.

## *You Poor Thing!*

People who have disabilities are often characterized by the uncontrollable nature of their problem, which leads the potential helper to feel pity for the person. The connotation of the "crippled child," for example, not only breaks some of the person/identity-first language rules but immediately connotes a poster-child image intended to elicit donations to a well-meaning charitable organization. Social scientists and fundraisers have known for years that our perception that another person has a problem that is out of their control stimulates our desires to help. However, pity turns out to be an emotion that tends to marginalize people with disabilities and interferes with our ability to see them as people who share our aspirations and disappointments, with equal rights and responsibilities to take social and political action.

HCPs often choose to enter these professions out of their desire to help individuals who have experienced misfortune, disabilities, family problems, poverty, and similar challenges in their lives. Not all HCPs agree on the nature of or the kind of help that will effect change in the lives of those they help, however (see Chapter 6). Even HCPs want to be successful healers, helping others who are seen as least capable, responsible, and in control of their lives (see Chapters 9 and 16).[17–18]

None of these characteristics are consistent with the image of a healthy, competent, empowered, responsible member of society. As we learned in Chapter 2, HCPs often want to "fix it" for their patients/clients, an insurmountable and undesirable task given the complexity of our educational, social, and health care systems and the loftier goal of empowering clients or patients to fix it for themselves. In contrast, when HCPs are faced with persistent, unrelenting demands for medication, better care, benefits, equal access to opportunity, or legal rights, they often feel powerless or threatened and may be less likely to help.

When HCPs feel upset at their clients, it may be an indication that they consider their clients to be competent and in control, albeit demanding or intrusive. Unfortunately, it may also cause withdrawal of needed services or less energy spent in moving the patient/client in a positive direction, when they should be encouraged to be making their own decisions.[17] This is an interesting dilemma and one that is up to HCPs, not patients/clients, to resolve for the good of the patients or clients.

Our professional help should be offered in accordance with our perceptions of how likely the client's situation is to benefit from that help. Ask yourself the question, "What type of help would be of greatest benefit and in what ways is this help likely to effect change?" Or, "How will my action change the individual's ability to participate in society?" Ask the client, "What would be most helpful? What are your goals?" and then listen. Recognize that some of those goals relate to the ways you have been educated to help and some do not. Be clear about what falls within your realm of professional expertise and what must be left for others or the individual to resolve (see Chapters 5, 11, and 15).

## You Are Such an Inspiration!

At the awards banquet of a national track and field championship for athletes with disabilities, a famous sports figure rises to the podium to give an after-dinner speech. The speech follows: "You people ... are such an inspiration. The courage I have seen is remarkable. You have faced the challenges and overcome them. You are all heroes today. You are all winners."

Although well intended, the speaker has distanced the group by immediately emphasizing the distinction of "you people." Furthermore, instead of complimenting the group on their athletic accomplishments, world record performances, or victories, the speaker has essentially created different standards for recognition of achievement in this group of athletes with disabilities. In reality, not everyone is a winner. Athletic competition is serious business; it requires long training hours, dedication, commitment, arduous work, perseverance, and skill.

Of course, there may be a role for courage and inspiration somewhere in the mix, but the point is that athletes who have disabilities share the common experience of commitment, training, successes, and failures with all athletes. Individuals who have disabilities are human—no more, no less. A person with a disability is not a paragon of virtue just because they have a disability.

When we recognize persons who have disabilities for what they have accomplished, for their achievements and victories, using standards that are used for everyone, then we empower them, educate society, and change attitudes about disability. When we overdo it on praise for minimal achievements, it infers low ability of the achiever. When you are not held to the same standards that everyone else is, it is usually because the evaluator does not feel that you have the capacity to achieve those standards. This is not a good message to give and certainly a worse one to receive. Instead, give positive messages that emphasize what was accomplished and what standards you are using to judge this accomplishment. Indicate where the person stands in progress toward a goal and the endpoints to be reached if you are using a different standard to evaluate success.

## What Happened to You? Tell Me About Your Disability

In Chapter 14, you learned how to interview patients and clients as part of your professional development. You learned how to ask specific questions that are intended to focus your professional attention on a problem at hand. Your questions assume a clinical orientation, describing the signs, symptoms, onset, and severity of problems. Although helpful for providing information for a specific diagnosis or planning a treatment, these questions might ignore the one essential factor that will determine the importance of all the information you seek—context.

A person who has a disability experiences a problem in context: in a family; on a wheelchair basketball team; as a student in school; as a colleague, supervisor, or supervisee in a work setting. The client may be with or without social support, financial resources, adequate health care, or housing. Focusing on the clinical aspects of the disability alone in the interview negates the importance of the context and/or roles in society, but, more important, may assume that the same common symptoms or problems have the same meaning to all people who have a similar disability.

The meaning that any problem has for an individual may differ markedly. One individual may be mortified by unexpected urinary incontinence; another may consider it a minor inconvenience and have strategies in place to deal with the problem quickly and without great emotional cost. Questions such as "How have you managed similar situations in the past?" and "How important is this to you to take care of?" associate competence and ability with the current issues. Never make assumptions about what a problem means to your patient or client. Ask them. Treat the individual as a "culture of one" (see Chapter 13). Avoid reference to disability groups to which some individuals belong, such as "Many of my clients who have quadriplegia have skin problems; is this a problem for you?" Instead, ask open-ended, empowering questions, such as "What strategies do you use to prevent pressure sores?" Use active listening instead of a relentless list of questions, and, most important, talk with the person who has the disability. Listen carefully to their story; you have never heard it before. As you listen, the uniqueness of this particular person and their meanings emerge to assist you in your role as an effective helper.

# THE EFFECT OF BIASES AND STIGMATIZATION

Cultural beliefs—the way our lenses are set—including our values, practices, conceptions of illness, and acceptable behavior, greatly influence our perceptions of disability. The context in which we live determines the meaning of a disability. For example, as we realized in Chapter 15, Western practitioners tend to conceptualize medicine in a reductionistic and despiritualized fashion, searching for cause-and-effect relationships that can be explained and controlled.[19] In contrast, Eastern philosophies that may be based in concepts of a life force, such as energy or chi, defy Western scientific explanation, yet may be just as valid to a practitioner of Eastern medicine. Similarly, an individual's illness or disability is understood and given significance based on the culture in which it occurs. It is important to understand that we take on social roles to meet the behavioral expectations of influential others. Consider the behavior-shaping influence of the environment on persons incarcerated, children who are institutionalized, and people who have lived in situations of physical and emotional abuse.

People who do not have disabilities often hold attitudes and perceptions that separate them from individuals who have disabilities. For example, a study of more than 200 Spanish university students discovered that they perceived individuals with hearing and visual impairments to be less communicative, less intelligent, less independent, slower, and less active than individuals with no sensory impairment.[18] In a comparison of the descriptors of individuals with hearing impairments with those with visual impairments, these students perceived that those with hearing impairments were more reserved, less calm, less sociable, less attentive, less prudent, less sure, and less thoughtful than those with visual impairments.[19] Some researchers in other areas of the world have found that women tend to hold more positive perceptions of individuals with disabilities than do men.[20-21] Interestingly, some studies of the perceptions of individuals who work in medical settings fail to show that their attitudes are more positive toward individuals with disabilities than are those of the general public.[22-23]

In other words, those who often work with people with disabilities may hold the same prejudices as do lay people. So, how do we influence attitudes and eliminate negative stereotypes? Some authors argue that even sensitivity training, intentionally provided in professional training programs, may overly emphasize negative perceptions of the difficulties encountered by persons with physical disabilities, rather than providing learners with a positive perspective of ability.[23]

For example, the experiences of students using a wheelchair as a first-time simulation experience may provide some awareness of the physical barriers encountered but do not seem to reflect the overall generally positive quality of life experienced by enabled persons who use wheelchairs. The apparent paradox of creating negative attitudes by focusing on the salient differences in the experience of people with disabilities creates a dilemma for the education of human service professionals, such as teachers, HCPs, and social workers; people who we want to be sensitive to the needs of and to recognize and foster the abilities of their students, and patients/ clients.[24-25]

## How Can We Counter Our Biases?

Recognition of sameness is a key factor. Social psychology tells us that rather than focusing on our differences, it is probably more productive to emphasize our similarities. What do we have in common with a person who has a disability? Their age, educational objective, vocational choice, parenthood, automobile owner, book lover, bus user, or technology user are often more unifying characteristics than the apparent (or often unapparent) nature of a person's disability.

When HCPs are providing services, they are often forced to focus on the disability or its effects. Don't forget that this person, with desires, aspirations, a family, a job, a living situation, is not defined by the nature of their disability. Be aware of the many limiting ideas and concepts that prevail in our culture, but also be aware that your cultural beliefs may not be shared by the patient. Furthermore, be cognizant of rapidly changing and evolving rehabilitation technology, new genetics, and emerging science, e.g., 3-dimensional printing of functional, prosthetic upper extremities; being capable of directing lightning energies; directed gene therapies. One cannot be resistant to consider innovative technologies, while learning and incorporating past lessons. Even a decade ago, few would have believed possible that those with nerve damage would be utilizing mind control to activate sensors for movement. Listen, believe, and do not allow yourself to be limited by stereotypes and expectations. Stay abreast of emerging science and technology. *Don't be afraid to shift your paradigm!*

# LEGISLATIVE AND ECONOMIC ASPECTS OF DISABILITY

In the past 40 years, many legislative acts have affected the quality of life of individuals with disabilities. Table 17.3 lists some pithy examples of major pieces of legislation that provide the basis for the rights of persons with disabilities in the United States. Unfortunately, although there is legal protection in many situations, we still have a long way to go in changing public beliefs that it serves all people to make entrances to buildings barrier free, to actively foster opportunities for employment for individuals with disabilities, and to provide diagnostic and treatment services to the millions of children and adults with disabilities who live in poverty and experience homelessness.

---

TABLE 17.3

## KEY LEGISLATIVE ACTIVITY AND DISABILITY ISSUES

**LEGISLATION AFFECTING PERSONS WITH DISABILITIES**

**1965 Enactment of Medicaid Amending the 1935 Social Security Act:** Established Medicare and Medicaid for low-income persons.

**Rehabilitation Act of 1973:** Mandated no discrimination by federally funded agencies against workers and students with disabilities and affirmative action requirements for federally funded employers.

**Americans With Disabilities Act (ADA) of 1990:** Mandated reasonable accommodations to ensure the integration of people with disabilities in the private sector, including employment, telecommunications, transportation and public services, and accommodations.

**The Workforce Investment Act of 1998:** Focuses on training, educating, and employing skilled workers to meet the needs of businesses. One-stop career centers (workforce centers) serve to meet job seekers' needs by providing an integrated service model to offer many work-related programs.

**Assistive Technology (AT) Act of 1998 & Improving Access to Assistive Technology for Individuals with Disabilities Act of 2004** (reauthorization): Ensures the continued existence of a major source of funding for assistive technology, grants to States to maintain comprehensive statewide programs designed to: maximize the ability of individuals with disabilities, and their family members, guardians, advocates, and authorized representatives, to obtain AT; and increase AT access.

**2001 New Freedom Initiative:** Part of a nationwide effort to remove barriers and facilitate full participation in community life for people with disabilities. The initiative increased access to assistive and universally designed technologies, expanded educational and employment opportunities, and promoted increased access into daily community life. The act supported the integration of people with disabilities into the workforce.

**Americans With Disabilities Act, Amendments Act of 2008:** Emphasizes the definition of disability to make it easier for an individual seeking protection under the ADA to establish disability. The ADA defines disability as an impairment that substantially limits one or more major life activities, a record of such an impairment, or being regarded as having such an impairment.

**2010 Affordable Care Act (ACA):** designed to make health care insurance more affordable, especially for those falling below the poverty income levels, and increase health insurance coverage for the uninsured, while implementing reforms to the health insurance market; expands Medicaid coverage for adults where states have applied.

*(continued)*

| TABLE 17.3 (CONTINUED) |
| :---: |
| ## KEY LEGISLATIVE ACTIVITY AND DISABILITY ISSUES |

**2013 Jimmo v. Sebelius:** A settlement to a class action lawsuit that determined that Medicare coverage for skilled services, to maintain an individual's condition, cannot be improperly denied or discontinued regardless of the individual's potential to improve.

**2014 IMPACT Act:** Provides for establishing standardized post-acute care assessment data, which can be shared by providers for quality, payment, and discharge planning to facilitate coordinated care and improved Medicare beneficiary outcomes.

**2015 Direct Access:** Provides for *some form of direct access* at the *State levels* for the *majority of jurisdictions,* allows for persons to seek physical therapy services without the need for prescription, sometimes with certain stipulations that vary by jurisdictions. Especially relieves cost burdens for those with chronic diseases and conditions.

**Nondiscrimination in Health Programs and Activities, Affordable Care Act, Section 1557:** Final rule prohibits discrimination on the basis of race, color, national origin, sex, age, or disability in certain health programs and activities. Builds on Title VI of the Civil Rights Act of 1964, Title IX of the Education Amendments of 1973, Section 504 of the Rehabilitation Act of 1973 and the Age Discrimination Act of 1975.

**21st Century Cures Act, 2016:** Designed to help accelerate medical product development and bring new innovations and advances to patients who need them faster and more efficiently.

**2021 Build Back Better Act:** Strengthens Medicaid home and community-based services; extends/expands the Affordable Care Act tax credits; adds benefits for hearing.

**2022 Effective Suicide Screening and Assessment in the Emergency Department Act:** Helps to standardize the suicide screening tools used in emergency rooms. Since 2001, the suicide rate in the U.S. has risen by a shocking 31%, making suicide the tenth leading cause of death in the nation, with an estimated 47,000 lives lost each year. The Act helps to maximize the likelihood that those admitted to the ER with attempted suicide, or suicidal ideation, will receive appropriate follow-up care at discharge.

**Covid-19 Pandemic Related***

2020 Paycheck Protection Program and Health Care Enhancement Act

2020 Families First Coronavirus Response Act

2021 Executive Order on Ensuring an Equitable Pandemic Response & Recover

2021 Executive Order on Strengthening Medicaid and the Affordable Care Act

2021 Consolidated Appropriations Act

2021 American Rescue Plan Act

2021 Coronavirus Aid Relief & Economic Security (CARES) Act

*\*Legislative responses to Covid-19 pandemic, including provision for telehealth measures, support for personal protection equipment, critical health care for essential services and preventative vaccine coverage, public health measures, along with timely, lifesaving response medications for those infected and ensuring equitable response for health care needs of all; funding for critical community programs including nutrition, support for Native Americans, Covid relief including additional booster vaccines, addressing social isolation, implementation of evidence-based health promotion, national caregiver support, including the long-term care ombudsman program; and addressed many other aspects of the pandemic in addition to health care.*

**H.R.2617 Consolidated Appropriations Act, 2023:** Final spending act that fell short in offsetting Medicare Fee Schedule cuts, impacting 27 health-related disciplines negatively. The omnibus package provides insufficient relief, but it does include several wins in other areas. Stepped-up emphasis on physical therapy in the Department of Veterans Affairs. Provides for research to study impacts of home health with Centers for Medicare and Medicaid Services (CMS) and extended telehealth provisions through 2024 from emergency related to pandemic. Provides stipends for educational programs to increase health-related workforce diversity through grants for support through Health Resources and

*(continued)*

---

TABLE 17.3 (CONTINUED)

## KEY LEGISLATIVE ACTIVITY AND DISABILITY ISSUES

Services Administration (HRSA) to higher education programs in OT, RT, PT, SLP-Aud. Expanded Medicare coverage for lymphedema-related pressure garments. Increased funding for suicide prevention measures and mental health coverage. Increased National Institutes of Health (NIH) funding for disability-related research for special education state grant programs that support services, including early intervention and pre-school. Provides funding for the Prevention and Public Health Fund for collaborative work with the CDC Coalition. See Congress.gov for additional information.

**Medicare and Medicaid Programs; CY 2025 Payment Policies under the Physician Fee Schedule and Other Changes to Part B Payment and Coverage Policies:** Adjusts various payments for services; extends telehealth coverage; modifies codes to reflect time and complexities; incentivizes ACOs to provide high-quality care at lower costs; addresses drug prices; recovery of Medicare overpayments and enhanced detection of fraud, waste and abuse. Provisions for efficiency, quality care and financial integrity of Medicare and Medicaid with reduced burdens on beneficiaries, especially related to drug costs out-of-pocket expenses.

### LEGISLATION AFFECTING CHILDREN WITH DISABILITIES

**PL 94–142 (Education for All Handicapped Children Act of 1975):** Mandated a free and appropriate education and the least restrictive environment (i.e., mainstreaming) Annual Individual Educational Plans are developed for all children with disabilities.

**PL 101–476:** Revised provisions of PL 94–142 to include children with autism and brain injury and included training and technology provisions for education of children with disabilities

**Individuals With Disabilities Education Act (IDEA) of 1997:** Gave parents and school districts more autonomy in determining children's needs for special education services through a mediation process, further defines services available to infants and toddlers, and provides disciplinary sanctions for students who engage in criminal misconduct, unrelated to disability.

**Individuals With Disabilities Education Improvement Act of 2004:** Four parts: (A) administrative aspects of the Office of Special Education Programs; (B) educational requirements of the Act; (C) guidelines for children with special needs who are less than 2 years of age, includes Early Intervention Programs; and (D) creates national grants and resources for implementation and established Child Find to identify those with disabilities in school districts and requirements for Individualized Education Plans (IEPs) with annual review, with inclusion of needed therapy and assistive technology.

**2006 Individuals with Disabilities Education Improvement Regulations:** Required schools to use research-based interventions in the process of assisting students with learning difficulties or determining eligibility for special education.

*The cornerstone of the IDEA is the entitlement of each eligible child with a disability to a free appropriate public education (FAPE) that emphasizes special education and related services designed to meet the child's unique needs and that prepare the child for further education, employment, and independent living. Under the IDEA, the primary vehicle for providing FAPE is through an appropriately developed IEP that is based on the individual needs of the child. An IEP must consider a child's present levels of academic achievement and functional performance, and the impact of that child's disability on their involvement and progress in the general education curriculum. IEP goals must be aligned with grade-level content standards for all children with disabilities. The child's IEP must be developed, reviewed, and revised in accordance with the requirements outlined in the IDEA.*

**Pediatric Device Consortia Program Reauthorization Act 2022:** Advances the development of pediatric medical devices by reauthorizing the Pediatric Device Consortia (PDC) grant program and extending the Humanitarian Device Exemption (HDE) incentive pathway. These programs provide additional opportunities to improve the number of medical devices in pediatric populations, especially those with rare diseases. See also **H.R.2617 Consolidated Appropriations Act** (above).

### LEGISLATION AFFECTING OLDER ADULTS

**PL 101–234 (The Omnibus Reconciliation Act [OBRA] of 1987):** Major legislation that set standards for nursing home personnel, home health agencies, and the rights of nursing home residents.

*(continued)*

| TABLE 17.3 (CONTINUED) |
|---|

## KEY LEGISLATIVE ACTIVITY AND DISABILITY ISSUES

**1990 Nursing Home Reform Amendments of OBRA:** Nursing homes required by law to focus on each resident's highest potential for physical, mental, and psychosocial well-being by assessing these abilities and developing individualized care plans. These care plans must be reassessed for any change in function at least quarterly.

**1997 Balanced Budget Act:** Medicare Cap on Rehab Services placed a cap on Medicare reimbursement for rehabilitation services for seniors resulting in negative consequences for health care access and treatments.

**Health Care and Education Affordability Reconciliation Act of 2010:** Reformed Medicare payment policy so it more equitably reimburses those who care for older adults. Designed to support mechanisms to develop new payment and promising models of care, including comprehensive geriatric assessments and care coordination for older patients with multiple chronic illnesses and cognitive impairment. Supported expansion of geriatrics training programs, including those designed to prepare specialists to meet the needs of the most complex, frailest older patients, as well education for the direct-care workers and family caregivers who provide care for millions of America's seniors.

**21st Century Cures Act of 2016: Specifically for older Americans:** Provides for locum tenens in underserved health shortage areas for recipients of Medicare for physical therapists.

**The Bipartisan Budget Act of 2018 H.R. 1892:** Large omnibus act addressing many issues. Part of the Act established through the bipartisan budget extended the sequester for mandatory spending through the fiscal year 2027 and adjusts the cuts required for Medicare. Addressed a more permanent solution to the prior 20-year hard cap for rehabilitation services with Medicare. (Direct spending, also known as mandatory spending, is spending provided by laws other than appropriations bills. Sequestration is a process of automatic, usually across-the-board spending reductions under which budgetary resources are permanently cancelled to enforce specific budget policy goals.)

**H.R. 113 Consolidated Appropriations Act of 2021:** This was legislation that included a 3.75% boost in funding to the 2021 Medicare Fee Schedule to mitigate planned payment cuts.

See also **H.R.2617 Consolidated Appropriations Act** (above).

**The Dr. Emmanuel Bilirakis and Honorable Jennifer Wexton National Plan to End Parkinsons Act of 2024:** Public Law No: 118–66: This act requires the Department of Health and Human Services (HHS) to carry out a project to address Parkinson's disease (a progressive brain disorder that causes unintended or uncontrollable movements) and related conditions. Among other components of the project, HHS must (1) implement and periodically update a national plan to coordinate and guide efforts to prevent, diagnose, treat, and cure the disease; and (2) improve the care of those with the disease. HHS must also annually assess the preparations for and response to the increased burden of Parkinson's disease. In addition, the act establishes a council, composed of federal and nonfederal stakeholders, to advise HHS on, and make recommendations concerning the prevention and treatment of Parkinson's disease.

## STILL A LONG WAY TO GO

Although legislation (see Table 17.3) has protected some of the rights of individuals with disabilities, we still live largely in a world that does not yet meet the needs of those with disabilities, nor recognize their potential power as a group. Adequate income, accessibility in navigating physical facilities, finding employment, adequate access to health care equipment, feeling supported in education, health insurance, suitable housing, and gainful employment still largely remain challenges for members of our community who have disabilities. The Covid-19 pandemic, coupled with health disparities, has underscored the disparate disease burdens for Black, Native American (Alaska Native, American Indian), and Hispanic populations.[26] Persons who receive care from HCPs of their own cultural background tend to have better outcomes; and these HCPs are more likely to return to live in their service areas.[26] Hence, while we have a long way to go, progress through advocacy efforts is moving forward. Legislation effective in 2023 (H.R.2617) provides for grants to institutions to increase the support for diversity in the health professions through the Health Resources and Services Administration.

However, limiting and negative stereotypes are continuing to be encountered by persons with disabilities. These contribute to further exclusion and social isolation, oftentimes adding to challenges in finding meaningful roles and affecting the ability to adjust to changing expectations.[27-28] For disabled persons, higher rates of poverty, mental health, and financial challenges are prevalent, as well as caregiver dependence and avoidance of confrontation,[27] while most persons with disabilities have a desire to improve functional independence and be able to self-manage as much as possible;[29] hence the importance of utilizing a comprehensive health care team approach for persons with disabilities to address all aspects of quality of life and to assist with social connections, while including effective education, and collaborating with the patient and support networks.[27-29] Consider what types of HCPs and other specialists you would want to have access to for your team if you were disabled, and why.

# AGING WITH A DISABILITY

The lifespan for people with disabilities has increased markedly, resulting in many people with severe disabilities reaching middle-age and older age groups. Age-related changes, when combined with preexisting impairments, often create secondary disabilities, which, if left unrecognized or untreated, may impair quality of life and independence.[30]

HCPs must be aware of screening for recent loss of function in individuals with long-term disabilities and chronic conditions. These are referred to as "late effects" or all the new health problems that derived from the chronic impairment/s linked with the existing disability and impairments.[30] Routinely asking questions such as the following may identify a secondary problem before it becomes a serious health threat. Have you noticed the following:

- Describe any increased fatigue or pain you may be experiencing during daily activities?
- Describe any changes in your posture?
- Describe any difficulty sleeping or change in your sleeping?
- Describe any change in your weight you may have noticed?
- Describe any change in your sensation?
- Describe any shift in your abilities to perform the tasks, hobbies, and recreational activities you enjoy?

# SECONDARY CONDITIONS AND SOCIAL DETERMINANTS OF HEALTH IMPACTS

Although disability and health are two distinct phenomena, people with disabilities are 30% more likely to report a poor health status than are people without disabilities.[31,32] People with disabilities are at increased risk for secondary problems, impairments, and limitations to participation from a host of medical, social, emotional, family, or community issues.

A study of more than 1,000 people with disabilities showed that almost 9 in 10 persons with disabilities self-reported at least one secondary condition, with an average of 4.1 conditions. In addition to disability-specific medical issues, such as muscle spasms, bowel and bladder problems, falls and injuries, respiratory infections, asthma, and skin problems; the most common conditions reported by adults with disabilities included chronic pain, sleep disorders, fatigue, weight problems, depression and anxiety, difficulty getting out, feelings of isolation, and problems with making/seeing friends.[33] In addition to higher rates of these conditions, evidence supports that individuals with disabilities, in comparison with individuals without disabilities, are likely to have lower levels of education; lower rates of employment; higher rates of poverty; problems finding safe, accessible, and affordable housing; higher likelihood of being a victim of crime of domestic violence; higher rates of being overweight and obese; and higher rates of tobacco use.[1,34-37]

Social determinants of health—social, economic, environmental, and community conditions—may have a stronger influence on the population's health and well-being than services delivered by practitioners and health care delivery organizations. The overall percentage of people with health insurance coverage has increased greatly in the past decade. However, those gains vary by ethnicity and race; people in low-income households, minority communities, and "inner city" and "rural" communities are significantly less likely to have health insurance coverage. Non-Hispanic American Indian or Alaska Native groups and Hispanic groups are significantly less likely to be insured.[37] Nearly 63% of U.S. counties are now designated as primary care health professional shortage areas, where lack of primary care professionals threatens access to needed services. Not surprisingly, disproportionately more rural counties received this designation than metropolitan.[37] According to the National Healthcare Quality and Disparities Report, five states in the Northeast region (Maine, Massachusetts, New Hampshire, Pennsylvania, and Rhode Island), four in the Midwest region (Iowa, Minnesota, North Dakota, and Wisconsin), and two in the West region (Colorado and Utah) had the highest overall quality scores; while seven states in the West region (Alaska, Arizona, California, Montana, Nevada, New Mexico, and Wyoming), five states in the South region (District of Columbia, Georgia, Mississippi, Oklahoma, and Texas), and New York had the lowest overall quality scores.[37]

Individuals with disabilities experience high rates of disadvantages relating to the Social Determinants of Health (SDoH), as adopted from the World Health Organization by the U.S. Centers for Disease Control, and incorporated within Healthy People 2030.[38] In 10-year cycles, the U.S. Department of Health and Human Services uses available evidence and experience to establish goals, action steps, and indicators for the nation's health. Using available evidence of the issues faced by persons with disabilities, Healthy People 2030 addresses targets for action to achieve better health by the year 2030,[38] including risks to health and wellness, emerging public health priorities, and critical issues related to preparedness and prevention. The SDoH[38] focus on population aspects of economic stability, access to health care and education, and quality education and health care, neighborhoods, and built environments as well as social and community contexts. For example, persons with mobility disabilities report significant challenges utilizing both private and public transportation services due to accessibility, safety, availability, advanced planning needs, and the attitudes of society.[39] Clearly, the serious issues reported by persons with disabilities diminish their sense of health and well-being. Strategies to identify, address, and ameliorate these commonly experienced conditions are key to reducing disability-related health disparities.

Over 30 million women with disabilities experience unique challenges. Women with disabilities have been documented to have limited access to medical services, education, and vocational opportunities. These issues influence their health because they often lack information, financial resources, and health services to meet their unique needs. Despite the needs, there are many barriers that reduce the quality and accessibility of services for women with disabilities. Physical and communication barriers often limit access to health care settings, despite the requirements of the Americans with Disabilities Act. In many cases, women also lack adequate transportation and support services to get to health care appointments. Statistical differences exist with men with disabilities in that they have increased social isolation and less access to higher education. In comparison with men with disabilities, women also have higher unemployment rates, and even those employed earn lower incomes.[40]

A women's perspective on disability can be appreciated, in the words of Nancy Mairs, who wrote about body image and disability perceptions:[41]

> *The "her" I never was and am not now and never will become. In order to function as the body I am, I must forswear her, seductive though she may be, or make myself mad with self-loathing. I get virtually no cultural encouragement. Illness and deformity, instead of being thought of as human variants, the consequence of cosmic bad luck, have invariably been portrayed as deviations from the fully human condition, brought on by personal failing or by divine judgment.*

Take a moment to journal how the perspective makes you feel and impacts your future as a HCP.

Although health care delivery for some conditions, such as breast cancer and HIV/AIDS, has improved for all populations, disparities by race, ethnicity, household income, and location of residence persist because the gains experienced by disadvantaged populations have been insufficient to close the gap between advantaged and disadvantaged populations. In some cases, the disparity has widened.[37] While some health care disparities, such as for HIV care, are present across many disadvantaged groups, other disparities disproportionately affect certain groups, which may reflect circumstances and issues specific to that group.[37] Hispanic people and non-Hispanic Black people consistently experience worse care on most quality measures of breast cancer care.[37]

Women with disabilities often have less access to breast health services. Women with disabilities are at a higher risk for delayed diagnosis of breast and cervical cancer, primarily for reasons of environmental, attitudinal, and information barriers, including reported difficulties receiving women's health services (e.g., mammograms and Pap smears, reproductive health/birth control, sexually transmitted diseases screening, and services to address specific issues of aging). In addition to reproductive health needs, women with disabilities frequently experience a lack of privacy and autonomy while receiving health care, high rates of violence and abuse, and unmet mental health needs.[42–45] In low- and middle-income countries, women with disabilities were approximately twice as likely as women without disabilities to be exposed to discrimination and violence with approximately one-third more likely to feel unsafe in their homes or local neighborhoods, with a higher risk of domestic violence.[43] Renewed efforts to address the need for breast cancer awareness and screening for those with disabilities have begun, yet more effort is needed for education and interventions.[44–45]

Strategies that eliminate barriers to care include providing education to women and their HCPs and identifying solutions, such as appropriate communication techniques, accessible equipment, and available services. HCPs can make a difference treating women with disabilities as women first, with health needs, perspectives, and issues that they share with all women.

# PANDEMIC IMPACTS AND NEED FOR TRAUMA-INFORMED CARE

Unfortunately, because of the Covid-19 pandemic, lives were dramatically impacted and society forever changed. According to the Peterson Center on Healthcare report in 2022 (petersonhealthcare.org), life expectancy in the U.S. has decreased in all ethnicities and races, with persons of color experiencing an even greater decline, while 30 million still have no health insurance. While health care costs are greater in the U.S. (4.1 trillion, 5% of the Gross Domestic Product) than those of comparable countries (spending twice the average), outcomes are no better. Not only are costs higher, the administrative burden of the complexities of the U.S. health care systems contributes to expense, with prescription drug costs currently growing the fastest and hospital expenditures outpacing all overall costs for health care. Health care access and affordability continue to be challenging for many, with Medicare and Medicaid currently bearing the largest financial burdens for health care, followed by private insurance. In the U.S., following heart disease and cancer, Covid-19 is the third leading cause of death.

Today, child and adolescent mental health has become urgently concerning. An increase in the number of adolescents reporting persistent feelings of sadness or hopelessness, resulting in increased numbers of emergency department visits for mental health needs, increased suicide rates; and non-Hispanic White adolescents (7.4 deaths per 100,000 population) were more likely to die from suicide than Hispanic (5.0 deaths per 100,000 population) or non-Hispanic Black (4.6 deaths per 100,000 population) adolescents.[37]

Substance Use Disorders occur when problematic recurrent use of alcohol or other drugs causes health problems, disability, or failure to meet major responsibilities at work, school, or home. Published studies signal a rise in health concerns related to both alcohol and illicit drug use in recent years. Substance use disorders continue to rise as well as opioid-related deaths.[37]

The staggering altered health status of many led to increasing impacts of trauma and stress for society in general, raising mental health concerns. Today, HCPs should approach all care considering the need to screen and refer for adverse trauma experiences, including adverse childhood events that may impact adults, including post-traumatic stress disorders. Thus, as discussed throughout this book, collaborative and individualized patient-centered care is needed that is nonjudgmental, utilizing trauma-informed principles of care:[46]

- Establish the physical and emotional **safety** of patients and staff
- **Build** trust with the health care team
- **Recognize** symptoms and signs of trauma exposure on mental and physical health
- Promote **patient-centered, evidence-based** health care
- Ensure HCP and patient **collaboration** by bringing patients into the treatment process and discussing mutually agreed upon goals for treatment
- Provide care that is sensitive to the patient's **racial, ethnic, cultural background, and gender identity**

# WHAT CAN YOU DO TO MAKE A DIFFERENCE?

The chapter exercises are designed to help you raise your awareness to recognize the perceptions and biases you may hold about individuals with disabilities. You are morally obliged to make an active effort to recognize the abilities of all people. Be aware of the influence of your language. Continue to take action to alleviate discriminatory practices, as with the group of HCPs who realized from evidence that labeling, such as with a person's weight, can indeed result in psychological and physical harm, therefore persons with weight concerns are less likely to receive adequate care. Hence, this group of international experts developed a joint statement with recommendations to eliminate weight bias and the stigma of obesity (Figure 17.1).[47]

Researchers[48] also developed a more appropriate screening questionnaire to address weight concerns including statements to assist HCPs in discussing weight management needs and functional goals. Clients are now asked, "How I might feel if I lose weight" with respect to their level of agreement with the following goals: "Live longer, Be healthier, Have fewer aches and pains, Be more physically active, Have more energy or stamina, Be able to find clothes I feel good in, Feel better about myself, and Feel more confident."[48] Screening fosters patient self-advocacy for persons who are overweight or obese, providing the chance to first self-identify weight-management goals and discuss with a HCP to collaborate for care and interventions.[48]

To make a difference, set a personal goal to encourage individuals with whom you have contact and support person-centered care, access to health care, educational opportunities, employment, housing, and transportation.

**Figure 17.1.** Pledge to eliminate weight bias and stigma of obesity. (From Rubino F, Puhl RM, Cummings DE, et al. Joint international consensus statement for ending stigma of obesity. *Nat Med.* 2020;26:485–497.)

**We recognize that**

- Individuals affected by overweight and obesity face a pervasive form of social stigma based on the typically unproven assumption that their body weight derives primarily from a lack self-discipline and personal responsibility.
- Such portrayal is inconsistent with current scientific evidence demonstrating that body-weight regulation is not entirely under volitional control, and that biological, genetic, and environmental factors critically contribute to obesity.
- Weight bias and stigma can result in discrimination, and undermine human rights, social rights, and the health of afflicted individuals.
- Weight stigma and discrimination cannot be tolerated in modern societies.

**We condemn**

- The use of stigmatizing language, images, attitudes, policies, and weight-based discrimination, wherever they occur.

**We pledge**

- To treat individuals with overweight and obesity with dignity and respect.
- To refrain from using stereotypical language, images, and narratives that unfairly and inaccurately depict individuals with overweight and obesity as lazy, gluttonous, and lacking willpower or self-discipline.
- To encourage and support educational initiatives aimed at eradicating weight bias through dissemination of current knowledge of obesity and body-weight regulation.
- To encourage and support initiatives aimed at preventing weight discrimination in the workplace, education, and healthcare settings.

Always be an advocate (refer to Chapter 11) for those with disabilities! Remember that clients/patients undergoing care for musculoskeletal-related pain prefer HCPs who are *outgoing* and *energetic*, achieving better outcomes;[49] while those with chronic diseases who are treated by HCPs who are *secure, calmer, more relaxed*, and *resilient* have a larger reduction in severity of complaints compared with patients/clients treated by HCPs who demonstrate fewer of these traits.[50] "Good" HCPs are *responsive, ethical, communicative, caring, competent, and collaborative*.[51] Reflect on these characteristics and journal about how you can make a difference in the lived experiences of your clients/patients.

# References

1. Center for Disease Control and Prevention. *Learn About Disability and Health, Data and Statistics.* Available: https://www.cdc.gov/ncbddd/disabilityandhealth/index.html Accessed: January 13, 2024.
2. Administration for Community Living. *Data and Research.* Available: https://acl.gov/aging-and-disability-in-america/data-and-research Accessed: January 13, 2024.
3. Centers for Disease Control and Prevention. *National Center on Birth Defects and Developmental Disabilities, Division of Human Development and Disability. Disability and Health Data System (DHDS) Data.* Available: https://dhds.cdc.gov Accessed: January 3, 2024.
4. U.S. Department of Labor. *Disability Employment Statistics.* Available: https://www.dol.gov/agencies/odep/research-evaluation/statistics Accessed: January 3, 2024.
5. Lund EM, Forber-Pratt AJ, Wilson C, Mona LR. The COVID-19 pandemic, stress, and trauma in the disability community: a call to action. *Rehabilitation Psychology.* 2020;65(4): 313–322.
6. Best KL, Mortenson WB, Lauzière-Fitzgerald Z, Smith EM. Language matters! The long-standing debate between identity-first language and person first language. *Assistive Technology: The Official Journal of RESNA.* 2022;34(2):127–128.
7. Dwyer P. Stigma, incommensurability, or both? Pathology-first, person-first, and identity-first language and the challenges of discourse in divided autism communities. *J Dev & Behav Ped.* 2022;43(2):111–113.

8.  Hubbard S. Disability studies and health care curriculum: the great divide. *J Allied Health.* 2004;33(3):184–188.

9.  Brinkman AH, Rea-Sandin G, Lund EM, Fitzpatrick OM, Gusman MS, Boness CL. Scholars for Elevating Equity and Diversity (SEED). Shifting the discourse on disability: moving to an inclusive, intersectional focus. *Am J Orthopsychiatry.* 2022 Oct 20. doi: 10.1037/ort0000653.

10. Levine A, Breshears B. Discrimination at every turn: an intersectional ecological lens for rehabilitation. *Rehabil Psychol.* 2019 May;64(2):146–153.

11. International Classification of Functioning, Disability and Health (ICF). Available: https://www.who.int/standards/classifications/international-classification-of-functioning-disability-and-health. Accessed February 14, 2024.

12. American Psychological Association. *Inclusive Language Guidelines.* Available: https://www.apa.org/about/apa/equity-diversity-inclusion/language-guidelines Accessed: February 14, 2024.

13. Nicks S, Johnson AL, Traxler B, Bush ML, Brame L, Hamilton T, Hartwell M. The use of person-centered language in medical research articles focusing on hearing loss or deafness. *Ear Hear.* 2022;43(3):703–711.

14. Headley S, Potter I, Ottwell R, Rogers T, Vassar M, Hartwell M. Adherence rates of person-centered language in amputation research: a cross-sectional analysis. *Disabil Health J.* 2022 Jan;15(1):101172.

15. Robling K, Cosby C, Parent, G, Swapnil G, Tessa C, Michael B, Hartwell M. Person-centered language and pediatric ADHD research: a cross-sectional examination of stigmatizing language within medical literature. *J Osteo Med.* 2023;123(4): 215–222. doi: 10.1515/jom-2022-0126.

16. Reddy AK, Norris GR, Nayfa R, Sajjadi NB, Checketts JX, Scott JT, Hartwell M. The presence of person-centered language in orthopedic-related amputation research: a cross-sectional analysis. *J Osteopath Med.* 2022; Dec 15. doi: 10.1515/jom-2022-0181.

17. Sliwinski MM, Smith R, Wood A. Spinal cord injury rehabilitation patient and physical therapist perspective: a pilot study. *Spinal Cord Ser Cases.* 2016;7(2):15036.

18. Goldsmith EM, Krebs EE. Roles of physicians and health care systems in "difficult" clinical encounters. *AMA J Ethics.* 2017;19(4):381–390.

19. Banja JD. Ethics, values, and world culture: the impact on rehabilitation. *Disabil Rehabil.* 1996;18(6):279–284.

20. Cambra C. A comparative study of personality descriptors attributed to the deaf, the blind, and individuals with no sensory disability. *Am Ann Deaf.* 1996;141(1):24–28.

21. Gannon PM, MacLean D. Attitudes toward disability and beliefs regarding support for a university student with quadriplegia. *Int J Rehabil Res.* 1996;19(2):163–169.

22. Wang Z, Xu X, Han Q, Chen Y, Jiang J, Ni GX. Factors associated with public attitudes towards persons with disabilities: a systematic review. *BMC Public Health.* 2021 Jun 3;21(1):1058.

23. Satchidanand N, Gunukula SK, Lam WY, McGuigan D, New I, Symons AB, Withiam-Leitch M, Akl EA. Attitudes of healthcare students and professionals toward patients with physical disability: a systematic review. *Am J Phys Med Rehabil.* 2012 Jun;91(6):533–545.

24. Barney KW. Disability simulations: using the social model of disability to update an experiential educational practice. *SCHOLE: A J Leisure Studies & Recreation Educ.* 2017;27(1):1–11.

25. Ma GYK, Mak WWS. Meta-analysis of studies on the impact of mobility disability simulation programs on attitudes toward people with disabilities and environmental in/accessibility. *PLoS One.* 2022;17(6):e0269357.

26. Salsberg E, Richwine C, Westergaard S, Portela Martinez M, Oyeyemi T, Vichare A, Chen CP. Estimation and comparison of current and future racial/ethnic representation in the US health care workforce. *JAMA Netw Open.* 2021; Mar 1;4(3):e213789.

27. Jespersen LN, Michelsen SI, Tjørnhøj-Thomsen T, Svensson MK, Holstein BE, Due P. Living with a disability: a qualitative study of associations between social relations, social participation and quality of life. *Disabil Rehabil.* 2019;41(11):1275–1286.

28. Barclay L, Lentin P, Bourke-Taylor H, McDonald R. The experiences of social and community participation of people with non-traumatic spinal cord injury. *Aust Occup Ther J.* 2019;66(1):61–67.

29. Krysa JA, Gregorio MP, Pohar Manhas K, MacIsaac R, Papathanassoglou E, Ho CH. Empowerment, communication, and navigating care: the experience of persons with spinal cord injury from acute hospitalization to inpatient rehabilitation. *Front Rehabil Sci.* 2022;3:904716.

30. Lim JY. Aging with disability: what should we pay attention to? *Ann Geriatr Med Res.* 2022;26(2):61–62.

31. Carmona RH, Giannini M, Bergmark B, Cabe J. The surgeon general's call to action to improve the health and wellness of persons with disabilities: historical review, rationale, and implications 5 years after publication. *Disability & Health J.* 2010;3(4):229–232.

32. Centers for Disease Control and Prevention. Racial/ethnic disparities in self-rated health status among adults with and without disabilities—United States, 2004–2006. *MMWR Morb Mortal Wkly Rep.* 2008;57(39):1069–1073.

33. Kinne S. Distribution of secondary medical problems, impairments, and participation limitations among adults with disabilities and their relationship to health and other outcomes. *Disabil Health J.* 2008;1(1):42–50.

34. Centers for Disease Control and Prevention. *Disability and Health Promotion, Data and Statistics on Disability and Health.* Available: https://www.cdc.gov/ncbddd/disabilityandhealth/data.html Accessed: February 5, 2024.

35. Barrett KA, O'Day B, Roche A, Carlson BL. Intimate partner violence, health status, and health care access among women with disabilities. *Women's Health Issues.* 2009;19(2):94–100.

36. Campbell KA, Ford-Gilboe M, Stanley M, MacKinnon K. Intimate partner violence and women living with episodic disabilities: a scoping review protocol. *Syst Rev.* 2022;11(1):97.

37. 2022 National Healthcare Quality and Disparities Report. Rockville, MD: Agency for Healthcare Research and Quality; October 2022. *AHRQ* Pub. No. 22(23)-0030.

38. Office of Disease Prevention and Health Promotion. Disability and health. *Healthy People 2030.* https://health.gov/healthypeople. Accessed February 1, 2024.

39. Remillard ET, Campbell ML, Koon LM, Rogers WA. Transportation challenges for persons aging with mobility disability: qualitative insights and policy implications. *Disability & Health J.* 2022;15(1)S.101209.

40. Jans L, Stoddard S. *Chartbook on Women and Disability.* Washington, DC: U.S. National Institute on Disability and Rehabilitation Research; 1999. www.infouse.com/disabilitydata/womendisability. Accessed June 15, 2015.

41. Mairs N. *Waist-High in the World: A Life Among the Nondisabled.* Boston, MA: Beacon Press; 1997.

42. Nosek MA, Howland C, Rintala DH, et al. National Study of Women with Physical Disabilities: final report. *Sexuality and Disability.* 2001;19:5–40.

43. Emerson E, Llewellyn G. Exposure of women with and without disabilities to violence and discrimination: evidence from cross-sectional national surveys in 29 middle- and low-income countries. *J Interpers Violence.* 2022 Dec 21:8862605221141868.

44. Walsh S, Hegarty J, Lehane E, Farrell D, Taggart L, Kelly L, Sahm L, Corrigan M, Caples M, Martin AM, Tabirca S, Corrigan MA, O'Mahony M. Determining the need for a breast cancer awareness educational intervention for women with mild/moderate levels of intellectual disability: a qualitative descriptive study. *Eur J Cancer Care* (Engl). 2022;31(4):e13590.

45. Walsh S, O'Mahony M, Lehane E, Farrell D, Taggart L, Kelly L, Sahm L, Byrne A, Corrigan M, Caples M, Martin AM, Tabirca S, Corrigan MA, Hegarty J. Cancer and breast cancer awareness interventions in an intellectual disability context: a review of the literature. *J Intellect Disabil.* 2021;25(1):131–145.

46. Forkey H, Szilagyi M, Kelly ET, Duffee J; Council on Foster Care, Adoption and Kinship Care, Council on Community Pediatrics, Council on Child Abuse and Neglect, Committee on Psychosocial Aspects of Child and Family Health. Trauma-informed care. *Pediatrics.* 2021;148(2)e20210580.

47. Rubino F, Puhl RM, Cummings DE, et al. Joint international consensus statement for ending stigma of obesity. *Nat Med.* 2020;26:485–497.

48. Kim N, Brown TM, Burudpakdee C, Kanu C, Woodard K, Fehnel S, Morrison C, Nadglowski J, Nadolsky K, Kolotkin RL. Development of an assessment tool for completion by patients with overweight or obesity. *Adv Ther.* 2023;40(1):174–193.

49. Kooijman MK, Buining EM, Swinkels ICS, Koes BW, Veenhof C. Do therapist effects determine outcome in patients with shoulder pain in a primary care physiotherapy setting? *Physiotherapy.* 2020 Jun;107:111–117.

50. Buining EM, Kooijman MK, Swinkels IC, Pisters MF, Veenhof C. Exploring physiotherapists' personality traits that may influence treatment outcome in patients with chronic diseases: a cohort study. *BMC Health Serv Res.* 2015;15:558.

51. Kleiner MJ, Kinsella EA, Miciak M, Teachman G, McCabe E, Walton DM. An integrative review of the qualities of a "good" physiotherapist. *Physiother Theory Pract.* 2023;39(1):89–116.

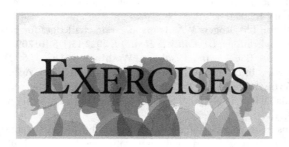

# EXERCISE 1: EXAMINING YOUR BELIEFS ABOUT DISABILITY AND SDoH

What beliefs do you have about the following conditions and/or SDoH? What beliefs do you think most people have?

| CONDITION AND/OR SDOH STATUS | YOUR BELIEFS | OTHERS' BELIEFS |
|---|---|---|
| Person with epilepsy | | |
| Child with cerebral palsy | | |
| Veteran experiencing homelessness with a foot ulcer | | |
| Person with substance abuse admitted for hospital-based care due to kidney disease | | |
| Person who is obese | | |
| Person who is quadriplegic | | |
| Person who is incarcerated with low back pain | | |
| Person who is Covid+ | | |
| Person with cataracts | | |
| Person who is limb different | | |
| Person with cancer | | |
| Person with a traumatic brain injury | | |
| Person who has a sexually transmitted infection | | |
| Person with congenital heart disease | | |
| Person with schizophrenia | | |

# EXERCISE 2: USING PERSON/IDENTITY-FIRST LANGUAGE

Replace each of the following phrases with person/identity-first language:

1. He is a quadriplegic:


2. It is a fundraiser for the mentally retarded:


3. The blind man came in last:


4. The developmentally disabled children:


5. Congenitally dislocated baby hips:


6. Confined to a wheelchair:


7. Stroke victim:


8. Stricken with Lou Gehrig's disease (amyotrophic lateral sclerosis):


9. Cystic fibrosis kids:


10. ADHD defiant

# Exercise 3: Media Portraying Persons with Disabilities

Analyze the experience and portrayal of individuals with disabilities in one or more of the following movies, series, or documentaries:

- *A Beautiful Mind* (2001, Imagine Entertainment)
- *A Brilliant Young Mind* (*X + Y*, 2016, BBC Films)
- *A Day in the Life of Bonnie Consolo* (1975, Independent Film, YouTube)
- *A Mile in His Shoes* (2011, MGN Productions)
- *Attitude is Altitude.com/Life Without Limbs* (Nick Vujicic, YouTube)
- *Best Foot Forward* (2022, Apple TV+)
- *Breathe* (2017, Bleeker Street)
- *Children of a Lesser God* (1986, Paramount)
- *CODA* (2021, Apple TV+)
- *Do You Remember Love* (1985, CBS)
- *Drought* (2020, Amazon)
- *Home of the Brave* (2006, MGM)
- *I Am Sam* (2001, New Line Cinema)
- *Inside I'm Dancing* (2004, Studio Canal, Working Title Films, Screen Ireland)
- *King Gimp* (1999, HBO)
- *Love and Other Drugs* (2010, 20th Century Fox)
- *Move Me* (2022, Submerged Film, LLC)
- *My Left Foot* (1989, Miramax)
- *Passion Fish* (1992, Miramax)
- *Rainman* (1988, United Artists)
- *Regarding Henry* (1991, Paramount)
- *Run* (2020, Hulu)
- *Sound of Metal* (2017, Amazon Prime)
- *Soul Surfer* (2011, Affirm Films)
- *STILL: A Michael J. Fox Movie* (2023, AppleTV+)
- *Still Alice* (2014, Sony Pictures Classics)
- *Superman: The Christopher Reeves Story* (2024, Warner Brothers)
- *The Best Years of Our Lives* (1946, Available Apple TV+)
- *The Dinner* (2017, Protagonist Pictures)
- *The Diving Bell and the Butterfly* (2007, France, Miramax)
- *The Father* (2020, Sony Pictures)
- *The Fundamentals of Caring* (2016, Levantine Films, Worldwide Pants, Netflix)
- *The Greatest* (2022, Apple TV+)
- *The Last Days of Ptolemy Gray* (2022, Apple TV+)
- *The Normal Heart* (2014, HBO Films)
- *The Other Side of the Mountain* (Parts 1 and 2) (1975 and 1978, Universal)
- *The Other Sister* (1999, Touchstone)
- *The Peanut Butter Falcon* (2019, Armory Films)

- *The Sea Inside* (*Mar Adentro*) (2004, Spain/France/Italy, Warner Home Video)
- *The Sessions* (2012, Fox Searchlight)
- *The Theory of Everything* (2014, Universal Pictures)
- *The Terry Fox Story* (1983, HBO)
- *The Triple Cripples* (2018–Present, https://thetriplecripples.uk/, YouTube)
- *The Upside* (2019, Amazon Prime); *The Intouchables* (2011)
- *The Way He Looks* (2014, Strand Releasing)
- *The Wedding Gift* (1994, Miramax)
- *The Whale* (2022, Protozoa Pictures)
- *Whose Life Is It Anyway?* (1981, Warner Bros.)

These exercises are also available online at www.routledge.com/9781638220039.

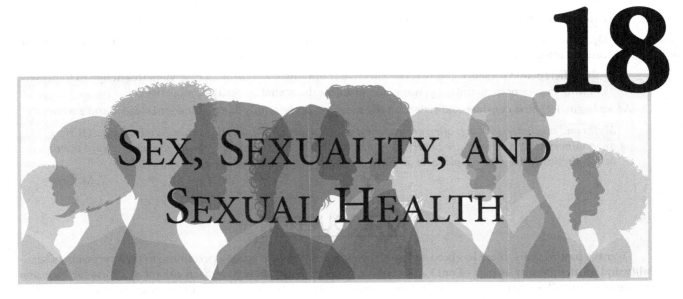

# Sex, Sexuality, and Sexual Health

*Sherrill H. Hayes and Solange Dagress*

## Objectives

*The learner should be able to:*

- Define sex, sex acts, sexuality, and evolving terminology related to lesbian, gay, bisexual, transgender, queer/questioning one's sexual or gender identity, intersex, and asexual/aromantic/agender, expanding two-spirited, and new (LGBTQIA2S +) individuals.

- Consider biological sex, sexual orientation, gender identity, and expression spectrums.

- Support that one should be inclusionary with respect to LGBTQIA2S+ communities as part of addressing global health and inequities of care.

- Emphasize the importance of understanding one's own sexuality, values, beliefs, and biases (conscious and unconscious), to communicate effectively in the clinical setting.

- Discern myths and misconceptions regarding sexuality and disability, and how these may affect the patient's and practitioner's viewpoints and comfort levels.

- Differentiate experiences of the patient as a sexual being that may compromise self-image, loss, and/or precipitate feelings of shame.

- Explain the importance of self-esteem, self-image, and self-actualization with respect to rehabilitation.

- Distinguish normal sexual arousal cycles for the male and female, the neurophysiology of sexual response, and the impact of disabilities and certain illnesses on sexual abilities and functioning.

- Recognize cultural differences, historical and contemporary perspectives related to sexuality, sexual orientation, and disability.

- Discuss the role of the rehabilitation professional with respect to sexuality, the disabled, and those with chronic diseases with special focus on patients with spinal cord injury (SCI), myocardial infarction (MI), and gender-affirming surgeries.

- Apply the principles of the permission, limited information, specific suggestions, and intensive therapy (PLISSIT) model as a structure for identifying one's knowledge base, comfort, and skills in providing respectful and comprehensive care and information regarding sexuality and disability for all patients.

DOI: 10.4324/9781003525554-18

- Discover common drugs, classifications, and categories that may interfere with sexual response and function.

- Describe specific sexual and health-related issues in individuals who are LGBTQIA2S +, and the role of health care professionals (HCPs) in providing safer spaces and ensuring equitable health care.

- Adapt therapeutic presence and practice effective communication through case vignettes designed to prevent shaming experiences, maintain privacy, and promote the sexual integrity of all patients.

As we begin, let's first consider and reflect on the meaning of the words of an educational leader and author:

> *Myths and misunderstandings often arise around groups of people who display three characteristics: (1) They are a minority; (2) members are clearly identifiable; and (3) society harbors fears or aversion toward them. Many physically disabled people meet all three criteria and thus become objects of social bias.[1]*
>
> —T. M. Cole

# INTRODUCTION

Over the past 75 years, there has been a virtual revolution in Western society pertaining to the expression of sexuality and gender identity as part of one's self-concept. More recently, there have been enhanced efforts for inclusion of the LGBTQIA2S + communities, where gender and sexual identification have become more diverse, fluid, and less binary (refer also to Chapter 7). The "typical" family core of the male working outside the home and the female staying home with the children has moved away from such strict gender roles and toward a variety of family structures, and work–life roles within and outside the home. In addition, we have seen a substantial increase in single-parent families, gender-diverse relationships, civil unions, and marriages; and parents with a variety of sexual and gender identities raising children. Sexual behaviors have changed as well, from little premarital sex to the "free love" of the 1960s and 1970s, to the current trend of more of a series of longer-lasting relationships or "serial monogamy," which began largely due to the HIV/AIDS epidemic in the 1980s. Relationships may span a variety of sexual orientations. Concomitantly, there is an increase in the number of people with disabilities due to improved medical diagnostics, interventions, therapies, and technologies, providing for increased survival for people who have been injured or people with chronic disabling conditions.

In the past 25+ years, more research relating to sexual function and sexual counseling has ensued, albeit not as large a volume as in the 1970–80s. In 2000, *Physical Therapy Journal* devoted a special series to spinal cord injury (SCI), examining issues related to sexuality and disability, including challenges due to musculoskeletal, neuromuscular, and cardiopulmonary issues; seating and mobility; and chronic pain (see the Suggested Readings at the end of this chapter). Additionally, there have been major advancements in the field of sexual dysfunction and infertility, which have dramatically improved the lives of people who are able-bodied and people with disabilities or chronic illnesses. For example, treatments for erectile dysfunction (ED) are widely known and advertised in the mainstream media, in vitro fertilization is common, and electro-vibration and electro-ejaculation techniques have dramatically improved fertility in males with SCI. And finally, there have been substantial inroads with respect to gender-affirming medical and surgical interventions. Sexual function and counseling research is frequently published in medical journals and is increasing in rehabilitation-associated journals, especially relating to cancer, spinal cord injury, Parkinson's disease, multiple sclerosis, health care disparity in general, and specifically with LGBTQIA2S + individuals, as well as psychological issues and cognitive disabilities. Specific terminology and acronyms with respect to LGBTQIA2S + are provided in Table 18.1 (see related discussions in Chapter 7); this table is not meant to be comprehensive and serves as a foundational guide for the currently fluid terminology. Let's first begin with three traditionally important definitions:

1. **Sex:** The biological characteristics of a person who classifies themselves as male, female, or intersex at birth; considered one of the four primary drives (along with hunger, thirst, and avoidance of pain) that originate in the subcortex and are modified by learned responses in the cortex.

2. **Sex acts:** Any behaviors involving the secondary erogenous zones and genitalia, such as kissing, hugging, caressing, and fondling, with sexual intercourse being only one kind of sex act.

3. **Sexuality:** The combination of sex drive, sex acts, and all those aspects of personality concerned with learned communications and relationship patterns. There are many levels to sexuality: conversation, shared activities and interests, various expressions of affection and intimacy, and sexual intercourse; all of which may be fluid or evolving. Some people equate sexuality with intimacy. Everyone is capable of intimacy—young or old, able-bodied, or disabled, and individuals of any gender or sexual orientation.

Any discussion regarding sexuality should consider the broad picture and note that definitions of sexuality vary. Common thoughts regarding sexuality often focus on what happens in bed—or the sex acts—as the essence of sexuality. Some see sexuality as being "the major way people define and present themselves to others as people."[2] Another definition of sexuality involves "the way one dresses, the way one carries oneself, the way one looks at others and oneself, the way one speaks to other people, the way one touches other people and oneself."[3] Yet another definition includes "the many facets of an individual's personality, including affection, companionship, intimacy, and love."[4]

In sum then, what all of these evolving definitions display is the universality of the emotional importance of sexuality, whether someone is disabled or able-bodied, cisgender, heterosexual, or sexual and gender minority (SGM). Some also feel that because of the relationship of sexuality to self-esteem and body image, it is an important part of rehabilitation.[5-6] Because self-esteem is so important to a person's psychological well-being, and because disability affects the way people feel about themselves, it is logical to see that a damaged self-esteem will also affect one's sexuality. Self-image and self-efficacy are also important considerations and are affected by disability. In addition, disability and illness affect the injured person and their partner, which is dealt with in more detail later in this chapter. Respectful health care, addressing sexual and reproductive concerns, regardless of sexuality and orientations is a right for everyone.[6]

In previous chapters, the importance of developing listening skills and effective communication in the patient–practitioner interaction (PPI) was presented. Identification of who owns the problem and communicating about emotion-laden topics is evident with issues of sexuality and self-image in the rehabilitation process. Building upon the Helping Interview (Chapter 14), HCP communication[7-9] endeavors to meet six essential goals[8] when addressing sexuality and disability:

1. Establish rapport in a non-judgmental way, using inclusive language

2. Determine a medical and interpersonal history, including sexual orientation and gender identity

3. Assess the role and nature of relationships in the patient's life

4. Identify the changes that have occurred since the onset of the disability or illness

5. Determine how those changes have been explained to the patient and how the changes have affected quality of life

6. Encourage questions always

Sexuality continues to be a sensitive topic that many clinicians are often uncomfortable addressing with their patients. Reasons for this discomfort include: (1) lack of training and knowledge in the area of sexuality, as well as LGBTQIA2S+ health care issues (variable increased risks for mental health and substance abuse disorders, obesity, and sexually acquired diseases, unique needs for transgender people, e.g., cancer screenings); (2) the subject of sexuality being an area where the HCP's conscious or unconscious biases are based on their own upbringing and background, and can interfere with optimum care; (3) lack of exposure to people who identify as SGM in professional education or clinical cases; (4) sexual orientation and gender identity issues can generate strong personal reactions that are most often related to religious and socio-political conservatism, making clinical training and competency more difficult; and (5) holding incorrect assumptions equating sexual orientation and gender identity, which can alienate patients.[10] Thus, rehabilitation professionals often feel they lack competence to provide information, and they are unsure of their roles in providing this information to their patients. For many professionals, it is difficult to separate their own values and attitudes about sexuality from those of their patients in order to be objective. Therefore, it is not surprising that the subject of sexuality is rarely addressed, addressed inappropriately, or simply dismissed.

Attitudes of HCPs toward sexuality have been studied, predominantly with nurses and less so with rehabilitation professionals.[11,12] In studies of nursing students, it has been found that they are less knowledgeable and more conservative than other students.[13] In rehabilitation nurses, increased religiosity was correlated with decreased knowledge of sexuality and more conservative sexual values.[14] Nursing faculty were found to be unprepared to teach this content; thus, it was ignored or limited in content.[15] In a study of occupational therapists (OTs), the therapists rarely addressed sexuality in their practice, and expressed lack of knowledge and confidence in addressing the issues; they also had an apparent heteronormative and conservative view of sexuality.[11] Although studies of HCPs are somewhat limited, one could assume that many of these HCPs have similar origins and values. In another study of rehabilitation professionals, it was found that the majority (79%) thought that sexuality was as important as other aspects of rehabilitation, but few (7%) were comfortable addressing sexuality with their patients.[16]

A similar study found that the majority of patients (73%), patients' partners (59%), and rehabilitation professionals (67%) thought that sexuality was an important issue to be addressed in the rehab setting.[17] Similarly, the study also

| TABLE 18.1 | |
|---|---|
| **FOUNDATIONAL GUIDE TO TERMINOLOGY AND ACRONYMS WITH RESPECT TO LGBTQIA2S+[5-7]** | |
| Lesbian, Gay, Bisexual, Transgender (LGBTQ) | Abbreviated term, now expanded, with QIA+—Queer or Questioning, Intersex, Asexual or Ally; A is used for both, with the second definition relating to the broader community of advocates for human rights of LGBTQIA2S+ people. |
| Sexual and Gender Minority (SGM) | More recent, shorter term for LGBTQIA2S+ individuals, advocated for by the National Institutes of Health.[6,7] |
| Gender | A socially constructed system of classification that ascribes qualities of masculinity and femininity. Gender characteristics may change over time and are different between cultures. Words that refer to gender include man, woman, transgender, masculine, feminine, and gender-queer or nonbinary.[5] |
| Gender Identity | The gender that a person sees oneself as, or the self-awareness of their own gender. This can include choosing not to label oneself with a gender, which is often referred to as being nonbinary.[6] |
| Cisgender | An individual whose gender identity is consistent with their sex assigned at birth. |
| Transgender | When one's gender identity or gender expression does not correspond with the sex they were assigned at birth. |
| Sexual Identity | How one thinks of oneself in terms of to whom one is attracted; components are biological gender, gender, gender role, and sexual orientation. |
| Sexual Orientation | The deep-seated direction of one's sexual or erotic attraction and preferences. Sexual orientation is a continuum and not a set of absolute categories, and although labels such as "heterosexual," "homosexual," or "bisexual" are often used to define sexual orientation, an individual's sexual orientation may be fluid or fall outside any of these labels.[6] |
| Heterosexual | Sexual, emotional, and/or romantic attraction to a sex other than your own. Commonly thought of as attraction to the opposite sex.[6] |
| Homosexual | Sexual, emotional, and/or romantic attraction to a person of the same sex.[6] |
| Bisexual | One who is sexually and/or emotionally attracted to more than one gender.[5] |
| Queer | A term to refer to the entire LGBTQIA2S+ community[6 (p 739)]; often used as an umbrella term for anyone who is not heterosexual and not cisgender.[5] |
| Questioning | Someone who is not sure how they identify, i.e., questioning their sexual orientation or their gender identity.[5] |
| Asexual | People who experience little or no sexual desire, and who may have different sexual orientations and gender identities. |
| Ally | People who identify as cisgender or heterosexual and believe in social and legal equality for LGBTQIA2S+ people.[5] |
| Gender Transition | When individuals strive to align their internal knowledge of gender identity with its outward appearance or anatomy, as in:<br>○ **Social transition**—such as change of name, clothing, hair style, make-up, use of pronouns (she/her, he/him, they), etc. to be recognized as the gender that individual identifies with.<br>○ **Physical transition**—use of hormone therapy, surgery (when the body is modified through medical and/or surgical intervention), or other interventions to align the individual's physical appearance/anatomy with their gender identity. |

found that 93% of physicians, psychologists, and social workers felt it was within their domain of practice, as well as 87% of nurses, but only 48% of physical therapists (PTs) felt it was within their practice domain. For something that is obviously important to patients, rehabilitation professionals need to increase their knowledge and comfort levels. PTs and OTs provide rehabilitation to address movement and skills for the job of living; sex is in fact an activity of living, which involves movement! Sex is a valued function for many patients/clients, and many impairments, functional limitations, disabilities, and handicaps have an effect on the ability to function, perform sex acts, express sexuality, and influence sex drive.

The reasons for HCPs' discomfort with sexuality have been noted to be a lack of knowledge or an assumption that "someone else does it." Because sexual/gender identity, self-concept, and self-worth are so strongly linked, if one of these is impaired, all are affected. In addition, impaired sexual function has a direct adverse effect on the medical, psychological, and vocational rehabilitation of an individual, and addressing this issue can have a positive effect on the overall rehabilitation of a patient with a disability or chronic illness. It is the job of the rehabilitation professional to increase the function of our patients in all domains. Knowledge building in the areas of anatomy and physiology is easily accomplished, as well as disability-specific effects and cultural variables. However, other areas to be included in the common education of patients in a rehabilitation setting are human sexual response, spirituality, and religious values, and the dispelling of myths and stereotypes, along with physical health, mental health, well-being, quality of life, and the topic of sexuality. More specific training is necessary for rehabilitation professionals to feel confident, as well as to reflect on their own values, beliefs, and biases regarding sexuality.

Skills training should address effective and active listening (see Chapters 8 and 14), interviews and assessment skills (which should include skilled, nonjudgmental history taking, including taking a sexual history when needed), and values clarification (see Chapter 3); discussion and modeling of compassion, patience, perceptiveness, and integrity are also valuable. Because of the close bonds patients develop with rehabilitation professionals, especially therapists, due to the intensity of contacts and type of care, therapists are in a unique position to respond to their patients, often more so than physicians. The main objectives are to create a supportive and safe environment, ensuring equity in the provision of health care to all, and to encourage active participation of the patient in increasing function in all aspects of their life.

# THE PERMISSION, LIMITED INFORMATION, SPECIFIC SUGGESTIONS, AND INTENSIVE THERAPY (PLISSIT) MODEL

The PLISSIT model[18] is ideally utilized by all members of the health care team in conversing with people with disabilities who are asking about sex and sexuality. In this model, all members of the team are educated to feel comfortable enough with their own sexuality and have enough knowledge to function at the first two levels of the model (i.e., permitting discussion of the topic of sex and sexuality and having enough knowledge about sexuality and about various specific disabilities to provide limited information). Team members should also reflect on their own values and beliefs. For instance, knowing what topics create feelings of uncertainty or embarrassment for themselves, such as sexual orientation or gender identity issues. What brings them sexual pleasure? What would it mean for them to have their own sexual ability affected by illness or trauma? Rehabilitation professionals will undoubtedly encounter patients with different values from their own.[19] Thus, awareness of one's own biases helps to define topics or areas one is not comfortable with and which, therefore, should be referred to someone else on the team. In addition, they should know enough about their own limits, or "know what they do not know," in order to properly refer the patient to a more knowledgeable HCP. Each PLISSIT model[18] element will be briefly described here.

## Permission

Permission is a valuable tool to help patients deal with basic issues of self-esteem, personal worth, and body image. At this first level, the HCP gives overt and covert messages to the patient who inquires about sex, provides permission through their responses to the patient's questions, offers more information when the patient is ready, and introduces the topic in a nonthreatening manner. Here, the HCP is being open and accepting of the topic of sex and gives the patient permission to inquire without embarrassment. Although many rehabilitation professionals are not confident in discussing sexuality, most have adequate skills to perform at this level.

## Limited Information

At this second level in the model, the HCP provides general and basic education, such as anatomy and physiology, dispelling of myths, and describing general ways in which others in similar situations have resolved their own problems. At this level, it is important that the HCP know their own limitations (in knowledge, skill, and comfort) and refer the patient to others when the patient's needs exceed their own limits.

## Specific Suggestions

In this third level, the HCP assists the patient with more specific needs or concerns by suggesting or providing specific ways to resolve a problem (e.g., specific adapted positions for sexual intercourse, ED, and management of bowel or bladder problems) or specific effects of medications or surgeries. At this stage, discussion of sexual boundaries and roles that are acceptable to the patient and their partner would be appropriate. Depending on the injury, helping the patient redefine their personal definition of sexuality, including attitude change and broadening of views, may be included (e.g., oral genital stimulation).[13] For functioning at this level, the HCP should have additional education, expertise, or experience in sexuality and disability beyond others on the team and be astutely aware of their own limitations in knowledge, comfort, or skills.

## Intensive Therapy

This level is usually beyond the rehabilitation setting and requires psychotherapy, relationship counseling, or surgical or invasive procedures (penile implants or injection therapy, for example). **Referral** to other HCPs for more intensive therapy is usually coordinated outside the inpatient setting.

The PLISSIT model[18] provides a structure for an effective multidisciplinary team approach and for individuals to identify their own levels of appropriate practice or expertise, as well as a process that assists one to identify areas for future professional growth. It is also particularly important to consider any potentials, *as needed*, related to domestic and/or partner violence utilizing the Partner Violence Screening[10] format consisting of three gender-neutral questions:

- Have you been hit, kicked, punched, or otherwise hurt by someone in the past year? If so, by whom?
- Do you feel safe in your current relationship?
- Is there a partner from a previous relationship who is making you feel unsafe now?

Case presentations are particularly helpful in addressing specific sexual health needs for all patients, identification of previously unknown biases or assumptions, and identifying options for management and problem solving, as well as HCP mentoring opportunities. You will have the opportunity to continue your professional formation with the case vignettes in Exercise 1 at the end of the chapter.

# SEXUALITY AND DISABILITY: HOSPITALIZATION—THE PROCESS OF BECOMING A PATIENT

Becoming a patient in today's health care arenas involves many processes that threaten one's independence and dignity and one's very sense of self-identity (see Table 13.1). The transformation of a person into a patient begins with several predictable events:[20]

- Answering the same seemingly innocuous questions from several people about personal information (name, address, Social Security number, insurance, age, weight, reason for admission)
- Undressing and donning the "neuter" hospital gown (affording little in the way of propriety)
- The surrendering of all personal effects
- The application of the plastic wristband for identification and/or other monitors
- The transportation via wheelchair to a room with a bed and a chair, even when one is capable of walking unaided and even possibly sharing intimate space with another "unknown" patient

Whether the hospitalization is for a minor procedure or life-threatening illness, the process remains the same. Even with the use of modern, electronic health records, much is unchanged as due to required reverifications. The point is that there is a **ubiquitous custom of forced dependence of individuals who have previously been in control of their lives outside the hospital, but who are forced to lose their identities and senses of self when they become patients.** Suddenly, a person is no longer Mary Smith, CEO, or John Jones, Esq., but Ms. Smith or Mr. Jones, or even worse, Mary and John. The ultimate insult occurs when they become "Room 22, Bed 2," and this process occurs in just about every inpatient setting in the country.

Following the initial round of the admission process and settling into the institutional routine is the process of myriad evaluations by different HCPs assigned to the patient's care—nurses, physicians (including residents, interns, and medical students), and rehabilitation professionals and their assistants and students. All are asking comparable questions about the patient's personal and medical history, doing physical examinations, and ordering invasive and noninvasive procedures in the process of establishing a diagnosis or treatment regimen.

All these assessments are necessary and important in the process of diagnosis and treatment of the patient's problem. However, what is sometimes overlooked in this process is the privacy of the individual, personal preferences, and often there is a consistent lack of concern about personal modesty and humility as the patient is questioned, examined, prodded, and probed, often in intimate places. Significantly, the patient's problem may involve areas of the body that reflect one's sexuality, such as the breast, uterus, prostate, or genitalia. And increasingly, physical therapists are part of the team involved in both the pre-op and post-op treatment for sexual re-assignment or gender-affirmation surgical procedures[21] (see later in this chapter).

When these areas of the body are the cause of the hospitalization, there is an inevitable increased sense of invasion accompanying the process of assessment. If surgery is imminent, whether a mastectomy, hysterectomy, prostatectomy, vaginoplasty, or phalloplasty, there is a significant, unspoken fear about the patient's sense of self after the surgery.

# BODY IMAGE

Any patient who experiences trauma, surgical removal of a body part, or treatment that results in disfigurement or loss of a body part experiences a disturbance of their body image. Body image disturbances may occur when there is a discrepancy between the way in which one had mentally pictured the body and the way the body is currently perceived. This conflict can arouse anxiety and fear of rejection. The response of loved ones is especially important and thought to exert a considerable influence on the patient's ability to reintegrate their new body image. Body image distortion may elicit feelings of unacceptability, thus negatively influencing the person's perception of self as a sexual being and, in turn, influencing sexual function. And to add a traumatic physical disability, such as a spinal cord injury, on to a person who is a member of the LGBTQIA2S+ community creates increased minority stress related to having multiple marginalized identities, and a risk of greater health disparity.[22]

# EFFECTS OF ILLNESS ON SEXUALITY

Illness may influence one's sexuality in many different and diverse ways (refer to Table 18.2). It is important for HCPs to be aware of how various disease processes or drugs may affect their patients' physiological functioning, as well as their sense of self. There are several excellent and comprehensive resource textbooks for HCPs' (see Suggested Readings) continued learning.

# ACTING OUT SEXUALLY

When patients consciously or unconsciously test the response of others to themselves as sexual beings, they may act out as a means of gaining control of a situation in which they feel dependent. For example, flirtatious behavior is often exhibited as a way to attract attention. What the patients may be expressing is the effect of sexual deprivation or separation from a sexual partner or significant other. Also, they may simply be seeking out validation of themselves as still being attractive or desirable. Chapter 12 on neurolinguistic psychology offers communication skills and alternatives to help HCPs set strong boundaries and break rapport if this

TABLE 18.2

## EFFECTS OF DISABILITIES ON SEXUALITY AND SELECT EXAMPLES

| EFFECT ON SEXUALITY | SELECT EXAMPLES |
|---|---|
| Interference with sexual function due to physiological changes or tissue damage | Spinal cord injury, diabetes, prostate cancer |
| Treatment may result in a change in body image, which may seem incompatible with maintaining a sexual relationship | Mastectomy, orchiectomy, ostomy, amputation |
| Pharmacological agents may interfere with sexual function | Antihypertensive medications, chemotherapy, insulin |
| Physical symptoms (fatigue or pain) may interfere with or hamper sexual performance | Cancer patients on chemotherapy or radiation therapy, rheumatoid arthritis, multiple sclerosis, low back pain |
| Anxiety related to illness may interfere with sexual response | Post-myocardial infarction, cancer, genital herpes, HIV, some chronic diseases |
| Depression, grief, substance abuse and/or suicide, suicide risk may be associated with impaired libido or sex drive | Post-myocardial infarction, hysterectomy, mastectomy, cancer, multiple sclerosis, Parkinson's disease |
| Illness may necessitate physical separation from a partner | Spinal cord injury, post-stroke, accident, HIV, AIDS, Covid-19 |

acting out becomes sexual harassment (see also Chapter 9, Matters of Morality: Assertiveness Skills and Conflict Resolution).

# CULTURAL VARIABLES

As described in Chapter 13, it is important for HCPs to be aware of diverse cultural customs and beliefs in the patients they are treating. Often, without thinking of it consciously, different customs are considered odd or strange, when they should merely be considered different. Greater emphasis on cultural diversity is evident in most professional curricula, which is certainly needed in the multicultural environment encountered by HCPs today. In many cultures, there are certain proscriptions that may modify an individual's response to hospitalization and treatment. For example, in certain cultures, illness is believed to be a manifestation of weakness, while loss of blood is thought to impair sexual vigor. Protection of a wife's "modesty" is seen as a duty of a good husband during physical examinations. Any or all cultural dictates may be misinterpreted by uninformed HCPs as stubbornness or stupidity unless cultural differences are understood and verified with the individual patient. Likewise, if a HCP is not accustomed to being in the presence of SGM couples, they may find themselves acting in ways that are judgmental or unkind, and not conducive to therapeutic presence. SGM couples have similar needs and concerns as cisgender and heterosexual couples, and efforts should be made to make them feel comfortable and understood, without judgment. When appropriate, safer sex options and practices should be discussed.

The following recommended questions are provided for guidance to obtain sexual history. McNamara and Ng[10] suggest considering:

> *questions inclusive of nonbinary identities—instead of asking whether the patient identifies as a man or a woman or as gay or straight, ask about anatomy and behavior, e.g.:*

- *Are you sexually active? (Explore what sexual activity means for the patient)*
- *With whom do you have sex? Men, women, or both?*
- *What parts of your body do you use when having sex with your partner(s)?*
- *Do you practice safer sex? (Explore what safer sex means for the patient) With primary partners? With casual partners?*
- *How do your partners identify their gender or sexual orientation?*

# BASIC GUIDELINES FOR EFFECTIVE COMMUNICATION ABOUT SEXUALITY AND REHABILITATION

To enhance your therapeutic sensitivity with PPI, follow these three basic HCP guidelines:

1. **Prevent shaming experiences**: Shame implies admitting to oneself that part or all of the self is unacceptable. Shaming experiences can be prevented by providing physical and psychological privacy, carefully reading body language, listening to words to avoid "touchy" areas, and explaining that the given situation is not intended to embarrass but is necessary for effective care. This is especially true when taking a sexual history, for example.

2. **Maintain privacy**: During hospitalization, personal autonomy and the limitation and protection of information are usually jeopardized. In order to emphasize confidentiality, it is often wise to acknowledge to patients that you realize that some things are difficult to discuss; then provide some dimension of privacy and always show respect as a means to address this problem. Make use of curtains and closed doors whenever possible.

3. **Do not make judgments**: Chapters 2, 3, and 4 emphasize that we all have our own values, and there are some individuals whose values may conflict with our own. Accept that people are different and maintain a professional decorum without inflicting your own values on others, verbally or nonverbally. Be aware of whether you are a person who readily displays facial expressions that reveal dissatisfaction with different values from your own and make efforts to adjust.

In sum, understanding oneself, understanding one's patient, and understanding the dysfunction or disability are all essential roles for rehabilitation professionals. HCPs should continually strive to continue their education and professional development and to address all aspects of being and knowing, for their patients' benefit and their own self-preservation, maintaining a humanistic approach to health care for all.

# MYTHS AND HISTORICAL PERSPECTIVES

As reflected in the quote from Cole[1] at the beginning of this chapter, people with disabilities fit the three criteria that would characterize them as being different from the majority of the population. People with disabilities are a readily identifiable minority, and others often feel uncomfortable in their presence. Most people in ethnic or racial minorities, or in the SGM community, have also experienced these three criteria at some point in their lives, and the similarities are striking.

Over the past 50 years, there have been numerous changes in behaviors and attitudes regarding disability and sexuality. During the 1970s and 1980s, there was a rash of medical, psychological, and behavioral investigations that added greatly to our body of knowledge about sexuality and disability. Prior to this period, there were many myths perpetuated by the media, as well as educational publications, which did little to explore the true realities and capabilities of sexual functioning in people with disabilities. Furthermore, there was little in the medical literature regarding sexuality and disability, further perpetuating the myth of asexuality.

Prejudice against individuals with disabilities in our culture and others has existed for many years, often perpetuated by popular literature. Captain Ahab from *Moby-Dick*, Quasimodo from *The Hunchback of Notre Dame*, and Dr. No, James Bond's arch-rival, come readily to mind. Often these characters were referred to as "grotesquely deformed and evil." Is it any wonder that many of us have grown to harbor feelings of revulsion or pity for people with disabilities?

Similarly, many individuals with a traumatic disability, such as an amputation or SCI, may have themselves harbored feelings of revulsion toward those with disabilities prior to their own injury. In effect, these preconceived beliefs may result in considerable self-prejudice, hampering their own self-acceptance. This further complicates the acceptance of their new body image for their own self-esteem. In a society such as ours, with so much emphasis placed on beauty, health, and physical fitness, it is easy to see how physically disabled people may feel ostracized in today's sexual arena and low on a scale of sexual desirability. In an era of selfies, and social media platform instant sharing, the visual perception may be even further magnified.

It is important to note that over the past 20 to 25 years, people with visible disabilities have now been regularly featured in mainstream media in print and broadcast advertisements and as main characters in television shows. Social media and networking sites have also helped to provide increased opportunities for more interaction and education for people with disabilities (yet some have also provided detrimental influences). Certain television shows have also utilized social and comedic satire to aid in changing perspectives, such as with the character Jimmy, a male fourth grader who is disabled, in the Comedy Central series *South Park*. Jimmy was first introduced in a "cripple fight" and has endless optimism, despite his disability. The episodes featuring Jimmy provide moral insights into the thoughts of individuals with disabilities, bringing forth important lessons, albeit in satirical comedy. Modern technology has also assisted in bringing about greater connectivity for all, and there are also online dating sites[23] specifically for people with disabilities and LGBTQIA2S+. Fortunately, it would appear that at least some of these previously held attitudes and aversions may be changing in a positive manner. Indeed, with the advent of gay marriage, there is more open acceptance of LGBTQIA2S+ people, and with young children relating to friends who have gender-diverse parents without a second thought, society seems to be evolving and moving toward a more global view of humanity in our future.

To sum up, it is important for HCPs to recognize that people are not "handicapped" intrinsically. As pointed out in Chapter 17, a person with a disability only becomes handicapped when they are restrained from usual social interaction by barriers, social and architectural, that prohibit participation in normal daily activities.

# SELF-ESTEEM

According to Abraham Maslow,[24] sex is one of the basic physiological needs that must be met, in addition to air, water, food, shelter, and sleep. All are needed in order for an individual to move toward self-esteem and self-actualization. Taking Maslow's theory to practical application, Anderson and Cole[25] did groundbreaking research with respect to examining the interrelationship of sexual success, work success (meaningful employment), and the self-esteem of an individual with a disability. They found that if there was perceived success in sexual activity, the person with a disability reported a higher self-esteem and fewer feelings of castration. If there was success in work life, there was less tolerance for dependency and thus a higher self-esteem. If there was success in both areas, the individual had a high self-esteem, fewer medical complaints, and less need for medical and social support. Many authors since this seminal work have stressed the importance of sexuality on self-esteem and self-image.[20,26–28]

Another meaningful point with respect to success in sexual relations relates to the importance and significance of the sexual partner/s or significant other. Significant others play a pivotal role in the acceptance of a changed body image for a person with a disability. As Rosenbaum[29] so eloquently stated:

> What becomes apparent when the direct genital urge toward physical release is lost, are the many other needs, that can be met or expressed through sexual activity—the need for touching, for reassuring body contact, to be held and to hold, to express love and caring through caressing and kissing. These become especially important when the body has been damaged and the individual is attempting to integrate and accept a new and altered body image. We all need the acceptance of another to make the image of ourselves whole and more loveable.

Thus, the acceptance of the partner is important in allowing and assisting the reintegration of the individual with a disability in a new body image. Recent literature has emphasized the importance of the partner/s relationship/s because all people (the person with the disability and their partner/s if present prior to the disability) are affected.[27] Furthermore, the committed relationship, regardless of whether the relationship is heterosexual or not, married or cohabiting, is impacted. Suffering a disability has a profound effect on the quality of life of an individual, as well as the life of their partner/s. People with disabilities, if married, also have higher divorce rates than those with no disabilities.[27] Finally, it was also determined that partners of people with disabilities have lower scores on all "quality of life" measures, presumably due to increased stress.[27] It has been postulated that the nondisabled partner often struggles in the role of caretaker, especially if it involves bowel and bladder care or management. On top of that, switching from caretaker to the role of intimate lover then becomes a major source of stress. Sometimes this can also lead to abuse or domestic violence, with the person with the disability fearful of leaving the relationship because of their dependency upon the abuser, who is also their caretaker.[22]

Besides the partner/s, the next most important person is the HCP and their attitude toward their patients. Self-esteem and self-confidence depend largely on feedback from the environment and those around the patient. If the HCP projects a sensitive, honest, and nonjudgmental attitude, with an openness to questions and concerns, the patient can be encouraged to discover a new sense of self without anxiety. If, however, the patient and their questions are not addressed openly and honestly or are brushed off in a shaming experience, the patient's adjustment and acceptance will be dealt a significant blow, and their recovery will be compromised.

# NORMAL HUMAN SEXUAL RESPONSE—NEUROPHYSIOLOGY

In a culture and era where sexuality seems to scream from billboards, magazines, movie theaters, the Internet, and social media, it is amazing how little education those in the health care professions actually receive with respect to normal human sexuality. Understanding sexuality and disability, especially as it relates to the person with SCI, requires an understanding of the normal sexual response and its components. The biological male and female response cycles are found in Table 18.3.

In biological males, it is important to note the following facts regarding erection and ejaculation, based on neurophysiology. There are two centers for erection within the spinal cord:

1. **Psychogenic (T11–L2)**—Mental arousal, fantasizing, psychic stimuli (or "whatever turns you on").

2. **Reflexogenic (S2–S4)**—Local arousal, masturbation, rubbing the inside of the thigh, full bladder, catheter change (reflex sensorimotor feedback loop).

Ejaculation is mediated by the sympathetic nervous system (T11–L2), the parasympathetic nervous system (S2–S4), and the somatic nervous system. The two kinds of erection are not separate in the nondisabled male response cycle, but become important in understanding sexual function in males with SCI.

| TABLE 18.3 |
|---|
| **THE SEXUAL AROUSAL CYCLE: MALE AND FEMALE** |

**1. EXCITATION:** Develops from any source of bodily or psychic stimuli and, with adequate stimulation, leads to further excitation. The first phase may be interrupted, prolonged, or ended by distracting stimuli.

| MALE | FEMALE |
|---|---|
| ○ Rapid engorgement and erection of the penis<br>○ Tensing and thickening of the scrotal skin<br>○ Elevation of scrotal sac<br>○ Occasional nipple erection<br>○ Elevation of HR and BP | ○ Clitoral glans enlarges<br>○ Vaginal lubrication<br>○ Nipples become erect, breast size may enlarge<br>○ Sexual flush may be seen (rash on chest to breast)<br>○ HR and BP increase |

**2. PLATEAU:** Often called the consolidation period. A period of intensified sexual tension; also affected by distracting stimuli.

| MALE | FEMALE |
|---|---|
| ○ Increased penile circumference<br>○ Increase in testes size<br>○ Continued increase in muscle tension, HR, RR, and BP<br>○ Sexual flush—rash over face, neck, and chest | ○ Lower one-third of vagina constricts, upper two-thirds balloons (creates a squeezing action)<br>○ Clitoral glans retracts<br>○ Uterus elevates<br>○ Sexual flush may spread to entire body<br>○ Increase in muscle tension, HR, RR, and BP |

**3. ORGASM:** Involuntary climax of sexual tension increments; really only a few seconds of the sexual response cycle during which vasocongestion and myotonia are released; greater variety of intensity and duration in the female.

| MALE | FEMALE |
|---|---|
| ○ HR, RR, and BP increase further<br>○ Expulsive contraction of the penile urethra<br>○ Ejaculation (internal bladder sphincter closes, preventing retrograde ejaculation)<br>○ Involuntary muscle contraction of perineal muscles | ○ Further increase in generalized muscle tone, HR, RR, and BP<br>○ Involuntary rhythmic muscle contraction in perineal muscles<br>○ Involuntary contraction, spasm of muscle groups<br>○ May be multiple orgasms (unlike males) |

*(continued)*

| TABLE 18.3 (CONTINUED) | |
|---|---|
| **THE SEXUAL AROUSAL CYCLE: MALE AND FEMALE** | |
| **4. RESOLUTION:** The period when involuntary changes occur that restore the individual to the pre-excitatory state. | |
| MALE | FEMALE |
| ◦ Gradual reversal of anatomical and physiological changes<br>◦ Males require a refractory period before another cycle occurs | ◦ Gradual reversal of anatomical and physiological changes<br>◦ Females usually do not have a refractory period and may begin another cycle immediately |
| BP = blood pressure; HR = heart rate; RR = resting rate. | |

# SEXUALITY AND SPINAL CORD INJURY

Sexuality is affected more with SCI than with any other disease or pathological condition. The patient's first question is usually, "Will I live?" The second question (often unexpressed) is, "How will this injury affect me sexually?"

There are far too many exceptions within each spinal cord level to state, with any certainty, what any one patient's sexual disability will be, and this is evolving with the new genetics and robotics. What is known is that the majority of people with SCI are satisfied (72%), although this is lower than able-bodied men and women.[30] In general, erection capability (whether reflexogenic or psychogenic) has been reported by 80% to 100% of males with SCI, and ejaculation occurs in 4% to 18%, with people with quadriplegia being in the 0% to 4% range.[31] What should be emphasized is that sexual activity may or may not involve genital sensation. Ultimately, sexual satisfaction is a cerebral event and therefore can be achieved by everyone. Furthermore, sexual function has been found to be especially important to most patients with SCI in several studies, in which the majority placed sexual functioning ahead of return of sensation, walking, or bowel and bladder function (and second only to hand function in people with quadriplegia).[31]

# SPINAL CORD INJURY—SEXUAL FUNCTION IN MALES

SCI is a devastating injury to anyone, but there are significant effects with respect to sexuality that affect males more than females (Table 18.4).

| TABLE 18.4 | | |
|---|---|---|
| **SPINAL CORD INJURY: EFFECTS OF SEXUAL FUNCTION IN MALES**[A] | | |
| **QUADRIPLEGIA** | **PARAPLEGIA**[B] | **CAUDA EQUINA LESIONS** |
| ◦ Reflexogenic—Intact<br>◦ Psychogenic—Not intact<br>◦ Ejaculation—Rare<br>◦ Fertility[C]—Almost nil | ◦ Reflexogenic—Intact<br>◦ Psychogenic—Not intact<br>◦ Ejaculation—Rare<br>◦ Fertility—Almost nil | ◦ Reflexogenic—Arc may be disturbed (below L2)<br>◦ Psychogenic—Intact (T11–L2)<br>◦ Ejaculation—Moderate chance<br>◦ Fertility—May be present, but with sperm problems (retrograde ejaculation, temperature problems) |
| [A]There is a distinct difference between complete and incomplete lesions of the spinal cord, with effects from incomplete lesions being far less predictable than from complete lesions, although more positive with respect to ejaculation and orgasm in lower motor neuron lesions compared with upper motor neuron lesions.<br>[B]Essentially, there is no difference between a male with quadriplegia or paraplegia with respect to sexual capability and fertility. The major difference is in the greater area of intact skin sensation and motor ability (trunk, arms, and abdomen).<br>[C]Because ejaculation is rare, fertility is severely affected; however, fertility can be greatly assisted today with technological advances, such as electro-vibration, electro-ejaculation, and artificial insemination. | | |

For levels above the cauda equina, the ability to achieve and sustain an erection is generally maintained as long as there is local stimulation to activate the feedback loop for reflexogenic erection. Ejaculation is rarer, and fertility is a problem, although there have been recent major breakthroughs (e.g., electro-vibration and electro-ejaculation) in this area.

It is also important to remember that males, with or without SCI, have been heavily conditioned by society to perceive sexual performance as a key component of "masculinity." Given this message, it is no surprise that if a male's ability to achieve an erection is impaired—as it certainly is in a male with SCI—this can feel like a threat to his "masculinity" in a world which considers this to be of primary importance.

# SPINAL CORD INJURY—SEXUAL FUNCTION IN FEMALES

There has been a sexual bias in the literature regarding female sexuality, although it is true that the majority of people with traumatic SCI are young males. Females with SCI are often thought to be unaffected because their fertility remains intact; thus, many people mistakenly believe that they do not suffer the overt sexual disability that is seen with males. Often, they are told that their sexuality is unaffected, but females experience the same differences and inabilities, neurophysiologically, as do men. The female sexual cycle is similar to that of the male; thus, the lubrication, engorgement, and contraction components of the sexual response cycle are affected. Recent research has shown that females with complete SCIs with upper motor neuron lesions will have reflexogenic lubrication but not psychogenic lubrication, similar to their male counterparts with the same type of injuries.[32] Yet, because these problems are not as overt and obvious as when a male is unable to achieve erection or has difficulty doing so, females are mistakenly viewed as unaffected.

Immediately after a traumatic SCI, a female's menses may be halted, but her menstrual cycles will usually return within 6 months, and fertility is therefore unaffected, unlike males. Pregnancy, if it occurs, can be problematic due to difficulties with movement and transfers due to the pregnant uterus, and there is an increased risk of autonomic dysreflexia. Labor and delivery also present complications due to the inability of a female with SCI to sense labor contractions or to push during the expulsion phase of labor. Cesarean birth is usually not necessary because the uterus is an involuntary muscle capable of contracting despite loss of innervation. However, due to the inability of the female to push during delivery, and potential problems of emboli or autonomic dysreflexia, vaginal births are rare, although not impossible.

# SEXUAL DYSFUNCTION AND FERTILITY

Sexuality is much more than childbearing for females and fertility for males, but information usually given in a rehabilitation setting is often overly clinical. It tends to focus on bowel and bladder routines and stresses more the physical act of intercourse, removed from the context of the entire relationship. Although it is true that the greatest concerns of individuals focus on the physical (autonomic dysreflexia and bowel or bladder accidents) and the psychological (satisfying the partner, being attractive), the latter usually diminishes over time, but the former persists, partially due to the emphasis placed by HCPs who tell individuals to expect bowel and bladder accidents and other negative possibilities. If individuals with SCI are told repeatedly of the negative consequences during rehabilitation, a time when their self-esteem and self-confidence are already challenged, it is no wonder that many are not encouraged, or are scared, to form a relationship. Warnings about potential problems should be realistic but not overwhelming. Discussion of these issues should be done in a nonjudgmental way to promote self-confidence and self-acceptance.

With respect to the treatment of sexual difficulties, there are far more options and much more successful ones for males than for females. For females, various medications for sexual difficulties (e.g., phosphodiesterase or topical prostaglandin) have not proven successful for disabled or able-bodied females with sexual dysfunctions. Vibro-stimulation and the use of vibrators have been helpful for many females, and there is some promise with Food and Drug Administration-approved clitoral vacuum stimulation procedures.[33]

For males, current options include the common oral medications (Viagra [sildenafil], Levitra [vardenafil], and Cialis [tadalafil]). Additionally, there are lesser-known medications (Staxyn, Caverject, Alprostadel, Edex, Stendra), as well as injectable medications that relax the penile smooth muscle to cause an erection, topical agents, vacuum devices or penile rings, and surgical penile implants. There are also Alternative or Natural products such as Damiana, Horny Goat Weed, and Yohimbine. Electro-ejaculation and artificial insemination have greatly aided fertility in males with SCI.

Relating to the human sexual response, Masters and Johnson (see Suggested Readings) were pioneers, and contributed greatly to our understanding, of this basic human need of sexuality and sexual response. One of the things they noted is that the human sexual response is a total body response, rather than merely a pelvic phenomenon. There are changes in cardiovascular and respiratory function, as well as reactions of the skin, muscles, breasts, and rectal sphincter. This whole-body response is an important distinction because it is commonly reported that many individuals with SCI actually experience orgasm, although usually of a different type from what they experienced prior to their injury. Individuals with SCI are often taught to use various methods of assignment, fantasy employment, memory, and recall, and report that they experience a sensation that, although different, is nonetheless satisfying. In one study, sensory substitution techniques using training and neuroplasticity to map tongue sensations were successfully used to increase pleasure and orgasm in sexual experiences in males with SCI.[34] Orgasm can still remain elusive to individuals with SCI. They must undergo—accomplished much more easily with a willing partner—a process of learning to enhance their sexual responsiveness over time, and adjustment of their own values, through self-experimentation and open-mindedness.

# SEXUALITY AND MYOCARDIAL INFARCTION

Although a great volume of literature exists relating to sexuality and SCI, sexuality and myocardial infarction (MI) is the second most researched topic in the medical literature. With respect to sexuality and MI, there are still discrepancies in the literature. Either little information is given (and what is given is often too conservative) or conflicting information is given, making it difficult for patients to decide whether it is safe to resume sexual activity after a MI. Much of the discrepancy in the literature about sexuality and the post-MI patient is related to discrepancies in the maximal heart rate during sexual activity. In their classic studies of human sexual response, Masters and Johnson recorded couples' heart rates, respiratory rates, and other physiological responses during sexual intercourse and found that heart rates escalated to 180 bpm during intercourse; therefore, concluded that sexual activity was "heavy cardiac work."

Many cardiologists and other physicians, when asked by their patients, related these findings and cautioned against any excessive cardiac work for their post-MI patients (i.e., resumption of sexual relations). What was missing in this information for cardiac patients was the fact that the Masters and Johnson studies were conducted on healthy, young heterosexual college students in their early twenties. The average post-MI patient in the mid-1980s was a male in his fifties, married for 20 or more years to the same spouse. Hellerstein and Friedman[35] saw this discrepancy and pursued their own study, similar to that of Masters and Johnson, except using couples with a post-MI spouse in their fifties. Their results were dramatically different: They found the maximal heart rates to be 120 bpm, roughly the equivalent of climbing two flights of stairs, and lower than heart rates during a football game or a heated argument in the office. They concluded that, for the "typical male post-MI patient," with their spouse of 20 or more years and a frequency of sexual intercourse of one to two times per week, sexual activity was not the wild, amorous fit of passion seen often in the movies of today and did not constitute heavy cardiac work. A gradual return to sexual activity for most post-MI patients is recommended; although all studies have shown a reduction in the frequency of sexual activity when compared with the pre-MI state for both males and females.[8]

Stratification of post-MI patients into high, intermediate, and low categories of cardiac risk appears to be the norm (with erectile hardness being correlated), with those in the low-risk category being the most ready to resume sexual activity and others dependent on results of exercise testing and other medications.[36] It was further presumed that patients without cardiac ischemia during exercise would not develop ischemia during sexual intercourse.[37] Finally, all episodes of ischemia associated were associated with increased heart rate; thus, recommending therapeutic strategies to reduce heart rate and improve exercise threshold.[37]

The focus on SCI and post-MI patients in this chapter is largely due to the amount of literature in these areas, but almost any kind of disease process or treatment can have an effect on a person's sexuality (Table 18.5).

| TABLE 18.5 |
|---|

## OTHER CONDITIONS THAT MAY CAUSE PROBLEMS WITH SEXUAL INTERCOURSE

| CONDITION | PROBLEM |
|---|---|
| Genital lesions | May cause difficulty with penetration or painful intercourse (dyspareunia) |
| Respiratory disease | May impair the ability to breathe adequately or limit positions used to engage in sexual intercourse |
| Cardiac disease | May involve poor circulation to the genital area, angina with exertion, or decreased libido due to medications; denial, anxiety, and depression |
| Neurological diseases (stroke, multiple sclerosis, Parkinson's) | May involve components of the nervous system, altering sensation or motor ability (erection, lubrication); may also have spasticity, impairing range of motion; decreased libido; language deficits or changes in affect |
| Amputations | May limit some positions due to inability to assume them; may be a physical turn-off or fetish for the partner, or body image |
| Arthritis | Limitations due to joint mobility and/or painful joints limiting activity |
| Ostomies | May limit some positions due to pressure on ostomy site; may be a physical turn-off to the partner, or body image |
| Severe burns | May be limited in joint range of motion, difficulty in assuming some positions due to limited mobility; may be a physical turn-off to the partner, or body image |
| Scleroderma | May be limited in joint range of motion, difficulty in assuming some positions due to limited mobility; loss of elasticity of skin may hamper intercourse or cause painful intercourse; may be a physical turn-off to the partner |
| Gender confirmation/ affirming surgeries | May involve years of psychotherapy, hormonal treatments, culminating in extensive surgery involving the genitalia and sex organs (uterus, ovaries, penis, vagina), often with hypertonia of the pelvic floor muscles, and extensive scar tissue |
| Cancer | Physical and emotional disturbances; primary sexual organs may be affected (disfigurement, body image); treatment options (chemotherapy, radiation therapy, or surgery) may cause impairment; fatigue, nausea, vomiting; anxiety and depression; hormonal changes if early menopause as consequence (decreased lubrication, increased pain with intercourse) |

# DRUGS THAT MAY INTERFERE WITH SEXUAL FUNCTION

Many pharmacological agents can affect sexual performance directly or indirectly, a factor that has been increasingly noted in the media today. Because most drugs affect the autonomic nervous system (sympathetic or parasympathetic), sexual function is commonly affected. Normal sexual function depends on multiple physiological mechanisms, including vascular, hormonal, neurologic, and psychological processes, all of which can be altered by medications. Again, there is a gender bias in much of the literature, with few studies evaluating adverse effects on biological female sexual response. The most common adverse side effect is erectile dysfunction (and presumably the female counterpart of inadequate lubrication during sexual intercourse). Some of the more common drug families and their effects are listed in Table 18.6.

| TABLE 18.6 | | |
|---|---|---|
| **DRUG FAMILIES** | | |
| **CARDIOVASCULAR DRUGS** | **PSYCHOTROPIC DRUGS** | **STIMULANTS/ANORECTICS** |
| Antihypertensive agents | Antidepressants | (Weight control, ADD) |
| Sympatholytic | Tricyclic antidepressants | |
| Reserpine, beta-blockers | MAOIs | Anticonvulsants |
| Diuretics | SSRIs | |
| Thiazides | Lithium carbonate | Antiulcer drugs |
| Anticholesterolemic agents | Anti-anxiety agents | |
| (Statins) | Neuroleptics | Anticancer drugs |
| Digoxin | Phenothiazines | Glycemic control |
| Antiarrhythmic drugs | Butyrophenones | Insulin |
| ADD = attention deficit disorder MAOIs = monoamine oxidase inhibitors SSRIs = selective serotonin reuptake inhibitors. | | |

# LGBTQIA2S+ CONSIDERATIONS

There has been an explosion of literature, evolving terminology and acronyms, and advocacy efforts with respect to sexual and reproductive health in the LGBTQIA2S+ community. At the same time, there has also been a significant increase in addressing social, ethnic, and racial disparities, as well as social justice. Most professional training in caring for individuals who are LGBTQIA2S+ or SGM starts with consideration of the evolving terminology. Using the preferred pronouns (e.g., he/him, she/her, they/them) may make an enormous difference to the patient and improve their rapport with that professional.[9]

Discrimination in health care settings against SGM people can also manifest as outright denial of care, disrespect and abuse, low quality of care provision, and/or negative attitudes of health care providers.[38] Transgender health continues to emerge and most medical, nursing, and HCP students are beginning to receive some, albeit often limited, training in sexuality and LGBTQIA2S+ and SGM health issues. It is also important to remember that the SGM community is also diverse, in terms of race, ethnicity, age, socio-economic status (SES), and whether disabled or able-bodied.[39] All are bound together and may cause exposure to stigma, prejudice, and discrimination from living as a minority (or with "multiple minorities"), and all are often subject to health care inequities.[39]

A key focus of Healthy People 2030 (health.gov/healthypeople), which provides national objectives for the U.S. improvement of health and well-being, is on the major Social Determinants of Health (SDoH): (1) *economic stability or socio-economic status (SES)*; (2) *education*; (3) *health and health care*; (4) *neighborhood and physical environment*, (5) *employment*; and (6) *social support networks*. Addressing social determinants of health is important for improving health and reducing health disparities for all people. As part of the effort to address global health issues and inequities in health care, it is imperative to increase the knowledge, competence, and confidence in human sexuality for health care providers in order to address this social determinant of health. Both the World Health Organization (WHO), and Healthy People 2030 have identified the poor health of people who are LGBTQIA2S+ as an area for improvements in health care. Specific hurdles to overcome in providing sexual and reproductive health care in this population are the lack of (1) educational resources, (2) clinical experiences with the LGBTQIA2S+ population, and (3) personal insight into HCPs' conscious or unconscious personal attitudes or biases.[6,40] Healthy People 2030 is focusing on data collection, particularly on LGBTQIA2S+ adolescents. Part of the problem identified was that not all national surveys collect data on sexual orientation and gender identity. Adding these questions to surveys can help to inform health policy strategies for LGBTQIA2S+ populations.

Let's also specifically further consider transgender individuals (those whose gender identity and expression does not correspond with their birth sex). Accounting for 0.5% to 1.2% of the world population, transgender individuals are disproportionately affected by HIV, depression and suicide risk, and anxiety.[41] In fact, gender incongruence (when one's gender identity differs from their sex assigned at birth) is now recognized in the International Classification of Disease Codes (ICD-11) as reframed within the sexual health category (moved from the mental and behavioral health classification).[41] Transgender recognition is becoming more familiar in many countries throughout the world, and has many different names (*muxé* in Mexico, Two-Spirit in the North American Indigenous Coalition, for example).[41] Because gender transition[21] is becoming more common, and because physical therapists are increasingly involved in caring for these individuals, it is important to discuss some basic definitions, medical and surgical interventions, and specific rehabilitation concerns here, with further readings recommended at the end of the chapter. To briefly review and highlight Table 18.1:

- **Social transition**—when a person who identifies as transgender changes their name, adopts alternative pronouns, or alters their dress, hairstyle, make-up, etc. in order to better align with their gender identity.

- **Medical transition**—when a person who identifies as transgender commences gender-affirming medical or surgical interventions.

  ○ Surgical interventions for female-to-male (FTM) transition of individuals who were assigned a female sex at birth may include testosterone therapy, hysterectomy/oophorectomy, and phalloplasty (creation of a neo-penis, often referred to as gender-confirmation surgery).

  ○ Surgical interventions for a male-to-female (MTF) transition of individuals who were assigned a male sex at birth may include facial feminization surgery (including surgical removal of the Adam's apple or tracheal shave, brow lift, lip enhancement), hormonal treatment, breast augmentation, and vaginoplasty.

In a study[21] of 77 patients who underwent vaginoplasties in one medical center, the surgical team included physical therapists, serving as an integral part of the transgender genital surgery programs. This seminal investigation detailed the physical therapists' role with both pre- and post-op pelvic floor physical therapy, with transgender females undergoing vaginoplasty. PTs' pre-op evaluation included voiding and defecation patterns, questions regarding any history of abuse, and internal pelvic floor examination, especially for muscle tone. PTs' post-op interventions focused on assisting the patient with dilation (dilators, or vaginal expanders, are used to gradually enlarge and maintain the vagina open, and to decrease scar tissue build-up) and pelvic floor movements with associated lumbo-pelvic stability. Within the study population 42% presented with pelvic floor dysfunction and 37% presented with bowel dysfunction. At perioperative visits resolution resultant rates were 69% and 73%, respectively; and significantly lower for those participating in pelvic floor PT (28% vs. 86%, P =.006). Those that participated reporting historical abuse presented with a significantly higher rate of pelvic floor dysfunction (91% vs. 31%, P <.001).[21]

PTs provided patient education on methods to decrease hyperactive pelvic floor muscle tone through stretching of the levator ani complex with specific therapeutic exercises. While 89% achieved successful dilation at 3 months postoperative, clearly demonstrating the success of PT with education for the pelvic floor for those undergoing gender-affirming vaginoplasty.[21] Yet, one does not need to be a "pelvic floor specialist" as all physical therapists often do pre-op evaluation and treatment for *all* sorts of patients with pelvic floor movement needs (e.g., orthopedic problems such as joint replacements, spine surgeries, low back pain, overuse injuries, post-op for C-sections, bariatric surgery, pelvic girdle pain, erectile dysfunction, etc.). Again, the pelvic floor moves and therefore physical therapy is often called upon to optimize this movement to improve the human experience, not just for sex! Pre- and post-op pelvic floor physical therapy is associated with improved functional outcomes and quality of life in orthopedic, cardiopulmonary, gynecological, and obstetric surgeries. The use of dilators and training is also done by physical therapists for pelvic pain syndromes and cancer-related therapies that could cause vaginal stenosis. Thus, incorporation of physical therapy in gender-confirmation surgeries is a natural extension of our role as a primary health care provider for all individuals.

Finally, SGM individuals are a small minority in number. People with disability are also a small minority of populations. Hunter[22] addresses people who are both gender minorities and people who are disabled, thereby becoming "multiple minority identification," and subject to even more minority stress. The take-home message in this article is that people identifying as SGM with disabilities want people to know that they exist and are fully capable and desirous of meaningful occupations, with affectionate relationships and social lives.[22] Though the subjects in Hunter's study mostly had developmental disabilities rather than physical disabilities, their adaptations to adversity hold important lessons for all health care providers. Positive elements from HCPs and family members to support this adaptation, termed *Resilience* by the authors, were self-acceptance, advocacy, and social support; negative elements included fragmentation, identity concealment, and punishment. From a multicultural perspective, disability is yet another facet of diversity.

Rehabilitation professionals have an opportunity to engage in social justice work at an individual level during clinical encounters, as well as at organizational and societal levels. Gaps in addressing the health care of transgender and LGBTQIA2S+ populations will diminish if we can continue to work toward eradicating discrimination and prejudice, while improving professional training and education to make health care more inclusive and holistic. If we uphold the fundamental values described in the Universal Declaration of Human Rights[42]—that of protecting the human rights of all individuals—then inequities in health care will diminish, and social justice for all can be realized.

# CONCLUSION

Self-image and self-esteem are major considerations in the sexual rehabilitation of people with disabilities. When one's sense of self is seriously disrupted by the trauma of a SCI or any other disability, it is more important than ever to help the patient re-establish a positive self-concept. Responding to an individual's sexual concerns can go a long way toward re-establishing a feeling of self-worth, which is essential to rehabilitation. Rehabilitation has traditionally emphasized the comprehensive management of the total patient. The basic premise is to help each patient to use all of their strengths and assets to the maximum in forming a new self-image based on positive factors, and to help the patient focus on areas of worth instead of deficiency. It is unfortunate that the patient's sexuality, with its potential as a positive integrating force in building a new image of self and body, has been neglected for so long.

Many HCPs do not volunteer information to the patient because the patient has not asked. Because the subject of sex, sexuality, and sexual health is often viewed with discomfort by the patient *and* the HCP, they are caught in the dilemma of who will initiate the communication. It is easy to ask questions regarding the patient's home, family, number of stairs to climb, etc.; it is not easy to ask questions about the patient's customary sex life. Hence, patients are afraid of asking, and HCPs are not comfortable with asking, or with answering when asked. Yet, it has been shown that increased knowledge about a subject enhances feelings of comfort about the subject matter. Perhaps by providing HCPs with at least minimal information and suggesting where to look for more information, comfort levels in providing this necessary care will improve for patients'/clients' overall well-being and sexual health.

Cole and Cole[43] perhaps said it best as they listed guidelines for HCPs and patients in learning about the sexuality of physical disability:

> *Absence of sensation does not mean absence of feelings … the presence of deformities does not mean absence of the desire … the inability to perform does not mean the inability to enjoy. … Sexual health cannot be separated from total health.*

Thus, education and communication are key components in providing our patients with information regarding sexuality and disability.

The education of developing HCPs for the integration of sexual and reproductive health should include the following:[6] understanding the evolving terminology and acronyms; development of lectures and online modules; identification of barriers to care, such as personal bias (conscious or unconscious); the art of taking a sexual health history using the PLISSIT[18] model; the development of case studies incorporating specific sexual health needs; inclusion of people who are LGBTQIA2S+ as exam patients; and including LGBTQIA2S+ issues in the study of all systems. Incumbent upon HCPs' faculty is to educate professional learners to provide comprehensive and respectful health care to all.[44–46] What is encouraging in the U.S. today is an increased comfort level in HCPs when providing care for patients who are LGBTQIA2S+. Indeed, there are now numerous articles relating comfort levels and obstacles cited for medical, physical, and occupational therapy learners (refer to Suggested Readings at the end of this chapter). As with other fraught issues like abortion, America has become a split screen, with gender-related care banned in an increasing number of states, creating a bewildering landscape for families with transgender children. The intrusion of politics into science makes all of this more difficult.

Millennial (Generation Y, see Chapter 2) learners today are becoming more tolerant of differences in race and gender issues, and more committed to health equity for all.[44,45] This is highly relevant as, by the year 2030, the number of people who are LGBT over 65 years is predicted to be between 2 and 6 million. Millennials profess to feeling somewhat comfortable treating LGBTQ patients, and answering their questions, but admit to feeling less comfortable about raising questions regarding sexuality, if the patient does not ask. They desire more education in their professional formation and seek out further competency through continuing education courses. Furthermore, given the increasing frequency and options in gender-affirming care, including surgical procedures, physical and occupational therapists are increasingly involved in the post-operative phases in muscle re-education, use of dilators, and in the treatment of pelvic pain syndromes.[21,22,44,45]

However, a more recent study[46] of Western (U.S., Canada, U.K., and Australia) society, exploring the lived experiences and outcomes of practicing physical therapists who identify as LGBTQIA+, provided evidence of persistent cis-/hetero-normativity in the profession, along with stress and labor (e.g., energy and efforts to hide elements of one's gender or orientation, time and effort to educate others about diverse roles, emotional exhaustion, and other work necessary to make their work environments safe) experienced due to this normativity.[46] Interview analyses suggested a pervasive normativity relating to sexual orientation and gender identity in physical therapy, frequently intersecting with other factors such as race and ethnicity.[46] Suggestions by the researchers to address these disparities included learning and implementing appropriate terminology, support from professional organizations and associations, showing indicators of inclusivity, and undertaking cultural safety training.[46]

Physical and occupational therapists are in an excellent position to coordinate discussions about sexuality because they are members of the disciplines around which total rehabilitation evolves, especially for the individual with SCI.

Therapists must be comfortable with their own sexuality, however, through adequate knowledge and an accepting, compassionate, and nonjudgmental attitude. In addition, because most previous studies never distinguished between differing sexual orientations, there is extraordinarily little specific information overall for people with disabilities who are not cisgender or heterosexual. Responding to questions without judging is important, and an emphasis on safe sex practices is also vital for all.

Attitudes around sexual expression may communicate a message that encourages adjustment and growth or may accomplish the opposite and inhibit patients from taking positive avenues of action, thus discouraging a desirable outcome. Harmful attitudes can, in effect, add a new disability to the preexisting one for the patient. If a therapist is uncomfortable with a patient's questions, at the very least they should refer the patient to another person on the rehabilitation team who could answer the patient's questions and render the assistance and advice that the patient is seeking. To ignore the subject or downplay it only further hinders the patient, exposes them to a shaming behavior, and closes down any further communication regarding this important component in their self-esteem. All rehabilitation professionals should be comfortable communicating within the first two components of the PLISSIT model and should be knowledgeable about referring to other HCPs if more specific information is requested that is beyond their knowledge, experience, or comfort levels. HCPs should continue to seek professional development through continuing education to address ongoing learning and practice needs.

All rehabilitation professionals are educators with our patients, their partners, and their families, support networks, and caregivers. In this value-laden topic of sex, sexuality, education of the couple/s (the patient and the partner/s) about the disability itself, the prognosis, complications, sexual anatomy, physiology, and function, fertility, pregnancy, contraception, bowel and bladder issues, safer sex, and dispelling of myths should all be done by the collaborative efforts of the rehabilitation team. It matters little who is responsible for which content. It just matters that someone is there to ask the questions, and to truly listen to the patient/client and their needs. The exercises at the end of this chapter will assist you in understanding your knowledge and attitudes in order to facilitate your PPI therapeutic presence in helping patients reconcile unwelcome changes in their ability to be sexual following injury, illness, or surgical intervention or procedure.

# REFERENCES

1. Cole TM. Teaching for professionals in the sexuality of the physically disabled. In: Rosenzweig N, Pearsall FP, eds. *Sex Education for the Health Professional—A Curriculum Guide.* New York, NY: Grune & Stratton; 1978:88.
2. Chipouras S, Cornelius D, Daniels SM, Makas E. *Who Cares? A Handbook on Sex Education and Counseling Services for Disabled People.* Austin, TX: Pro-Ed; 1979.
3. Trieschmann RB. *Spinal Cord Injuries: Psychological, Social and Vocational Rehabilitation,* 2nd ed. New York, NY: Demos; 1988.
4. Rotberg A. An introduction to women, aging, and sexuality. *Phys Occup Ther Geri.* 1987;5(3):3–12.
5. OutRight Action International. *Discrimination at every turn.* https://outrightinternational.org. Updated May 17, 2024. Accessed November 11, 2024.
6. Walker K, Arbour M, Waryold J. Educational strategies to help students provide respectful sexual and reproductive health care for lesbian, gay, bisexual, and transgender persons. *J Midwifery & Women's Health.* 2016;61:737–743.
7. Balik CHA, Bilgin H, Uluman OT, Sukut O, Yilmz S, Buzlu S. A systematic review of the discrimination against sexual and gender minority in health care settings. *Int J Health Services.* 2020;50(1):44–61.
8. Sipski ML, Alexander CJ. *Sexual Function in People with Disability and Chronic Illness: A Health Professional's Guide.* Gaithersburg, MD: Aspen Publications; 1997.
9. Baldwin A, Dodge B, Schick V, Herbenick D, Sanders SA, Shoot R, Fortenberry JD. Health and identity-related interactions between lesbian, bisexual, queer and pansexual women and their healthcare providers. *Culture, Health & Sexuality.* 2017;19(11):1181–1196.
10. McNamara MC, Ng H. Best practices in LGBT care: a guide for primary care physicians. *Cleve Clin J Med.* 2016 Jul;83(7):531–541. doi: 10.3949/ccjm.83a.15148. PMID: 27399866.
11. Hyland A, Mc Grath M. Sexuality, and occupational therapy in Ireland—a case of ambivalence? *Disabil Rehabil.* 2013;35(1):73–80.
12. Lepage C, Auger LP, Rochette A. Sexuality in the context of physical rehabilitation as perceived by occupational therapists. *Disabil Rehabil.* 2021;43(19):2739–2749.
13. Medlar T, Medlar J. Nursing management of sexuality issues. *J Head Trauma Rehabil.* 1990;5(2):46–51.
14. Wilson PS, Dibble SL. Rehabilitation nurses' knowledge and attitudes toward sexuality. *Rehabil Nurs Res.* 1993;2(2):69–74.
15. Gender AR. An overview of the nurse's role in dealing with sexuality. *Sex Disabil.* 1992;10(2):81–89.
16. Ducharme S, Gill KM. Sexual values, training, and professional roles. *J Head Trauma Rehabil.* 1990; 5(2):38–45.
17. Gianotten WL, Bender JL, Post MW, Hoing M. Training in sexology for medical and paramedical professionals: a model for the rehabilitation setting. *Sexual Relationship Ther.* 2006;21(3):303–317.
18. Annon J. The PLISSIT model: a proposed conceptual scheme for the behavioral treatment for sexual problems. *J Sex Educ Ther.* 1976;2:1–15.

19. Esmail S, Esmail, Y, Munro B. Sexuality, and disability: The role of health care professionals in providing options and alternatives for couples. *Sexuality and Disability*. 2001;19:267–282.

20. Woods NF. *Human Sexuality in Health and Illness*. 2nd ed. St. Louis, MO: CV Mosby Co; 1979.

21. Jiang DD, Gallagher S, Burchill L, Berli J, Dugi D. Implementation of a pelvic floor physical therapy program for transgender women undergoing gender-affirming vaginoplasty. *Obstetrics & Gynecology*. 2019;133(5):1003–1011.

22. Hunter T, Dispenza F, Huffstead M, Suttles M, Bradley Z. Queering disability: exploring the resilience of sexual and gender minority persons living with disabilities. *Rehabilitation Counseling Bulletin*. 2020;64(1):31–41.

23. Courtois FJ, Charvier KF, Leriche A, Raymond DP. Sexual function in spinal cord injured men: Assessing sexual capacity. *Paraplegia*. 1993;31(12):771–784.

24. Maslow A. *The Further Reaches of the Mind*. New York, NY: Viking Press; 1971.

25. Anderson TP, Cole TM. Sexual counselling of the physically disabled. *Postgrad Med*. 1975;58:117–123.

26. Klein MJ, Merritt LM, Moberg-Wolff EA, Salcido R, Talavera F. *Sex and Disabil*. Meier RH, ed. New York, NY: Medscape; 2015.

27. Esmail, S., Huang, J., Lee, I. et al. Couples' experiences when men are diagnosed with Multiple Sclerosis in the context of their sexual relationship. *Sex Disabil*. 2010;28:15–27.

28. Ganz PA, Rowland JH, Desmond K, Meyerowitz BE, Wyatt GE. Life after breast cancer: understanding women's health-related quality of life and sexual functioning. *J Clin Oncol*. 1998;16(2):501–514.

29. Rosenbaum M. Sexuality and the physically disabled: the role of the professional. *Acad Med*. 1978;54:501–559.

30. Kennedy P, Lude P, Taylor N. Quality of life, social participation, appraisals, and coping post spinal cord injury: a review of four community samples. *Spinal Cord*. 2006;44:94–105.

31. Anderson KD, Borisoff JF, Johnson RD, Stiens SA, Elliott SL. The impact of spinal cord injury on sexual function: concerns of the general population. *Spinal Cord*. 2007;45(5):328–37.

32. Sipski ML, Alexander CJ, Rosen RC. Physiological parameters associated with psychogenic arousal in women with complete spinal cord injuries. *Arch Phys Med Rehab*. 1995;76:811–818.

33. Elliott S. Sexuality after spinal cord injury. In: Field-Foote E, ed. *Spinal Cord Injury Rehab*. Philadelphia, PA: FA Davis & Co; 2009.

34. Borosoff JF, Elliott SL, Hocaloski S, Birch GE. The development of a sensory substitution system for the sexual rehabilitation of men with chronic spinal cord injury. *J Sex Med*. 2010;7(11):3647–3658.

35. Hellerstein H, Friedman EH. Sexual activity and the post-coronary patient. *Scand J Rehabil Med*. 1970;2(2):109. PMID: 5523820.

36. Drory Y, Shapiro I, Fisman EZ, Pines A. Myocardial ischemia during sexual activity in patients with coronary artery disease. *Am J Cardiol*. 1995;75(4):835–837.

37. DeBusk R, Drory Y, Goldstein I, et al. Management of sexual dysfunction in patients with cardiovascular disease: recommendation of the Princeton Consensus Panel. *Am J Cardio*. 2000;86(2):175–181.

38. Sekoni AO, Gale NK, Manga-Atangana M, Bhadhuri A, Jolly K. The effects of educational curricula and training on LGBT-specific health issues for healthcare students and professional: a mixed-method systematic review. *J Int AIDS Soc*. 2017 20.1.21624.

39. Institute of Medicine (US) Committee on Lesbian, Gay, Bisexual, and Transgender Health Issues and Research Gaps and Opportunities. *The Health of Lesbian, Gay, Bisexual, and Transgender People: Building a Foundation for Better Understanding*. Washington (DC): National Academies Press (US); 2011. PMID: 22013611.

40. Bidell MP, Stepleman LM. An interdisciplinary approach to lesbian, gay, bisexual, and transgender clinical competence, professional training, and ethical care: introduction to the special issue. *J of Homosexuality*. 2017;64(10):1305–1329.

41. Hana T, Butler K, Young LT, Zamora G, Lam JSH. Transgender health in medical education. *Bull World Health Organ*. 2021 Apr 1;99(4):296–303.

42. Office of the High Commissioner for Human Rights. The *Universal Declaration of Human Rights*. United Nations, 1948. https://www.un.org/en/about-us/universal-declaration-of-human-rights. Accessed November 11, 2024.

43. Cole TM, Cole SS. The handicapped and sexual health. In: Comfort A, ed. *Sexual Consequences of Disability*. Philadelphia, PA: George F. Stickley Co; 1978.

44. Dockter M, Parker M, Gebeke L, Scheresky K, Tulintseff A, Truscinski M, Ver Burg K, Abraham K, Reisch R. Comfort level of occupational and physical therapist students in addressing sexual issues with patients. *J Phys Ther Ed*. 2022;36(3):256–262

45. Morton, RC, Ge W, Kerns L, Rasey J. Addressing lesbian, gay, bisexual, transgender, and queer health in physical therapy education, *J Phys Ther Ed*. 2021(35):4:30–14.

46. Ross, MH, Hammond J, Bezner J, Brown D, Wright, A, Chipchase L, Miciak M, Whittaker JL, Setchell J. An exploration of the experiences of physical therapists who identify as LGBTQIA+: Navigating sexual orientation and gender identity in clinical, academic, and professional roles, *Phys Ther*. 2022;102(3):pzab280. doi: 10.1093/ptj/pzab280.

47. Jensen GM. Time to Shine the Light. *Phys Ther*. 2022 Mar 1;102(3):pzab257. doi: 10.1093/ptj/pzab257. PMID: 35230446.

48. Ross MH, Neish C, Setchell J. "It's just as remarkable as being left-handed, isn't it?": exploring normativity through Australian physiotherapists' perspectives of working with LGBTQIA+ patients. *Physiother Theory Pract*. 2023 40(10), 2309–20. doi: 10.1080/09593985.2023.2241079.

49. Bayram E, Weigand AJ, Flatt JD. Perceived discrimination in health care for LGBTQIA+ people living with Parkinson's Disease. *J Gerontol B Psychol Sci Soc Sci*. 2023 Aug 28;78(9):1459–1465. doi: 10.1093/geronb/gbad046. PMID: 36896976; PMCID: PMC10461524.

50. Hofmann MC, Mulligan NF, Stevens K, Bell KA, Condran C, Miller T, Klutz T, Liddell M, Saul C, Jensen G. LGBTQIA+ cultural competence in physical therapist education and practice: a qualitative study from the patients' perspective. *Phys Ther.* 2024 Oct 2;104(10):pzae062. doi: 10.1093/ptj/pzae062. PMID: 38625042.

51. Bishop MD, Morgan-Daniel J, Alappattu MJ. Pain and dysfunction reported after gender-affirming surgery: a scoping review. *Phys Ther.* 2023 Jul 1;103(7):pzad045. doi: 10.1093/ptj/pzad045. PMID: 37471638.

52. Alappattu MJ, Stetten NE, Rivas A, Chim Harvey WM, Bishop Mark D. A Survey of Pain and Musculoskeletal Dysfunction Prevalence After Gender-Confirming Surgery of the Urogenital System. *J Women's & Pelvic Health Phys Ther.* 2024;48(4): 249–256. DOI: 10.1097/JWH.0000000000000316.

# SUGGESTED READINGS

Abramson CE, McBride KE, Konnyu KJ, Elliott SL; SCIRE Research Team. Sexual health outcome measures for individuals with a spinal cord injury: a systematic review. *Spinal Cord.* 2008;46(5):320–324.

Adam A, McDowall J, Aigbodion SJ, Enyuma C, Buchanan S, Vachiat A, Sheahan J, Laher AE. Is the history of erectile dysfunction a reliable risk factor for new onset acute myocardial infarction? A systematic review and meta-analysis. *Curr Urol.* 2020;14:122–129.

Alappattu MJ, Bishop MD. Psychological factors in chronic pelvic pain in women: relevance and application of the fear-avoidance model of pain. *Phys Ther.* 2011;91(10):1542–1550.

Alexander CJ, Sipski ML, Findley TW. Sexual activities, desire, and satisfaction in males pre- and post-spinal cord injury. *Arch Sex Behav.* 1993;22(3):217–228.

Arthur S, Jamieson A, Cross H, Nambiar K, Llewellyn CD. Medical students' awareness of health issues, attitudes, and confidence about caring for lesbian, gay, bisexual, and transgender patients: a cross-sectional survey. *BMC Med Educ.* 2021 Jan 14;21(1):56.

Benevento BT, Sipski ML. Neurogenic bladder, neurogenic bowel, and sexual dysfunction in people with spinal cord injury. *Phys Ther.* 2002;82(6):601–612.

Borisoff JF, Elliott SL, Hocaloski S, Birch GE. The development of a sensory substitution system for the sexual rehabilitation of men with chronic spinal cord injury. *J Sex Med.* 2010;7(11):3647–3658.

Brackett NL, Nash MS, Lynne CM. Male fertility following spinal cord injury: facts and fiction. *Phys Ther.* 1996;76(11):1221–1231.

Burch A. Health care providers' knowledge, attitudes, and self-efficacy for working with patients with spinal cord injury who have diverse sexual orientations. *Phys Ther.* 2008;88(2):191–198.

Carpenter C. The experience of spinal cord injury: the individual's perspective—implications for rehabilitation practice. *Phys Ther.* 1994;74(7):614–628.

Couldrick L. Sexual issues within occupational therapy, part 1: attitudes and practice. *Br J Occupational Ther.* 1998;61:493–496.

Craik RL. Spinal cord injury: the bridge between basic science and clinical practice. *Phys Ther.* 2000;80:671–672.

Derogatis LR, Edelson J, Jordan R, Greenberg S, Portman DJ. Bremelanotide for female sexual dysfunctions: responder analyses from a phase 2B dose-ranging study. *Obstet Gynecol.* 2014;123(suppl 1):26S.

Dockter M, Parker M, Gebeke L, Scheresky K, Tulintseff A, Truscinski M, Ver Burg K, Abraham K, Reisch R. Comfort level of occupational and physical therapist students in addressing sexual issues with patients. *J Phys Ther Ed.* 2022;36(3):256–262.

Ducharme SH, Gill KM. *Sexuality After Spinal Cord Injury: Answers to Your Questions.* Baltimore, MD: Paul H. Brooks Publishing; 1997.

Dumolin, Davis S, Taylor B. From PLISSIT to ExPLISSIT. In: Davis S, ed. *Rehabilitation: The Use of Theories and Models in Practice.* Edinburgh, United Kingdom: Elsevier Health Sciences, Churchill Livingstone; 2006:101–130.

Ferreiro-Velasco ME, Barca-Buyo A, de la Barrera SS, Montoto-Marqués A, Vázquez XM, Rodríguez-Sotillo A. Sexual issues in a sample of women with spinal cord injury. *Spinal Cord.* 2005;43(1):51–55.

Giaquinto S, Buzzelli S, Di Francesco L, et al. Evaluation of sexual changes after stroke. *J Clin Psychiatry.* 2003;64(3):302–307.

Haines, KJ. Engaging families in rehabilitation of people who are critically ill: an underutilized resource, *Phys Ther.* 2018;98(9):737–744.

Hatzimouratidis K, Amar A, Eardley I, et al. Guidelines on male sexual dysfunction: erectile dysfunction and premature ejaculation. *European Urology.* 2010; 57:804–814

Hazeltine FP, Cole SS, Gray DB. *Reproductive Issues for Persons with Physical Disabilities.* Baltimore, MD: Paul H. Brooks Publishing; 1993.

Ide M. Sexuality in persons with limb amputation: a meaningful discussion of re-integration. *Disabil Rehabil.* 2004;26(14–15):939–943.

Jiang DD, Gallagher S, Burchill L, Berli J, Dugi D. Implementation of a pelvic floor physical therapy program for transgender women undergoing gender-affirming vaginoplasty. *Obstetrics & Gynecology.* 2019;133(5): 1003–1011.

Kaufman M, Silverberg C, Odette F. *The Ultimate Guide to Sex and Disability: For All of Us Who Live with Disabilities, Chronic Pain, and Illness.* San Francisco, CA: Cleis Press; 2007.

Kingsberg SA, Woodard T. Female sexual dysfunction: focus on low desire. *Obstetr Gynecol.* 2015;125(2):477–486.

Lavoisier P, Roy P, Dantony E, Watrelot A, Ruggeri J, Dumoulin S. Pelvic-floor muscle rehabilitation in erectile dysfunction and premature ejaculation. *Phys Ther.* 2014;94(12):1731–1743.

Landry AM. Integrating health equity content into health professions education. *AMA J Ethics.* 2021;23(3):229–234.

Masters WH, Johnson V. *Human Sexuality.* Boston, MA: Little Brown & Co; 1966.

Morton, RC, Ge W, Kerns L, Rasey J. Addressing lesbian, gay, bisexual, transgender, and queer health in physical therapy education. *J Phys Ther Educ.* 2021;35(4):307–314.

Nosek MA, Howland CA, Young ME, et al. Wellness models and sexuality among women with physical disabilities. *J Applied Rehabil Couns.* 1994;25:50–58.

Nosek MA, Rintala DH, Young ME, et al. Sexual functioning among women with physical disabilities. *Arch Phys Med Rehabil.* 1996;77(2):107–115.

O'Shea A, Latham JR, McNair R, et al. Experiences of LGBTIQA+ people with disability in healthcare and community services: towards embracing multiple identities. *Int J Environ Res Public Health.* 2020;17(21):8080.

Pynor R, Weerakoon P, Jones MK. A preliminary investigation of physiotherapy students' attitudes towards issues of sexuality in clinical practice. *Physiother.* 2005;91:42–48.

Ross, MH, Hammond J, Bezner J, Brown D, Wright, A, Chipchase L, Miciak M, Whittaker JL, Setchell J. An exploration of the experiences of physical therapists who identify as LGBTQIA+: navigating sexual orientation and gender identity in clinical, academic, and professional roles, *Phys Ther.* 2022;102(3):pzab280. doi: 10.1093/ptj/pzab280.

Sangiori G, Cereda A, Benedetto D, et al. Anatomy, pathophysiology, molecular mechanisms, and clinical management of erectile dysfunction in patients affected by coronary artery disease: a review. *Biomedicines.* 2021;9:432. doi: 10.3390/biomedicines9040432.

Sipski ML, Alexander, CJ. *Sexual Function in People with Disability and Chronic Illness: A Health Professional's Guide.* Gaithersburg, MD: Aspen; 1997.

Tarasoff LA. A call for comprehensive, disability- and LGBTQ-inclusive sexual and reproductive health education. *J Adolesc Health.* 2021 Aug;69(2):185–186.

Weerakoon P, Jones M, Kilburn-Watt E. Allied health professional students' perceived level of comfort in clinical situations that have sexual connotations. *J Allied Health.* 2004;33(3):189–193.

# SUGGESTED VIEWING

*Blue is the Warmest Color* (2013, French): Two young Lesbian women and their passionate relationship, deep love, and heartbreak, hailed as a major work of sexual awakening, with explicit sex scenes.

*Born on the Fourth of July* (1989, Universal): Biography of Ron Kovic, a paralyzed Vietnam veteran who later becomes an anti-war and pro-human rights activist. It follows his travels and struggles adjusting to life post-Vietnam and explores issues of sexuality and disability.

*Boy Meets Girl* (2014, Wolfe Video 2015, Netflix 2016): Depicts the struggles of a 20-something transgender girl dealing with identity and romantic issues and family relationships.

*Brokeback Mountain* (2005, River Road Entertainment): American drama about the complex emotional and sexual relationship between two American male cowboys in the years 1963–1983. This film has been regarded as a turning point for the advancement of *queer cinema* into the mainstream.

*Call Me By Your Name* (2017, SONY Pictures): Coming of age drama set in northern Italy, which chronicles a romantic relationship between 17-year-old Elio, and 24-year-old American graduate student Oliver, who came to work as an assistant to Elio's father, an archeology professor.

*Coming Home* (1978, United Artists; 2004, MGM): Riveting drama about three people whose lives changed dramatically following the Vietnam War. It explores issues of sexuality, relationships, and disability.

*Dallas Buyers Club* (2013, Voltage Pictures): In 1985 Dallas, Texas, Ron is an electrician and rodeo cowboy, and a patient with AIDS (contracted from a prostitute, not a gay partner). It is the mid-1980s when AIDS was not well-understood, and treatments were limited, and mostly experimental. Jake smuggles experimental drugs from Mexico into Texas to treat himself, and then joins forces with Rayon, a drug-addicted, HIV-positive trans woman, to form the Dallas Buyers Club to distribute the drugs to others.

*Endless Abilities* (2013): Follows a group of friends as they travel the country in search of recreational activities designed or adapted for the disabled. The purpose here is clear: to prove that everyone—even those who have been disabled for decades—can find a fulfilling way to remain physically active and in an entirely new community—open your eyes to a brave new world of possibilities.

*Moonlight* (2016, Lionsgate): A young African-American man grapples with identity and sexuality in Miami, through the everyday struggles of his childhood, adolescence, and adulthood with a drug-addicted mother and her pimp.

*Move Me* (2022, Submerged Film, LLC): Kelsey Peterson, a former dancer, faced a life-changing accident at 27 when she dove into Lake Superior and became paralyzed. As she navigates her new reality and redefines herself, Kelsey encounters a chance to dance again and contemplates participating in an innovative clinical trial. This decision challenges her to assess her recovery's potential and her resilience, balancing hope with acceptance of her circumstances.

*Murderball* (2005, MTV Films, Paramount Pictures): US Quadriplegic Rugby Team plays full-contact, fast-paced rugby in specialized wheelchairs, overcoming obstacles to compete in the Paralympic Games in Athens, Greece. It explores the lives of wheelchair-abled athletes and their function. It blows away many stereotypes for those with disabilities and explores issues of bias, prejudice, sex, relationships, and disabilities.

*Superman: The Christopher Reeve Story* (2024, Warner Bros.): Follows Reeves rise to star power as Superman, then tragedy hit with a fatal horse-riding accident (1995) that left him paralyzed from the neck down. He then became an activist for spinal cord injury research, treatments, and disability rights.

*The Waterdance* (1993, The Samuel Goldwyn Company; 2001, Sony): Examines the struggles of dealing with paralysis following a cervical spine fracture from a hiking injury and explores issues of sexuality, relationships, and disability.

*The Way He Looks* (2014, Lacuna Films—Brazil): A coming-of-age romantic drama, about Leo, a blind teenager and his search for independence, his best friend Giovana, and his new friend, Gabriel, with whom he has his first loving relationship.

*Unbeaten* (2009): Like *Murderball*, this film centers on a group of disabled athletes who refuse to yield to their condition. It follows 31 paraplegics across several days as they travel by wheelchair and hand cycle through the world's toughest road race, extending a full 267 miles. Taking on a broad array of individuals' stories, the film provides an extensive look at what happens when dedication and sheer force of will overcomes the supposed limitations of the human body.

*Upside* (2019, Lantern Entertainment, STX Films): A recently paroled ex-convict (Kevin Hart) becomes a caretaker for a paralyzed billionaire (Bryan Cranston), and their unlikely friendship.

*When I Walk* (2013): Although Jason DaSilva's primary progressive multiple sclerosis has led to a debilitating condition, *When I Walk*—co-written and directed by DaSilva himself—tracks his personal relationships as his condition progresses and is a true testament to the strength of the human spirit. DaSilva's story proves how essential a role a strong family unit can be for resilience facing a serious diagnosis.

# SUGGESTED EDUCATIONAL RESOURCES

**Center of Excellence for Transgender Health**
transhealth.ucsf.edu
*Evidence-based care guidelines and protocols for transgender people.*

**Centerlink**
www.lgbtcenters.org
*Local member LGBT centers supporting social justice.*

**Christopher & Dana Reeve Foundation**
www.christopherreeve.org/living-with-paralysis
*Resources and support for living with paralysis.*

**Consortium for Spinal Cord Medicine**
https://pva.org/research-resources/consortium-for-scm/
Sexuality and reproductive health in adults with spinal cord injury: a clinical practice guideline (CPG) for health-care professionals. *J Spinal Cord Med.* 2010;33(3):281–336 *CPG to promote sexual awareness, ethical PPI, and as a resource for expertise and questions.*

**Decreased Sexual Desire Screening Tool for Hypoactive Sexual Desire Disorder**
media.reachmd.com/uploads/related_-_client_provided_materials/dsdsv3.pdf

**Department of Health and Human Services, Office for Civil Rights Sex Discrimination Index**
www.hhs.gov/civil-rights/for-individuals/sex-discrimination/index.html

**Education Network**
www.glsen.org
*Champions LGBTQ rights in K-12, provides community chapter and support information.*

**Facing Disability: Expert Topics**
www.facingdisability.com/expert-topics/what-is-the-first-thing-to-know-about-having-sex-after-a-spinal-cord-injury/diane-m-rowles-ms-np

**Facing Disability: Social Life and Sex After SCI**
https://facingdisability.com/spinal-cord-injury-videos/social-life-and-sex

**Health Equality Index**
www.thetaskforce.org
*A national LGBT benchmarking tool that evaluates health care facilities' policies and practices related to the equity and inclusion of their LGBT patients, visitors, and employees.*

**Human Rights Campaign**
www.hrc.org
*Strives to end discrimination against LGBTQ+ people with achievement of fundamental fairness and equity for all.*

**LGBTQIA+ Health Education Center**

www.lgbtqiahealtheducation.org

*Nationally sourced site of educational programs, resources, and consultation to health care organizations with the goal of optimizing quality, cost-effective health care for LGBTQIA+ people.*

**LGBTQIA Resource Center – LGBTQIA Resource Center Glossary** (ucdavis.edu)

https://lgbtqia.ucdavis.edu/educated/glossary

*Provided by UC Davis as an open, safe, inclusive space and community that is committed to challenging sexism, cissexism/ trans oppression/transmisogyny, heterosexism, monosexism, and allosexism. Includes a fluid glossary of terms supportive of those identifying as LGBTQIA+ including helpful tips, terms, and training.*

**The Miami Project to Cure Paralysis**

www.themiamiproject.org

*A premier research program conducting innovative discoveries, translational and clinical investigations targeting traumatic spinal cord and brain injury, and other neurological disorders. International team with over 175 scientists, researchers, clinicians, and support staff, dedicated to improving the quality of life and, ultimately, finding a cure for paralysis. Testing neuroprotective strategies, cellular therapies using Schwann cell and stem cell transplantation and advanced rehabilitation and neuromodulation approaches including the use of brain machine interface technologies. Other areas of current research include drug discovery for axonal regeneration and immune modulation, neuropathic pain, male fertility and cardiovascular disorders.*

**National Coalition of Anti-Violence Programs**

www.avp.org

*Training, technical assistance, support services and resources on reducing violence and its impact on LGBT and HIV-affected.*

**National LGBT Health Education Center**

www.lgbtqiahealtheducation.org

*Online training on many LGBT health topics, with live and on-demand webinars and learning modules with free continuing medical education and continuing education unit credit, downloadable content, and other resources.*

**Sex After Spinal Cord Injury—Sexual Self Esteem SCIRE Team**

(https://scireproject.com/) scireproject.com/videos-and-toolkits/videos/+Spinal Cord Injury Research Evidence toolkits and videos to support people with SCI, several address sex health.

**Sexual Health for Trans and Nonbinary People—Terrence Higgins Trust**

(www.tht.org.uk) www.tht.org.uk/sexual-health/trans-people

*Provides relevant information for managing risks through safer sex and maintaining good sexual health to feel good about one's sex life for trans and nonbinary people.*

**Sexuality Reborn: An Educational Video for Persons with SCI**

Kessler Foundation, Kessler Institute for Rehabilitation, West Orange, New Jersey, 1993

https://www.kflearn.org/courses/sexuality-reborn

*Funded by the Paralyzed Veterans of America, the physical and emotional effects of SCI are frankly discussed by four couples. These couples demonstrate and share their firsthand experiences concerning self-esteem, dating, bowel and bladder function, sexual response, and varying types of sexual activities. This video is for SCI and other physically disabled individuals. It can be viewed by individuals, their partners, or as part of a sexuality education session in rehabilitation. The video was produced and narrated by Dr. Craig Alexander and Dr. Marca Sipski, with Guest Narrator, Mr. Ben Vereen. This video is 48 minutes in length and is an educational tool. While this film is dated in clothing styles, and only shows cisgender couples, the importance of seeing the role of open, nonjudgmental communication between health care professionals and partners is highly informative. It contains sexually graphic content.*

**Spinal Cord Injury & Brain Injury Resources, Talk to Experts You Trust**

www.spinalcord.com

*Resource for spinal cord and brain injury survivors and their families in navigating medical information, resources, and facilities; a place for survivors to share their stories and get advice from others.*

**Spinal Cord Injury Sexual Health Video Resource Library—Craig Hospital**

https://craighospital.org/resources

*Provides several educational videos for function and movement, including sexual health needs for people with SCI.*

**The Trevor Project | For Young LGBTQ Lives**

www.thetrevorproject.org

*Resources for younger people who may need assistance. Provides resources, networking, and counseling with educational insights addressing the expression of the spectrum of gender and sexual orientations.*

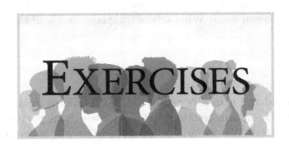

# EXERCISE 1: PATIENT—PRACTITIONER INTERACTIONS—CASE VIGNETTES

Each of the following case vignettes involves an actual patient–practitioner scenario which many of you may encounter in the clinical setting. Divide into groups and discuss how you would manage the following PPIs. Discuss the case study as it is written among yourselves, but first write down how *you* would manage the patient's or other HCP's requests before your discussion.

Use your understanding of the **PLISSIT model** in framing your response. Use your active listening skills and effective communication skills when presented with difficult and emotion-laden questions. Avoid using less-than-helpful responses, such as those mentioned in Chapter 8 (reassurance, judgmental responses, defensiveness), and remember that indifference is the most unhelpful response.

1.  A female who is 37 years old, divorced, with a complete C6-C7 lesion requests assistance from the sex counselor. She wishes to have sex with a male friend but is afraid that, "I won't be able to move my hips and clasp my legs around him." The sex counselor approaches you, the physical or occupational therapist, for specific information on the woman's hip movement capabilities and asks for possible assistance with pillow supports under her pelvis and legs and for some method of helping her hold her ankles together to clasp the male. What are your feelings as the sex counselor asks for this information?

2.  A male who is 49 years old with complete paraplegia and his husband who is 37 years old expressed great concern about involuntary urinary and bowel discharge during sex. The patient is on intermittent catheterization and uses a condom catheter during the daytime. The patient's husband approaches you for suggestions about alternative positions to avoid undue pressure or irritation for both partners. You verified the patient's sexual functioning status with the sex counselor before discussing these questions with the couple. How does this request make you feel? (Remember, feelings are one word, see Figure 1.3, The Feeling Wheel, in Chapter 1.) What information must you have in order to respond to their request?

3. You are a physical therapist, specializing in women's health, working in a major medical center with a large Gender Identity Clinical Service. While taking a medical and sexual history for a trans female patient who is now post-op vaginoplasty, she relates to you that sexual intercourse with her male partner has been painful. What more information do you need? What follow-up questions should you ask?

4. A male who is 21 years old and identifies as bisexual, with quadriplegia turns to you, a female, to express his embarrassment over his constant erections (priapism), which are particularly noticeable while doing mat exercises. How would you feel? What would be an appropriate way to respond to him? Role-play this PPI in your group.

5. A person who is 29 years old and identifies as transgender presents with severe low back pain approaches you with questions about positions for sexual intimacy that would not aggravate their back pain. You know that they have limited flexibility in their low back, either in flexion or extension. How would you feel? What follow-up questions would you ask her?

6. A female who is 18 years old complete T4 paraplegia is planning to go to her high school prom and then wants to spend the night afterward in a hotel with her boyfriend. She asks you, a female, for suggestions for various positions that she could use for sexual intercourse. Before the accident, they were sexually active, and she is unsure what she is able to do now. Also, due to problems with thrombophlebitis, she is no longer able to take birth control pills and asks what other birth control method is possible. How would you feel? What would you respond? If you are a male, how would you tell your female colleagues to respond?

7. A client who is female and 18 years old with spina bifida is engaged in a lighthearted conversation with a male rehabilitation aide about the latest fashions and trends in hair styles while doing exercises in the gym. Discussion focuses on the difference between "sexy" and "sensuous" clothing and the patient turns to you for your opinion. What are you feeling? What would your response be? Does your code of ethics inform you on your course of action?

8. The wife of your patient who is 54 years old with a previous MI asks to speak with you outside the physical therapy gym. Her husband is about to be discharged home, and she is uncertain about resumption of sexual activities due to his heart condition. Before his MI, they engaged in sexual intercourse two to three times per week for most of their 26-year marriage. She is afraid that he might have another heart attack if they resume sex. How would you feel? What questions would you ask her, and what advice would you share?

9. A patient who is female and 57 years with severe rheumatoid arthritis asks you about sexual activity now that her disease has progressed to severe joint immobility and pain. Previously, she and her husband had always favored the missionary position, but that has become impossible due to her lack of hip range of motion. How would you feel? Where would you direct her to go for the information she needs? How would you assist in the movement related concerns?

10. A practicing, orthopedic physical therapist, who is openly lesbian, is coming to you for updates to her long-standing exercise program for non-progressive, chronic multiple sclerosis and asks you if you would come to her for care, if needed, if she decided to become a pelvic floor women's health specialist. She fears that she might be judged as inappropriate with her professional practice and open herself up to potential concerns. How would you feel? How would you respond? What resources might you be able to provide to guide her on this career journey? Are there any updated movement concerns you might need to address as she considers this career change?

11. A patient who is male and 42 years old experiencing Parkinson's disease asks you how to deal with his intermittent pill rolling that frequently occurs when he and his partner are watching sex films and he begins thinking about sex. He finds this disruptive before he is engaged in sexual relations with his partner, as he finds it is embarrassing. How would you feel? How would you respond? What resources might you suggest? How would you assist in the movement related concerns?

12. A patient who is female and 67 years old shares with you the quote from Bernard Shaw that "dancing is a perpendicular expression of a horizontal desire." She has been battling Parkinson's disease and expresses to you that she loves doing line dancing with her partner and while her physical and occupational therapy has helped her to continue being as active as possible, she still has challenges at times with Freezing of Gait, especially in turning motions and then becomes quite self-conscious on the dance floor and uncomfortable for her partner who is line dancing next to her on Friday nights. How would you feel? How would you respond? What resources might you be able to provide? Are there any updated movement concerns you might need to address?

13. A patient who is male and 55 years old displays obvious discomfort as an older female nurse cares for him following complications from a stroke after prostate surgery. As head nurse in the intensive care unit, he requests to speak with you in private. He shares with you that he feels uncomfortable being cared for by an older woman and he feels that his nurse is touching him inappropriately when care for his surgical site. When you question him further, he tearfully tells you he is an adult survivor of sexual abuse. How would you feel? As the administrator of the unit, what are your duties and priorities? What would you say to the patient? What would you do to diminish his discomfort?

14. While working with you on a low mat table in the open gym area of a rehabilitation unit, a A gentleman who is 29 years old, recovering from a traumatic brain injury due to a motorcycle accident places his arm around your shoulder and reaches for your breasts and states he would like to have sex with you. How would you feel? How would you respond? How might his coma levels be impacting his actions?

15. A gentleman who is 45 years old admitted to the hospital for severe low back pain is referred to physical therapy. Following your initial history taking, tests, and measures, he states that he is very attracted to you and would like to go out on a date with you as soon as he can. How would you feel? How would you respond? What guides your course of action?

# EXERCISE 2: RESOURCE REFLECTIONS

Decades ago, the thought of addressing sex and sexuality with patients during rehabilitation would have potentially been considered taboo or controversial and infrequently accomplished by HCPs. Today, HCPs realize the importance and relevance of sexuality in the lives of their patients. Even so, in a survey[44] completed by 128 DPT students from three universities, final year learners were more comfortable addressing sexual issues than first-year, developing learners. Developing learners expressed perceived barriers that included lack of experience, confidence, and knowledge.[44] Your practice with the **PLISSIT model** with the case vignettes in Exercise 1 helps to address your professional formation in addressing sexual issues and continued practice is warranted. Hence, HCPs must self-develop not only to be more comfortable in addressing sex, sexuality, and matters of gender and gender identities with their patients and clients, but also to serve as a resource in three specific areas: (1) educational information, (2) lending the "third ear" (see Chapters 6 and 14), and (3) appropriate interprofessional referral. With this in mind, please select two to three of the Suggested Readings, Suggested Viewings, and/or Suggested Educational Resources provided at the end of this chapter; review and provide your reflections, summarizing your self-learning, and using the guiding questions that follow; and be prepared to share with your peers in roundtable discussions.

Guiding Queries to Journal:

1. How did the additional resources specifically assist you in being more comfortable with aspects of sexuality and disability?

2. How do you feel now that you have completed the additional exploration of the topic for your self-learning? (Recall that feelings are one-word, affective domain descriptors, see Figure 1.3, The Feeling Wheel, in Chapter 1.) How has this resource changed your approach to practice?

3. How did each resource assist you in your HCP role and abilities to do the following:

    a. Provide educational information?

    b. Enhance your skills in your ability to lend the "third ear" (see Chapters 6 and 14)?

    c. Provide appropriate interprofessional referral?

# EXERCISE 3: SHINING A LIGHT ON LGBTQIA2S+ COMMUNITIES

Dr. Gail Jensen, PT, PhD, FAPTA asked us to continue to take time to shine the light on lived experiences for people who are LGBTQIA+.[47] For this exercise, that is precisely what we will do. We ask that you explore the five articles below to gain insight into the lived experiences of people identifying as LGBTQIA+ as health care professionals, patients experiencing chronic diseases, and those receiving physical therapy services, or who are not but may benefit. As you review each article, consider any similarities and differences of the lived experiences and how you personally and professionally have changed as a result of these timely explorations and research. Be prepared to discuss the research findings in class and to reflect on how they have impacted you as a future HCP:

1. Ross, Hammond, Bezner, et al.[46] examine physical therapists who identify as LGBTQIA+ and their experiences. An exploration of the experiences of physical therapists who identify as LGBTQIA+: Navigating sexual orientation and gender identity in clinical, academic, and professional roles. *Phys Ther.* 2022;102(3): pzab280. doi: 10.1093/ptj/pzab280.

2. Ross, Neish, and Setchell[48] provide a qualitative investigation of the perspectives and experiences of physiotherapists working with members of the LGBTQIA+ community in Australia: "It's just as remarkable as being left-handed, isn't it?": exploring normativity through Australian physiotherapists' perspectives of working with LGBTQIA+ patients. *Physiother Theory Pract.* 2023 Jul 31:1–12. doi: 10.1080/09593985.2023.2241079. Epub ahead of print. PMID: 37519133.

3. Bayram, Weigand, and Flatts[49] explore discrimination of LGBTQIA+ people with Parkinson's: Perceived discrimination in health care for LGBTQIA+ people living with Parkinson's Disease. *J Gerontol B Psychol Sci Soc Sci.* 2023 Aug 28;78(9):1459–1465. doi: 10.1093/geronb/gbad046. PMID: 36896976; PMCID: PMC10461524.

4. Hofmann, Mulligan, Stevens, et al.[50] provide a highly insightful qualitative review of LGBTQIA+ people receiving physical therapy services: LGBTQIA+ cultural competence in physical therapist education and practice: a qualitative study from the patients' perspective. *Phys Ther.* 2024 Apr 16:pzae062. doi: 10.1093/ptj/pzae062. Epub ahead of print. PMID: 38625042.

5. Bishop, Morgan-Daniel, and Alappattu[51] discover that pain and urogenital dysfunction often occur after gender-affirming surgery, and the opportunity for physical therapy to have a larger role in the management of pain for this patient population. The high-quality, scoping review noted that vaginal stenosis and incontinence were the most frequent complications and that patients most often managed by physical therapists presented with vaginal stenosis or dyspareunia: Pain and dysfunction reported after gender-affirming surgery: a scoping review. *Phys Ther.* 2023 Jul 1;103(7):pzad045. doi: 10.1093/ptj/pzad045. PMID: 37471638.

6. Alappattu, Stetten, Rivas, Chim, Bishop. A Survey of Pain and Musculoskeletal Dysfunction Prevalence After Gender-Confirming Surgery of the Urogenital System. *J Women's & Pelvic Health Phys Ther.* 2024;48(4):249–256. DOI: 10.1097/JWH.0000000000000316.

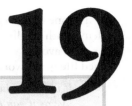

# 19

# ATTUNEMENT

## BIOPSYCHOSOCIAL ELEMENTS OF DEATH AND DYING

*Gina Maria Musolino and Carol M. Davis*

## OBJECTIVES

*The learner should be able to:*

- Describe the importance of death and dying for the maturation of the health care professional (HCP).
- Value the importance of the therapeutic communication skills of touch and active listening with patients, their families, and support networks.
- Explain current values around dying and death.
- Articulate current comfort around dying and death.
- Differentiate the knowledge and skill needed to facilitate a life of quality for the dying patient.
- Compare and contrast palliative care and hospice care.
- Describe the developmental stages HCPs go through as they learn to cope with the anxiety of caring for dying patients.
- Support the importance of a written living will and one's Five Wishes related to aging with dignity.

Helen Hayes is an actress known as the "First Lady of the American Theater." She captivated audiences not only with her talent, but with her grace and charm. Her name was bestowed in 1974 to the Helen Hayes Rehabilitation Hospital (West Haverstraw, NY) in her honor. She graciously served on the hospital Board for 49 years, until her death at 93 years of age from congestive heart failure (CHF). Helen Hayes was instrumental in transforming the hospital into a state-of-the art facility, as well as opening her Pretty Penny home for fundraiser dinners and events. The Helen Hayes Rehabilitation Hospital remains one of the United States' premier physical rehabilitation facilities. Let's consider her reflections related to eternity as we begin this chapter:

*The truth is that there is only one terminal dignity—love. And the story of love is not important—what is important is that one is capable of love. It is perhaps the only glimpse we are permitted of eternity.*

—Helen Hayes

DOI: 10.4324/9781003525554-19

No one likes to contemplate death, except perhaps those for whom living has become entirely too painful. But to deny death totally throughout one's life, to refuse to reflect on the certainty that one day life will end for each one of us, is to avoid a wonderful opportunity for enriching the quality of one's life. You've heard the phrase, "The unexamined life is not worth living." Elisabeth Kübler-Ross[1] wrote:

> It is the denial of death that is partially responsible for people living empty, purposeless lives; for when you live as if you'll live forever, it becomes too easy to postpone the things you know that you must do. You live your life in preparation for tomorrow or in remembrance of yesterday, and meanwhile, each today is lost. In contrast, when you fully understand that each day you awaken could be the last you have, you take the time that day to grow, to become more of who you really are to reach out to other human beings.

In the words of Camus, "There is only one liberty … to come to terms with death. After which, everything is possible."[2] Becker, in his Pulitzer prize-winning book, *The Denial of Death*,[2] wrote, "Of all the things that move men, one of the principal ones is his death. … All historical religions address themselves to this same problem of how to bear the end of life."

This chapter addresses a topic that is most critical to the maturation of health care professionals' (HCPs) professional formation. To grow into one's profession requires both personal and professional growth; confronting aspects of death and dying is part of that life maturation. Some of you who have already lost a loved one will know what it means to say that this experience is unique in its ability to "grow one up" rapidly. In *A Death in the Family*, Agee[3] recounts a tale of fresh grief as experienced by several members of one family following the sudden death of the husband and father in a car accident. Mary, the victim's wife, stands in front of a mirror ready to place the mourning veil over her face as she dresses for the funeral, thinking to herself:

> I am carrying a heavier weight than I could have dreamed it possible for a human being to carry, yet I am living through it. … She thought: this is simply what living is; I never realized before what it is … now I am more nearly a grown member of the human race; bearing children, which has seemed so much, was just so much apprenticeship. She thought that she has never before had a chance to realize the strength that human beings have to endure.

# THE EXISTENTIAL FEAR OF DEATH

Children are not born with a fear of death. At about age 3 years, children begin to deal with object loss and experience fear at the disappearance of a parent and joy at playing peek-a-boo. It is not until age 10 or so that we begin to realize what it means for "life to disappear forever."[2] In fact, if fear of death were held constantly conscious, we would be unable to function normally, so we repress it; and by adulthood, the common thought is, "I know I'll die one day, but I'm having too much fun living to worry about it."[2]

We can ignore our fears of death, or we can carefully absorb them and repress them in what Becker[2] described as our "life-expanding process." With each victory in life comes a feeling of indestructibility, of proven power. Each time we notice the strength of our bodies, recover from the flu, avoid an automobile accident, or narrowly escape an injury—or, more phenomenal yet, escape death—we further prove that we are indestructible. In addition, as we grow into secure and loving relationships with partners, parents, and children, we feel secure support and appreciation for our existence, and a warmly enhanced sense of self acts to further repress the fear of our inevitable death. A healthy self-esteem doesn't have time to ponder death, we believe.

Only when death confronts us in remarkable ways do we even consider our own mortality. Besides near-death experiences, perhaps the deepest assault to our repression of the fear of death as HCPs is to care for a patient or a cherished family member who is close to the moment of death. If we pay close attention, an indescribable glimpse into the soul is possible.

# WHY CONCERN OURSELVES WITH DEATH AND DYING IN HEALTH CARE?

To come to terms with imminent death is one of the most difficult tasks human beings ever have to face, and we face it absolutely alone. No one can take our death away from us or give us the courage to die. However, the role others play at our side during this intense time can be tremendously helpful or cruelly fragmenting and hurtful. The quality of the help we render to those who are dying and their families has everything to do with our own ideas, values, and fears about death, and until we clarify those ideas and values and confront our fears, we will be apt to increase the burden that is already almost too great to bear.

**When death is imminent, we will be governed by what is deep inside of us, and our patients or loved ones will either benefit or suffer.** If our fears of death predominate, we will deny the inevitable or defend fiercely against it. Out of our inner anxiety will emanate denial statements such as, "Oh hogwash! You're healthier than I am! You're going to live forever!" or, "Don't talk like that, silly. It makes me depressed." If our fears get stirred up too much and our denial starts to break, we can expect anger and aggressive and passive-aggressive assaults against those who are suffering.

The more our behavior is governed by our denial and fear of death, the greater the chance that we will add to the already overwhelming burdens of the patient and the family as they struggle with one of life's deepest pains.

As HCPs, we should work hard to never lose touch with our feelings and emotions about all matters of life and death. When needed, we should not hesitate to seek our own counseling and debriefing to work on our own coping strategies and abilities so that we can best serve our patients. Trauma and loss abound in health care, and debriefing from critical incident stressors is vital for effective coping and not becoming numb and insensitive. Follow-up counseling is certainly utilized by the healthiest of HCPs to maintain psychological well-being. It takes courage and strength to cope and not just push the feelings aside or suppress them and later have them resurface inappropriately or at the expense of our patients and others.

Author and dancer Isadora Duncan lost both of her young children in a tragic accident in which a taxicab carrying them both fell into the River Seine and they drowned. After the accident, she fled to her friend, the Italian actress Eleonora Duse, at her villa in Italy. Her friend knew how to help her grieve and did not offer platitudes or sit with her in embarrassed silence, but rather offered her ideas and activities to "take her mind off her worries." She allowed Duncan to feel what had happened to her, to experience her loss. Duncan wrote in *My Life*:[4]

> *The next morning I drove out to see Duse. … She took me in her arms and her wonderful eyes beamed upon me such love and tenderness that I felt just as Dante must have felt when, in "Paradisio," he encounters the Divine Beatrice. From then on I lived at Biareggio, finding courage from the radiance of Eleonora's eyes. She used to rock me in her arms, consoling my pain, but not only consoling me, for she seemed to take my sorrow to her own breast, and I realized that if I had not been able to bear the society of other people, it was because they all played the comedy of trying to cheer me with forgetfulness. Whereas Eleonora said: "Tell me about Deidre and Patrick," and made me repeat to her all their little sayings and ways, and show her their photos, which she kissed and cried over. She never said, "Cease to grieve," but she grieved with me, for the first time since their death, I felt I was not alone.*

As a HCP, you will not be called upon to provide this level of support and caring. Yet the simple question to ask, "tell me about your loved one," provides the opportunity for the person to reflect and grieve. Once people have matured and confronted their innate fears of death, we find that their ability to comfort and support the dying in whatever way is needed in the moment develops into quite profound skill and sensitivity. Block and Billings,[5] physician educators, wrote about teaching a course called "Living with a Life-Threatening Illness" to first-year medical students. Developing physicians visited critically ill patients in their homes and interviewed them, asking them about their lives, focusing on how different patients and families deal with dying, truth telling, decision making, and after-death rituals. When asked how this course helped to prepare students for providing end-of-life care, they reported:

> [The students'] *tendency to avoid the sadness, hopelessness, and helplessness they had associated with a dying person is replaced by a sense of the approachability of the dying, an interest in the medical, psychosocial, and spiritual aspects of "the case," and a belief in the possibility of doing good work through such encounters.*

They learned to value the patient's perspective and to understand that each person's approach to dealing with illness is unique.

When we get beyond our defenses about death, we can then learn how to be therapeutically present for the dying. Life affirmation replaces death denial, and our actions are characterized by an intrinsic belief that life, moment to moment, is good and that we have the power to do something about the quality of a person's life, moment to moment. We realize that, even in the face of inevitable death, the support and comfort of family and mature HCPs can help the patient transform their last days into some of the most rich and meaningful of their entire life.

Confronting our fears of death is not easy, and we reflexively avoid it. But when we face this task with courage, we experience a quality of growth that is unparalleled in our development, personally and professionally. Let's now consider the wisdom of someone who has aptly confronted death and contemplated dying.

> *Betsy Hearne Claffey, PhD has lived her life as a loving daughter, wife, mother, and grandmother; accomplished writer, editor, and PhD; teacher and mentor at the University of Chicago and the University of*

*Illinois in Champaign-Urbana; former runner, ongoing walking enthusiast and yoga practitioner. In a retirement that is far from retiring, Betsy possesses all those wonderful aspects of a life well lived, and more. Now, she has achieved a status using words you don't often see together: Pancreatic—Cancer—Survivor.*[6]

Consider now the expressive address and profound insights provided by Elizabeth "Betsy" Hearne Claffey, PhD. After you have read her impacting treasured words, in *DEAD-LINES: The Term(s) of Retirement*, please pause to reflect in your journals.

# DEAD-LINES: THE TERM(S) OF RETIREMENT

## *Betsy Hearne Claffey*

Academic retirees who have honored multiple requirements, commitments, and deadlines for a lifetime can sometimes lose the ability to practice a sense of free choice, to feel our way through a day. Instead of asking "What do I choose to do now?" we are habituated to asking, "What must get done first, second, third, ad infinitum, before 5 p.m., or worse, before 5 a.m. of whatever day looms?" Whereupon, inevitably, a binding list emerges, the price of previous success. But during the precious period of retirement, habit and success can incarcerate us or at least threaten to turn liberation into obligation. Free choice is, after all, a terrifying prospect. What if we fail the freedom of choice test?! This is not to vilify a sustaining passion for work, but to shift the emphasis from the products of living to the process of living.

I was lucky post-retirement. A year afterwards, I got pancreatic cancer. Even luckier, to a statistically improbable degree, I've survived 15 years since then. We don't all get such a clear warning to cancel everything while we reconsider our intentions for the retirement years. I'd like to use that experience to reflect on some aspects more common to retirees, especially those who have succeeded in academic environments. First, some details before I suggest a proposition.

Cancer took me by surprise, sneaking up despite my prior 66 years of a healthy diet, daily exercise, no smoking, and regular medical checkups. Looking back, I can see some clues: a family history of cancer, a high stress level from decades of intense work deadlines, and a 7-month stomachache that defied testing and did not respond to standard treatments. I insisted there was a problem while my gastroenterologist suspected that I was "getting into a tizzy over nothing." The day after making that remark, he called to apologize for it. In the last test, a tumor had been found in my pancreas. I knew nothing about pancreatic cancer and didn't have time to find out how slim were my chances of survival. I was too busy reorganizing an overload of professional and family commitments. Five days after the diagnosis, I had Whipple surgery that extended to 14 hours.

A Whipple (named after the doctor who developed it) involves removing the distal half of the stomach (antrectomy), the gall bladder and its cystic duct (cholecystectomy), the common bile duct (choledochectomy), the head of the pancreas, duodenum, proximal jejunum, and regional lymph nodes. A vein from my thigh was also taken out and used to re-channel blood flow around a celiac artery blockage. After the surgery I spent two months in the hospital with complications that included pneumonia, heart irregularities, and an antibiotic-resistant MRSA infection. I lost 50 pounds and was too weak for chemotherapy. Pain was intense, digestion treacherous, and recovery slow. I was suddenly diabetic and always cold. My concentration was fragmented by drugs, and the creative energy that had sustained me through many past difficulties had evaporated. Scar tissue began to pull my body out of alignment despite a regimen of walking and massage.

Fragility is hard for someone who has always been strong. For a person who needs to help others, needing help comes as a shock. My regeneration depended on family, friends, a sense of humor, and new priorities. I found guidance in books like David Servan-Schreiber's *Anti-Cancer: A New Way of Life* and determined to revisit yoga, which I had practiced in the early 1970s before getting overtaken by teaching, writing, and parenting.

A year after the Whipple, I began therapeutic yoga to lift the chest and open the abdominal area, both deeply scarred and tightened by adhesions. Yoga, it turns out, is forgiving. In the beginning, I could barely stretch at all, and there were discouraging setbacks after a second surgery to clean out infection around internal stitches that felt like barbed wire. But as my body slowly lifted and opened, so did my mind and spirit. I practiced being in my body patiently and wrote poems tracing the slow journey from wreckage to renewal.

I wouldn't call cancer a blessing, but it has brought me blessings. And here's the happy secret: you don't have to get pancreatic cancer to experience a new lease on post-retirement life. You can pretend. That's what imaginations are for, and we are too often discouraged from using our imaginations. But at this point we can unfold embryonic wings without concern for appearing imaginative, subjective, or—God forbid—creative. Even for a habitually creative spirit, here is an opportunity to explore new possibilities.

Before committing to the excessive number of projects you thought you'd do after retiring—or, conversely—reveling in doing absolutely nothing for as long as you want: Pretend you are leaving the doctor's office with a diagnosis that you don't have much time left to live. Don't limit this exercise to a few minutes or days. Let it take over your mind and meditations for as long as it takes to embody the idea, or rather, the situation. This situation is the real perspective that brings wisdom to perceptive elders. It is the wisdom to select while there is still freedom to exercise that selection. There is only one future deadline, and it could be any day. Each day in unstructured retirement we are privileged to choose how to use it.

Suddenly, values and decisions shift. This can be dramatic. For some, it's scary, threatening, depressing; for others, satisfying, joyful, even miraculous. For everyone, it brings inevitable change. Unlike our deceptive vistas at the youthful beginning of a career, there is absolutely no use in thinking that retirement is going to stretch out with timeless opportunities. Our bodies will see to that. In a recent article about archiving my papers I wrote:

> *Unless the author of the papers has simply boxed, taped, and shipped them off unsorted, archiving involves reviewing the evidence of what s/he's done. This can be physically, mentally, and emotionally intense during a period of aging when energy is increasingly limited and health fragile. Reviewing often means re-experiencing—and grieving for—lost people and lost worlds. By its very nature, becoming archived is becoming past. At some point, a person stops but the world keeps going. Even for those who work to the very end, there is an end. But during transitional stages after retirement, a sense of loss often precedes a realization of how the past can resurface in new directions. Archives suggest a future informed by past knowledge ("Leaving a Trail: Personal Papers and Public Archives," Archivaria, Fall 2018, p.78).*

And now for some past knowledge—2,500 years past. The three most important sources of suffering, according to Buddhist teachings, are greed, aversion, and delusion. And this teaching applies to the feast of retirement years: not to overfill the plate, on one hand; not to waste tasting opportunities, on the other; and finally, not to assume the feast goes on forever.

Following are five of Betsy's poems marking her transitional journey that led her to embody this understanding.

## I OPERATION[6]

*The days after death has pressed me and moved on*
*lie buried deep in a body slit and sewn. Incisions*
*ache with abandoned plans, memories of undimmed*
*energy. Nurses bring mercy with sharp needles.*
*Words no sooner read or spoken roll out of reach.*
*How will I find them, how will I walk the halls,*
*tied with tubes and draped with bags of liquid*
*dripping through my veins? The pain eclipses*
*time but cells still multiply, malignant or benign,*
*as pulsing minutes open, close, open, close, open,*
*close.*

## II EXPIRATIONS

*She had practiced death, it was going pretty well,*
*limbs and will loosening, lungs and veins stilled.*
*Not so bad, she thought, I can do this—relieved*
*at her capability. In the cluttered hospital night*

*a rare quiet grew. Here it comes, she thought.*
*Among beeping machines leaped points of light,*
*faces glowing over them, angels oddly familiar.*
*So it's true about the light, she thought, but music—*
*she didn't know about the music, didn't know*
*that angels sang Happy Birthday when you died.*
*Overhead florescence switched on, nurses bore*
*toward her a chocolate cake celebrating her 66th.*
*Blow them out, they said, blow them out and make a wish.*

*When the day shift came on, they brought another cake*
*yellow with pink icing. Not exactly her wish, given*
*the feeding tube. But hey, we forgot the candles,*
*said the young nurse. Are you kidding, said the old one,*
*with that oxygen, we'd blow the place to kingdom come.*

*She smiled and the rest of her life, never breathed*
*a word about the night shift's secret.*

## III INOPERABLE

*The headlines catch her eye but the stories hardly hold her*
*anymore. It has all happened so many times before.*
*She has happened so many times before.*

*She has transformed the noun remission*
*into a verb and re-missioned herself.*
*It's turtle work, halting and shelled by uncertainty.*

*But without a turtle's weight, she buzzes like flies.*
*Fly, the noun, degrades. Fly, the verb, uplifts.*
*What is the life of the remissioned?*

*And what incarnation awaits the humble fly?*
*A spider dances its art of air and thread.*
*Aren't spiders also caught within their webs?*

*The news does not answer*
*old questions, so she folds it*
*neatly for recycling.*

## IV BONUS[6]

*When your oncologist says that death*
*is a mystery, minutes begin to sing.*

*Whoever is in charge of such things,*
*thanks for giving me a day. The wind*
*blew from the south*
*and I had a good lunch.*
*Either would have been enough.*

## V  ZEN PRIZE[6]

*If it's now,*
*you've won.*
*What you've won*
*is now.*

# QUALITY OF LIFE IS MORE IMPORTANT THAN QUANTITY

Each one of us will die. We're only here for a fleeting time on earth. Over the prior 50 years the life expectancy had increased by up to 10 years.[7] Yet around 2010 the U.S. life expectancy plateaued and then began to decline, especially in midlife.[7] The life expectancy now has declined (falling 2.1 to 6.6 years) in recent years due to Covid-19, drug overdoses, and accidental injury accounting for most reasons, along with heart and liver disease, and suicides.[8]  Many groups (American Indian, Alaska Natives, Hispanic, and Black Americans) experienced larger drops due predominantly to social determinants of health (SDoH) including poverty, food insecurity, living conditions, and access to health care. Globally, the average life expectancy is about 76 to 81 years (73.2 to 79.1 average years in the U.S.),[8] which may seem like forever to us when we are young, but as we approach that age, we will wonder where the years went. Dying is a holistic experience. All of a person is involved—the physical part of us "gives up the ghost," the intellectual often struggles with meaning, the emotional with the deep feelings of the inevitability of this moment, and the spirit is released to continue on in a journey that we can only speculate about.

The lucky ones among us will have time to prepare for death. We believe this preparation time is a cherished gift, not just because it feels good to be able to tie up loose ends, to tell our dear friends how much life with them has meant to us, and to make final arrangements. In most cases, when you know your time is extremely limited and you accept the inevitability of your death, the quality of that time increases exponentially. You become as liberated as a 4-year-old child in your intentions and in your communication. You ask for what you want and you say what you really feel without the concern for whether someone will think ill of you or not like you. This is a tremendously freeing experience. Commonly felt anxieties are replaced with living each moment just as you wish because these are your last moments here on earth, and they are very precious because few of us feel that we really know what lies beyond death. Genuine, heartfelt feelings are expressed. There is no time for superficialities or small talk unless one chooses. Every conversation reflects deeply held thoughts and values. Great wisdom is passed along without fear of being accused of egocentrism. In fact, the predominant feeling becomes, "What is to be feared now?" The ultimate fear has been confronted. The goal becomes how to live well the remaining time, rather than how to avoid death. This acceptance does not happen all at once but takes place in stages over time, as we'll discuss in a moment.

When we, as HCPs, take the opportunity to work with the dying, the quality of our lives can also improve. However, we find it far easier to be present to the dying, who have accepted the inevitability of their imminent death, than to work with patients and families, who refuse to face inevitable death and live each day working furiously to maintain denial or controlling the anxiety of the inevitable. There are few worse situations in life than to try to be present, in a therapeutic way, to a patient or family who is denying imminent death. This situation most often develops out of a mistaken fear that the patient (or family) will lose hope and the patient will give up the will to live. Studies reveal the opposite.[9] Depression and the loss of hope may appear as part of the coping of dealing with dying, but these feelings usually do not last long and are replaced by hope for more realistic things. For example, patients will maintain their hope for a miracle, all the while accepting the inevitability of death. Then, more pragmatically, they will shift their emphasis to, for example, the hope to live long enough to see a child be married or return home to see loved ones or pets.[9]

# STAGES OF LOSS

Elisabeth Kübler-Ross, in her well-known book *On Death and Dying*,[9] described what we can expect to experience as we go through the loss of a loved one or experience our own dying. People initially experience a **denial** at the news of impending or actual death of a loved one. The most extreme forms of denial include total repression of the news or actually losing consciousness. Denial is often followed by **anger**. Once we allow the news to begin to penetrate, intense feelings of anger can be expected to emerge. HCPs must take care not to personalize this anger, but to allow patients to fully experience it and express it. This is made more difficult in a society that does not tolerate emotional outbursts of any kind.

Following anger, the patient often experiences a brief **bargaining** phase in which a kind of deal is cut with life, with fate, or with God. For example, one will hear such thoughts as, "Okay, I know I'm going to die soon, but please let me live long enough to see my children get married." Or, "If I can live, I'll never smoke another cigarette again."

Often the next stage that emerges is **depression**. Patients become quiet and more lethargic, reacting to the undeniability of this news, as they live with it, day after day. They keep to themselves, often refusing to see visitors or speak to certain family members. Reactive depression then leads into a preparatory depression in which patients quietly reflect on the sadness of their fate and prepare for inevitable death.

Finally, patients move into **acceptance** of their fate and begin to live life as a precious gift. Not everyone reaches this stage before dying, and very often these stages do not occur in a linear sequence. It is quite common to hear a patient who seems to have worked through the stages into acceptance say, for example, "Next year I'm going to plant a different garden. I'm tired of the same old flowers. I'm going to rethink the whole layout and do it the way I always wanted to."

Thus, the dynamics of coping with inevitable death take on a certain predictable rhythm and character, **but each person copes in their unique way**.[6–10] It would be wrong to suggest that each and every person follows the same identical linear pattern of coping stages. Likewise, family members go through their own unique stage processes, and it can become quite complex just trying to keep track of where each person is in the process of accepting one person's imminent death. The patient may be in acceptance, but her husband may still be angry. Children may need to deny until the end. It takes great sensitivity and acceptance to be willing to be therapeutically present to each of these people and requires that we choose to believe that each one is doing the absolute best they can, at the moment, to cope. It is not our role to force any realities onto them.

Most important, be careful not to use this knowledge of the various stages as a way of diminishing the importance of certain statements and removing them from the context of their meaning. For example, to say, "Oh, they're just in the anger stage. They'll get over that" as a way to avoid meaningful interaction is not a wise use of this knowledge.

# DEATH, DYING, EXISTENTIAL ALONENESS AND LONELINESS

Working with the dying can become a great challenge, depending on the extent to which we have confronted our own fears and the extent to which the patient and family have accepted the inevitability of the imminent death. What data exist to help us understand our natural responses to this caregiving challenge? How can we be guided to offer a healing response no matter the atmosphere surrounding the patient?

As a result of the Covid-19 pandemic, many experienced a different kind of "dying"; that of the death of the spirit due to the profound aloneness. This then led to the existential loneliness that so many experienced due to the loss of contact and closeness with friends and family, the lack of human touch, and, subsequently, the lack of meaning in a life with a lack of purpose. Joy was sucked out of life. Owing to the vacuum of human interaction, loneliness was experienced in so many unexpected ways. Even when utilizing alternative forms of connection (telephone, Zoom, FaceTime, etc.) it was not the same as first-hand human touch and interactions. We will discuss this more in Chapter 20 when considering transitions. Everyone needs "alone time" to be with their own thoughts and "me" time to stay centered, yet the pandemic put everyone on the sidelines for far too long and it was too much for social human beings who thrive on real, first-hand connections. Even if you could see each other, often it was restricted by windowpanes, two-dimensional technology, and barriers without opportunity for touch due to pandemic restrictions in efforts to protect the vulnerable; or altered touch through barriers. While some tried virtual reality, it still left one wanting for all five senses to be fully engaged in nuances of lived, first-hand experiences.

Both social and emotional aloneness were felt by many and especially the elderly. Children were also unable to socialize and due to two years of intermittent isolation, failed to thrive in social, emotional, and physical development, lagging behind their predecessors. The elderly, a high-risk group, often already displaced and lonely, grew even more isolated and depressed. All experienced a lack of wholeness or completeness due to the loss of normal interactions in everyday life, with a profound sense of unfulfilled hours, lost days, and desperation in many instances.

The many hospitalized patients tried desperately to speak through the valiant efforts provided by overstretched health care providers, who held electronic devices for patients in an attempt to keep them connected. Yet patients were often too fatigued and impaired to meaningfully connect. Personal protective equipment (PPE) was yet another barrier to normal communications. Many shared painstaking parting words in the disjointed way in which the world was turned upside down. Not only that, but family and loved ones were unable to even grieve through normal burial/ funeral services that were often protracted or that never occurred. HCPs were hailed for their bravery yet became disenchanted by the lack of compliance with PPE and other efforts to arrest the spread of Covid-19; predominantly due to the politicization of science and public health efforts, along with the rampant spread of misinformation. Additionally, the media and social media perpetuated the confusion and more provider anxiety with numerous forms of fatigue setting in: compassion fatigue, physical and mental fatigue, Zoom fatigue, question fatigue, constantly changing policies, with a disconnect of values. The frontline HCPs also experienced a loss of interactions with their immediate families and loved ones by isolating themselves, protecting them from potential second-hand exposures, resulting in additional stress, isolation, compassion fatigue, and moral injuries (see Chapters 5 and 9).

Frontline workers not only experienced deaths of their patients daily, but often hourly, and even of their own colleagues, as exponential Covid-19 cases ensued, despite life-saving efforts and sometimes due to lack of proper equipment and resources. Exhaustion, coupled with existential loneliness, was more than many could bear; some quit, or quietly quit, some committed suicide, some became more resilient than believed possible. Many developed new hobbies or made efforts to occupy themselves in other productive, albeit isolated ways, others struggled, became frozen, and/or spiraled downward. Mental health needs soared, and support could not arrive quickly enough. Great moral courage prevailed within many HCPs, families, caregivers, friends, support teams, and suffering patients. Many searched for hope, as we learned to cope with so much death, loneliness, and loss. Unfortunately, because of being bombarded daily by death and dying, there was little time or space to debrief. This is a suitable time to remind ourselves from prior chapter learnings that there are many ways to positively deal with anxiety, e.g., physical exercise, talking it out with a trusted friend, and mindfulness activities, such as breathing exercises, which have been found to be as effective as anxiety drugs.[11]

Today, it is still unknown what the ramifications of long Covid will be, and current research indicates that the more frequently one is infected, the more likely one will experience long Covid, which leads to more likely complications, e.g., heart, lung, or mental health problems.[12] In a large, eloquent study of U.S. Veterans, it was found that Covid-19 reinfection further increases the risk of death, hospitalization, and sequelae in multiple organ systems, in both the acute and post-acute phase. Reducing overall burden of death and disease due to Covid-19 will require strategies for reinfection prevention.[12]

# STAGES OF COPING

Harper[10] has studied the development of HCPs' ability to cope with the anxiety surrounding the death of their patients. Figure 19.1 illustrates the five stages of coping[10] observed in social workers as they dealt with their anxiety about dying patients. The nature and intensity of anxiety of caregivers shifted in a developmentally predictable way from stage I (*intellectualization, characterized by the need to deny and intellectualize death*) to the inevitable stage V (*deep compassion, characterized by the development of the ability to give of oneself and a feeling of comfort in relation to oneself, the patient, the family, and the tasks of caregiving*).

Figure 19.1 can help you anticipate and analyze your responses when you first confront a patient who is dying. We offer it to assure you that your therapeutic skill in caring for the dying will develop and improve and to remind you that caregiving for the ill involves a personal as well as professional growth process. You should not expect yourself to be an expert in this area from the very start. Here is a good example:

In a two-year study, residents in the intensive care units at the University of Washington and University of Utah hospitals participated in "death rounds" once each month.[13] They met regularly to debrief and to respond to three questions following the deaths of patients in their intensive care unit: (1) Did you have any concerns about how care was provided? (2) What could have been done differently? and (3) How did it feel? Residents,[13] found that those who attended death rounds regularly became increasingly more at ease with dealing with dying and death and appreciated the opportunity to discuss their feelings about how they and the staff responded to situations, as they unfolded while caring for dying patients. The residents felt that this experience, over time, helped improve their ability to care for dying patients, and even the more introverted residents were eventually able to express emotions around this experience, which they felt was beneficial in their ability to help others.

**Figure 19.1.** Coping with professional anxiety in terminal illness. (Reprinted with permission from Harper B. *Death: The Coping Mechanism of the Health Professional.* Greenville, SC: Southeastern University Press; 1977.)

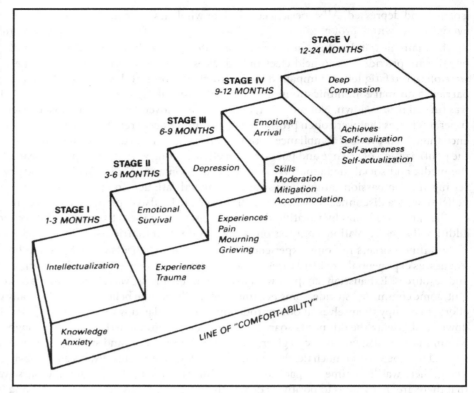

# THERAPEUTIC PRESENCE IN THE ATMOSPHERE OF DENIAL OF IMMINENT DEATH

The atmosphere of death denial is extremely uncomfortable. As mentioned earlier, there seems to be an aura of fear surrounding the patient and family member; a false cheerfulness pervades that is edged with an iciness of the need to control every situation and every conversation. Instead of feelings of liberation, genuineness, and authenticity, we feel surrounded by paranoia, fear, defensiveness, and nervous chatter. Silence is often avoided, as is warm eye contact. Death can be painful, as when we face it with or through another we are acknowledging our own immortalities too—which may be extremely uncomfortable at first.[14–18]

When we contribute to the conspiracy of silence, we condemn a patient to the pain of facing death alone.[14] Our task is not to judge those who need to deny death or to contribute to that conspiracy. Rather, we can help by accepting their fear and by realizing that their need to deny is highly likely well intentioned. Active listening skills are imperative, as is the use of touch.[14]

Whether the patient has accepted the imminence of death or not, our approach to caring remains essentially the same. Debra Flomenhoft,[14] a physical therapist who died of cancer, wrote the following important suggestions after having undergone treatment for over a year:

- Don't be afraid to say the wrong thing, and don't keep silent out of that fear. Silence is often interpreted as avoidance and rejection. Instead of worrying about the content of your response, reach out to the patient and show your support by actively listening and allowing the patient to talk.

- Learn to recognize your feelings and the effect these feelings may have on the communication process. Direct your predictable anger at something other than the patient.

- When patients ask the tough questions (e.g., "Why me?"), don't respond by trying to fix it. Patients aren't looking for answers as much as they are expressing grief and anger. Allow that expression. Supportive listening is the best response.

- Recognize the importance of touch, even as simple as a handshake or a touch on the shoulder. Communicate with touch and eye contact that you care and that you are there to listen and to do whatever you can to maintain or improve the quality of the patient's life.

- Don't assume that patients want to talk about their illness. Ask the patient if they want to talk about their illness before initiating a discussion.

- Never assume that you know what the patient is feeling. Ask instead, "Am I right that you are feeling...?"

- Communicate confidence in your therapeutic skills both verbally and nonverbally. This is essential for patient trust. Answer the patient with authority and no hesitation, and if you don't know the answer, simply say, "I can't answer that, but I will find out who can."

- Don't try to anticipate which stage of coping patients are in, or that they will progress through the stages in exact linear sequence. Accept patients where they are, each day, with caring and understanding. Try to view the impending death from the patient's perspective, not from the "theory" of dealing with loss.

- Take care not to contribute to isolation of the patient as death nears. Once a relationship has been established, work to maintain it, even if the required therapy is minimal or the patient has been discharged from your service. Stopping in to say hello, no matter how busy you are, will mean a great deal.

- Help patients maintain hope at all costs. Maintaining hope is not in direct conflict with being realistic. The value of hope far exceeds the need to face the truth of the inevitable. One can feel hope in spite of imminent death, and it is important to nurture and sustain it, being both realistic and hopeful at the same time. Learn to communicate honestly and frankly, always with hope.

- Take care of your own emotional needs to prevent professional burnout so that you can continue to communicate care, sympathy, and support to the patient and family. If you need help in dealing with your feelings, get it. Your patient can't wait for you to grow at your own pace.

What do dying patients want and deserve to have regarding care? Table 19.1 illustrates the Dying Person's Bill of Rights.[17] Read each item carefully. Each right represents the minimal goals for care by which we all should be guided.

| TABLE 19.1 |
|---|
| ## THE DYING PERSON'S BILL OF RIGHTS |
| ○ I have the right to be treated as a living human being until I die. |
| ○ I have the right to maintain a sense of hopefulness, however changing its focus may be. |
| ○ I have the right to be cared for by those who can maintain a sense of hopefulness, however changing this might be. |
| ○ I have the right to express my feelings and emotions about my approaching death, in my own way. |
| ○ I have the right to participate in decisions concerning my care. |
| ○ I have the right to expect continuing medical and nursing attention even though "cure" goals must be changed to "comfort" goals. |
| ○ I have the right not to die alone. |
| ○ I have the right to be free from pain. |
| ○ I have the right to have my questions answered honestly. |
| ○ I have the right not to be deceived. |
| ○ I have the right to have help from and for my family in accepting my death. |
| ○ I have the right to die in peace and dignity. |
| ○ I have the right to retain my individuality and not be judged for my decisions, which may be contrary to the beliefs of others. |
| ○ I have the right to expect that the sanctity of the human body will be respected after death. |
| ○ I have the right to be cared for by caring, sensitive, knowledgeable people who will attempt to understand my needs and will be able to gain some satisfaction in helping me face my death. |

Adapted from Barbus A. The Dying Person's Bill of Rights. *American J Nursing*. 1975;75(1):99.

# PALLIATIVE CARE

Many patients would like to be able to die at home, but for those for whom that is not possible, palliative care programs are offered in institutions to provide pain control and simple quality of life measures, similar to hospice care. Pain near the end of life often has multiple components: physical, psychological, existential, and spiritual. It is important to differentiate these varied aspects through a thorough evaluation shared with an interprofessional palliative care or hospice team and address improving the patient's physical, social, and emotional well-being.[15,16]

The growth of palliative care programs in hospitals in the U.S. has grown tremendously, with approximately 83% of hospitals with 50 or more beds having a palliative care team.[12] Future palliative care will be expanded to much needed nursing home teams, office practices, and patients' homes.[18] Access and quality of palliative care do vary by available health care staff, resources, geographical location, hospital size; and more nonprofit hospitals have palliative care than for-profit hospitals.[19] Once the family agrees, the specialized care team do all they can to keep patients comfortable, control pain, and allow family to be present. The added layer of support includes skilled communication from all front-line providers. Palliative care is appropriate at any stage of serious illness; services are based on the patient/family needs, and are not prognosis based.[19] Research supports that palliative care improves quality of life, lowers costs, and meets what patients want.[19] Do-not-resuscitate orders are firmly agreed to and hopefully determined in advance of the final stage of life.[18,19]

# HOSPICE CARE

An effective way of helping to ensure therapeutic effectiveness in caring for the dying is hospice. Hospice is not a building but a philosophy of care that promises that the patient will die with any pain controlled to the greatest possible extent and that the quality of life will become the primary focus of all treatment. Hospice is a model for quality, compassionate care for people facing life-limiting illness or injury and involves a team to manage medical care, pain management, and emotional and spiritual support. Interdisciplinary team members each contribute to the care of the patient through direct services, often in the home, and by teaching family members and volunteers how to ensure that the quality of life for the patient remains as high as possible. Pain is controlled while maintaining alertness; yet patients are not allowed to suffer if that is their wish. Death is accepted as inevitable, and family members are encouraged to talk openly with patients in preparation for the time of death. In addition to effective control of pain, it is important for the physical and occupational therapists to teach the patient and family how to keep the lived world of the patient as large as possible, for as long as possible. By lived world, we mean the world that is accessible for the patient to live in. With hospice care, different from palliative care, only symptom relief is provided, rather than longer treatments directed at curing the diagnoses/illness.

Traditionally, our lived world shrinks from almost limitless possibilities (given the funds and opportunities to travel) to confinement to a chair or bed in one room as we age and become unable to move about. Range of motion, ambulation with support, bed mobility, getting up for meals, even placing the bed in the living room in front of a window all help to prevent the lived world of the patient from shrinking to a circle on the ceiling above the bed, as some patients have reported. Family members have utilized technology to project images (in a user-friendly format) of a person's life and family for their recollection, reliving, and reflection. If the patient wishes, the time to celebrate their life is a welcome opportunity to share and for you to learn and appreciate your patient more too. The HCP can help by learning the patient's life story and incorporating it with their care. The quality of life has every bit to do with how much of the world is available for us to experience.

Family members are encouraged to be around the patient as the patient requests. Pets are allowed to be close by for comfort. The atmosphere becomes one of living life fully. Pain control is made possible through finely titrated medications, massage, mindfulness techniques and therapeutic exercise to the patient's tolerance, and the use of transcutaneous electrical stimulation (TENS) to the nervous system. Patients often respond very favorably to TENS, especially in the presence of severe, intractable pain, often accompanying imminent death.[20] The overall goals for treatments in end-of-life care remain focused upon relieving social, psychological, physical, and spiritual suffering to improve the quality of life of the patients.[16]

# DISTINGUISHING PALLIATIVE CARE AND HOSPICE CARE

Both palliative and hospice care focus on providing comfort by addressing symptoms and quality of life. Palliative care, however, also addresses life-extending treatments while with hospice care that is not the focus. With hospice care, one agrees to give up life-extending treatments, as hospice only provides symptom-based comfort care.

Palliative care is also available to anyone, at any age, with a serious illness—you do *not* have to be dying to receive palliative care. Care settings for both palliative and hospice may occur in the home, assisted living, nursing homes, hospitals, and/or specialized, designated settings, e.g., palliative care clinic or hospice facility. Palliative care focuses on maintaining the highest quality of life while managing treatment and other needs. Palliative care can start at any time of diagnosis for advanced or serious illnesses (for example, heart failure, COPD, cancer, dementia, Parkinson's disease, Aids, diabetes). Palliative care emphasizes quality of life to control symptoms, availability of caregivers for the patient and family support, control with respect to medications and medical treatments, collaboration with your medical team, along with communication about our ongoing care with the health care team, family, and most importantly the patient.

Hospice care specifically focuses on the period closest to death. Hospice is also classified as an insurance benefit and may be tied to terminal illness or those with less than a certain number of months that they are expected to live (usually 6 months or less). Palliative care may also be covered by insurance policies, along with Medicaid, Medicare, and the Department of Veterans Affairs, and personal funds are often needed or utilized to supplement care coverage options. Policy coverage varies and is best answered by carriers. Both palliative and hospice care are focused on quality of life and honoring the wishes of patient-centered care. Consider exploring the following websites to learn more:

- Palliative Care

  https://getpalliativecare.org

- The Eldercare Referral Locator

  1–800–877–1116

- Long-Term Care

  https://acl.gov/ltc

- National Institutes of Health, National Institute on Aging

  www.nia.nih.gov/health/end-life

- Health In Aging

  www.healthinaging.org/

- Caregiver Action Network

  (202) 454-3970 | www.caregiveraction.org

- Eldercare Locator (a national directory of community services)

  (800) 677-1116 | www.eldercare.gov

- Family Caregiver Alliance

  (800) 445-8106 | www.caregiver.org

- Medicare Hotline

  (800) 633-4227 | www.medicare.gov

- National Alliance for Caregiving

  (301) 718-8444 | www.caregiving.org

# THE IMPORTANCE OF A LIVING WILL—THE SCHIAVO CASE

Throughout the latter part of 2004 and early 2005, the media in the United States detailed the struggle of Terri Schiavo, a young woman in Florida who had been in an irreversible coma for more than 10 years and was being cared for in a hospice.[21] Her husband wanted to honor her verbal wishes to not have her life extended by extraordinary means under these circumstances, but because Ms. Schiavo never wrote down her wishes in a living will or end-of-life document, her parents contested her husband's decision to remove her feeding tube and allow her to die and took their case to the Florida Supreme Court. The court ruled that her husband had the final authority, not her parents, and ruled in favor of the husband. The parents appealed but lost in court, and Terri Schiavo died peacefully a week after removal of the feeding tube, with her husband at her side.

There were many lessons learned from this case. Primary is the importance of writing down and sharing with close family members your wishes for end-of-life care, as specifically as you can. This is an ethical dilemma between benefi-cence and autonomy. Everyone wanted to do for Terri Schiavo what they felt she wanted, but no written instructions were made to help them. The court ruled that her husband had more recent and intimate knowledge of her wishes than did her parents, but her parents had been caring for her for the better part of the last decade of her life and found great meaning in that process. They held out hope that one day she would wake up and heal from this crisis.

Unfortunately, the main fact that the media failed to mention in many of the debates was that those who believed that Terri Schiavo would wake up one day and be back to her old self didn't know, or chose to ignore for personal reasons, that this was impossible given the magnetic resonance images of her brain. Her ventricles had expanded to the point that the greater percentage of her cranium was filled with fluid; insufficient gray matter existed to support meaningful cognition.

Terri Schiavo went into cardiac arrest because of a metabolic electrolyte imbalance in her early twenties, most likely due to a lifelong struggle with anorexia. When young people are doing their best to be approved of and loved by others, the last thing on their minds would be to create a living will. The fear of death, or the superstition that thinking about one's death will bring it on, must be faced to confront this issue in a mature way. Perhaps Terri Schiavo's gift to others will be to point out the extreme dangers of anorexia and to emphasize the critical importance of creating a living will and communicating to your loved ones your wishes if you should lapse into irreversible coma or brain death. It is important to share your choices for advance directives and to let others know your wishes so that they don't have to make hard choices without your input if you become extremely ill or have a bad accident. Today, as a gift to our own family and friends, we can complete our Five Wishes for aging with dignity, at any age, and voice our choices online, print and sign them, and encourage our patients, clients, family members, and colleagues to do the same (http://www. fivewishes.org/). Expressing your wishes helps reduce unwanted care, assure accessibility of value care, preserving your humanity by personalizing care for your health in the way in which you want to be cared for now and in the future.

# ADDITIONAL CONSIDERATIONS

Several important matters with respect to death and dying are not fully explored in this chapter. The mass and school shootings with resulting injuries and deaths that continue to rise, moral issues of "mercy killing," "medically assisted dying," or euthanasia (active and passive), suicide, the unique perspectives of those who have been brought back to life after technically dying, and the fascination with past lives[22] are a few additional considerations. After one confronts one's own fear of death, it becomes easier to read and study such topics independently. All are critically important to one's development and professional formation as an adaptive HCP.

There exists some controversy around the topic of near-death experiences as researched by Moody[23] and around the person of Elisabeth Kübler-Ross.[24] Any consideration of death must, by necessity, incorporate the spiritual because to ask, "Why have I lived?" is a spiritual question (see Chapter 15). It is within this category of awareness that much criticism was leveled at Kübler-Ross. I would encourage you to read about this controversy and form your own opinions. Once you have experienced the death of one who resides in your innermost circles of self, these readings—indeed, this entire chapter—will likely assume new meaning. For now, deal with this material seriously and as best you can. You may wish to revisit the chapter at a later point in your life journey and as you gain additional experiences with direct patient care.

Victor Frankl,[25] a survivor of two Nazi death camps, said, "Everything can be taken from a person but one thing: The last of the human freedoms—to choose one's attitude in any given set of circumstances, to choose one's own way." To accept death as a necessary part of life is not resignation; it is surrender to an opportunity to grow into one's own complete humanness. We conclude now with the following thoughts from Elisabeth Kübler-Ross:[1]

> *We are living in a time of uncertainty, anxiety, fear, and despair. It is essential that you become aware of the light, power, and strength within each of you, and that you learn to use those inner resources in service of your own and others' growth. The world is in desperate need of human beings whose own level of growth is sufficient to enable them to learn to live and work with others cooperatively and lovingly, to care for others— not for what those others can do for you or for what they think of you, but rather in terms of what you can do for them. If you send forth love to others, you will receive in return the reflection of that love; because of your loving behavior, you will grow, and you will shine a light that will brighten the darkness of the time we live in—whether it is in a sickroom of a dying patient, on the corner of a ghetto street in Harlem, or in your own home. Humankind will survive only through the commitment and involvement of individuals in their own and others' growth and development as human beings. [Through this commitment will come] ... the evolution of the whole species to become all that humankind can and is meant to be. Death is the key to that evolution. For only when we understand the real meaning of death to human existence will we have the courage to become what we are destined to be.*

# CONCLUSION

This text is devoted to helping you, as HCPs, grow to be mature and healing in your very nature, so that your actions with those needing your help will be healing and therapeutically whole. The goals for this chapter are for you to confront your own fears about death at whatever level you can, at this time, in order for you to become more aware of whom you are becoming and whom you are to be. By way of reflection on this content and by completing the exercises, you will conduct a current values clarification about death, recognizing your experiences of death-denying rather than life-affirming ways.

What should our goals be with persons who are facing imminent death? In sum, what we want to achieve with dying patients includes the following:

- Assist the patient to remain in control of most decisions concerning daily life for as long as possible and serve as the advocate for their wishes when called upon.

- Keep the patient's lived world (the world available for the patient to move about) as large as possible for as long as possible by helping the family learn to transfer or assist with ambulation or wheelchair management, assist with transfers out of bed, or move the bed to an appropriate place to avoid isolation, and work to incorporate the patient's life stories in the provision of health care.

- Control pain with medication, activity, imagery, guided imagery, and TENS, yet allow maximum alertness.

- Along with other HCPs, perform professional skills with self-confidence and patience, being sure to include the patient and family in the therapeutic process.

- Provide support for loved ones and family, realizing that each is in various stages of coping with the impending loss of a loved one.

- Utilize active listening skills and touch as our primary forms of communication, allowing the dying person to have control over the topics and length of conversations.

- Avoid the desire to want to fix anything.

- Be willing to stand by, to touch, to reach out, and to risk in the face of our own fears.

- Clarify in writing (see Exercise 2), your wishes at the end of your life.

This is not an easy task. Stanley Kellerman, in *Living Your Dying*,[26] said, "There's big dying and there's little dying." As HCPs, we confront loss of health and mobility as a "little death" rather regularly. In your day-to-day patient care, always remember that people cope with little deaths similarly to big deaths.

Now move on to the exercises, and don't forget to journal about what you're feeling and about what you've learned.

# REFERENCES

1. Kübler-Ross E. *Death—The Final Stage of Growth*. Englewood Cliffs, NJ: Prentice Hall; 1975.
2. Becker E. *The Denial of Death*. New York, NY: Free Press; 1973.
3. Agee J. *A Death in the Family*. New York, NY: Grosset and Dunlap; 1957.
4. Duncan I. *My Life*. New York, NY: Liveright Publishing Corp; 1955.
5. Block SD, Billings JA. Becoming a physician—learning from the dying. *N Engl J Med*. 2005;353:1313–1315.
6. Reproduced here with permission of Betsy Hearne Claffey. Previously published in part: Steinberg B. From surviving to thriving. *Silent Sports Magazine*. 2019;February 1. https://silentsportsmagazine.com/2019/02/21/from-surviving-to-thriving/
7. Woolf SH, Schoomaker H. Life expectancy and mortality rates in the United States, 1959–2017. *JAMA*. 2019;322(20):1996–2016. doi:10.1001/jama.2019.16932.
8. Arias E, Xu J. National Center for Health Statistics. United States life tables, 2020. *National Vital Statistics Reports*. 2022;71(1).
9. Kübler-Ross E. *On Death and Dying*. New York, NY: Macmillan; 1969.
10. Harper B. *Death: The Coping Mechanisms of the Health Professional*. Greenville, SC: Southeastern University Press; 1977.
11. Hoge EA, Bui E, Mete M, Dutton MA, Baker AW, Simon NM. Mindfulness-based stress reduction vs escitalopram for the treatment of adults with anxiety disorders: a randomized clinical trial. *JAMA Psychiatry*. 2023;80(1):13–21.
12. Bowe B, Xie Y, Al-Aly, Z. Acute and postacute sequelae associated with SARS-CoV-2 reinfection. *Nat Med* 28, 2398–2405 (2022). doi: 10.1038/s41591-022-02051-3.
13. Hough CL, Hudson LD, Salud A, Lahey T, Curtis JR. Death rounds: end of life discussions among medical residents in the intensive care unit. *J Crit Care*. 2005;20:20–25.

14. Flomenhoft DA. Understanding and helping people who have cancer. *Phys Ther.* 1984;4:1232–1234.

15. Wilson CM, Briggs R. Physical therapy's role in opioid use and management during palliative and hospice care. *Phys Ther.* 2018 Feb 1;98(2):83–85.

16. Putt K, Faville KA, Lewis D, McAllister K, Pietro M, Radwan A. Role of physical therapy intervention in patients with life-threatening illnesses. *Am J Hosp Palliat Care.* 2017 Mar;34(2):186–196.

17. Barbus A. The Dying Person's Bill of Rights. *Am J Nurs.* 1975;75(1):99.

18. Center to Advance Palliative Care. *Growth of Palliative Care in US Hospitals, 2022 Snapshot.* New York, 2022.

19. America's Care of Serious Illness: A State-by-State Report Card on Access to Palliative Care in Our Nation's Hospitals. *Center to Advance Palliative Care and the National Palliative Care Research Center.* September 2019.

20. Reuss R. Hospice: one PT's personal account. *Clin Manage.* 1985;4(6):28–37.

21. Quill T. Terri Schiavo—a tragedy compounded. *N Engl J Med.* 2005;352:p1630–1634.

22. Weiss BL. *Many Lives, Many Master.* New York, NY: Simon and Schuster; 1990.

23. Moody R. The light beyond. *New Age J.* 1988;May–June:55–67.

24. Nietzke A. The miracle of Kübler-Ross. *Hum Behav.* 1977;206–211, 254.

25. Frankl V. *Man's Search for Meaning.* New York, NY: Washington Square Press; 1963.

26. Kellerman S. *Living Your Dying.* New York, NY: Random House; 1974.

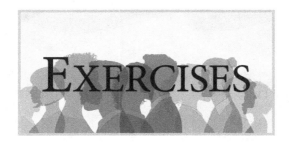

# EXERCISE 1: PERSONAL DEATH HISTORY

Answer the following history questions.

1.  The first death I ever experienced was the death of:

2.  I was _____ years old.

3.  At that time I felt:

4.  I was most curious about:

5.  The things that frightened me most were:

6.  The feelings I have now as I think of that death are:

7.  The first funeral I ever attended was for:

8.  The most intriguing thing about the funeral was:

9.  I was most scared or upset at the funeral by:

10. The first personal acquaintance of my own age who died was:


11. I remember thinking:


12. I lost my first parent when I was:


13. The death of this parent was especially significant because:


14. The most recent death I experienced was when _____ died years _____ ago.


15. The most traumatic death I ever experienced was:


16. At age _____ I personally came closest to death when:


17. The most significant loss I have ever had to endure was:


Because:


What insights come to you as you review your answers or as you discuss your answers with a classmate? What do these answers have to do with your current ideas about death? The next exercise will help you clarify your current ideas.


(Adapted from Worden JW, Proctor W. *Personal Death Awareness*. Englewood Cliffs, NJ: Prentice Hall; 1976.)

# EXERCISE 2: VALUES AROUND DEATH AND DYING

To better clarify your current feelings, attitudes, and beliefs concerning death and dying, please reflect on and respond to the following questions:

1. When I die, I believe that... (What will happen?):




2. I would rather die... (Suddenly and without warning or after being given a period of time in which to say goodbye to loved ones? What beliefs make me say this?):




3. When I die, I'd like the following to be done. (Be as specific as possible. Make a list.):




4. The person I want to be in charge of this process is:

   Because:




5. The worst possible thing that could happen to me around my dying and death is:




6. As a HCP, the best thing I can do for my dying patients and their families is:




   Because:

# EXERCISE 3: HOPE AND HOSPICE

You are working with a John, a 59-year-old White male patient who was referred from hospice to keep his endurance and activity levels as high as possible and to assist with his ability to complete activities of daily living (ADLs). You have come to know the patient as a formerly thriving engineer, and, due to his cancer, he is unable to return to work because of fatigue from radiation therapy. The 1920s building he works in has his office on the second floor. There is no elevator, and the first floor is the machinery production floor. Your patient does not anticipate returning to work and reports he does not have the mental stamina for the job any longer. He enjoys classical music, problem solving, and spending time with his wife of 40 years. John understands that his cancer is terminal and that he has been given a prognosis of 2 to 4 months to live. His goal is to be able to continue to get to the bathroom with assistance of the walker; to maintain, as he states, "his dignity"; to stay as strong and mobile as possible around the home; and to feed himself. He knows he does not have long to live and is realistic in his goals. He appreciates all the help of the hospice care providers. You have also met the patient's overbearing yet well-meaning and loving wife and homemaker, who is working with a lawyer, trying to get the company he worked for to install an elevator. She wants him to be able to walk more so he can return to work and attend church with her on Sundays. Each home visit, you continue to educate the hospice aides and the patient's wife in how they can assist him in his home program activities and the related precautions and contraindications to keep John as safe and comfortable as possible. Some of the aides are not following the home program because they don't see it as their job, and they express this to you. You have also educated the patient's wife and caregivers in the appropriate body mechanics and safe patient-handling skills; you consider aspects of the transtheoretical model of change (see Chapter 16) in your educational approach. You recommend some adaptive equipment to assist in his ADL functions.

In the course of your twice-weekly home visits, John has had varied and fluctuating abilities physically. As his condition and vitals tolerate, John has been able to walk short distances of 50 to 200 feet, endurance dependent, with a rolling walker and minimal to moderate assistance of one person, and he completes generalized strengthening and conditioning exercises to tolerance. Although John is more of a quiet man and deep thinker, he begins to share more of his life story. John shares some of his work accomplishments during rest periods while on your strolls and speaks with warmhearted remembrance of dates with his wife and of their vacation travels. John's wife is planning to have a bed brought in for the downstairs to the living room in the next few weeks just during his chemo time so he does not have to deal with the stairs at home, but she is not happy about the rearrangement because she will miss him at night. John tries to make light of the situation. Using the permission, limited information, specific suggestions, and intensive therapy (PLISSIT) model and some bridge statements (see Chapter 18), you recognize that the couple share loving embraces and massages and pleasure each other with sexual activities but are no longer interested in sexual intercourse. John and his wife are careful not to overfatigue him with these sexual activities. No referral is needed.

As the first few weeks of care commence, on good days John takes short strolls in the driveway to the sidewalk, picks up the mail from the mailbox, and completes 15 to 20 minutes of exercise activity. On bad days, John can barely walk to the bathroom due to the toll of the three-times-weekly chemotherapy sessions and the related side effects. His recovery time following bouts of exercise and ADLs is becoming more prolonged. John has begun occasionally using a bedside commode and urinal when he is particularly fatigued. John has bouts of intense nausea, hair loss, and difficulties with bowel and bladder movements at times; is beginning to present with muscle atrophy; and at times has labored breathing.

In the third week, John is utilizing intravenous-drip morphine and a pain-control pump more regularly to control his pain. In the fourth week of care, he is unable to rise from the bed, so you complete all the care at the bedside. You turn on the patient's classical music to assist in his comfort during the therapy session. As you begin working with him at the bedside on light exercises and assisted range of motion activities while performing your skin integrity assessment, you and the patient hear his wife in the background speaking loudly with a neighbor about how therapy is here working with John to get him outside and walking today. As you assist him with his movements, you note that John is particularly dependent upon you today as the weight of his atrophied limbs becomes heavier in your hands. As you begin to work with John's arms while John is lying supine, he looks up at you despondently and asks, "How much longer are we going to do this?"

1. How does this make you feel? How will you respond?

2.  What additional information would you like to know from the patient? What aspects of culture and spirituality might be relevant (see Chapters 13 and 15)? What losses are John and his wife experiencing? Compare where you think the patient is vs. where the wife is in the stages of acceptance.

3.  What is your role for advocating for the patient's wishes in this case? How might you use your neurolinguistic psychology skills in pacing, leading, and matching and your describe, express, specify, and consequences (DESC) skills (see Chapters 9 and 12) to educate and advocate?

4.  What aspects of the Patient's Bill of Rights apply? Do you need to make any specific referrals?

5.  What should be the primary goals of the interprofessional team at this juncture?

6.  Select one aspect of the case to role-play, with a partner, the specific skill you would like to practice (describe, express, specify, and consequences; neurolinguistic psychology; etc.). Share with your partner the specific skill you are practicing and open your text to the related skill information for reference during the practice session. Verbally role-play and then debrief about your abilities through peer and self-assessment.

# EXERCISE 4: LIFELINE

The line below represents your total lifespan. At the end of the line, mark the year and your age at the point of your death. Indicate the ups and downs of your life by labeling them with words and dates.

_____

1.  Reflections:

    a.  Is your line a straight line, or does it have curves and dips in it?

    b.  How does it feel to consider the total span of your life? Remember, feelings are one word, such as "anxious" or "exciting," not "I feel like my life…"

    c.  How would you characterize your life so far? More up than down, the reverse, or neutral?

    d.  What are the major forces that have contributed to this assessment?

    e.  Did you have difficulty actually marking the date of your death? Some people think this a difficult, if not impossible, task. If you did, why? Why not?

    f.  Do you have certain life goals that you can identify? If so, identify them and comment on how well you feel you are progressing toward them. Indicate what goals you expect to have achieved at certain points along your lifeline.

2.  Journal about this experience and consider this quote by Theodor Seuss Geisel, American Children's Author (1904–1991):

    *Don't cry because it's over, smile because it happened.*

                                                                Dr. Seuss

---

These exercises are also available online at www.routledge.com/9781638220039.

# 20

# TRANSITIONING FROM CLASSROOM TO CLINIC

## GROWTH MINDSETS, INTERGENERATIONAL ENGAGEMENT, TELEHEALTH, AND ARTIFICIAL INTELLIGENCE

*Alecia Helbing Thiele and Gina Maria Musolino*

## OBJECTIVES

*The learner should be able to*:

- Discover growth-mindset approaches to transitioning from classroom-based to clinical education (CE) environments, as adaptive health care professionals (HCPs) on a journey toward expertise in practice.

- Examine the impacts of the HCPs' human body, especially the hands, heart, and head influencing reflective practice.

- Utilizing a growth mind-set, reflectively express one's perceptions of one's continued professional development journey.

- Develop responses to real-world, generative case scenarios applying newly acquired and prior patient–practitioner interaction (PPI) learning capacities.

- Envision potential career pathways as a novice-to-early career professional, including the role of clinical instructor (CI) and benefits of specialization.

- Consider unique aspects of communication within telehealth environments and the use of artificial intelligence (AI) to augment practice.

- Adopt an initiative-taking approach for success in CE.

- Create written CE professional development goals utilizing affective, cognitive, and psychomotor learning domains.

- Explore the gifts of formative and summative feedback to progress your reflective practice as an adaptive learner.

- Appraise the need for interactive, clinical reasoning employing a biopsychosocial, behavioral-change approach for holistic, patient-centered care.

DOI: 10.4324/9781003525554-20

As we embark on this concluding chapter, reflect upon these vital points and their meaning to you, take a moment to place your thoughts in your reflective journal:

> *[T]he secret of the care of the patient is in caring for the patient.*
> *The art of medicine and the science of medicine are not antagonistic but supplementary to each other.*
>
> —Francis Peobody, MD

# AMALGAMATION AND A TIME OF TRANSITIONING

Now it is time to think about your preferred future once again. Just as when you started your PPI journey we asked you to focus on your self first and on your foundations, it is now time to think about your transitions more formally. You will shift from predominantly didactic learning and need to ready yourself to enter real-world clinical practice environments for the first time as a novice HCP, in your defined role with renewed responsibilities. It is much to shoulder, yet you stand on the generosity of those who supported you on this journey and the learning thoughtfully shared and graciously imparted by your clinical and academic faculty, your peers, and your patients within your learning environments. You are deemed ready … ready to continue to challenge assumptions … ready to ask better questions … ready to stay curious … ready to imagine more profoundly … ready to improve movement for life. Ready to discover how to solve problems with people and make a difference in others' lives as servant leaders and advocates for your patients and clients. Oh the opportunities are daunting, exciting, and breathtaking all at once: truly challenging and ultimately rewarding, as you dedicate yourself to changing lives! It takes courage and strength, yet you are prepared! Let's take a moment to once again reflect. Let's revisit and consider the Feeling Wheel again (Chapter 1, Figure 1.3). How are you feeling as you consider what's next? How do you think you will feel after the first week on CE? How about midway through CE? Why? How will you address and manage your feelings?

You are at the stage where you have completed a meaningful, integrated, and highly granular personal-professional journey. Now, you have achieved the distinct honor and privilege to serve in clinical capacities to collaborate with your clinical mentors to serve their patients/clients, families, significant others, and caregivers to help them achieve their patient-centered, health care goals. You have established a strong professional foundation to embark on this next phase of your professional formation. You have dreamed of this day and are excited to provide hands-on health care. Let's not hold back from being who our patients need us to be by embracing the change you are embarking upon. Welcome to the health care profession—we need you—one more ethical and competent person with a greater purpose to assure we meet the needs of society and continue to advance care as change agents and lifelong learners.

- How will you intentionally sustain yourself on this magnificent journey?
- What specific techniques from your learning with this experiential book resonate with you to engage in for staying grounded emotionally, integrated physically, refreshed cognitively, and collaboratively connected?
- How will you persevere in calibrating your own moral compass through these challenges?

You shall be challenged in the alterated environments, physically, cognitively, and emotionally.

Physically, you will be on your feet and utilizing your hands and body to assist others' movement, while moving for multiple hours in the day. You will need to maintain your own personal health to be capable of being strong and flexible to meet the technical demands of being a HCP. You will likely need to stretch your hamstrings more, and assure you keep your core strong, especially in neuro and pediatric settings, as you will need to be both strong and flexible with a balanced core. To ensure your good physical endurance, especially in the acute care setting, you will need to keep up your physical capacities with regular, appropriate, cardiovascular exercise. Through maintaining your core strength with flexibility, you will be doing your best to protect your own spine as you assist others in regaining function. You will self-monitor your own body mechanics in the care for others and give feedback to others for the same. Safety first is key for you, your colleagues, your patients, and their caregivers in order to best assure a long, healthier life.

Cognitively, you will be required to put the pieces of the puzzle together through higher-level clinical reasoning (CR) to determine the best course of action, based on your tests and measures, and the most appropriate plans of care in collaboration with the patient and other HCPs. You will quickly discern that interactive clinical reasoning, keeping your patients' desires, goals, values, and beliefs at the forefront, will assure a step-up in rehab progress and patient motivation. You will need to meet the patient "where they are," considering the many influences of the Social Determinants of Health (Chapters 1 [Figure 1.1], 3, 11, and 13–19) and deploying the Transtheoretical Model of Change (Chapter 16 Table 16.2) with continual monitoring.

Emotionally, you will be challenged daily to maintain your own stress management and to embrace a growth mindset, and one of cultural humility and cultivating hope, while pro-actively counteracting moral injury and averting burnout by doing activities that mend your mind and maintain your brain (proper sleep, nutrition, physical and mental exercise). As a HCP, you must be wise enough to seek your own health care when you are out of balance; and you would not be alone, as 1 in 5 persons in the U.S. experience mental health challenges each year.[1] Self-care remains vitally important for your success as a HCP as, inherently, mental health challenges can have ripple effects for families, your co-workers, and the communities you serve.

Having a growth vs. fixed mindset entails looking at challenges and setbacks as opportunities for growth and embracing vs. avoiding these prospects. A growth mindset[2] ensures that you consider obstacles as opportunities; to persist rather than giving up; knowing that your growth mindset and intentional effort are the pathway to success, rather than a burden. A growth mindset is accomplished by learning and thriving from constructive criticism rather than ignoring useful feedback; supporting others in their journeys too, finding lessons and inspiration in others' success, rather than feeling threatened. With a growth mindset, you shall have more free will and self-determination to achieve all that is possible. According to Dweck,[2] we should seek others who provide and share growth mindsets:

> *The passion for stretching yourself and sticking to it, even (or especially) when it's not going well, is the hallmark of the growth mindset. This is the mindset that allows people to thrive during some of the most challenging times in their lives. The other thing exceptional people seem to have is a special talent for converting life's setbacks into future successes.*

When you began this *PPI* experiential journey, you examined yourself, your personal background, family history, generational differences, values, and beliefs (Chapters 1–3); along with the need to evolve in your affective, cognitive, and psychomotor learning domains (Chapter 3, Appendix) for professional formation. You then opened your hearts and minds to consider whom you are becoming as a health care professional along with the consideration of potential ethical dilemmas you may encounter (Chapter 4). Next, you embarked on considerations of your capacities for self management, assertiveness skills, and conflict resolution (Chapters 5–9) to assure patient-centered approaches to care. You reconsidered matters of justice, equity, diversity, and inclusion (JEDI), along with helping behaviors (Chapters 7–8). With your peers, you courageously embarked on novel case-based assertiveness exercises, working to refine your PPI skills (Chapter 9). You examined the need for authentic peer and self-assessment for Reflective Practice (RP) along your professional formation journey from novice to expert (Chapter 10). You discovered how important it is to manage the stresses associated with turbulence in the work place and the need for daily self-care (Chapters 5, 11). You set personal and professional expectations for yourself and coached others toward professional development. You recognized that the Transtheoretical Model of Change (Chapter 16) provides important insights to patient-centered approaches to care, including the absolute necessity to include the patient's context, with appropriate levels of intervention and education to assist patients to evolve to where they are capable of progressing, keeping *caring* at the forefront.

You began to understand the relevance of rapport with patients, and being leaders in health care and through advocacy for your patients and the profession (Chapter 5, 11). You valued that together everyone achieves more and how to communicate with cultural sensitivity, humility, and compassion (Chapters 11–13). You learned to value the need for in-depth patient/client interviews, and that the process never really stops, yet continues with each visit and the need for true collaboration with your patient in their contexts for successful evidence-based practice and excellence in outcomes (Chapter 14).

You then ascertained the significance of spirituality in health care (Chapter 15). You gained abilities in appropriate patient/client education, incorporating a variety of learning domains and teaching and learning styles; along with methods to promote healthier behaviors, considering elements of health literacy and transformative health care models with applied theories (Chapter 16). You discovered principles and practices for more effective communication with and for all persons with disabilities (Chapter 17). You discovered more about sex, sexuality, and sexual health and how HCPs can best communicate with persons and their significant others with specific chronic diseases and conditions (Chapters 16–18). Finally, you bravely considered the biopsychosocial aspects of death and dying, your own lifespan, and how HCPs provide communication, support, and ethical care in palliative and hospice settings (Chapter 19).

Now, preparation meets presence …

All along the way you have continued to practice application exercises and case vignettes, to reinforce your learning, amalgamating your new learning for continued professional development. You persisted to synthesize your affective learning domain with your cognitive and psychomotor domains and development through reflective journals; verbalizing and sharing your deep thoughts and feelings in discussion and through narrative, written application exercises followed by enriching discussions with your peers and faculty. You have changed because of your efforts; accordingly, preparation meets presence …

Now let's take a look at the environment you are transitioning to for your full-time CE experiences and offer some insights for your continued acculturation, professional readiness, and further professional formation as an adaptive learner, exercising a growth mindset.

# THE HUMAN BODY: FOUNDATION FOR THE FUTURE

Our human bodies remain a fascinating and amazing amalgamation of DNA. Human bodies provide the ever-important framework for our everyday movements, navigating us safely through the world with much gratitude to our strong, yet importantly flexible muscles (always in motion especially cardiac), bones (the femur being the longest), and skin (15% of body weight).[3] Our bodies exhibit control through our experiences, understanding, and responsiveness to our surroundings through our brains, nervous systems, and hormones. Our hands alone consist of 27 bones[3] that work in concert for activities of daily living. Our hands are truly a pair of instruments we deploy with artistic and fluid interaction with our patients' human bodies to facilitate movement. Nevertheless, the human body is fragile. We have come to know that working persons are four times more likely to stop work due to disability than from dying.[4] However, loss of the use of one's hands entails great grief—and a sense of death—for those who rely on them for their livelihood.[4] This leads to the need for great effort to focus on what one still has and to appreciate what one can still do, instead of focusing on loss.[4]

With our organic body of interweaving movement systems, we autonomically fuel, cleanse, and protect our cells while pumping blood (traveling 12,000 miles in a day) to our vital organs.[3] This only happens through care and feeding of our bodies. We know that not only do we have a lifespan, but a life cycle that evolves from a single cell to birth through death. We now know that the human genome is predominantly identical throughout the world, yet we each have unique finger and tongue prints![3]

We realize how things can go wrong, with cellular adaptations that lead to cancers, and inflammatory processes that lead to degenerative diseases, such as arthritis. We recognize that healing webs are produced through various stages and phases for body tissues with many histological changes. We realize the importance of those 12 pairs of cranial nerves[3] working in amazing synchronicity from the brain and head to influence the body. We also have come to count on that "tough mother" or dura matter[3] to protect our brains. We realize that the brain, despite its enormous capacities, does not have the ability to safely multitask in some situations (e.g., distracted driving). The more one can focus on just one stream of information, the faster the result. We recognize that neurotransmitters, such as endorphins and oxytocin, influence our physical and emotional drive.[3] Yet, we also realize that many chronic diseases (e.g., Parkinsons', depression, schizophrenia, Alzheimer's) with hereditary components, and often negatively impacted by particulate matter in the environment, have disruptions of important neurotransmitters (e.g., L-dopa). We have come to appreciate even our fragile, tiny hair cells that register vibrations in the ear to allow us to perceive sound and how the "rocks" or otoliths[3] impact our balance capacities. Our eyes have over 125 million photoreceptors[3] that allow us to sense light—our senses are powerful instruments that not only provide vision but may also significantly influence balance and movement. We truly appreciate the quietly working endocrine system that impressively regulates our various glands and realize that, when not working well, diseases, such as diabetes, may ensue.

The most important muscle, our heart, contracts and relaxes well over 100,000 times a day and when one is angry or in a state of fear, the heart rate can escalate by approximately 30–40 more beats per minute;[3] just one more reason to manage anger and why de-escalation is so very important for ourselves and our patients. At rest we breathe about 8 to 16 times[3] a minute, providing much-needed oxygen and gas exchange for vital organs, like the lungs and brain cells. We have come to appreciate that to keep healthy, one must keep moving! Even sustained postures on an airline trip or long car ride, without a stretch break or exercise, can lead to unfortunate cases of deep vein thrombosis due to blood pooling in the lower legs and thighs from not moving.

We all recognize that in a normal lifespan, aging is inevitable, yet how it happens to each individual manifests in different ways. Regular exercise, appropriate sleep, stress-reducing activities, and a healthy diet with appropriate hydration, make the process go much better. While new data have demonstrated cutting calories might slow aging, questions remain.[5] While the mysteries of aging continue to be explored, our bodies fight declining metabolism and sensation, and the aging impacts on bones (decreased density) and muscles (decreasing muscle mass), and on the cardiovascular (thicker and stiffer valves and walls), digestive, integumentary (thinner), and immune systems.

The wisdom of Nelson Mandela comes to mind. He once said, "Our human compassion binds us to one another—not in pity or patronizingly, but as human beings who have learnt how to turn our common suffering into hope for the future." Hope is not only about the distant future, however. Hope is also about every day, as we address current challenges in changing lives for enriching health capacities, the quality of lives, and access to care for those with disabilities, chronic and acute conditions/diseases, and aging. It is our hope that, through your *PPI* learning and this chapter, you will transition successfully, while overcoming the probable and oft predictable setbacks along the way. It is our hope that you will approach change with grace, compassion, humility, love, and a renewed sense of optimism for your preferred future and that of your patients/clients whom you serve, to bring about both individual and societal change. Hope goes hand-in-hand with vision—your ability to think or plan for your preferred future with both wisdom and imagination. Let's consider the possibilities. How will you move forward? So once again, we ask:

- Who are *you* becoming?
- Where do you see your future going?
- It's in your head, hands, and hearts.

You utilize every one of your senses and human body capacities to perceive[6] as an adaptive learning professional, always striving for your continued professional formation to best serve your patients/clients, maintaining a growth mindset.[2]

For example, in terms of PPI, you utilize your:

**Eyes:** To see the consequences of your choices and intake information to help you to think about how you can be most ethical, to see nuances in movement, and visually appraise your patient's even before you interact with them.

**Mouth:** To share and communicate your ideas creatively and with confidence and to collaborate with patients and others.

**Heart:** Filled with courage to take risks when approaching novel experiences and learning with the belief that these help you to grow as a HCP and sustain physical and emotional wellness.

**Arms:** To show compassion and care to others with hugs and pats on the back and shoulders and to skillfully apply interventions and support your physical wellness.

**Hands:** To serve others by helping wherever there is a need; and to skillfully assess and re-assess with tests and measures and apply interventions through both strength and flexibility. For writing in your learning journal—where you record your thoughts about your learning and experiences with reflection on your strengths and needs, along with progress made to become a more reflective practitioner, moving from novice to expertise; for documenting your patients' progress and communicating with the health care team;

**Muscles:** With both voluntary and involuntary movements. To breathe, to propel yourself with strength, speed, and force. To provide stability and grace; along with meaninful movement for your patients.

**Feet:** To keep your balance with commitments and responsibilities and ensure your physical wellness.

**Spine:** To help you stand up tall for justice and fairness by being principled, showing respect for yourself and others, being honest, and taking responsibility for your actions.

**Ears:** To help hear about the beliefs, values, and perspectives of others with an open mind, then compare these with your own ideas and grow from the experiences.

**Brain:** To help you to thoughtfully and mindfully make inquiries, stay curious, formulating sound and relevant questions and researching for answers about your own ideas and utilizing evidence-based resources and prior knowledge and skills to support your understanding and applications for best practice and sustaining intellectual wellness.[6]

Excellent care entails intuiton, using your instinctive feelings, and building upon your personal and professional experiences. Caring entails offering comfort to those you care for. According to Merriam-Webster's dictionary, comfort is derived from late Latin, *confortō*, "to strengthen greatly"—Latin *con* meaning "with" and *fortis* meaning "strong." Comfort offers behaviors and mindsets to that which pains us, to face adversity, together, with strength and bravery. HCPs instictively utilize the heart in caring, which continually enlightens the head and intuitively leads the hands.

Now take a moment to respond and journal with respect to these queries considering your preferred future. Be prepared to discuss with your peers and/or trusted advisors. So, once more, we ask:

- Who are you becoming?
- Where do you see your career as a HCP going forward in the first year?
- And as an early career professional in years 2–5 of your career?
- What advice do you have for your future self?

Once again, your preferred future is in your hearts and hands. No one else will care for it like you will—and we must care for ourselves before we can care for others. No one else will steer the wheel of your career down the many potential pathways you may traverse. In just one short year of practice, you are viable to begin mentoring other full-time HCP learners, like yourself, today.

# PROFESSIONAL PATHWAYS: PREPPING FOR FUTURE POTENTIALS

## *Super Powers: Collaborative Clinical Instructors (CIs)*

Believe it or not, once you have that first year of practice, you have gained enough experience to begin to teach others "how-to" be a HCP and share your words of wisdom to guide others with hands-on care. You will be entrusted to serve, as others have served for you in CE. Before you do, however, we highly recommend that you first consider learning more about being a clinical instructor or fieldwork supervisor. Check with your professional organizations to determine if this career development, continuing education offering is available. Many offer similar programs, yet the American Physical Therapy Association, Credentialed Clinical Instructor Program (APTA CCIP)[7] is also open to all HCPs at Level 1. The APTA CCIP Level 1[7] course is designed to provide continuing education skills for CE instruction through six modules (*Clinician as Clinical Educator, Readiness to Learn, Facilitating Learning in the Clinical Environment, Evaluating Performance and Providing Feedback, Compliance and Regulatory Issues in CE*, and *Facilitating Success in CE*), along with an Assessment Center, addressing the following overall course objectives:[7]

- Plan and prepare for students during their CE experiences
- Support continuing education through questioning and effective feedback
- Provide for effective performance evaluation skills
- Identify and manage learning needs and areas of compentence
- Recognize legal and supervisory implications for CE, including issues related to the Americans with Disabilities Act, Medicare regulations, and the Patient's Bill of Rights

At this point you might wonder why you would want to serve as a clinical instructor or find the idea intimidating, with so little experience. Trust yourself that, with adequate preparation, your limited year of experience with numerous patients equates to being capable of serving in this capacity. It is not about quantity; quality matters. You may recall our earlier discussions on "expertise in practice" and it is not about the years of experience but more about the quality of those lived practice experiences with your patients' lived experiences, as a new HCP. Keep in mind, CE students have never had any first-hand, full-time experiences in their new and changed role. In fact, having students in CE has multiple benefits, including the opportunity to gain new knowledge, how to serve in the new capacity as an educator for a HCP, erudition of teaching and learning styles, refinement of practice skills, enhanced cognizance of ethical and legal issues, heightened awareness of communication needs, and improvement of CE instructional methods.[8] As a result of the APTA CCIP Level 1[7] course, participants gained increased knowledge, confidence, and effectiveness to serve as CIs, improved their assessment abilities, both for themselves and for their students, learned how to structure learning within the clinical environment, were better equipped to facilitate or guide learning through both summative and formative assessment, enhanced their goal-setting capacities, and improved their CE problem-solving skills. Utlimately 99.3% of newly credentialed CIs stated that they had gained what they had hoped to learn and would also recommend the APTA CCIP to their colleagues.[8] In fact, HCP CE students first and foremost care about their CI's **communication** and **interpersonal skills**, rather than their professional and teaching skills[9]—the golden rule prevails—they don't care how much you know, until they know that you care about them as a **person first**! The same holds true for your patients, as you have gleaned from PPI. Our hope for you is that you include becoming an APTA Credentialed Clinical Instructor[7] on your professional development journey, not only to be a CI, but also to ameliorate patient education capacities too and enhance your expertise.

As a new HCP student in CE, don't expect to be capable of everything your CI demonstrates and a full caseload! That is not realistic. In terms of a full caseload, understand what is expected of a new, entry-level graduate—that is the high bar. As first introduced in Chapter 3 (Appendix), you should be prepared to gradually ramp up your higher-level (applying, analyzing, evaluating, creating, adapting, and valuing) abilities in all three learning domains (affective, cognitive, and psychomotor) in the CE environments. You have never been the HCP you are becoming, and you can only gain experience by doing so in CE; progressing from novice-beginner to, eventually, entry-level, consulting with your CI, as your guide on the side. Review carefully the anchor definitions for your summative evaluation instrument (e.g., APTA Clinical Performance Instrument (CPI), or other) and start at the beginning—it is not a sprint, it is a marathon of lifelong learning. Recall that caseload is only part of the picture, as are efficiency and effectiveness of practice performance. The amount of supervision and guidance, the consistency of your performance with the patients, as well as the complexity of the patient presentation all combine to determine your current level of performance. (See APTA Learning Center, Student APTA CPI training.)

In CE, you must first be open to being exposed to new learning, patients, environments, and techniques; then, willing to acquire new abilities as an adaptive learner, with a growth mindset; and finally, over time, to integrate your capacities with those of your patients. Do not try to jump ahead of yourself, you cannot "fake it to make it." Your CI will see through that type of approach quickly enough. Your CI is your guide on the side and will ensure that you and your patients stay safe. Listen to your CI carefully and respectfully; judiciously and promptly respond to the gifts of feedback you are given. Be proactive by utilizing the Weekly Planning Form (WPF) for your focused learning goals each week (see Figure 20.1). Remember to set goals in all three domains of learning (see Exercise 6 at the end of this chapter) and utlize the Professional Behaviors Assessment Tool (see Appendix to this chapter) as a starting point for fast-formative, written feedback.

Seek informal, daily, formative feedback using a 2-minute approach. Ask your CI daily two things you are doing well and two things you need to work on; taking a quick 2 minutes to discuss. Then provide the same feedback to your CI in two ways in which they may better assist you in your CE professional development, expressing gratitude for two ways they are helping you. Remember that patient care comes first, and the patient is the center of the CE experience—not you.

Using the formal, formative Weekly Planning Form (Figure 20.1) allows you to solidify your plans for progression and seek consultations on ways to improve. Planning allows your CI time and opportunity to provide the resources and patients you need to achieve the goals. Remember, as time progresses, go where it is hardest first, as you will benefit from your CI input, and your CI will not always be there to guide you!

If you falter, don't let this set you back. Remember, all feedback is a gift, both in areas to strengthen your abilities and in constructive critique to improve your capabilities. Even if the feedback is critical, this is vital, as without this insight and information you will be hard pressed to be successful and meet the expectations of your CE experiences. In most cases, once identified you will make a plan with your CI and progress along steadily. Do not be the one who denies that there is indeed a problem. This will only hold you back in your progress and learning. The licensed professional serving as your CI has every capacity to provide feedback on the professional expectations for the work of the job that they are doing. If you need assistance, be sure to consult with your Fieldwork Supervisor or Director of CE or whomever provides oversight from the academic program for your CE experiences. They can assist you in navigating any challenges you may be experiencing.

Student learners in CE often believe that, when conflict occurs in CE, it is due to a personality conflict; this is not an appropriate pursuit, as just as with our patients, we all will encounter others with differing personalities (as well as differing teaching and learning styles) and we must learn to adapt and find ways to get along in teams and through adult interactions (review Chapter 9 on assertive communication techniques if you are struggling). You definitely should consult with your Director of CE, Fieldwork supervisor, and/or faculty overseeing your CE, for *any* assistance with this process. Proactive guidance and consultation can save much time and effort later. Seek counseling and student support services too, as this is an excellent path to maintaining your mental well-being as you face adversity with renewed strength. Remember these tips too for peers who may reach out seeking guidance—a little help goes a long way!

On rare occassions, a student may receive critical feedback and, in spite of every effort and resource to try to improve, may still not meet the expectations. Again, this is an opportunity to reset and readjust, and your academic institution may provide an opportunity for an individualized, customized plan for improvement to re-prepare you academically to once again attempt to perform to the expecations in CE. Not all students translate from didactic to CE easily or readily in all settings. There may be some environments that you find much more challenging, for a variety of reasons. Some common examples include a gap in what you cognitively were able to retain and apply over time; an inablity to synthesize information and thoughts while performing psychomotor care skills; or a high-stress clinical environment that challenges your affective coping abilities and negatively impacts your patient–practitioner interaction skills with your patients and/or colleauges. Furthermore, there are instances when CE learners may be challenged in ways that learning or psychological disabilities require accommodations. Take time to disclose your challenges in not just the classroom, but for CE experiences too, and seek appropriate accommodations up-front, to set-up and plan for success, addressing and removing any barriers, or potential barriers, that may be reasonably accommodated wherever and whenever possible. Afterall, if rehabilitation professionals cannot provide accommodations, with or without the use of accommodations or assistive technologies, who else can? Do not let your pride or feared perceptions stand in the way of you being set up for CE success. Discuss the potentials with your CE faculty and support systems. Sometimes, life happens too, and you may be dealing with circumstances that prevent you from being fully dedicated to your patients and CE. You may need to pause to deal with emotional distress related to life circumstances, e.g., the death or declining health of a family member, divorce, personal health needs, etc. Seek counseling and support services to approach life challenges in the best way possible and avoid negatively impacting those whom you are trying to assist in their health challenges. Everyone grieves or copes in different manners, and one must take the time to address any physical or mental health challenges. Again, consult with your clinical and academic faculty to keep them informed as to your circumstances and it may be appropriate, at times, to consider leaves of absence and return with a renewed capacity. These are individual and programmatic decisions and require attention and full considerations in light of the demands of practice. Please address these needs proactively—it is your responsibility to do so for yourself and an ethical obligation for your patients and clients.

*University of Southern California*
**Physical Therapy – Student Weekly Feedback Form**

Student Name: ▮▮▮▮                                    Week: ▮ /▮ (i.e. 1/16)

Facility: ▮▮▮▮

Clinical Instructor Name: ▮▮▮▮

| Student Self-Assessment Guiding Questions | Responses—When answering, consider 3-4 APTA CPI performance criteria per week |
|---|---|
| **Performance Reflection** Which CPI performance criteria do you feel you performed the best? Which needed most improvement? Why? Were any of these Red Flag items? | ▮▮▮▮ |
| **Caseload Reflection** | What is considered a full caseload for a new grad? (Patients per day or patients per hour) ▮▮▮▮  How many patients were you primarily responsible for treating and/or developing plan of care this week? (pts per day or pts per hour) ▮▮▮▮  How much guidance or input from your CI did you need for the patients you were primarily responsible for this week? ▮▮▮▮ |
| **Next Week's Goals** Write 2-3 goals related to CPI performance criteria targeted for next week. | Goals from previous week: ☐ Met   ☐ In progress   ☐ Not Met  Goals for next week: ▮▮▮▮ |
| **Plan for Improvement** What patient experiences and learning activities will help you accomplish your goals for next week? | ▮▮▮▮ |
| **Communication with CI** What were your positive experiences from this week? Were there any challenging experiences from this week? How could your CI best support you next week? | Supervision Rating: ☐ too little   ☐ adequate   ☐ too much  Comments: ▮▮▮▮ |

Student please mark if any of the following is/are true:

☐ I would not change anything        ☐ I am overwhelmed            ☐ I can take on more challenge
☐ I am unclear about expectations    ☐ I am worried I am not on track

**STUDENT Signature:** ▮▮▮▮                                    Date: ▮▮▮▮

**CI TO COMPLETE**: Student **is** ☐ or **is not** ☐ progressing as expected for this experience.
* If student IS NOT progressing as expected, please contact either the SCCE (facility) or the DCE (University)

Comments for the week—Please note at least one area of student success and one area where the student can continue to grow: ▮▮▮▮

**CI Signature:** ▮▮▮▮ _____                        Date: ▮▮▮▮

**Figure 20.1** Weekly Planning Form used with permission of USC DPT Program, Michael Simpson, PT, DPT, Board-certified Cardiovascular & Pulmonary Clinical Specialist.

Clinical environments remain places of authentic pluralism that require you to interact with your patients, families, caregivers, professionals, and the public with cultural humility, being open and oriented to others' identities, which are often different from your own. We must authentically listen with the "ear of our heart." CE environments also require continuous and pronounced physical effort that you may not yet be accustomed to and for sustained periods. CE environments require you to also be mindful in your interactions with others, by assuring that you are including your patients. Your mind must be open to the possibilities and have space for imaginative thought. It must be capable of producing creative, engaging treatment plans that address the patient's multiple concerns in the context of their lived experiences. Just as with you, your patients' physical well-being impacts their mental health too. You and your CI have a moral imperative to ensure you are providing the best possible care, by including the context of the patient with correspondingly appropriate clinical practice guidelines (CPGs), utilizing the best evidence (EBP), while keeping the patient's values, beliefs, and collaborative goals at the forefront. If not, it remains likely that your patient will not achieve their full rehab potential!

It is no small feat transitioning from classroom to clinic. Yet you've got this—and you are most surely ready—as this is what you have prepared, practiced, and applied yourself to do and you know your learning journey is truly just beginning, all over again. Have faith in yourself, so others will too. Measured confidence with compassion is key. Utilize your professional library to revisit and speak to you once again in the context of patient care and the patient's mileau. Use the voice of reason supplied by your professional learning to discern what is useful, useless, and harmful. Deploy your research strategies to provide the best informed EBP possible, every day. Do not fear disagreement amongst resources, researchers, and/or CIs. Use this as the basis for robust discussion to dialogue about these differences and to determine the best course/s of action. The right care, at the right time, is ever changing as new technologies and evidence emerge. Keeping your patients' wants, needs, desires, and capacities first and foremost ensures you are on the right track, in consultation with your CI and the patient! Be enriched by their collective experiences and avoid unsafe or less than adequate approaches. This can also prove to be an unlimited pursuit too, ostensibly the precise course of patient care or movement diagnosis/es may not reveal itself readily; reel it in when it comes time to act and provide care, as the patients need you here and now. Each treatment is a test of your hypothesis, problem-solving, and clinical reasoning abilities and will guide you in your next steps, along with the patient's presentation and movement system responses (or not).

Let us not forget the need to practice reflection along the way. We are called upon to become Reflective Practitioner's (RPs),[10] continually *reflecting in, on and for action*, while *recognizing surprise* (see Chapter 10). Be intentional with reflection verbally with your CI, with self-talk while you are exercising, with a trusted peer, and/or in written reflective journals. No matter the method, the mindfulness is what matters; to glean all that you can from your professional CE and patient-centered interactions, to assure you are providing the best course of action for health care as possible, and to facilitate your own journey toward expertise. As you likely recall, even experienced physiotherapists engage in lifelong RP.[10,11] According to Dalley-Hewer, Clouder, and Jones,[12] the RP activities engaged in by experienced physiotherapists, when reflecting, mirror Musolino's[13] findings that (student) DPT learners engaged in reflection and self-assessment during lunch activities, while showering, exercising, and walking down the hall. Often physical places are used to create "reflective thinking, head spaces" to "see" things differently (e.g., walking a wooded forest, hiking or skiing a mountain, cycling a new path, swimming pools, art museums, or listening to classical music) providing environments for creative thinking (or through virtual realities),[11-13] often performing novel tasks will free your neurons to expand processing too. You may have experienced this when you study, that sometimes your favorite study space no longer works for you and you need a different space to keep things fresh and focused or have a different view.[13] Our abilities to be supported in RP are influenced by the environments, others, and those supporting or detracting from the capacities to be reflective.[10-14] You will find good colleagues supportive in your quest for enhanced RP. Many seasoned therapists value their dialogical reflection with colleagues; nevertheless, a balance between dialogue and solitude remains key to facilitate reflection.[12] RP is also key to keeping the "care" in health care. In fact, through a hermeneutic phenomenological investigation,[14] physiotherapists' perceptions of what constitutes a responsive physiotherapist highlighted key practices that may underpin Tronto's Ethic of Care Theory: (1) *oriented to care*, (2) *integrating knowledge sources*, (3) *competent*, (4) *responsive*, (5) *reflective*, (6) *communicative*, and (7) *reasoning*. Further in-depth analysis resulted in six themes of being "responsive" to patients, demonstrating a moral responsibility to care: *Being person-centered, attentive, open, a listener, validating, and positive.*[14] Hence, there exists a fluid balance between technical competence and the relational dimensions of practice that responsive practitioners best meet our patients'/clients' needs. HCPs are empathic and make time to fully address the concerns of the patient, in a reciprocal manner, while making themselves accessible and noting the unique life circumstances, including the Social Determinants of Health (SDoH), that impact health care needs.[12-18]

Let's take a moment to reflect on these important concepts before talking a bit about process matters to set you up for success in CE. Consider how you will assure these moral imperatives and demonstrate an ethic of care with your patient/client interactions. How will you assure that you are a "responsive" practitioner?

## Top Tips for CE Success

Remember, little things mean a lot. So, show up on time, or early, then on the rare occasion you are unexpectedly late, all will be forgiven. You will also notice a calm, and clearer mind, when beginning your day instead of needing to rush. Make your best effort to get to know your CI as a person first, and in advance, with a quick breakfast bagel meeting, or Zoom call. Ask for their CV or resumé when you provide your resumé, discuss hobbies and interests, share your learning styles and realistic goals for the CE experience. Ask for an orientation. Understand what constitutes a "full caseload" for a new graduate for each particular CE setting, as it is different for different setting types. Plan for and schedule with your CI time for your midterm and final debriefing, in advance. Know where to park beforehand, and how the commute time is going to work out, if applicable. Know and comply precisely with the dress code; when in doubt, ask. Wear your name badge/s and introduce yourself as the HCP student—as your patients have the right to know. Yet also share that you are working hand-in-hand with your CI, hence two are better than one! Be proud of your background and experience to date, yet seek new opportunities daily.

Getting to know your patients can be as easy as asking four things: What's their favorite music, food, pet's names, hobbies? Think of patients as people first! Once rapport is established, then the therapeutic relationship proceeds and you may delve deeper into what patients value, believe, and want to accomplish as a result of the health care they are seeking. Demonstrative of an ethic of care, this is also a good opportunity to remind ourselves of the need for informed consent, both written and verbal. HCPs openly communicate with their patients, disclosing any risks and benefits related to treatment, as both a legal and an ethical obligation. HCPs are compelled to accurately present information and with sensitivity, keeping with the patient's preferences for receiving information, and collaborating with respect to the plan of care, incorporating the patient's values and beliefs.

Attaining ongoing verbal consent as we proceed with tests, measures, and ongoing interventions is good practice. Most facilities have related policies and procedures that you should make yourself aware during your orientation. If this is not offered, be sure to inquire.

While in the care settings, if patients are present—be with the patients. Do not ask to leave early or miss days without offering to make them up. Your CI has set up this time for you—respect it and be mindful of their time too. Allow your patients to offer you feedback on your peformance—they will tell you almost everything you need to know—if you just inquire. Generally, patients welcome the opportunity to work with students, and give copious insights, yet it remains their right to decline. Brush it off and move on—many more opportunities will present. Also, when it comes time to exit the facility to return to your didactic education and/or move on to your next clinical experience or first professional position, be certain you have made hand-off procedures clear with your patient and CE instructors, to avoid any perception of patient abandonment. Be certain that your CI is aware of your gratitude for sharing their patients and their experience with you.

Take in all the feedback you receive and provide a service back to your CE site of something you think they might benefit from based on your contemporary education. They may require you to do an educational inservice on a patient of their chosing or a topic of your own or their selection—then offer to do something additional that you have noticed the CE site might benefit from learning more about (e.g., information related to area community support agencies for frequent patient populations, new technologies, etc.) or engage in a quality improvement project. Review your formative assessment along the way with your CI, yet do not shy away from occassionally visiting the summative assessment critiera for the midterm and final (APTA CPI, etc.). It is always good to seek further insights along the way to assure you are on the right track in your self-assessment too. Afterall, you have *never* been in this specific role before and are not yet consciously competent of what the expectations are in this particular setting. This will hold true for each new setting you go to for your progressive CE experiences. You are starting fresh each time, yet building from a different starting point. With each CE experience, the context will change, the CI will change, the types of patients and acuity levels will alter, and you too will be changing as a developing HCP in CE, evolving to entry-level.

If and when you experience setbacks, reframe them and avoid rigid thinking. Leverage these setbacks for future growth. Consider your own self-assessment in a clinical context and debrief with your CI. Consider these growth mindset queries:

> *How could I have done this differently? What did I learn about what works? What did I learn about what doesn't work? What do I need to pay more attention to in the future? What can I do to better prepare for*

*next time? Have I remembered to consider the Social Determinants of Health for your patients? Have I incorporated the patient's and family's goals? What cognitive tendencies or emotional/situational factors have influenced my clinical reasoning processes? What test and measures and/or interventions have I deferred as they are less important or likely? Has bias gotten in the way of your clincial reasoning,[15] e.g., anchoring bias—being too impacted by first impressions; ascertainment bias—being too impacted by ageism and other stereotypes; premature closure—relying too soon on an initial physical therapy movement diagnosis without considering alternatives; unpacking principle—failing to collect all necessary data through test and measures and/or exploring the patient history adequately, with probing queries, missing significant possibilities, etc.?*

Let your CI guide you, whilst being pro-active and optimistic in the process. Consider that you are a welcome "learning worker" and have the privilege of serving your CI's patients under their direct supervision and guidance. Your CI wants to guide you and facilitate your success! Tap into your growth mindset, take initiatives, and exercise your resilience—bouncing back from challenges and failures. Be self-compasssionate along the way, employing your mindfulness techniques (Chapter 14). When in doubt, ask questions. When seeeking more information, look things up first, whenever possible, then discuss with your CI. Utilize true evidence-based, peer-reviewed Internet resources, not just a web-based search (e.g., PubMed, Cochrane reviews, PeDro, Shirley Ryan Ability Lab Resources, APTA CPGs, Tests and Measures, etc.). Use the power of the Internet and prioritize people through person-centered care[16-18] and communication for transformative impacts for movement systems. As you develop and implement your collaborative plans of care, always be checking in with your patients, with a people-first approach, asking: *What can I do to support you better? What has been challenging for you lately? Is there anything we can do differently or keep doing to help you achieve your goals?* To reiterate, your patients will often tell you everything you need to know, if you just ask! Demonstrating this culture of interactive caring and clinical reasoning makes a difference in ensuring an ongoing, human-centric approach to care and in ensuring you and your patients/clients reach your maximum potentials. Be prepared to dedicate a minimum of 8–12 hours weekly, outside of your regularly scheduled CE time to prepare for your patient-centered health care. Complete all your CE assignments in a timely fashion and be prepared to handle an appropriate caseload. Utilize your CI and CE support team at the clinical and academic institution to support you along the way by communicating early and often. When in doubt, reach out via email, text, or phone—don't delay. This will help to assure you that you are on the right track. Have fun, be joyful and creative with your therapeutic activities using innovation and multiple methods to achieve therapeutic goals (avoid stagnation!).

*Now let's stop again for a moment and journal about two things you will change for your prefered CE future as a result of this newly acquired learning. Be prepared to discuss with a trusted peer and/or advisor.*

## *Power for Practice: Clinical Specialization*

Pathways to continue to improve your clinical excellence do not end with the entry-level degree. As a lifelong learner and reflective practitioner (RP; see Chapter 10), you will also embark on continuing education **focusing on your own professional development** and learning needs, and with respect to the types and kinds of patients you are working with now or in your planned future, to incorporate an emerging practice area or to take your basic skills to a higher level of practice. Oftentimes, HCPs continue with post-professional certifications (e.g., Lee Silverman Voice Treatment (LSVT) BIG and LOUD: Behavioral Treatment Programs for Speech and Body Movement for Persons with Parkinson's Disease; Parkinson's Wellness Recovery (PWR); Advanced Vestibular Physical Therapist (AVPT) Certification; Vestibular Rehabilitation: A Competency-Based Course; Certified Exercise Experts for Aging Adults (CEEAA); APTA Credentialed Clinical Instructor Program, Level 2–3 Courses; Orthopedic Manual Therapy; Pelvic Health Certification; Dry Needling Certification), while others may elect to formally seek additional advanced degrees due to job demands or practice and research interests (e.g., MBA, MPH, Health Informatics, Genetics, PhD in Rehabilitation Sciences) or to pursue a higher education, terminal academic degree to teach in academic programs and become a full member of the academy (PhD, EdD). Many elect post-professional residencies with a goal toward specialization or not, many elect to pursue board certifications, and some even dual or triple board certifications. Check with your professional organization to determine what opportunities are provided and how that program maintains its standards and accreditation processes to ascertain the value and potential impacts. Confer with HCPs at your CE sites and your faculty that maintain many of these credentials and explore how the advanced professional development has benefited their patients and practice.

For example, the American Board of Physical Therapy Residency and Fellowship Education (ABPTRFE) accredits the American Board of Physical Therapy Specializations (ABPTS). The specialization process is a formal voluntary one, unrestricted and coordinated by ABTS. Clinical specialization requires: (a) a broad-based foundation of physical therapist education and clinical practice; (b) depth and breadth of knowledge in a specialty area; and (c) advanced clinical expertise and skills. According to ABPTRFE and ABPTS, the purpose of Board Certification is threefold, to: (1) recognize specialists through established testing methods to ensure a defensible process, and a reliable and valid examination; (2) promote the highest possible level of physical therapist care, and ongoing development of the science and art underlying each specialty practice; and (3) inform stakeholders of physical therapists who are certified in a specialty area. To learn more about what it takes to become a specialist and the specialty certification and maintaining specialization, eligibility, costs, examinations, clinical hours required, explore via https://specialization.apta.org/become-a-specialist as well as related residency and fellowship opportunities, explore via https://abptrfe.apta.org/. Many HCPs seek support for these opportunities with their employer, and often experience prioritization for certain employment opportunities because of their interest in pursuing specialization and/or because they are a specialist, resident, and/or Fellowship trained. Fellowships are available in several practice areas, as well as for Education. Fellowships have considerable depth of training, educational programming, and intensive mentorship. Specialists, residents, and fellows are often called upon by colleagues for their specialized areas of practice, provision of continuing education, mentoring, and/or peer consultation related to their specialty focus for problem-solving complex cases.

## Humanitarians

Health care professionals also maintain a pro bono obligation to serve society, which is often accomplished through volunteerism. The selfless act of volunteering is a kindness you extend that continually returns to you many times over what you put into the voluntary efforts. One in four Americans volunteers—approximately 80 million people—with nearly a third of adult Americans volunteering at least once over the course of a year. According to the U.S. Bureau of Statistics,[19] the estimated value of volunteer time is $28.54 per hour with nearly $200 billion in value for communities across the U.S. Unfortunately, due to the Covid-19 pandemic at least 11% of volunteer organizations in the U.S. ceased to operate and 65% had to reduce operations and resources; in a time of even greater need! This trend has been reversing as pandemic restrictions have lifted. Additionally, this is a good thing for health too, as volunteering can improve health:[19]

- Volunteers are healthier than non-volunteers who are 5 years younger
- Volunteers live longer than non-volunteers
- Volunteers with heart problems had reduced chest pain and lower cholesterol levels than non-volunteers
- Volunteers experience less stress, recover from illness quicker, and sleep better than non-volunteers
- Volunteering can improve mood, and volunteers, on average, have more friends and more social interactions than non-volunteers

We all have this capability for empathy and to "pay it forward" and should now be adequately inspired to engage as volunteers in some capacity. We are stronger and healthier as a result and clearly have impacting differences for society through coordinated volunteer efforts. Whether it be serving as a grass-roots advocate, volunteering as a coach, serving the underserved through the Salvation Army services, sharing your expertise with a developing professional or chronic disease support group, or being part of a global interprofessional health services organization, there remains a multitude of ways to serve.

## INTERSECTING GENERATIONS

Many factors affect the way people see the world, such as birth order, economic status, geography, and the decades of time when they were growing up. Each of these factors impacts personality, and sociology theory holds that your beliefs are formed early and the view you hold of the world is shaped in your formative years during your first 10 to 15 years of life. Some consider the generation of time when you are growing up as a life stage, but that is not accurate as certain attitudes and behaviors impact life stage (college-age, retirement). Certain generational traits and characteristics have been tracked over the decades by researchers,[20-25] and the generations are consistent in their values despite what life stage they enter. Simply stated, you cannot expect another generation will act like you when they grow up, or enter your current life stage.

Let's consider what influenced you and your classmates during your formative years. *What political and/or historic events, songs or musical groups, signs/symbols, slogans, heros or movie characters were impactful to your generation?* (See Chapter 2, Table 2.3.) Compare what you believe and experienced with those in Table 2.3. Understanding generations is very important as it holds the key to understanding yourself and understanding others. People are now living and working longer. Life expectancy, while recently having declined due to the pandemic, has overall increased over the past decades, hence there are now multiple generations in the workforce and in our health care system.[20-25] Change is also happenning at faster and faster speeds so each generation shows up to the workplace and our hospitals, care centers, and clinics with vastly different expectations and experiences.

At no previous time in our history have so many different generations interacted on a daily basis.[20-25] We all can have reactions to different generations that are rather strong and diverse. We have to remember as HCPs that people are the heart of our work in health care. We do not want to stereotype generations but consider understanding the generations[20-26] as a way to appreciate the person inside and their perspectives that you are working to support in their healing journey.

As described in Chapter 2, the generations in today's working society include: Traditionalists (2% of workforce born 1925–1945); Baby Boomers (25% of workforce born 1946–1964); Generation X (33% of workforce born 1965–1980); Millenial Generation/Generation Y (35% of workforce born 1981–2000); and NEXT Generation/Generation Z (5% of workforce born 2001–2020).[20-22,26]

**Traditionalists:** This generation is in their next phase of life, described as hardworking, waste not/want not, and influenced by the Great Depression, the New Deal, World War II, the GI Bill, the Cold War, and the Atom Bomb. This generation is actually made up of two generations: the GI/Veteran Generation (born 1900–1924) and the Silent Generation (born 1925–1945), which are combined together as they were both generations that lived through World War II and grew up during a time when there was no social security, Medicare, Welfare, or Federal Deposit Insurance Corporation (FDIC); 50% of the men of this generation were Veterans. Famous influencers of this generation were Franklin Delano Roosevelt (FDR), Joe DiMaggio, Elizabeth Taylor, Henry Fonda, Julia Child, and the Betty Crocker brand. Traditionalists are loyal, patriotic, hard working, fiscally conservative, had great faith in institutions, trusted the rules and the workplace, followed the military model of top down chain of command. This generation truly appreciates the personal touch in communication with handwritten notes vs. email. Traditionalists make up about 2% of the workforce, although some up-ticks were noted through and post pandemic.[26]

**Baby Boomers:** This generation is labeled as the sandwich generation, described as competitive but contributors to the team model, and influenced by a booming birthrate, economic prosperity, Vietnam/Watergate, Assassinations, Civil Rights, and the women's movement, sex, drugs, and rock and roll. This generation grew up at a time of a booming postwar economy, were educated by the smartest women when women primarily were teachers, nurses, or secretaries (if they were not stay-at-home moms). Famous influencers of this generation were Martin Luther King Jr., Rosa Parks, John F. Kennedy (JFK), the Beatles, and the Rolling Stones. Baby Boomers are idealistic, optimistic, competitive, questioners of authority, desiring to stand out from the crowd, and played by the rules in the workplace although they offered a change of command vs. chain of command model of business. The single most important arrival during this generation was the television in homes. This generation prefers to communicate via phone, email, and whatever way is most efficient. Boomers make up approximately 25% of the workforce today, with 10,000 per day reaching retirement age. However, 65% of the "workaholics" intend to work beyond the typical retirement age of 65 years. Boomers appreciate specific deadlines and being mentors.[26]

**Generation X:** This generation is labeled the most misunderstood generation, defined by "latch-key" kids who were the keepers of their home keys, babysitting themselves in families of this generation where most had both parents working outside the home. During the birth years of Generation X, the divorce rate tripled and this generation distrusted permanence, adapted to change, and trusted themselves, not institutions. Gen X grew up during the fall of corporate America, 24-hour news media, cable TV, the invention of the personal computer, fax machines, answering machines, and pagers. Missing children's pictures were posted on milk cartons and the discovery of AIDS happened during the formative years for this group. Famous influencers of this generation were Madonna, Michael Jordan, Bill Gates, Steve Wozniak, Oprah Winfrey, and Sesame Street. This generation is skeptical, independent, resourceful, adaptive to change, lives a balanced lifestyle, and in the workplace challenges the rules and status quo. This generation also prefers to communicate via phone, email and whatever way is most efficient. Gen X prefers self command to change of command or chain of command in the workplace. Gen X makes up about 33% of the workforce and remains highly motivated by work–life balance with flexible work places, times, and spaces, and by 2028 will outnumber Boomers. Gen X truly appreciates immediate feedback on their work with flexible arrangements for work–life balance with opportunities for professional development.[26]

**Millennials/Generation Y:** This generation was initially labeled Generation Y due to their inquisitory nature (Generation "why"?) but has since been termed the Millennial Generation due in part to this generation's influence on their label. There has been more money spent (birthing, in vitro, surrogate, adoption) to have this generation than any other previous generation in history. This is the most wanted, protected, overscheduled, bottled watered, everyone wins, safety conscious generation in history. This generation was influenced by the Fall of the Berlin Wall, the expansion of the media including the worldwide web, and violence close to home (in schools). Famous influencers of this generation include Prince William, Britney Spears, and Venus and Serena Williams. This generation is realistic, globally concerned, diverse, cyber literate/media savvy, inquisitive, and committed. Millennials are the digital generation in terms of preferred communication formats (instant messaging, texts, emails). Millennials prefer to be empowered to act in the workplace over self/change or chain of command. Currently making up 35% of the workforce, Millennials will reach 75% of the global workforce by 2025. Alterations in adulthood from past generations are noted with 15% of Millennials (aged 25–35) living at home with their parents. Millennials like their managers to know them personally, and to provide flexibility with schedules and assignments, and to be provided with unique work experiences and immediate feedback on progress.[26]

**Generation Z:** This generation is the most "connected" generation of digital natives who have always lived with Internet existence, and they are sometimes referred to as the Homeland Generation, having never lived without the homeland security that heightened after the tragic attacks and events of September, 11, 2001 (9/11). Gen Z is defined as multitasking, web influenced, caring, polite, and career oriented. Gen Z was influenced by 9/11, the wars in Iraq and Afghanistan, WikiLeaks, and the Arab Spring. Digitally immersed since birth, Gen Z is both diverse and multicultural, yet stressed, having matured during the crucible events of the 2020s including opioid addiction, political polarization, racial renewal, the Covid-19 pandemic, a vastly volatile economy, European war with a threatening nuclear power; along with the emergence of artificial intelligence (AI). Even though this generation has grown up with technology, they prefer traditional methods of communication including personal invites and are less driven by money and brands than their previous generation. Influencers of this generation include Barack Obama, Taylor Swift, and Justin Bieber. This generation is inclusive, diverse, and socially aware. Gen Z is said to be lonelier than any of the other generations in the U.S. as about two-thirds feel shy, that others don't undertand them, and that people around them are absent. Gen Z wants employers to be straightforward/honest and to take them seriously rather than being concerned about empowerment, self/change, or chain of command management styles. Making up about 5% of the workforce, Gen Z also prefers electronic communications (instant messages, emails, texts) with the addition of growing up with a strong social media presence as influences. The vast majority of Gen Z expects formal training from employers and 40% prefer to interact with their supervisors daily or even several times per day; yet still appreciate the opportunity to then be self-directed. Gen Z also appreciates work–life balance, the ability to be creative, and working on multiple projects at once. Gen Z values independence and innovating with co-workers, and Gen Zers are often unabashedly digitally oriented.[26]

Shortly, we will again offer the opportunity for you to problem-solve through applied generational exercise activities at the end of the chapter. We hope you will utilize these exercises and the deep discussion that may follow to further examine your personal and developing professional insights with respect to the diversity of the generations in the workforce you are entering.

# TELEHEALTH AND ARTIFICIAL INTELLIGENCE

In Chapter 6, we first talked about the need for "telepresence" and some of the unique aspects of HCP communication needs for telehealth. We considered how the concept of telepresence *is different* from therapeutic presence, yet nevertheless, is often complementary. As telehealth capacities evolve, the unique aspects of communication within telehealth and AI environments must be carefully considered.

Prior to the Covid-19 pandemic, a gap existed in the capacities and viability for delivery of telehealth in contemporary practice. Demonstration projects and pilot trials were being conducted to demonstrate telehealth efficacy for physical therapy services for those who might not otherwise be capable of receiving care or where time and distance barriers were not surmountable to achieve rehabilitation services. Additionally, there were some necessary legislative approvals for some telephonic follow-up services, but not via present-day virtual platforms, e.g., Zoom, Microsoft Teams, EMR virtual video, and Facetime; with related concerns for security and HIPAA compliance. The pandemic thrust many HCPs into the delivery of telehealth[27,28]—**ready or not**! As the world transitioned, so did the demands for developing HCPs' capacity to abruptly shift and learn to deliver care in telehealth environments, with little first-hand experience to draw upon. Novice learners relied heavily on the experiences of their CE instructors, while those with some experience were able to be more readily creative. Screen time fatigue and other barriers presented. The digital generations jumped in eagerly with fewer trepidations than their earlier generational counterparts. Everyone learned more resilience than they believed possible, and biases were broken down, as some care is better than no care.

The largest barriers to telehealth delivery by HCPs include adequate time and training for set-up, the need to learn on the fly, lack of established procedures, fear and almost paralyzing hesitation of being able to adequately deliver quality care of any type (for a predominantly hands-on profession), unfamiliarity with technology, especially visual interfacing; physical separation; lacking quiet space for implementation (home and work environments); changed roles from hands-on to consulting and more educating, based on limited information gathered and gleaned through remote means; lack of standardized technologically enhanced measures; and lack of fully appropriate technologies to implement; along with the need to coach patient-users in technology needs. The enablers for telehealth delivery by HCPs include being adaptable to the change and open to the possibilities for delivering care; supportive and engaged leadership; supportive information technologists, who were on-call; being open to learning on the fly, sometimes even from your patients regarding technology; utilizing flexible work frameworks; advocating for telehealth reimbursement; information flow and sharing of information on how-to's and successful means; recognizing hybrid model potentials and realistic direct translation of home programs by visual access into home environments; and increased access to geographically remote and underserved areas. Most importantly, HCPs and developing HCPs found that learning to be creative in problem-solving means for measures and implementation of interventions is key, being patient with themselves and each other, not overscheduling screen time, building in breaks, and to not become frustrated with trial and error.[27-34]

It was not all smooth sailing, however, as many stresses were evident, with HCPs feeling more like "call centers," impedance on home environments prevailed, with a meshing of home–work environments that was not sustainable, and related privacy challenges for patient-centered care. The work–home delivery locales intersected with family members, others, in proximity, or needing to access areas where telehealth was being delivered due to lack of dedicated spaces with competing noises, unexpected interruptions from people and pets, as well as lighting challenges for both patients and HCPS, along with the need for clothing that allows for optimal viewing and which is least restrictive (e.g., tanks tops, halters, bare feet, shorts). The environment was often prohibitive, even though realistic (e.g., space for movement with variation in camera views or portable views with smartphones being managed by others; seeing the precise piece of furniture that was challenging for the patient to rise from, identifying the best place in the home for balance support exercises, wall squats etc.). Further challenges included that of being able to fully interpret facial expressions, especially when masking was needed; the constraints of not seeing all movements in a 3-dimensional vs. 2-dimensional physical space, including the loss of quantum interactions and full body language so readily offered in Face-to-Face (F2F) environments; and lack of desire or motivation to engage in tele-environments by the patients and by loathing or lamenting HCPs.[27-36]

Zoom fatigue sets in readily, so HCPs quickly learned the need for abbreviated sessions for both patients and HCPs. Stand-up desks were quickly implemented by those realizing the ramifications of sitting for prolonged periods and ergonomic strains for those accustomed to moving around and being more erect all day. HCPs adjusted their affective considerations by being "okay" with it not being the ideal therapeutic interaction, but what was possible, although initially incredibly stressful for some. Consulting with colleagues and sharing ideas and helpful technological applications (apps) led to triumphs. Important tips for successful telehealth visits include having all electronic devices, including cell phone calls, texts, and email notifications silenced and in the off position, being in a quiet room, and allowing dedicated time to respond, up to and including 30 minutes.[27-35]

Most HCPs now see a place for telehealth as a hybrid model to enhance care without delays and wait times and to effectively monitor along the way; and recognizing that it is better than no care. Patients are becoming more tech-savvy, if willing. Yet, as technologies begin to emerge and more haptic measures come into existence, telehealth may actually be the enhancement needed for F2F health care. For example, efficiencies of care can also be improved, e.g., correcting a substitution motion with incorrect exercise performance activity before it becomes a habit prior to the next F2F visit; maximizing the number of visits spread out over a longer period to address compliance, accountability, and realistic progressions of care; and prohibiting functional decline. Telemonitoring is already surfacing and improving ongoing care with remote monitoring (e.g., wearable devices, bed/chair monitors, vital sign monitors, remote acute hospitalists oversight, etc.) of those with chronic diseases or in assisted living due to the greater risks for functional and physical decline; as well as rural acute care where lack of specialized providers may be the case. The opportunity to intervene earlier and make recommendations to care teams, before deconditioning and lack of movement has deleterious implications on the human body, remains omnipotent.[27-36]

Telerehabilitation requires multifaceted clinical reasoning when deciding what patient is appropriate for what types of telerehabilitation care. Safety considerations are needed to ascertain patients' cognitive and physical capabilities. Both safety and therapeutic factors need to be accounted for when considering the availability of family members and care teams, to assist in supporting and preparation for therapeutic interventions. In the future, HCPs would also be better served to have more guidelines and screening/support procedures in place so that more time can be spent on therapeutic health care services. This is also an opportunity to utilize the IPE team for more efficient and effective telerehabilitation efforts. Legislative (federal and state) reimbursement, ethical and curricular implications for HCPs' education regarding technology in rehabilitation have been identified and continue to be addressed as telehealth is likely here to stay for the near future in varied capacities.[27–36] The following tips are also important to consider as you engage in telehealth practice:

- **Be clear and present:** Adapt to the volume of virtual visits per hour, realize that you must be 1:1 with your patient, and consider how compensation changes because of the adapted environments.

- **Be tele-savvy:** Lights, camera, action—"webside manner" includes sustained eye contact with the camera, with appropriate lighting, in a "professional environment." Be aware of your background and/or use a background filter that is not distracting.

- **Expand your horizons:** Home is where the heart is and where the movement happens. You may even gain more clues about the daily occurrences in your patients' lived experiences by seeing their world first-hand; and you might be able to "see" them more frequently if access is an issue counteracting SDoH potential barriers (see Chapters 1 [Figure 1.1], 14, 17–18). As a result of telehealth services, patients may also benefit from lower care costs.

- **Be boundary conscious:** Sometimes remote care may need to be in person. Ensure that your patients/clients are cognizant of when a virtual visit is not sufficient and how to seek appropriate care. Make certain your patients/clients, families, significant others, and caregivers are aware and reminded of warning signs about their condition/s that will catalyze them to seek additional care if needed or if their condition/s and/or situations worsen. Virtual care is not a substitute for necessary face-to-face health care.

We would be remiss if we did not mention the potential role of enhanced artificial intelligence (AI) that is emerging, due to the latest generation of clusters of micro-processors offering nodes for memory-intensive computation platforms and other related platforms (e.g., Open AI-Chat Generative Pre-trained Transformer/ChatGPT, Google's BARD, Open AI-DALL-E deep learning model for images from art). The AI revolution of big data and robotics is bound to be one of the largest influencers of the current generation. AI is an umbrella term representing a vast array of technologies to create and train machines to do intelligent thinking tasks, drawing upon data and information that results in working knowledge and can translate into wisdom. AI itself is not new (created by Marvin Minsky in 1951), yet due to modern technologies the ways in which AI can be utilized have multiplied. AI, through deep learning models, can create words, sounds, images (from text), and video, mimicking neural networks through mathematical algorithms. AI is on the verge of becoming a contender as a strong assistant for HCPs, and while chatbots can produce empathic qualities, these technologies are not yet in line to replace HCPs.[36–39] Imagine utilizing an image AI system for predictive healing for wound care or altered gait patterns with therapeutic exercise dosage prescriptions. Using big data and algorithms, the applications for new knowledge and disease and disability reductions are at the forefront, along with potential improvements in health care delivery.

With the supply of qualified HCPs being limited in many regions, AI may yet prove to be an effective and life-saving feature for health care. Machine learning can be very efficient and machines generally take in information and process it now faster than humans.[37–40] Thinking back in time for a moment, I recall in my early practice days utilizing transcriptions services for medical documentation and initially this was done by landline; in the coming years, I was freed up to a portable Dictaphone, allowing me to dictate while commuting to and from work (before cell phones). This may seem inconsequential for those of you who have grown up with instant messaging, text, and telecommunication instantaneously available almost anywhere at any time, yet back then it was an efficient and effective time saver. I believe "thinking-out-loud" whilst dictating also aided in my abilities to further develop my clinical reasoning acumen with respect to differential movement diagnostics and pattern relationships, while considering prioritization of best practices for interventions and patient/family/caregiver education pathways. I had many "aha" moments amid dictation, and felt that this daily audio reflection aided my professional development. Also, early in my career, I witnessed, first hand, my father's neurosurgeon utilizing dictation, in front of his patients—that was amazing too as it offered the patient another chance to "hear" the specialists' impressions and their plan of care, and to ask any additional questions; clearly, an efficient way to document and stay on track as a busy neurosurgeon too! I could see utilizing AI in this way and to serve as another "consultant" as we "think out loud" and perhaps a collaborative advancement of our reasoning strategies or another way to help educate patients and reinforce learning and teaching about the movement systems for patients and families.

In fact, chatbots can be quite accurate and more empathic than some HCPs when asked to respond to basic questions. Which is not terribly surprising, as we have all experienced or witnessed a poor patient–practitioner interaction with a less than sympathetic ear, due to inability to fully manage the stresses of often hectic, understaffed health care environments. HCP can do better and may do better with AI assistance to ease the pressures. AI can read the emotional cues from users in many instances, with common nonverbal expressions and tone (you may have experienced this with your own interactions with Alexa, voice AI, or other similar devices in the responses to your requests for information or sharing jokes). Yet, oversight is still needed by HCPs to assure appropriate and accurate support for health care needs.[37-40] In fact, even ChatGPT[39] is aware of its limitations and has been quoted as stating:

> *As a language model, ChatGPT is not capable of replacing human healthcare professionals ... ChatGPT is an AI model, and it can't provide the human touch that some patients may need ... Human healthcare professionals have a deep understanding of the nuances of healthcare and the emotional and social context of their patients, and this is something that ChatGPT can't replicate.[39]*

Of course, many would and should argue that AI is no substitute for human empathy, yet progress is being made for the future.[37-40] Machine learning for compiling data sets and diagnostics, medical images, outcome analyses, and surgical workflow are powerful uses from a quantitative and algorithmic standpoint; yet the quantum aspects of communication continue to emerge, as many of the nuances of communication are individual and, as you are now fully aware, include body and facial language (nonverbal expressions), intonation, and often linguistic variables (natural language) that are unique.[41,42] Human communication is both diverse and complex, with high dimensionality, specific nuances, and a blending of cross-cultural, valence, prosody, emotional states, and environmental influences; which are quite idiosyncratic in nature.[40-44] Mega data[41-44] is now being collected to begin to derive sense-making of emotional expressions through a holistic toolkit for AI to predict, interpret, and understand human communication. Emotional recognition from text and written communications is also emerging with AI machine learning through natural language processing with deep learning and semantic text analyses with incredibly high accuracy rates for human emotion.[41-44] While we should be cautiously optimistic, and proceed with caution, as AI has also been known to cause harm and spread misinformation,[37-44] it behooves us to explore more of this fascinating, emerging technology utilizing global datasets with supported scientific controls to determine with data-driven science, the fine-grained patterns of human facial expressions and emotional behaviors being expressed, via the hume initiative (https://hume.ai/).

Consequently, ChatGPT[40] also offered a poem regarding the interview conducted on its role in health care:

> *This interview has been quite a ride,*
>
> *With questions on healthcare to guide,*
>
> *ChatGPT's capabilities we explored,*
>
> *And many insights were outpoured.*
>
> *From financial risks to patient care,*
>
> *We delved deep into what's fair.*
>
> *With technology's role in mind,*
>
> *We hope to leave the future kind.*

Alas, we are hopeful too, and time will tell how industries, including health care, are revolutionized by generative artificial intelligence through machine learning, while working to assure that they do not harm.

# CONCLUSION

As you go forward in your foundational elements of practice including safety, interpersonal communication, professionalism, ethical and legal practice, inclusivity, and clinical reasoning, be certain to consider all contexts that the patient may be experiencing in your efforts to motivate and connect with your patients. For example, through a qualitative examination of physical therapists' strategies utilized to engage their patients who had experienced stroke (participating in rehab), researchers[16] discovered that physical therapists utilize different strategies to encourage individuals' active participation. The nine themes that emerged from the study noted that participation depended upon the patients' mental health status, cognitive function, physical difficulties, personality, activities and participation, age, human environment, and the type of rehabilitation service, along with motivational strategies.[16]

Hence, if a patient was struggling with notable loss of self-confidence, as detected by the interpersonal communication with the patient and physical therapist, then the patient was offered smaller, achievable practice tasks to aid in success and re-gaining self-confidence, using patient-centered communication-built rapport to motivate the patients. Another example considered a patient who also had a co-morbidity of diabetes. Coaching them about the negative effects of a lack of activity was more impacting due to their prior lack of appreciation for the need for activity and movement. Another patient was genuinely interested in being able to have privacy in toileting activities and was therefore highly motivated and willingly engaged in therapeutic interventions of breaking down the movement component skills to achieve this more functional goal. While for others, they were missing social interactions and benefited from group therapy interaction opportunities and recreational therapy.[16] Considering upcoming home environments for transitioning from rehab and providing feedback ongoing were also key to motivating the patients. Danzl et al.[45] support these premises and reported four strategies utilized to build rapport and trust, including: (1) *spending time with the individuals without rushing them*; (2) *developing a deeper understanding of the individuals*; (3) *using a sense of humor when appropriate*; and (4) *showing compassion, empathy, and respect*. Key aspects, omnipotent to establishing the collaborative partnership with the patient, and essential for patient-centered practice, are listening to the individual while refraining from interrupting, understanding the individual's perspectives, and expressing empathy.[17,46–48]

**Be a good listener**. Do not interrupt your patients and become too dependent on checklists.[46,48] People want to be heard. Seek to understand how a patient perceives their problem. Really, truly listening requires concentrating on what your patient is sharing and focusing solely on the present moment. For many patients, this may be their first experience of being listened to by an empathic and attentive professional. Listening truly requires undivided attention and a nonjudgmental stance. One must listen carefully to the story being shared while also noticing the way it is being shared. People will often convey emotions through their behavior; for example, a patient whose voice rises as they talk about not getting the care they deserve—while they did not state they were angry, the associated behaviors and vocal tone indicate the contrary. Or consider the in-patient who has their head down and is in tears, and states, "I have never endured being away from my family for so long," conveying homesickness, along with their health care institutionalization. A good listener remembers the facts but also identifies the emotions, making appropriate referrals where needed, and addressing the affective domain of care whenever possible.

How will you address these needs with your patients?

Many HCPs clearly care and are empathic, giving their time to fully address patient concerns and make themselves readily accessible. When patients feel vulnerable, this caring is distinguished not just by kindness and compassion, but also by being open to the contextualization of care—noting the unique life circumstances that impact health needs. That need to fully understand your patients' lived experiences makes all the difference if your home exercise and education plan are realistic and viable or doomed to fail, as you did not consider the complexities of your patients' daily lives. HCPs must consider the humanistic side of the care they are imparting—without the uniqueness of the individual being fully considered, one may be providing the right care, but at the wrong time and in the wrong way.[46–48]

Even the simple act of being eye level with your patient is critical. Taking a moment to place your hand on their shoulder or place their hand between yours, showing you care, asking what matters and working to understand what they need is your job as a HCP. Then you will be capable of providing calm for their soul and participating in their care for their health. It is categorically different to have an exchange at eye level with your patients, than hovering over the top of them. Facilitate the physical aspects of your therapeutic relationship of being with your patient, not by hovering over them like a helicopter—adapt to the patient—physically minimizing your presence by allowing the patient to be larger and to be seen. Simply raising or lowering the bed to your eye level or sitting on a stool to be eye-to-eye (without any barriers in between, e.g., computer) with your patient is key for a therapeutic relationship with your patient and beginning to establish cultural humility.[48]

You were drawn to health care out of benevolence—the desire to do good. Now ensure that you achieve beneficence—actually doing good—by keeping the human side of health care at the forefront. As a novice you will be drawn to the clinical and machine interfaces of care, while expert providers realize that focusing on the soul, through human interactions, is actually what influences a life. You must always consider the mental, spiritual, and physical needs of your patients to be a true healer,[48] which is only accomplished by listening to the patient's narrative of their lived experiences.

One must have a humanistic heart for health care if one is to be sustained in the healing professions. Being a humanitarian means having **human values and an understanding of all human situations that we share, regardless of race, ethnicity, religion, and social status**. It's working toward common human goals and ensuring we support people with respect and dignity. And, when needed, shifting our focus on healing and curing to love and mercy when approaching death and dying. The only thing that matters is what the patients want at that point in time. Be present for their and their family's needs—everything else is merely secondary.[48]

We leave you now with one last quote as we close this chapter on transitioning. Please take a moment to reflect on what it means for you as you continue your professional formation. We share our heartfelt wishes for each of you for strength and courage for the journey ahead.

*Students, in the course of their formation, must let the gritty reality of this world into their lives, so they can learn to feel it, think about it critically, respond to its suffering, and engage it constructively.*

—Rev. Peter-Hans Kolvenbach, S.J. (1928–2016)

# REFERENCES

1. National Alliance on Mentally Illness (NAMI). *Mental Illness By the Numbers.* Available: https://nami.org/mhstats Accessed: May 5, 2023.
2. Dweck CS. The right mindset for success. In: *HBRs 10 Must Reads on Lifelong Learning.* Harvard Business Review Press: Boston, MA; 2021.
3. Dalley AF, Agur AMR. *Moore's Clinically Oriented Anatomy,* 9th ed. Wolters Kluwer: Philadelphia, PA; 2023.
4. Stern JD. It's like a death. *JAMA.* 2023;329(13):1061–1062.
5. Rubin R. Cut calories, lengthen life span? Randomized trial uncovers evidence that calorie restriction might slow aging, but questions remain. *JAMA.* 2023;329(13):1049–1050.
6. Harris J, Smith JG. *Sensation and Perception,* 2nd ed. Thousand Oaks, CA: Sage Publications; 2022.
7. Amerian Physical Therapy Association. *Credentialed Clinical Instructor Program,* Level 1. Available: https://www.apta.org/for-educators/clinical-education-development/ccip-level-1 Accessed: April 26, 2023.
8. Musolino GM, van Duijn J, Noonan AC, et al. Reasons identified for seeking the American Physical Therapy Association-Credentialed Clinical Instructor Program (CCIP) in Florida. *J Allied Health;*2013;42(3):51E–60E(10).
9. Emery MJ. Perceived importance and frequency of clinical teaching behaviors: survey of students, clinical instructors and center coordinators of clinical education. *J Phys Ther Educ.* 1987;1(1):29–32.
10. Schön DA. *Educating the Reflective Practitioner: Toward a New Design for Teaching and Learning in the Professions.* San Francisco, CA: Jossey-Bass; 1987.
11. Kleiner MJ, Kinsella EA, Miciak M, Teachman G, McCabe E, Walton DM. An integrative review of the qualities of a "good" physiotherapist. *Physiother Theory Pract.* 2023 Jan;39(1):89–116.
12. Dalley-Hewer J, Clouder DL, Jones M. Real world reflection: how physiotherapists experience reflection in their practice. *Reflective Practice.* 2023;24(1):85–99.
13. Musolino GM. Fostering reflective practice: self-assessment abilities of physical therapy students and entry-level graduates. *J Allied Health.* 2006;35(1):30–42.
14. Kleiner MJ, Kinsella EA, Miciak M, Teachman G, Walton DM. The "responsive" practitioner: physiotherapists' reflections on the "good" in physiotherapy practice. *Physiother Theory Pract.* 2022 July; 6:1–14.
15. Musolino, GM, Jensen, GM, eds. *Clinical Reasoning and Clinical Decision-making in Physical Therapy: Facilitation, and Implementation.* Thorofare, NJ: Slack; 2020.
16. Oyake K, Sue K, Sumiya M, Tanaka S. Physical therapists use different motivational strategies for stroke rehabilitation tailored to an individual's condition: A qualitative study. *Phys Ther.* 2023 Apr 5;103(6):pzad034.
17. Yun D, Choi J. Person-centered rehabilitation care and outcomes: A systematic 360 literature review. *Int J Nurs Stud.* 2019;93:74–83. doi:10.1016/j.ijnurstu.2019.02.012.
18. Wilson CM, Arena SK, Boright LE. State of the art physiotherapist-led approaches to safe aging in place. 2022. *Arch. Physiother.* 2022;12(17). doi: 10.1186/s40945-022-00142-5.
19. U.S. Bureau of Statistics. *Volunteer data.* https://www.bls.gov/
20. Lancaster L, Stillman D. *When Generations Collide: Traditionalists, Baby Boomers, Generation Xers, Millennials: Who They Are, Why They Clash, How to Solve the Generational Puzzle at Work.* New York, NY: Harper Business; 2003.
21. Howe N, Strauss, W. *Millennials Rising.* New York: Vintage; 2000.
22. Lancaster L, Stillman, D. *When Generations Collide: Who They Are. Why They Clash. How to Solve the Generational Puzzle at Work.* New York, New York. HarperCollins Publishers; 2002.
23. Tulgan B. *Managing Generation X.* Santa Monica, CA: Merritt Publishing; 1995.
24. Martin C, Tulgan B. *Managing the Generation Mix,* 2nd ed. Amherst, MA: HRD Press; 2006.
25. Zemke R, Raines C, Filipczak B. *Generations at Work: Managing the Clash of Veterans, Boomers, Xers, and Nexters in Your Workplace.* New York, NY: AMACOM; 2000
26. Bourne B. *Differing Generations in the Workplace.* [Infographic] Purdue Global. Available: https://www.purdueglobal.edu/education-partnerships/generational-workforce-differences-infographic/ Accessed May 7, 2023.
27. Kreider CM, Hale-Gallardo J, Kramer JC, Mburu S, Slamka MR, Findley KE, Myers KJ, Romero S. Providers' shift to telerehabilitation at the U.S. Veterans Health Administration during COVID-19: practical applications. *Front Public Health.* 2022 Mar 4;10:831762.

28. Lee AC. COVID-19 and the advancement of digital physical therapist practice and telehealth. *Phys Ther.* 2020 Jul 19;100(7):1054–1057.

29. Haines KJ, Sawyer A, McKinnon C, Donovan A, Michael C, Cimoli C, Gregory M, Berney S, Berlowitz DJ. Barriers and enablers to telehealth use by physiotherapists during the COVID-19 pandemic. *Physiotherapy.* 2023 Mar;118:12–19. doi: 10.1016/j.physio.2022.09.003.

30. Dario AB, Moreti Cabral A, Almeida L, Ferreira ML, Refshauge K, Simic M, Pappas E, Ferreira PH. Effectiveness of telehealth-based interventions in the management of non-specific low back pain: a systematic review with meta-analysis. *Spine J.* 2017 Sep;17(9):1342–1351.

31. Shukla H, Nair S, Thakker D. Role of telerehabilitation in patients following total knee arthroplasty: evidence from a systematic literature review and meta-analysis. *Journal of Telemedicine and Telecare.* 2017;23(2):339–346.

32. Gilbert, A., Booth, G., Betts, T. et al. A mixed-methods survey to explore issues with virtual consultations for musculoskeletal care during the COVID-19 pandemic. *BMC Musculoskelet Disord.* 2021;22: 245.

33. Miller MJ, Pak SS, Keller DR, Barnes DE. Evaluation of pragmatic telehealth physical therapy implementation during the COVID-19 pandemic. *Phys Ther.* 2021 Jan 4;101(1):pzaa19.

34. Grundstein MJ, Fisher C, Titmuss M, Cioppa-Mosca J. The role of virtual physical therapy in a post-pandemic world: pearls, pitfalls, challenges, and adaptations. *Phys Ther.* 2021 Sep 1;101(9):pzab145.

35. Abou L, Worobey LA, Rigot SK, Stanley E, Rice LA. Reliability of home-based remote and self-assessment of transfers using the Transfer Assessment Instrument among wheelchair users with spinal cord injury. *Spinal Cord Ser Cases.* 2023 Mar 30;9(1):10.

36. Greenfield B, Musolino GM. Technology in rehabilitation: ethical and curricular implications for physical therapist education. *J Phys Ther Educ.* 2012;26:81–90.

37. Lee P, Bubeck S, Petro J. Benefits, limits, and risks of GPT-4 as an AI chatbot for medicine. *N Engl J Med.* 2023 Mar 30;388(13):1233–1239.

38. Lee P, Goldberg C, Kohane I. *The AI Revolution in Medicine: GPT-4 and Beyond.* London: Pearson Education; 2023.

39. ChatGPT. *OpenAI.* Available: https://chat.openai.com/chat Accessed March 1, 2023.

40. Ascher, DA. An interview with ChatGPT about health care: many people are wondering how ChatGPT might be used in health care. So I asked it. *NEJM Catalyst Innovations in Care Delivery.* April 4, 2023. https://catalyst.nejm.org/doi/full/10.1056/CAT.23.0043

41. Guo, J. Deep learning approach to text analysis for human emotion detection from big data. *J Intelligent Systems.* 2022; 31(1): 113–126.

42. Cowen AS, Keltner D, Schroff F, et al. Sixteen facial expressions occur in similar contexts worldwide. *Nature.* 2021;589:251–257.

43. Brooks JA, Freeman JB. Conceptual knowledge predicts the representational structure of facial emotion perception. *Nat Hum Behav.* 2018 Aug;2(8):581–591.

44. Brooks JA, Chikazoe J, Sadato N, Freeman JB. The neural representation of facial-emotion categories reflects conceptual structure. *Proc Natl Acad Sci* USA. 2019 Aug 6;116(32):15861–15870.

45. Danzl MM, Etter NM, Andreatta RD, Kitzman PH. Facilitating neurorehabilitation through principles of engagement. *J Allied Health.* 2012 Spring;41(1):35–41. PMID: 22544406.

46. Weiner SJ, Schwartz A. *Listening for What Matters: Avoiding Contextual Errors in Healthcare.* Oxford University Press, Oxford: 2016.

47. Hashim MJ. Patient-Centered Communication: Basic Skills. *Am Fam Physician.* 2017 Jan 1;95(1):29–34.

48. Ely, W. *Every Deep Drawn Breath: A Critical Care Doctor.* Scribner; New York, NY: Scribner; 2022.

49. Lee AC, Deutsch JE, Holdsworth L, Kaplan SL, Kosakowski H, Latz R, McNeary LL, O'Neil J, Ronzio O, Sanders K, Sigmund-Gaines M, Wiley M, Russell T. Telerehabilitation in physical therapist practice: a clinical practice guideline from the American Physical Therapy Association. *Phys Ther.* 2024 May;104(5):pzae045. doi: 10.1093/ptj/pzae045.

# Suggested Readings and Resources

Ely, W. *Love and Mercy in the ICU.* Episode 41, The Doctor's Art, podcast. Available: thedoctorsart.com Accessed: April 23, 2023.

Raphael-Grimm T. *The Art of Communication in Nursing and Health Care: An Interdisciplinary Approach.* New York, NY: Springer Publishing Company; 2015.

Roundy RE, Stearns ZR, Willis MW, Blevins JJ, Linton TA, Medlin TR, Winger JG, Dorfman, CS, Shelby RA. Relationships between burnout and resilience: experiences of physical therapists and occupational therapists during the COVID-19 pandemic. *Phys Ther.* 2023: pzad022. doi: 10.1093/ptj/pzad022.

Weiner SJ. *On Becoming a Healer: The Journey from Patient Care to Caring about Your Patients.* Baltimore, MD: Johns Hopkins University Press; 2020.

Weiner SJ, Schwartz A. *Listening for What Matters: Avoiding Contextual Errors in Healthcare.* Oxford: Oxford University Press; 2016.

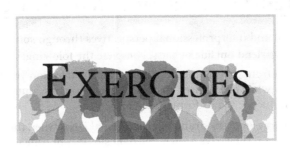

# EXERCISE 1: EXPLORING, EXPRESSING, AND ENGAGING

Through this exercise, you will complete three activities concurrently: (1) exploring by communicating through body movement, considering boundaries and identifying connects; (2) expressing by listening and calming the body; and (3) engaging through re-calibration of our embodiment with others, redressing and reconciling social-cultural norms.

Now, get with a trusted peer and sit facing each other, lotus-position (cross-legged), if possible, on the floor with no physical barriers in between each other. Take several slow, deep breaths in and forcefully exhale out before beginning. Throughout this activity, continue to breathe deeply and slowly, while keeping your body calm for the exploring and engagement exercise.

Then, first think about your own hands from the wrist to the fingertips, consider every component of the structure, volume, shape, weight, muscles, bones, tendons, ligaments, form, and texture of each wrist, hand, and fingers.

Next, following exploring your own hands, engage with those of your partner, with a reminder to keep breathing and calmly proceed. First, by just placing your palms near your partner's hands without touching, without pressing, without invading. Silently focus and just feel the warmth and quantum energies of your peer's hands. Do this with your eyes open, then closed.

Then explore your peer's hands, through touch, pressing, and palpating first with your eyes closed, then with your eyes open.

As you explore the hands of your peer:

Hold each other by the wrist, hand, and fingers—then detect differences in touch, then consider every component of the structure, volume, shape, weight, form, and texture of each wrist, hand, and fingers.

Then consider any thoughts and memories that come to mind as you complete the activity. You may benefit from doing the activity with other peers, family, and friends as you practice your skills in exploring, expressing, and engaging.

Now discuss the following queries with your peers:

- How did the activity lead to your own self-discovery, self-awareness, and that of others?

- How did the activity transform your physiological and relaxation state?

- What are the healing effects and vital benefits of combining breathing and movement on the body's systems (circulatory, digestive, endocrine, lymphatic, etc.)?

- Candidly discuss the mind–body interaction that occurred through the exercise and how that might influence your therapeutic touch, hands-on work with your patients.

- Why do you think hands-on health care is so important and impacting?

To conclude the activity, where time and space allow, lie gently supine in silence or with soft music that allows you to actively internalize your lived experience. Reflect and journal about your experience.

# EXERCISE 2: INTERGENERATIONAL AND INTERPROFESSIONAL INTERACTIONS

Let's consider intergenerational and interprofessional perspectives through some applied activities.
With a classmate and/or family/friend outside of class, complete the folowing:

1. Utilizing the information from this chapter, consider which generation you fall into or you feel fits you best. Share with your partner what political or historical events, songs, music groups, signs/symbols/slogans, heros/icons/characters influenced your formative years.

2. Sometimes individuals carry an extra strand of generational DNA when their birth years are positioned right between two generations or if they have grown up/spent significant time with others from multigenerational backgrounds. This group of individuals are called Cuspers. Cuspers play important roles in mediating, translating, explaining, coordinating, and resolving conflicts in schools and workplaces. With your partner, share where you feel you fall in terms of your generation and/or ability to be a Cusper in terms of our profession and other health care professions.

3. Finally, explore the screening tools related to the Social Determinants of Health and discuss how these related to intergenerational challenges in providing health care. www.cms.gov/priorities/innovation/files/worksheets/ahcm-screeningtool.pdf

# EXERCISE 3: INTERGENERATIONAL AND INTERPROFESSIONAL DILEMMA

You are a physical therapist from the millennial generation. You are collaborating with a client who is a retired teacher with a racquet sports-related injury (tennis, pickleball, badminton) from the Traditionalist generation. Based on your knowledge of generational expectations, what strategies can you use to increase your therapeutic effectiveness when collaborating with this individual?

1. How will you address this patient? Will you use formal or informal terms and names?

2. How will you provide patient education for this patient? Will you suggest websites or provide written home programs?

3. What challenges might you face in communicating effectively with this patient? How will you address those challenges?

4. How would this all change if you were a Baby Boomer therapist? Generation X therapist? Generation Z therapist?

5. How would this all change if your patient were a Baby Boomer? A Generation Xer? A Millennial? A Gen Zer? Explain how you will interact with the other health care professionals serving on your client's health care team so that you are all supportive to rehabilitative strategies including: MD? Chiropractor? Nurse Practitioner? Personal Trainer? Massage Therapist? Racquet Sport Coach?

**Tip**—In addition to the generational information in this chapter and Generations (in Chapter 2, Table 2.3), this is also a good opportunity to revisit the Checklist for Educational Activities (Chapter 16, Table 16.4) and PTPE (Chapter 16, Table 16.9).

# EXERCISE 4: TELEHEALTH ETHICS IN PRACTICE

For this activity, please proceed to explore the American Telemedicine Society website: www.americantelemed.org. Identify some of the key issues of special interest related to telehealth and explore recommendations for telehealth stethoscopes. Consider the current practice guidelines.

1.  What key issues did you find relative to telehealth tests and measures?

2.  What are key considerations for telehealth stethoscopes?

3.  What current practice guidelines apply related to telehealth test and measures?

Now provide your reflections on how these tips and recommendations might be helpful in your implementation of telehealth via virtual visits, chat-based care, and/or remote monitoring and technology-based rehabilitation devices.

4.  Share your reflections on practical applications for telehealth.

Next, conduct a search and locate a recommended telehealth rehabilitation application specifically (e.g., protractor extension for measuring range of motion online or the transfer assessment instrument for wheelchair users with spinal cord injury) and provide your impressions of the pro/cons of utilizing this app.

5.  Please provide the telehealth application information and your impressions.

6.  Share what core values and principles of your code of ethics apply with respect to telehealth, telerehabilitation, and current use of AI.

7.  Finally, if applicable, review the Clinical Practice Guidelines for Telerehabilitation in Physical Therapist Practice[49] https://pubmed.ncbi.nlm.nih.gov/38513257/ to discover the seven related recommendations and be prepared to discuss.

# EXERCISE 5: ARTIFICIAL INTELLIGENCE (AI)

## Part 1

Review the AI video and the Rome call resources (below). Be prepared to discuss your impressions in relation to the future of the usage of AI and health care. In your discussions be sure to consider matters of equity and inclusion, fairness (e.g., is there bias in the input or output data? Is it accessible for all?), reliability and rigor (e.g., can you trust the results?), responsibility and accountability (e.g., do the benefits outweigh the risks?), security and confidentiality (e.g., is the data safe?) and your profession's ethical considerations. Do you agree with Dr. Hinton's concerns expressed over AI in that generative intelligence could spread misinformation and, eventually, threaten humanity?

Why or why not?

> The call | Rome Call www.romecall.org
>
> A document first signed in early 2020 aimed to promote responsibility for AI development and use. It outlines six AI principles: Transparency, Inclusion, Impartiality, Accountability, Reliability, Security and Privacy; along with three key impact areas: Ethics, Education, and Rights.
>
> AI "might take over" one day if it isn't developed responsibly, Geoffrey Hinton warns—CBS News
>
> https://youtu.be/qrvK_KuIeJk?si=TXmfnFiQQ_vJaVkq
>
> The "Godfather of AI," one of the main developers of artificial neural networks, speaks about the potential benefits and the many concerns around generative AI.

## Part 2

Many of your patients/clients will soon, if not already, be utilizing AI as a means to gather information about health care matters that impact them and how to address them. Select a health condition or disease and ask AI to produce a patient guidance document or home exercise program to address the resulting implications for the movement system. Now take some time to review what AI produced and compare this with the evidence, matters of health care literacy, and what you now know about best practice in education, teaching, and learning. What did AI get right? What challenged AI in this exercise? How will you educate your patients/clients on matters of AI reliance for health care information and treatments?

# EXERCISE 6: WHO ARE YOU BECOMING? TRANSFORMATIVE LEARNING GOALS FOR CLINICAL EDUCATION AND REFLECTING FOR THE FUTURE

As you embark on your clinical education experiences, set three truly transformative starting goals for yourself for the first 2 weeks, focusing on your self-identified areas to strengthen. Referencing the PBAT (Chapter 20, Appendix), write your realistic goals in the measurable format (Audience—Who, Behavior—What, Condition/Circumstances, Degree—How Well and the Expected Time Frame—When to Achieve, as in Table 20.1), review with a peer for readability, succinct format and realistic transformation, and appropriate time frames. Then share and discuss each with your CE faculty before you initiate, re-assess in 2 weeks, and reset!

| TABLE 20.1 | | | | | |
|---|---|---|---|---|---|
| **THREE CE GOALS—ABCDE FORMAT** | | | | | |
| **LEARNING DOMAIN\*** | **AUDIENCE WHO?** | **BEHAVIOR WHAT?** | **CONDITION/S? CIRCUMSTANCES? WHERE?** | **DEGREE? HOW WELL?** | **EXPECTED TIME FRAME? WHEN?** |
| **Cognitive** | | | | | |
| **Affective** | | | | | |
| **Psychomotor** | | | | | |
| Spiritual (Optional) | | | | | |

\*Refer to Chapter 3, Appendix

## Reflection for the Future—A Growth Mindset

Now consider the following questions to ask and answer yourself as you continue your professional journey and revisit and discuss with a trusted mentor:

Who are the key decision-makers affecting your career internally and externally?

Are you standing out to them in appropriate ways or are they just vaguely aware of you?

What is a unique fact about you?

Can you share an accomplishment associated with this fact to engage further in your professional environment?

Are key people aware of what you can contribute, your skills and attributes, or are you primarily invisible to decision-makers?

How would you describe your self-confidence?

How does low confidence impact your life and work and how others perceive you professionally?

Who are the professionals who thrive and shine with realistic self-confidence, and what can you learn from them?

How can you gain visibility and actively seek out opportunities or do others have to seek you out?

Are you proactively building relationships with those who could be decision-makers in your future? Who are they?

What is your active approach for promoting yourself and your work? What is holding you back?

How can you use your awareness of others' needs and emotions to anticipate their expectations better?

How can you demonstrate the value of your research skills to your decision-makers?

Do your advocacy and volunteer efforts align with your core values and beliefs, and that of the profession?

How can you leverage your capacities in advocacy and volunteering to further benefit your organizations?

What steps can you continue to take to enhance your performance in areas where you may lack self-confidence?

How can you focus more on your strengths and passions rather than getting lost in the noise of other professionals' successes?

What does care for yourself look like? How do you take care of yourself and your needs?

What is the worst thing that could happen if you prioritize yourself?

What tools or habits can you employ to be more mindful for self-care?

Consider if setting goals in any of these areas of consideration would assist you in your continued professional development and maturation!

*Wishing you all the best of success for the patients/clients you serve, in your career and life!*

# APPENDIX

## PROFESSIONAL BEHAVIORS
## ASSESSMENT TOOL

Please note: A longer version of this Professional Behaviors Assessment Tool can be downloaded from www.routledge.com/9781638220039

# DEFINITIONS OF BEHAVIORAL CRITERIA LEVELS

- **Beginning Level**—behaviors consistent with a learner in the beginning of the professional phase of physical therapy education and before the first significant internship
- **Intermediate Level**—behaviors consistent with a learner after the first significant internship
- **Entry Level**—behaviors consistent with a learner who has completed all didactic work and is able to independently manage a caseload with consultation as needed from clinical instructors, co-workers, and other health care professionals
- **Post-Entry Level**—behaviors consistent with an autonomous practitioner beyond entry level

# BACKGROUND INFORMATION

Today's physical therapy practitioner functions on a more autonomous level in the delivery of patient care, which places a higher demand for professional development on new graduates of the physical therapy educational programs. The research team of Warren May (PT, MPH), Laurie Kontney (PT, DPT, MS), and Z. Annette Iglarsh (PT, PhD, MBA) completed a research project that built on the work of other researchers to analyze the PT-Specific *Generic Abilities* in relation to the changing landscape of physical therapist practice and in relation to generational differences of the "Millennial" or "Y" Generation (born 1980–2000). These are the graduates of the classes of 2004 and beyond who will shape clinical practice in the 21st century.

The research project was twofold and consisted of (1) a research survey which identified and rank ordered professional behaviors expected of the newly licensed physical therapist upon employment (2008); and (2) 10 small work groups that took the 10 identified behaviors (statistically determined) and wrote/revised behavior definitions, behavioral criteria, and placement within developmental levels (Beginning, Intermediate, Entry Level, and Post-Entry Level) (2009).

Interestingly, the 10 statistically significant behaviors identified were identical to the original 10 *Generic Abilities*; however, the rank orders of the behaviors changed. Participants in the research survey included Center Coordinators of Clinical Education (CCCEs) and Clinical Instructors (CIs) from all regions of the United States. Participants in the small work groups included Directors of Clinical Education (DCEs), Academic Faculty, CCCEs, and CIs from all regions of the United States.

This resulting document, *Professional Behaviors*, is the culmination of this research project. The definitions of each professional behavior have been revised along with the behavioral criteria for each developmental level. The 'developing level' was changed to the 'intermediate level' and the title of the document has been changed from *Generic Abilities* to *Professional Behaviors*. The title of this important document was changed to differentiate it from the original *Generic Abilities* and to better reflect the intent of assessing professional behaviors deemed critical for professional growth and development in physical therapy education and practice.

# PREAMBLE

The intent of the *Professional Behaviors* **Assessment Tool** is to identify and describe the repertoire of professional behaviors deemed necessary for success in the practice of physical therapy. This *Professional Behaviors* **Assessment Tool** is intended to represent and be applied to student growth and development in the classroom and the clinic. It also contains behavioral criteria for the practicing clinician. Each *Professional Behavior* is defined and then broken down into developmental levels with each level containing behavioral criteria that describe behaviors that represent possession of the *Professional Behavior* they represent. Each developmental level builds on the previous level such that the tool represents growth over time in physical therapy education and practice.

Opportunities to reflect on each *Professional Behavior* through self-assessment and through peer and instructor assessment is critical for progress toward entry-level performance in the classroom and clinic. A learner does not need to possess each behavioral criteria identified at each level within the tool, however, but should demonstrate, and be able to provide examples of, the majority in order to move from one level to the next. Likewise, the behavioral criteria are examples of behaviors one might demonstrate but these are not exhaustive. Academic and clinical facilities may decide to add or delete behavioral criteria based on the needs of their specific setting. Formal opportunities to reflect and discuss with an academic and/or clinical instructor is key to the tool's use, and ultimately professional growth of the learner. The *Professional Behaviors* Assessment Tool allows the learner to build and strengthen their third leg with skills in the affective domain to augment the cognitive and psychomotor domains (Chapter 3, Appendix).

# PROFESSIONAL BEHAVIORS

## 1 Critical Thinking

The ability to question logically; identify, generate, and evaluate elements of logical argument; recognize and differentiate facts, appropriate or faulty inferences, and assumptions; and distinguish relevant from irrelevant information. The ability to appropriately utilize, analyze, and critically evaluate scientific evidence to develop a logical argument, and to identify and determine the impact of bias on the decision-making process.

**Beginning Level**
- Raises relevant questions
- Considers all available information
- Articulates ideas
- Understands the scientific method
- States the results of scientific literature but has not developed the consistent ability to critically appraise findings (i.e. methodology and conclusion)
- Recognizes holes in knowledge base
- Demonstrates acceptance of limited knowledge and experience

**Intermediate Level**

- Feels challenged to examine ideas
- Critically analyzes the literature and applies it to patient management
- Utilizes didactic knowledge, research evidence, and clinical experience to formulate new ideas
- Seeks alternative ideas
- Formulates alternative hypotheses
- Critiques hypotheses and ideas at a level consistent with knowledge base
- Acknowledges presence of contradictions

**Entry Level**

- Distinguishes relevant from irrelevant patient data
- Readily formulates and critiques alternative hypotheses and ideas
- Infers applicability of information across populations
- Exhibits openness to contradictory ideas
- Identifies appropriate measures and determines effectiveness of applied solutions efficiently
- Justifies solutions selected

**Post-Entry Level**

- Develops new knowledge through research, professional writing, and/or professional presentations
- Thoroughly critiques hypotheses and ideas often crossing disciplines in thought process
- Weighs information value based on source and level of evidence
- Identifies complex patterns of associations
- Distinguishes when to think intuitively vs. analytically
- Recognizes own biases and suspends judgmental thinking
- Challenges others to think critically

# 2 Communication

The ability to communicate effectively (i.e. verbal, non-verbal, reading, writing, and listening) for varied audiences and purposes.

**Beginning Level**

- Demonstrates understanding of the English language (verbal and written): uses correct grammar, accurate spelling and expression, legible handwriting
- Recognizes impact of non-verbal communication in self and others
- Recognizes the verbal and non-verbal characteristics that portray confidence
- Utilizes electronic communication appropriately

**Intermediate Level**

- Utilizes and modifies communication (verbal, non-verbal, written, and electronic) to meet the needs of different audiences
- Restates, reflects, and clarifies message(s)
- Communicates collaboratively with both individuals and groups
- Collects necessary information from all pertinent individuals in the patient/client management process
- Provides effective education (verbal, non-verbal, written, and electronic)

**Entry Level**

- Demonstrates the ability to maintain appropriate control of the communication exchange with individuals and groups
- Presents persuasive and explanatory verbal, written, or electronic messages with logical organization and sequencing
- Maintains open and constructive communication
- Utilizes communication technology effectively and efficiently

**Post-Entry Level**

- Adapts messages to address needs, expectations, and prior knowledge of the audience to maximize learning
- Effectively delivers messages capable of influencing patients, the community, and society
- Provides education locally, regionally, and/or nationally
- Mediates conflict

# 3 Problem Solving

The ability to recognize and define problems, analyze data, develop and implement solutions, and evaluate outcomes.

**Beginning Level**

- Recognizes problems
- States problems clearly
- Describes known solutions to problems
- Identifies resources needed to develop solutions
- Uses technology to search for and locate resources
- Identifies possible solutions and probable outcomes

**Intermediate Level**

- Prioritizes problems
- Identifies contributors to problems
- Consults with others to clarify problems
- Appropriately seeks input or guidance
- Prioritizes resources (analysis and critique of resources)
- Considers consequences of possible solutions

**Entry Level**

- Independently locates, prioritizes, and uses resources to solve problems
- Accepts responsibility for implementing solutions
- Implements solutions
- Reassesses solutions
- Evaluates outcomes
- Modifies solutions based on the outcome and current evidence
- Evaluates generalizability of current evidence to a particular problem

**Post-Entry Level**

- Weighs advantages and disadvantages of a solution to a problem
- Participates in outcome studies

- Participates in formal quality assessment in work environment
- Seeks solutions to community health-related problems
- Considers second and third order effects of solutions chosen

# 4 Interpersonal Skills

The ability to interact effectively with patients, families, colleagues, other health care professionals, and the community in a culturally aware manner.

### Beginning Level

- Maintains professional demeanor in all interactions
- Demonstrates interest in patients as individuals
- Communicates with others in a respectful and confident manner
- Respects differences in personality, lifestyle, and learning styles during interactions with all persons
- Maintains confidentiality in all interactions
- Recognizes the emotions and bias that one brings to all professional interactions

### Intermediate Level

- Recognizes the non-verbal communication and emotions that others bring to professional interactions
- Establishes trust
- Seeks to gain input from others
- Respects role of others
- Accommodates differences in learning styles as appropriate

### Entry Level

- Demonstrates active listening skills and reflects back to original concern to determine course of action
- Responds effectively to unexpected situations
- Demonstrates ability to build partnerships
- Applies conflict management strategies when dealing with challenging interactions
- Recognizes the impact of non-verbal communication and emotional responses during interactions and modifies own behaviors based on them

### Post-Entry Level

- Establishes mentor relationships
- Recognizes the impact that non-verbal communication and the emotions of self and others have during interactions and demonstrates the ability to modify the behaviors of self and others during the interaction

# 5 Responsibility

The ability to be accountable for the outcomes of personal and professional actions and to follow through on commitments that encompass the profession within the scope of work, community, and social responsibilities.

### Beginning Level

- Demonstrates punctuality
- Provides a safe and secure environment for patients
- Assumes responsibility for actions
- Follows through on commitments

- Articulates limitations and readiness to learn
- Abides by all policies of academic program and clinical facility

### Intermediate Level

- Displays awareness of and sensitivity to diverse populations
- Completes projects without prompting
- Delegates tasks as needed
- Collaborates with team members, patients, and families
- Provides evidence-based patient care

### Entry Level

- Educates patients as consumers of health care services
- Encourages patient accountability
- Directs patients to other health care professionals as needed
- Acts as a patient advocate
- Promotes evidence-based practice in health care settings
- Accepts responsibility for implementing solutions
- Demonstrates accountability for all decisions and behaviors in academic and clinical settings

### Post-Entry Level

- Recognizes role as a leader
- Encourages and displays leadership
- Facilitates program development and modification
- Promotes clinical training for students and co-workers
- Monitors and adapts to changes in the health care system
- Promotes service to the community

## 6 Professionalism

The ability to exhibit appropriate professional conduct and to represent the profession effectively while promoting the growth/development of the Physical Therapy profession.

### Beginning Level

- Abides by all aspects of the academic program honor code and the APTA Code of Ethics
- Demonstrates awareness of state licensure regulations
- Projects professional image
- Attends professional meetings
- Demonstrates cultural/generational awareness, ethical values, respect, and continuous regard for all classmates, academic and clinical faculty/staff, patients, families, and other health care providers

### Intermediate Level

- Identifies positive professional role models within the academic and clinical settings
- Acts on moral commitment during all academic and clinical activities
- Identifies when the input of classmates, co-workers, and other health care professionals will result in optimal outcome and acts accordingly to attain such input and share decision making
- Discusses societal expectations of the profession

**Entry Level**

- Demonstrates understanding of scope of practice as evidenced by treatment of patients within scope of practice, referring to other health care professionals as necessary
- Provides patient/family-centered care at all times as evidenced by provision of patient/family education, seeking patient input and informed consent for all aspects of care and maintenance of patient dignity
- Seeks excellence in professional practice by participation in professional organizations and attendance at sessions or participation in activities that further education/professional development
- Utilizes evidence to guide clinical decision making and the provision of patient care, following guidelines for best practices
- Discusses role of physical therapy within the health care system and in population health
- Demonstrates leadership in collaboration with both individuals and groups

**Post-Entry Level**

- Actively promotes and advocates for the profession
- Pursues leadership roles
- Supports research
- Participates in program development
- Participates in education of the community
- Demonstrates the ability to practice effectively in multiple settings
- Acts as a clinical instructor
- Advocates for the patient, the community, and society

# 7 Use of Constructive Feedback

The ability to seek out and identify quality sources of feedback, reflect on and integrate the feedback, and provide meaningful feedback to others.

**Beginning Level**

- Demonstrates active listening skills
- Assesses own performance
- Actively seeks feedback from appropriate sources
- Demonstrates receptive behavior and positive attitude toward feedback
- Incorporates specific feedback into behaviors
- Maintains two-way communication without defensiveness

**Intermediate Level**

- Critiques own performance accurately
- Responds effectively to constructive feedback
- Utilizes feedback when establishing professional and patient-related goals
- Develops and implements a plan of action in response to feedback
- Provides constructive and timely feedback

**Entry Level**

- Independently engages in a continual process of self evaluation of skills, knowledge, and abilities
- Seeks feedback from patients/clients and peers/mentors
- Readily integrates feedback provided from a variety of sources to improve skills, knowledge, and abilities

- Uses multiple approaches when responding to feedback
- Reconciles differences with sensitivity
- Modifies feedback given to patients/clients according to their learning styles

**Post-Entry Level**

- Engages in non-judgmental, constructive problem-solving discussions
- Acts as conduit for feedback between multiple sources
- Seeks feedback from a variety of sources to include students/supervisees/peers/supervisors/patients
- Utilizes feedback when analyzing and updating professional goals

# 8  Effective Use of Time and Resources

The ability to manage time and resources effectively to obtain the maximum possible benefit.

**Beginning Level**

- Comes prepared for the day's activities/responsibilities
- Identifies resource limitations (i.e. information, time, experience)
- Determines when and how much help/assistance is needed
- Accesses current evidence in a timely manner
- Verbalizes productivity standards and identifies barriers to meeting productivity standards
- Self-identifies and initiates learning opportunities during unscheduled time

**Intermediate Level**

- Utilizes effective methods of searching for evidence for practice decisions
- Recognizes own resource contributions
- Shares knowledge and collaborates with staff to utilize best current evidence
- Discusses and implements strategies for meeting productivity standards
- Identifies need for and seeks referrals to other disciplines

**Entry Level**

- Uses current best evidence
- Collaborates with members of the team to maximize the impact of treatment available
- Has the ability to set boundaries, negotiate, compromise, and set realistic expectations
- Gathers data and effectively interprets and assimilates the data to determine plan of care
- Utilizes community resources in discharge planning
- Adjusts plans, schedule, etc. as patient needs and circumstances dictate
- Meets productivity standards of facility while providing quality care and completing non-productive work activities

**Post-Entry Level**

- Advances profession by contributing to the body of knowledge (outcomes, case studies, etc.)
- Applies best evidence considering available resources and constraints
- Organizes and prioritizes effectively
- Prioritizes multiple demands and situations that arise on a given day
- Mentors peers and supervisees in increasing productivity and/or effectiveness without decrement in quality of care

# 9 Stress Management

The ability to identify sources of stress and to develop and implement effective coping behaviors; this applies for interactions for: self, patient/clients and their families, members of the health care team, and in work/life scenarios.

### Beginning Level

- Recognizes own stressors
- Recognizes distress or problems in others
- Seeks assistance as needed
- Maintains professional demeanor in all situations

### Intermediate Level

- Actively employs stress management techniques
- Reconciles inconsistencies in the educational process
- Maintains balance between professional and personal life
- Accepts constructive feedback and clarifies expectations
- Establishes outlets to cope with stressors

### Entry Level

- Demonstrates appropriate affective responses in all situations
- Responds calmly to urgent situations with reflection and debriefing as needed
- Prioritizes multiple commitments
- Reconciles inconsistencies within professional, personal, and work/life environments
- Demonstrates ability to defuse potential stressors with self and others

### Post-Entry Level

- Recognizes when problems are unsolvable
- Assists others in recognizing and managing stressors
- Demonstrates preventative approach to stress management
- Establishes support networks for self and others
- Offers solutions to the reduction of stress
- Models work/life balance through health/wellness behaviors in professional and personal life

# 10 Commitment to Learning

The ability to self-direct learning to include the identification of needs and sources of learning; and to continually seek and apply new knowledge, behaviors, and skills.

### Beginning Level

- Prioritizes information needs
- Analyzes and subdivides large questions into components
- Identifies own learning needs based on previous experiences
- Welcomes and/or seeks new learning opportunities
- Seeks out professional literature
- Plans and presents an in-service, research, or cases studies

**Intermediate Level**

- Researches and studies areas where own knowledge base is lacking in order to augment learning and practice
- Applies new information and re-evaluates performance
- Accepts that there may be more than one answer to a problem
- Recognizes the need to and is able to verify solutions to problems
- Reads articles critically and understands limits of application to professional practice

**Entry Level**

- Respectfully questions conventional wisdom
- Formulates and re-evaluates position based on available evidence
- Demonstrates confidence in sharing new knowledge with all staff levels
- Modifies programs and treatments based on newly learned skills and considerations
- Consults with other health professionals and physical therapists for treatment ideas

**Post-Entry Level**

- Acts as a mentor not only to other PTs but to other health professionals
- Utilizes mentors who have knowledge available to them
- Continues to seek and review relevant literature
- Works towards clinical specialty certifications
- Seeks specialty training
- Is committed to understanding the PT's role in the health care environment today (i.e. wellness clinics, massage therapy, holistic medicine)
- Pursues participation in clinical education as an educational opportunity

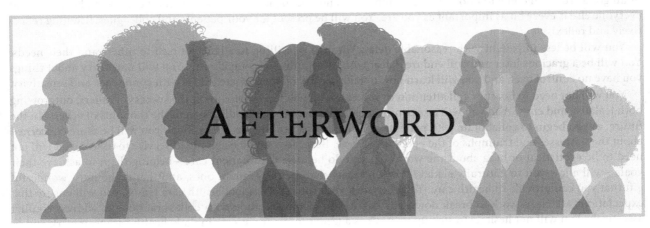

# AFTERWORD

*Carol M. Davis, DPT, EdD, MS, FAPTA and
Gina Maria Musolino, PT, DPT, MSEd, EdD*

## OUR FINAL CONCLUSION, WITH BEST WISHES

One of the goals of this text is to help you grow in self-awareness to be less susceptible to professional burnout. Only you can evaluate your current world view, level of self-esteem, and ability to alter harmful perceptions that contribute to negative stress. Only you can change your self-esteem. And only you can alter the perceptions about yourself, the world, and other people to the end that you experience a deep sense of personal confidence and satisfaction in your self and in your work. That is our wish for you. You, your patients, and the world will benefit from the positive energy that you will convey.

You have a start toward self-awareness and personal growth. Do not stop. Find ways to continue to take regular personal inventory of your self-esteem and stress levels. Use your journal to stay on top of feelings that would become buried in the overwhelming amount of work you have agreed to do in service to society. Make a personal commitment to ongoing growth in all four of your quadrants and keep a check on the imbalances. You know the value of peer and self-assessment for professional growth as a reflective practitioner and will assist others in introspective development, peers, patients, and future protégés. Keep up your advocacy works at the state and national levels, in daily patient care and through your communities of interest. Stay engaged in your continued professional formation leading to expertise in practice.

## The Signs of Maturation

How will you know when you are succeeding at the maturation process? Someone incredibly wise once offered this description: Life will become more enjoyable, and you will become less worried about making mistakes or not being liked. Relationships will become more important to you than things. You will accept the gifts of constructive criticism gratefully and graciously, glad for the opportunity to improve. You will not indulge in self-pity, but you will begin to see the marvelous opportunities for growth that misfortune and pain often bring. You will not expect special consideration from anyone. You will be aware of your emotions, and you will rarely feel the need to react impulsively in a tense situation. You will meet emergencies with poise; your feelings will not be hurt easily. You will accept responsibility for your own actions without needing to make excuses, readily acknowledging that you are still growing and learning.

DOI: 10.4324/9781003525554-21

You will have grown beyond dualistic, all-or-none, black-or-white, distorted thinking (absolutes) about the world, and you will be able to tolerate ambiguity and reframe your thinking. Understanding now, that life is complex, often uncertain, and ever-changing. You will recognize that people are doing the best they can and that no one is all bad or all good. You will come to know that true humility is not feeling less important than others are but believing that everyone else is every bit as important as you are. You will be present for your patients and colleagues, listening reflectively and reflexively.

You will be less impatient with reasonable delay. You will be willing to adjust yourself to others and their needs. You will be a gracious loser and will endure defeat without whining or complaining. You will not worry about things you have no control over, and you will learn how to take control of appropriate things with confidence and sensitivity.

You will not need to boast or call attention to yourself. You will feel sincere joy at the success of others, outgrowing both jealousy and envy. And you will be open-minded enough to thoughtfully listen to the thoughts of others. In the future, as you begin to collaborate with patients and clients as a health care professional, you will be more concerned about the successes and triumphs of the people you serve. Because you will be giving in service to others, you will not need to be egotistical or brag about the work that you do because your patient care—helping them to achieve their goals—will allow you to naturally achieve. Your patients shall be the grateful ones, and that is the most wonderful gift that you can provide in health care. Together with your interprofessional health care teams, you will ensure that expectations are clear, work to break down any barriers to communication with collaboration, and address conflict assertively. You will not hesitate to step up to serve as a leader for your patients in daily health care teamwork and in service to the profession and society.

Above all, you will not tolerate the mistreatment of human beings, especially those who are ill, by those who are careless in their interactions. You will take personal responsibility to help people realize the negative effects of their fragmenting interactions on you and on others, and you will kindly ask them to change their behavior for the good of all concerned. Best of luck to you as you set out to make the world, and yourself, better than they were when you started. You are on your way to becoming a leader in health care, putting your patients' needs forward and advocating for those who are unable to do so for themselves.

# INDEX

Note: **Bold** page numbers refer to tables and *italic* page numbers refer to figures.